NEUROLOGY FOR THE NON-NEUROLOGIST

Fifth Edition

NEUROLOGY FOR THE NON-NEUROLOGIST

Fifth Edition

Edited by

William J. Weiner, M.D.
Professor and Chairman
Department of Neurology
Director, Maryland Parkinson's Disease
and Movement Disorders Center
University of Maryland School of Medicine
Baltimore, Maryland

Christopher G. Goetz, M.D.
Professor of Neurological Sciences
and Associate Chairperson
Department of Neurological Sciences
Rush Medical College
Rush-Presbyterian–St. Luke's Medical Center
Chicago, Illinois

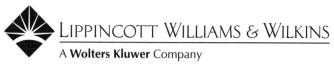

LIPPINCOTT WILLIAMS & WILKINS
A **Wolters Kluwer** Company
Philadelphia • Baltimore • New York • London
Buenos Aires • Hong Kong • Sydney • Tokyo

Acquisitions Editor: Anne M. Sydor
Developmental Editor: Tanya Lazar
Production Editor: Thomas Boyce
Manufacturing Manager: Benjamin Rivera
Cover Designer: David Levy
Compositor: Lippincott Williams & Wilkins Desktop Division
Printer: Maple-Press

© 2004 by LIPPINCOTT WILLIAMS & WILKINS
530 Walnut Street
Philadelphia, PA 19106 USA
LWW.com

1st edition, © 1981, Harper & Row; 2nd edition, © 1984, JB Lippincott; 3rd edition, © 1989, JB Lippincott; 4th edition, © 1999, Lippincott Williams & Wilkins

Printed in the USA

Library of Congress Cataloging-in-Publication Data

Neurology for the non-neurologist / edited by William J. Weiner, Christopher G. Goetz—
5th ed.
   p. ; cm.
   Includes bibliographical references and index.
   ISBN 0-7817-4631-0
      1. Neurology. 2. Nervous system—Diseases. I. Weiner, William J.
   II. Goetz, Christopher G.
   [DNLM: 1. Nervous System Diseases. 2. Diagnosis, Differential. 3. Diagnostic
Techniques, Neurological. WL 140 N4928 2004]
   RC346.N453 2004
   616.8—dc22
                                                                2004040838

10   9   8   7   6   5   4   3   2

To Maynard Cohen, M.D., Ph.D.

Friend, mentor, and neurologist

Contents

Contributing Authors

Neelum T. Aggarwal, M.D.
Assistant Professor
Department of Neurological Sciences
Rush Alzheimer Disease Center
Rush-Presbyterian–St. Luke's Medical Center
Chicago, Illinois

David A. Bennett, M.D.
Associate Professor
Department of Neurological Sciences
Director, Rush Alzheimer's Disease Center
Rush-Presbyterian–St. Luke's Medical Center
Chicago, Illinois

Meriem K. Bensalem, M.D.
Department of Neurology
University of Kentucky College of Medicine
Lexington, Kentucky

Donna C. Bergen, M.D.
Associate Professor
Department of Neurological Sciences
Rush University
Senior Attending Neurologist
Department of Neurological Sciences
Rush-Presbyterian–St. Luke's Medical Center
Chicago, Illinois

Joseph R. Berger, M.D.
University of Kentucky
Department of Neurology
L445 Kentucky Clinic
Lexington, Kentucky

Thomas P. Bleck, M.D.
Louise Nerancy Eminent Scholar in Neurology
Professor of Neurology, Neurological Surgery, and
  Internal Medicine
Chair, Critical Care Subcommittee
Director, Neuroscience Intensive Care Unit
The University of Virginia
Charlottesville, Virginia

Peter A. Calabresi, M.D.
Associate Professor of Neurology
Johns Hopkins Hospital
Pathology Building 627A
Baltimore, Maryland

Larry E. Davis, M.D., F.A.C.P.
Professor and Vice Chair
Department of Neurology
University of New Mexico School of Medicine
Chief
Neurology Service
New Mexico VA Health Care System
Albuquerque, New Mexico

Stewart A. Factor, D.O.
Parkinson's Disease and Movement Disorders
Albany Medical Center
Albany, New York

Morris A. Fisher, M.D.
Professor
Department of Neurology
Loyola University of Chicago
Stritch School of Medicine
Attending Physician
Department of Neurology
Hines VA Hospital, Hines
Attending Physician
Department of Neurology
Loyola University Medical Center
Maywood, Illinois

Russell H. Glantz, M.D.
Associate Professor
Department of Neurology
Rush Medical College
Chicago, Illinois
Neurologist
Parkview Musculoskeletal Institute
Palos Heights, Illinois

Christopher G. Goetz, M.D.
Professor of Neurological Sciences and Associate
  Chairperson
Department of Neurological Sciences
Rush Medical College
Rush Presbyterian–St. Luke's Medical Center
Chicago, Illinois

James A. Goodwin, M.D.
University of Illinois Eye & Ear Infirmary
Chicago, Illinois

Deborah Olin Heros, M.D.
Assistant Professor
Department of Neurology
University of Miami School of Medicine
Attending Physician
Department of Neurology
Jackson Memorial Hospital
Miami, Florida

Judd M. Jensen, M.D.
Penobscot Bay Physician's Building
Rockport, Maine

Roger E. Kelley, M.D.
Professor and Chairman
Chief of Service
Department of Neurology
Louisiana State University Health Sciences
  Center
Shreveport, Louisiana

William C. Koller, M.D.
Professor
Department of Neurology
Mount Sinai Medical Center
New York, New York

Katie Kompoliti, M.D.
Rush-Presbyterian–St. Luke's Medical Center
Department of Neurological Sciences
Chicago, Illinois

Ružica Kovačević-Ristanović, M.D., M.S.
Associate Professor
Department of Neurology
Feinberg School of Medicine
Northwestern University
Chicago
Medical Director of Sleep Disorders Center
Department of Neurology
Evanston Hospital (E.N.H.)
Evanston, Illinois

David S. Kushner, M.D.
20601 Old Cutler Road
Miami, Florida

Steven L. Lewis, M.D.
Associate Professor
Department of Neurological Sciences
Rush Medical College of Rush University
Section Head, Section of General Neurology
Department of Neurological Sciences
Rush-Presbyterian–St. Luke's Medical Center
Chicago, Illinois

Michael J. Makley, M.D.
Assistant Professor
Department of Neurology
University of Maryland School of Medicine
Medical Director
Brain Injury Unit
Kernan Hospital
Baltimore, Maryland

Alireza Minagar, M.D.
Assistant Professor
Department of Neurology and Anesthesiology
Louisiana State University Health Sciences Center
Shreveport, Louisiana

Hans E. Neville, M.D.
Professor
Department of Neurology
University of Colorado Health Sciences Center
Director, Outpatient Practice
Department of Neurology
University of Colorado Hospital
Denver, Colorado

Lois Margaret Nora, M.D., J.D.
Northeastern Ohio Universities College of Medicine
Rootstown, Ohio

Robert E. Nora, Esq.
Oak Park, Illinois

Neil C. Porter, M.D.
Department of Neurology
University of Maryland School of Medicine
Baltimore, Maryland

Dianna Quan, M.D.
Assistant Professor
Department of Neurology
University of Colorado Health Sciences Center
Director, Electromyography Laboratory
Department of Neurology
University of Colorado Hospital
Denver, Colorado

Steven P. Ringel, M.D.
Professor
Department of Neurology
University of Colorado Health Sciences Center
President, Medical Staff
Director, Neuromuscular Unit
University of Colorado Hospital
Denver, Colorado

Todd D. Rozen, M.D.
Neurologist
Michigan Head-Pain and Neurological Institute
Ann Arbor, Michigan

Joel R. Saper, M.D., F.A.C.P., F.A.A.N.
Clinical Professor
Department of Medicine–Neurology
Michigan State University
Lansing, Michigan
Director
Head Pain Treatment Unit
Chelsea Community Hospital
Chelsea, Michigan

Kathleen M. Shannon, M.D.
Associate Professor
Attending Physician
Department of Neurological Sciences
Rush-Presbyterian–St. Luke's Medical Center
Chicago, Illinois

Lisa M. Shulman, M.D.
Associate Professor
Department of Neurology
University of Maryland School of Medicine
Baltimore, Maryland

M. J. B. Stallmeyer, M.D., Ph.D.
Director of Radiology
Department of Diagnostic Radiology
University of Maryland School of Medicine
Baltimore, Maryland

Tricia Y. Ting, M.D.
Assistant Professor
Department of Neurology
University of Maryland School of Medicine
Baltimore, Maryland

Jordan L. Topel, M.D.
Associate Professor
Department of Neurological Sciences
Rush Medical College
Senior Attending Physician
Department of Neurological Sciences
Rush-Presbyterian–St. Luke's Medical
* Center*
Chicago, Illinois

Winona Tse, M.D.
Assistant Professor
Department of Neurology
Mount Sinai School of Medicine
Assistant Professor
Department of Neurology
Mount Sinai Medical Center
New York, New York

William J. Weiner, M.D.
Professor and Chairman
Department of Neurology
Director, Maryland Parkinson's Disease
Movement Disorders Center
University of Maryland School of Medicine
Baltimore, Maryland

Robert S. Wilson, Ph.D.
Department of Neurological Sciences
Rush Alzheimer's Disease Center
Rush-Presbyterian–St. Luke's Medical
* Center*
Chicago, Illinois

Gregg H. Zoarski, M.D.
Associate Professor of Diagnostic Radiology
University of Maryland
Baltimore, Maryland

Preface

This edition of *Neurology for the Non-Neurologist* maintains the basic focus of the previous editions and emphasizes the neurological education of health care professionals who deal with nervous system disorders regularly, but who have committed themselves primarily to other fields: internists, family practitioners, psychiatrists, geriatricians, rehabilitation specialists, and advanced nurses. As neurologists, we are conscious of the changing health practices that have emerged from managed care and new practice models, and we realize that non-neurologists are increasingly seeing neurologically impaired patients at the beginning, middle, and end stages of their diseases. At the same time, the increasing breadth of neurological knowledge places an ever-increasing responsibility on the non-neurologist to understand the basic elements of neurological pathophysiology, diagnosis, and treatment. The resultant need for interactions between neurologists and non-neurologists has reached a new level of importance, because often even with a neurologist's input on a patients care, the non-neurologist manages daily patient care.

In this light, we have compiled chapters on the common neurological diagnoses that non-neurologists will face in regular patient practice and outlined their neuroanatomical background, differential diagnosis, and evaluation recommendations. We have provided up-to-date treatment strategies that cover educational resources, and pharmacological and surgical treatments. New to this edition are discussions on rehabilitation efforts and alternative interventions that have enough scientific background to be recommended. Also, for each general topic, we have included discussions that address two continually posed questions: "When should a non-neurologist refer a patient to a neurologist" and "What are the special considerations for hospitalized patients".

The authors who have contributed to this book are noted neurologists who are involved in daily neurological teaching to medical students, community physicians, and other neurologists. Many of them have contributed to the prior editions of this book and some authors are new. All of them are experts in their field and are eminently equipped to guide non-neurologists in the evaluation and treatment of the neurological problems that they are likely to encounter. Many of these authors have participated in educational efforts such as conferences directed to non-neurologists, and in fact the original idea of creating *Neurology for the Non-Neurologist* grew out of a continuing medical education course that the two editors organized over twenty years ago in Chicago. This effort still goes on annually, and has been a model for similar educational venues.

Because of these many considerations, we consider this new edition a particularly important text for non-neurologists. The book can be read in multiple manners: read from cover to cover, it will serve as an up-to-date treatment of neurology as it affects non-neurological professionals; kept in the patient examination room or doctor's office, it can be quickly referenced to answer specific questions and treatment recommendations; reliance on the index and numerous tables and figures provide for rapid verification of information and efficiency of communication; finally, for CME review and self-assessment, each chapter is accompanied by clinically based questions that assess the reader's acquisition of the chapter material.

The editors especially thank four people for the smooth completion of this edition: Nandy Yearwood and Cheryl Grant-Johnson from the University of Maryland, Marilynn Payton from Rush University, and Anne Sydor from Lippincott Williams & Wilkins. Their organizational and administrative skills provided us the freedom to develop the book and work with authors efficiently and thereby provide this updated version of *Neurology for the Non-Neurologist* in a timely fashion.

William J. Weiner, M.D.
Christopher G. Goetz, M.D.

1

The Neurologic Examination

Neil C. Porter and William J. Weiner

The neurologic examination is the foundation of the practice of neurology, encompassing the patient interview and physical examination (Table 1.1). Unlike other medical disciplines that often emphasize ancillary studies, the neurologic investigations are guided wholly by the information gleaned from the neurologic interview and examination. The neurologic examination itself is guided by the information obtained from the interview. Every patient does not require a complete neurologic examination. The information obtained in the interview directs the examiner to the relevant parts of the examination.

The examination starts when the examiner enters the room with the patient. Observation is key. The examiner needs to observe who is in the room besides the patient, who is providing the history of the patient, the language used in the history, and the body movements of the patient during the interview. All of this information is potentially relevant to the neurologic examination and diagnosis. The information obtained in the history should be used to formulate a hypothesis and direct the neurologic evaluation.

The neurologic interview/history should be obtained with great care. The nature of the problem and its onset, time course, duration, associated symptoms, and exacerbating and alleviating factors should be elicited. Anatomic regions that are affected should be defined.

TABLE 1.1. *Organization of the Neurologic Examination*

I. The mental status examination
II. Cranial nerve examination
III. Motor examination
IV. Deep tendon reflex (DTR) testing
V. Sensory testing
VI. Coordination and gait assessment

In some instances, the history must be obtained from others. The patient who has a generalized seizure or an episode of impairment of consciousness will not be able to provide a complete history of the event. The patient with cognitive deficits or speech difficulties also will be unable to provide adequate historical information. It is important to question the spouse, a relative, or witnesses to a specific event to obtain a more complete and often more accurate story.

The neurologic examination is divided into several components. These include examination of the mental status, cranial nerves, sensory system, motor system, coordination, gait, and reflexes. Each of these components has several parts that will be addressed in this chapter. The depth of the examination of these components is directed by the information obtained in the history of the problem. If the patient is complaining of numbness and weakness of the hands, the examination concentrates on the peripheral nervous system. If, however, the patient is complaining of dysarthria and weakness on one side, the examination is directed at the central nervous system. The tempo of these neurologic changes also becomes important. If the deficits were of sudden onset, a vascular event is suspected, whereas slowly progressive deficits would suggest a space-occupying lesion such as a tumor. The following description of the neurologic examination is written for use by non-neurologists.

Certain neurologic conditions commonly are associated with a normal neurologic examination (e.g., primary generalized epilepsies, transient ischemic attacks [TIAs], migraine, and other headaches). In these and other disorders, initial diagnostic considerations depend on obtaining a complete history.

If the neurologic examination detects abnormalities, additional diagnostic alternatives may be raised. For example, a positive Babinski sign days after a grand mal seizure suggests that the seizure may have been of focal onset; therefore, a search for a structural brain lesion has to be considered. The finding of mild hand clumsiness after an acute event points to a stroke rather than a TIA. Therapeutic choices may differ depending on whether the patient suffered a TIA or a completed cerebrovascular accident (CVA).

Because the neurologic examination is often crucial in establishing the correct diagnosis, it is important for all physicians to be able to perform a complete, albeit often brief, evaluation of the nervous system. The often-written chart note for the neurologic examination found on non-neurology services (neuro: WNL, meaning within normal limits) should be avoided; most often, WNL is interpreted as "We never looked." The neurologic examination should be conducted with a consistent routine so that portions of the evaluation are not forgotten.

MENTAL STATUS

The mental status examination provides an assessment of the patient's general cognitive status, measuring the integrity of the cerebral hemispheres. The mental status examination includes assessment of the patient's appearance, speech, mood and affect, thought form and content, perceptions, cognition, judgment, insight, level of consciousness, and those thought processes believed to have localizing value. Many clinicians use the mini-mental status examination (MMSE; see later in this chapter), a set of standard questions that assesses a wide variety of cognitive domains, as a brief substitute for the full mental status evaluation. A number of the questions used to assess cognitive function can be woven into the interview so that the patient does not feel that he is being critically examined.

When the history suggests memory dysfunction or changes in behavior, historical information from relatives, friends, coworkers, and employers may be required. Often patients with early, mild dementing processes still may be smarter than their evaluators, and they often use various tricks of social grace and convention to evade specific questions. Patients may become belligerent if deficits are revealed, and this should be done cautiously. For example, specific mental status testing may be performed by telling patients in a non-threatening manner that silly questions have to be asked and by asking them to cooperate.

Appearance and Behavior

The patient's appearance and general behavior are important indicators of general level of function. The well-dressed, well-organized patient probably is functioning at a higher level than the disheveled, unkempt patient. Additionally, a patient's dress and demeanor are important indicators of underlying psychiatric and psychological disturbances, such as the patient who is inappropriately dressed for the weather or the patient who is clearly responding to unseen stimuli.

Speech and Language

The character of the patient's speech provides the examiner valuable insight into the patient's mental state. Important aspects of speech include the amplitude or loudness, volume or amount (paucity versus over abundance), and prosody or fluidity. Often patients with end-stage dementia will have paucity of speech. The patient with Parkinson's disease often will speak with a hypophonic, hushed quality.

Language can be assessed quickly by evaluating spontaneous speech, repetition, comprehension of spoken and written material, and the ability to write. Speech may be fluent or non-fluent, and this observation may be very useful in localizing a potential cortical lesion. Non-fluent speech (Broca's aphasia) is localized to the dominant posterior inferior frontal region and often is associated with a hemiparesis, whereas fluent aphasic speech (Wernicke's aphasia), which sounds normal in delivery but makes little or no sense, is localized to the posterior temporal area and is not associated with a marked paresis. The presence of aphasia may prevent adequate memory and other cognitive testing.

Mood and Affect

Mood refers to a person's persistent emotional state; the term affect denotes more immediacy. Mood and affect can be assessed by observing the patient's body language and behavior as well as by verbal report. Persistently depressed mood is characteristic of depression. A brief screen for depression includes inquiries about reduced "spirits," reduced energy, poor self-attitude, poor appetite, disturbed sleep, anhedonia, thinking difficulty, suicidal ideation, and psychomotor retardation. Conversely, a persistently elevated mood, increased energy, and heightened self-attitude in association with delusions of grandeur, pressured speech, and flight of ideas are indicative of mania. Depression is seen in a number of neurologic disorders including Parkinson's disease, Huntington's disease, and strokes affecting the dominant hemisphere; mania may be seen occasionally with cerebral lesions of the nondominant cerebral hemisphere.

Perceptual Disturbances

Patients who are psychotic or delirious often report bizarre sensory experiences such as hallucinations and illusions. Hallucinations are perceptions in the absence of stimuli. These can be elicited by asking the patient if they have seen (or heard) things that "weren't really there" or "that others couldn't see (or hear)." Illusions are misperceptions, whereby the patient mistakes an object for something else, such as a coat for an intruder. Both hallucinations and illusions are seen in patients who are delirious or encephalopathic.

Thought Form and Content

Abnormalities of thought form and content are "psychotic features" associated with delir-

ium, dementia, schizophrenia, and severe affective disorders. Abnormalities of thought content consist of bizarre beliefs such as delusions, obsessions, compulsions, and phobias. Delusions are fixed, false, idiosyncratic beliefs tenaciously held by the patient. Obsessions are intrusive, recurring thoughts that disturb the patient. Similarly, compulsions are acts that the patient feels compelled to perform over and over again. Phobias are irrational fears held by the patient. Abnormalities of thought content can be ascertained by simply asking the patient if they have any strong beliefs or practices that others do not share, such as any "special powers." Paranoid delusions can be specifically detected by asking the patient if "anyone is after them" or if "anyone is out to get them."

Abnormalities of thought form consist of disordered thought processes such as "thought blocking," "loosening of associations," and "flight of ideas." Thought blocking is evidenced by patients being unable to complete their thoughts. Loosening of associations is seen when patients jump from one subject to another with little connection. Flight of ideas is manifested by the patient speaking at a rapid pace, on any number of subjects, without easily identifiable connections. Detecting abnormalities of thought form involves noting the manner in which patients volunteer information and respond to questions. Responses that are clear and concise are easily distinguishable from answers that are difficult to follow or do not make sense.

Sensorium and Cognition

Level of consciousness is a crucial part of the mental status examination. One should note and document whether the patient is awake, alert, and attentive versus unresponsive or barely able to arouse. A reduced level of consciousness is seen in myriad neurologic conditions including metabolic derangements, infections, and structural lesions.

A brief assessment of cognition is an important measure of global cerebral function.

The MMSE represents a simple screen for abnormalities of cognition. It is a highly reliable and validated 30-point instrument assessing orientation, language, recall, concentration, and some visuomotor skills. Briefly, 10 points are awarded for varying degrees of orientation in time and space. Three points are given for registration (correctly repeating the names of three objects). Five points are given for concentration, which is tested by having the patient spell "WORLD" backwards or sequentially subtracting 7 from 100 five times (e.g., 100, 93, 86, 79, 72, 65). Three points are given for correctly naming two objects and repeating the phrase "No ifs, ands, or buts." Three points are given for following a three-step command. Three points are given for reading and enacting the sentence "close your eyes," writing a sentence, and copying a figure comprised of two interlocking pentagons. Finally, three points are given for recalling the three objects mentioned for testing registration.

Many clinicians substitute the MMSE for the full mental status evaluation. The MMSE can be very helpful in detecting isolated problems with language such as subtle aphasias and isolated disturbances of recall as is seen in Korsakoff's syndrome. The MMSE is notoriously insensitive, however, in detecting dementia.

Judgment and Insight

A person's judgment relies on their value system, making assessment of judgment the most subjective component of the mental status examination. Assessment of a patient's insight into their disorder, however, is much more straightforward. For judgment, clinicians routinely ask questions such as "What would you do if you found a stamped envelope lying on the ground" with the expected answer being "Place the envelope in a mailbox." Such questioning is probably most helpful in the patient who is demented or cognitively impaired. For insight, one simply inquires into the patient's understanding of their condition. The patient with Alzheimer's disease, for example, will have very little insight into their memory loss, often denying that they have any problems with their thinking.

CRANIAL NERVES

There are twelve pairs of cranial nerves, each of which serves specific functions as illustrated in Table 1.2. A systematic examination of each pair of cranial nerves is an essential part of the neurologic examination, providing information on the integrity of the medulla, pons, midbrain, and limbic and vi-

TABLE 1.2. *Cranial Nerves and Their Functions*

Cranial Nerve	Name of Cranial Nerve	Function
I	Olfactory	Smell
II	Optic	Vision
III	Oculomotor	Elevate, depress, and adduct the eye; pupillary constriction
IV	Trochlear	Depression, adduction, and intorsion of the eye
V	Trigeminal	Sensation of the face and motor control of the muscles of mastication
VI	Abducens	Abduction of the eye
VII	Facial	Muscles of facial expression, taste for anterior two-third of tongue, sensation from ear
VIII	Vestibulocochlear	Hearing and balance
IX	Glossopharyngeal	Taste posterior one-third of tongue, sensation from ear, gag reflex, contraction of stylopharyngius muscle
X	Vagus	Gag reflex motor to soft palate, pharynx, larynx; autonomic fibers to esophagus, stomach, small intestine, heart, trachea; sensation from ear; viscera
XI	Spinal accessory	Motor control of the sternocleidomastoid and trapezius muscles
XII	Hypoglossal	Motor control of the tongue

sual systems. A superficial examination of the cranial nerves should be incorporated into any neurologic examination and can be done in just a few minutes. Of course, if any abnormality is found on the cursory examination, a more detailed study of that area is necessary.

CN I. THE OLFACTORY NERVE

Although reduced olfaction most often is attributable to advancing age, the loss of the sense of smell can be seen in pathologic states such as head trauma, tumors affecting the base of the skull, and certain inflammatory disorders such as sarcoid. The olfactory nerve (cranial nerve I [CNI]) is usually not tested during the screening neurologic examination unless the patient complains of loss of smell. Olfaction is assessed by having the patient identify a fragrant substance such as coffee or cloves. A small vial of the aromatic substance is held under one nostril while the other nostril is occluded. The patient is asked to breathe through the unobstructed nostril and identify the odor. The exercise is repeated on the other side with a different aromatic substance. Noxious substances such as ammonia or "smelling salts" should be avoided because of the concomitant stimulation of cranial nerve V, the trigeminal nerve.

CN II. THE OPTIC NERVE

Because it is a visible part of the central nervous system (CNS), the optic nerve represents a unique opportunity to appreciate CNS pathology. Evaluation of the optic nerve (cranial nerve II) includes examination of visual acuity, visual fields, the pupillary light response (discussed with CN III Functions), and the fundus. Visual acuity is tested most easily at the bedside with a "near-card." With their glasses or contact lenses in place (if needed), the patient is instructed to hold the card in one hand at a comfortable distance in front of one eye while the examiner covers the other eye. The patient then is asked to read the smallest numbers discernible on the card. The visual acuity listed on the card next to that line (e.g., 20/30) then is recorded. For the second eye the patient should read the numbers in reverse to reduce their ability to use recall (because one's reverse digit span is shorter than their forward digit span). For the pupillary light response the patient is asked to look at a distance while a strong light is directed repeatedly into each eye. For each eye, the examiner first looks for constriction of the pupil viewing the light (the direct response) and then constriction of the pupil opposite the light (the consensual response). Normally both pupils should react equally to light shone in either eye. A lesion of one optic nerve may cause both pupils to react poorly when light is shone in that eye. Such a "relative afferent pupillary defect" may be most evident when the flashlight is swung quickly from eye to eye.

Visual fields are tested by confrontation. The examiner faces the patient, points to his own nose, and asks him to concentrate on it. The examiner then holds up some of his own fingers briefly in each of the four quadrants of the visual field and asks the patient to count them. If an abnormality was seen on the initial screening, the visual fields of both eyes are examined separately (by covering the other eye). Visual field defects of one eye suggest that the lesion is localized to that globe or in the prechiasmatic optic nerve. A defect in both eyes suggests lesions involving the optic chiasm, tract, radiations, or visual cortex. Defects involving the temporal half of one eye and the nasal portion of the other eye (homonymous hemianopsia) suggest a lesion of the optic radiation or occipital cortex, whereas a bitemporal field defect is found in a lesion of the optic chiasm.

The optic nerve head is evaluated during the funduscopic examination. Items to be evaluated include the optic disc, the retinal vessels that traverse the center of the optic nerve head, and the retina. The optic disc is evaluated for clarity and depth. Papilledema is associated with swelling of the optic disc and is visualized as indeterminate disc margins and loss of venous pulsations in the optic veins. It is bilateral and associated with preserved visual acuity except for extremely advanced cases. The presence of papilledema suggests increased intracranial pressure and can be seen with brain tumors, occlusions of the cerebral venous drainage, and benign intracranial hypertension. Glaucoma is associated with a deep optic disc, but all deep optic discs do not denote glaucoma. Optic neuritis is a common neurologic condition associated with some eye pain, decreased visual acuity that is not corrected by lenses, and an afferent pupillary defect (Marcus-Gunn pupil). Light shown into the affected pupil causes minimal or no pupillary restriction because the inflamed optic nerve is unable to transmit the light stimulus fully or at all. This results in the seeming paradox of the affected pupil dilating in response to a light stimulus. Light shown in the non-affected eye does cause papillary constriction in the opposite eye because of the consensual pupillary reflex (see later). Optic neuritis may be bilateral, and in that case the patient would have bilateral papillary defects.

CN III. OCULOMOTOR CN IV. TROCHLEAR CN VI. ABDUCENS NERVES

The oculomotor (cranial nerve III), trochlear (cranial nerve IV), and abducens (cranial nerve VI) primarily control the movements of the extraocular eye muscles, which are yoked in their actions. Contraction of the right lateral rectus and the left medial rectus causes the eyes to move toward the right, whereas contraction of the superior rectus muscles causes the eyes to deviate superiorly. The oculomotor nerve supplies the superior, inferior, and medial rectus and inferior oblique muscles. These muscles elevate, depress, and adduct the eye. The levator palpebrae muscle also is innervated by this cranial nerve. Denervation of this muscle would result in ptosis of the superior eyelid. The oculomotor nerve also carries parasympathetic fibers to the pupilloconstrictor and ciliary muscles, which cause constriction of the pupil to light and thickening of the lens during accommodation, respectively.

The trochlear nerve supplies the superior oblique muscle. Contraction of this muscle results in depression, adduction, and intorsion of the eye. The abducens nerve supplies the lateral rectus muscle. Contraction of this muscle results in abduction of the eye.

These three cranial nerves are tested together. The examiner first notes the position of the eyes in primary gaze. Are both eyes looking forward, or is one (or are both) deviated from the primary gaze position? The examiner asks the patient to follow his finger as he moves it in the four peripheral quadrants. He notes whether each eye is able to move in all four quadrants of gaze and whether the eye movements are conjugate (symmetric) or dysconjugate. If the eye movements are dysconjugate, each eye's movements are tested individually. Nystagmus may be noted during this examination.

Pupillary function is under the control of the parasympathetic and sympathetic nerves. The parasympathetic fibers are carried on the oculomotor nerve, whereas sympathetic fibers are carried on the carotid and intracranial blood vessels. Pupillary size and equality should be observed during the examination of the eyes and extraocular muscles. A difference of up to 1 mm in the size of the pupils is considered normal. Pupillary reaction to light and accommodation is tested. A bright light is shone into one eye first, and the pupillary response is observed in both eyes. The direct response is the response of the pupil that had the light shone in it. The constriction of the opposite pupil when light stimulates only one eye is called the consensual light reflex. These responses are usually equal. Pupils that are not reactive to light stimulus but that do constrict with accommodation are seen in light-near dissociation. These pupils, called Argyll Robertson pupils, are seen in conditions such as neurosyphilis, diabetes, and autonomic neuropathies. Lesions of the sympathetic pathway, either central or peripheral, result in miosis and ptosis of the affected eye (Horner's syndrome).

Involvement of cranial nerves III, IV, and VI, or of the muscles they serve, almost invariably is accompanied by diplopia except in longstanding squints and progressive external ophthalmoplegia (a rare muscular disorder). Involvement of cranial nerve III distal to its nucleus may present with unilateral ptosis and deficits of adduction, depression, or elevation of the eye with or without associated mydriasis. Bilateral asymmetric extraocular movement deficits without pupillary involvement may represent disease of the ocular muscles (Graves' disease) or the neuromuscular junction (myasthenia gravis). A lesion of cranial nerve VI will result in a deficit of abduction of the eye on straight-ahead gaze. A lesion of cranial nerve IV will result in a deficit of intorsion (internal rotation) of the eye (superior oblique weakness) when the effected eye is attempting to look down and in.

Impairment of conjugate eye movements implies pathology of the cerebral centers controlling eye movements. This may be seen in cerebral hemisphere strokes or basal ganglia degenerative diseases (e.g., progressive supranuclear palsy). These disorders are not accompanied by diplopia.

CN V. THE TRIGEMINAL NERVE

The trigeminal nerve is responsible for conveying sensory information from the skin of the face and anterior scalp, providing motor innervation to the muscles of mastication (masseter, temporalis, pterygoid), and mediating the jaw jerk reflex. The trigeminal nerve is divided into three branches, designated V1 (ophthalmic branch), V2 (maxillary branch), and V3 (mandibular branch) as shown in Fig. 1.1. V1 innervates the forehead and anterior scalp down to the lateral epicanthus of the eye; V2 innervates the cheek down to the corner of the mouth; and V3 innervates the jaw including the underside of the chin but excluding the angle of the jaw. The sensory function of the trigeminal nerve can be tested easily using a safety pin for pain sensation, a cool tuning fork for temperature sensation, and a fingertip or cotton swab for light touch. Testing of proprioception on the face is not practical, and testing of vibration measures CN VIII more effectively than CN V. The main focus for this portion of the examination is assessment of symmetry, with the examiner asking whether the stimuli feel the same or different on the two sides of the face. The corneal reflex also can be used to evaluate CN V function. A wisp of cotton is touched to the cornea while the patient is looking away from the examiner. Normally both eyes blink when either side is stimulated, but in the setting of a

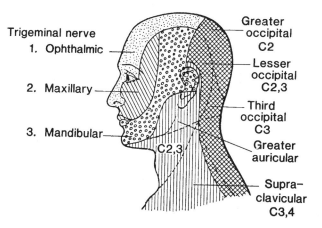

FIG. 1.1. Distribution of the three divisions of the trigeminal nerve. The sensory portion of the trigeminal nerve has three divisions: I, ophthalmic; II, maxillary; III, mandibular. Their approximate locations are illustrated. (From members of the Department of Neurology, Mayo Clinic, and Mayo Foundation for Medical Education and Research, *Clinical examinations in neurology,* 6th ed. St. Louis: Mosby Year Book, 1991:270, with permission.)

unilateral lesion of the trigeminal nerve, neither eye blinks when the abnormal side is stimulated. The motor function of CN V is tested by assessing the strength of jaw closure. This can be performed by having the patient forcibly clench his or her teeth against the resistance of the examiner or forcibly opening the jaw against resistance. In the latter case the jaw will deviate toward the weaker side in pathologic states. (Neither test is performed routinely as part of the screening neurologic examination.) It is interesting that the jaw jerk is mediated solely by the trigeminal nerve and is elicited by placing one's index finger across the relaxed jaw of the patient and tapping that finger with a reflex hammer. A normal response is a brisk but slight contraction of the muscles of mastication causing partial jaw closure. An exaggerated response is a sign of cerebral pathology (an upper motor neuron sign originating above the foramen magnum). An unelicitable response has little clinical significance.

CV VII. THE FACIAL NERVE

The facial nerve provides innervation to the muscles of facial expression and also supplies taste to the anterior two thirds of the tongue via the chorda tympani. Integrity of the facial nerve can be assessed by having the patient perform various maneuvers such as forcibly closing his or her eyes, smiling, puffing air into the cheeks, and wrinkling the forehead muscles. Weakness is indicated by unequal visibility of the eyelashes, an asymmetric smile, inability to hold air fully in the cheeks, and reduced forehead wrinkling, respectively. Facial weakness also can be assessed by simple observation. A down-turned mouth, sagging cheek (flattened nasolabial fold), or sagging lower eyelid (widened palpebral fissure) are all reliable indicators of facial weakness. Lesions of the facial nerve produce eyelid retraction and not ptosis, so that the eye on the affected side appears "larger" than the normal eye.

Facial weakness can occur on the basis of disturbances in the central or peripheral ner-vous systems. Involvement of the frontalis muscles (responsible for wrinkling the forehead) can reliably distinguish between these two possibilities. The forehead is spared with central lesions such as strokes but is affected by peripheral lesions such as Bell's palsy. The sense of taste may be affected by peripheral disturbances, if the lesion is proximal to the chorda tympani. To test the sense of taste, the patient is asked to protrude his or her tongue and identify sweet or sour substances without retracting the tongue. This testing is not performed routinely.

CN VIII. THE ACOUSTIC NERVE

The acoustic nerve (cranial nerve VIII) is a compound nerve comprised of the cochlear nerve that is responsible for hearing and the vestibular nerve that is involved in balance. Although a number of techniques can be used to assess hearing, a simple screen consists of gently rubbing one's fingers together near the patient's ear while performing a similar, mock action near the contralateral ear and having the patient identify from which ear the sound is heard. Normally, the patient should be able to hear the rubbing equally on both sides. A hearing defect would necessitate a stronger stimulus being used on the side of the impairment.

Additional methods to test function of cranial nerve VIII include the Rinne and Weber tests. A tuning fork (256 vibrations per second) is used for the Rinne. The vibrating tuning fork is held against the mastoid bone, and the patient is instructed to tell the examiner when he can no longer hear the noise. The head of the fork then is placed beside the patient's ear. The test result is normal when the patient can hear the vibrating tuning fork much longer when it is placed beside the ear (air conduction is greater than bone conduction). An abnormal Rinne, with bone conduction being greater than air conduction, could be the result of a blockage in the external canal or a lesion in the ossicles of the middle ear. In the Weber test, a vibrating tuning fork is pressed firmly against the middle of the forehead. Normally, sound is perceived equally in both ears and the sound of the vibration is appreciated as being in the midline. With a conductive hearing defect the sound lateralizes to the abnormal ear. In contrast, with a sensorineural hearing loss the sound lateralizes to the opposite ear with the intact nerve.

Dysfunction of the vestibular component of the acoustic nerve is suggested by complaints of vertigo and findings of nystagmus on examination of extraocular eye movements. For routine testing, the vestibular nerve is assessed only indirectly through testing of coordination.

CN IX. GLOSSOPHARYNGEAL NERVE

The glossopharyngeal nerve is responsible for providing sensation to the pharynx and taste to the posterior tongue, but only the former function is tested routinely. Cranial nerve IX mediates the sensory arm of the gag reflex and is tested by taking a cotton swab or tongue blade and gently stimulating the soft palate, looking for palatal elevation or gagging. Each nerve (right and left) can be tested by stimulating each side of the soft palate individually. Normally a gag response is elicited by stimulating either side. In contrast, a unilateral lesion prevents a response with stimulation from one side but not the other. Bilateral lesions prevent responses with stimulation from either side but do not preclude palatal elevation when the patient is prompted to say "aah."

The gag reflex need not be performed in every patient. There are a wide range of responses to this test, and many normal people are hypersensitive to it. Some patients will start to gag as soon as they see the tongue blade. The gag reflex also may be almost absent in a normal patient. A history of swallowing difficulties and speech changes and assorted neurologic abnormalities need to be present before the gag reflex assumes meaning. Isolated reports that the gag reflex is hypersensitive or absent are usually meaningless.

CN X. VAGUS NERVE

The vagus nerve performs a number of functions within the body, including supplying parasympathetic innervation to the heart and gut and contributing to the normal motor function of the oropharynx. As might be expected, CN X mediates the motor limb of the gag reflex and, therefore, also is tested via the gag reflex. Normally, the soft palate and uvula elevate symmetrically with stimulation of the soft palate or when a subject says "aah." With a unilateral lesion of the vagus nerve the uvula and palate deviate away from the lesion. With bilateral lesions no movement or reduced movement is seen. A unilateral lesion of the vagus nerve may not result in swallowing difficulties, whereas bilateral lesions result in regurgitation and dysphagia. A lesion of the recurrent laryngeal nerve, a branch of the vagus, causes unilateral paralysis of vocal cords in the abducted position, resulting in hoarseness.

CN XI. SPINAL ACCESSORY NERVE

The accessory nerve provides innervation to the trapezius and sternocleidomastoid muscles. It arises from the upper five cervical segments of the spinal cord, ascends through the foramen magnum, and exits through the jugular foramen. The accessory nerve is tested by having the patient shrug his or her shoulders or turn his or her head against resistance (the examiner's hand pressed against the subject's jaw). A unilateral lesion causes weakness of shoulder shrugging on the ipsilateral side or impaired head turning to the contralateral side.

CN XII. HYPOGLOSSAL NERVE

The hypoglossal nerve (cranial nerve XII) provides innervation to the tongue. Examination of the tongue includes looking for bulk of the muscle, midline protrusion, and rapid movements from side to side and in and out of the mouth. Unilateral lower motor neuron lesions will cause ipsilateral wasting of the tongue and protrusion toward the weaker side. Bilateral lower motor neuron lesions result in bilateral atrophy of the tongue, poor protrusion, and poor lingual sounds such as "la la la." Bilateral upper motor lesions cause a decrease in the rapidity of tongue movements, whereas unilateral upper motor neuron lesions cause deviation of tongue protrusion away from the side of the lesion.

SENSORY SYSTEM

The sensory examination is very dependent on the subjective responses of the patient. If the patient is confused, demented, or aphasic or has an altered state of consciousness, the responses will be invalid and this portion of the neurologic examination can be omitted. However, if the patient is anxious, seems to have limited tolerance to testing or a limited but not totally impaired attention span, and the history suggests that the sensory examination will be important in reaching a diagnosis, the examination should begin with sensory testing. The patient does not need to undress for the examination, but the legs below the knees and arms below the elbows should be exposed. If a spinal cord problem is suspected, the trunk should be accessible.

The sensory examination is divided into primary sensations and cortical sensations. The primary sensations, including pain, light touch, temperature, vibration, and joint position, are carried on two different tracts. The sensations of pain and temperature are transmitted to the ventroposterior lateral nucleus of the thalamus by the crossed spinothalamic tract. Vibration, joint position, and two-point discrimination are transmitted via the uncrossed posterior columns to the same thalamic nucleus. Both the spinothalamic and posterior columns transmit light touch. The combined sensations then are transmitted to the primary sensory cortex via the fibers of the posterior limb of the internal capsule. Cortical sensations include double simultaneous simulation, stereognosis, and graphesthesia. These sensations can be evaluated only in the presence of intact primary sensory modalities.

The sensory system should be evaluated in a organized manner. Side-to-side and proximal-to-distal comparisons should be made. Hemibody loss of all primary sensory modalities is the result of lesions in the contralateral sensory pathways of the brainstem or cerebral hemispheres. A useful examination technique is to quickly compare the patient's appreciation of pinprick from proximal to distal and from side to side. If a particular area of decreased sensation to pinprick is identified in a part of a limb, careful attention to its boundaries will suggest root (dermatomal), plexus, or peripheral nerve involvement (Fig. 1.2). Temperature can be tested by comparing the touch of a cool tuning fork or by using cold and warm test tubes. A cursory survey of temperature discrimination involves touching the three divisions of the trigeminal nerve with the warm and cool objects, followed by testing the dorsum of the hands and feet. If the patient lacks temperature discrimination in any of these areas, a more detailed examination of that area is required. If any loss of temperature sensation is found, it should be determined if there is a corresponding loss of pinprick sensation because these are carried on the same spinothalamic pathway. The pinprick test includes discrimination between sharp and dull sensations. The patient's response should be immediate, either "sharp" or "dull." A delayed response may suggest either inattention to the activity or that the sensation is traveling along the more diffuse polysynaptic pathway through the reticular formation. Testing of pain and temperature is quite useful, especially when looking for a spinal cord level, because spinothalamic fibers cross within a few segments of entering the spinal cord. The examination should be conducted with disposable pins so that they are not used from patient to patient.

Vibratory sense and joint position are sensations carried in the dorsal columns that do not cross until the cervicomedullary junction. Vibratory sense is tested by placing a vibrating tuning fork (either 128 or 256 Hz) on the nail

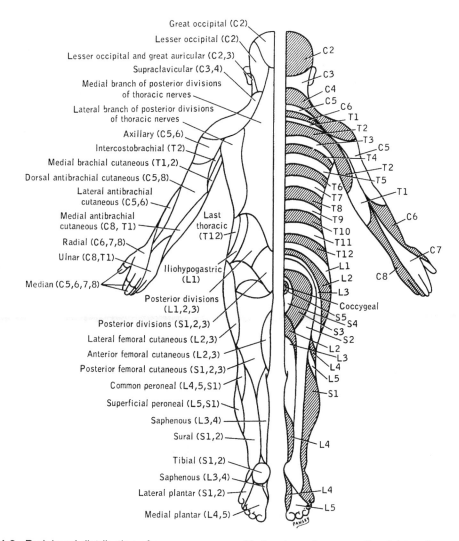

Great occipital (C2)
Lesser occipital (C2)
Lesser occipital and great auricular (C2,3)
Supraclavicular (C3,4)
Medial branch of posterior divisions of thoracic nerves
Lateral branch of posterior divisions of thoracic nerves
Axillary (C5,6)
Intercostobrachial (T2)
Medial brachial cutaneous (T1,2)
Dorsal antibrachial cutaneous (C5,8)
Lateral antibrachial cutaneous (C5,6)
Medial antibrachial cutaneous (C8, T1)
Radial (C6,7,8)
Ulnar (C8,T1)
Median (C5,6,7,8)
Last thoracic (T12)
Iliohypogastric (L1)
Posterior divisions (L1,2,3)
Posterior divisions (S1,2,3)
Lateral femoral cutaneous (L2,3)
Anterior femoral cutaneous (L2,3)
Posterior femoral cutaneous (S1,2,3)
Common peroneal (L4,5,S1)
Superficial peroneal (L5,S1)
Saphenous (L3,4)
Sural (S1,2)
Tibial (S1,2)
Saphenous (L3,4)
Lateral plantar (S1,2)
Medial plantar (L4,5)

C2
C3
C4
C5
C6
T1
T2
T3
C5
T4
T2
T5
T6
T7
T8
T9
T10
T11
T12
L1
L2
L3
Coccygeal
S5
S4
S3
S2
L2
L3
L4
L5
S1
L4
L4
L5
C6
C7
C8
T1

FIG. 1.2. Peripheral distribution of sensory nerves with the dermatomes on the right and cutaneous nerves on the left. (From House EL, Pansky B. *A functional approach to neuroanatomy.* New York: McGraw-Hill, 1960:286, with permission.)

or knuckle of the fingers and toes while the examiner places his or her finger under the patient's digit. In this way the examiner can tell when the vibration has ceased. The patient is asked to tell the examiner if the vibration is felt and when it stops. In this way, a difference in sensory discrimination can be noted if present. The examiner also should use a null stimulus such as a non-vibrating tuning fork for an accurate assessment of this sensory modality.

Gripping the digit by the sides and moving it up, down, or into the neutral position tests joint proprioception. The digits on either side of the digit to be tested should be spread apart so that they do not touch the digit being tested. Using three choices for the answer reduces the possibility of guessing and thus is more reliable. A normal test of joint position would have no incorrect responses. If there is evidence of loss of joint-position sensation in the digits, then testing of the more proximal joints of wrist and ankle is indicated.

Testing higher sensory functions (graphesthesia, stereoagnosia, two-point discrimination, and simultaneous sensation) can reveal information about cortical sensory association areas. It is essential that the primary modality of sensation be present prior to testing these higher cortical functions. Graphesthesia is the patient's ability to recognize written numbers or letters. With the patient's eyes closed, the examiner traces numbers or letters on the patient's palm using a blunt object. A normal test in an educated patient has few errors. Stereoagnosia is the patient's ability to recognize forms. Various objects such as safety pins, keys, coins, or pencils are placed in the patient's hand after the patient closes his eyes. He is allowed to move the object around in his hand to fully appreciate the form. A normal examination has few errors.

Two-point discrimination is the patient's ability to recognize two distinct pressure points. This ability changes, with areas of the face and hand being far more sensitive and the back being less sensitive. This sensory test is dependent on the patient having a mental image of body parts. Double simultaneous stimulation is a useful test in patients in whom inattention to body parts is suspected such as those with right parietal lesions. The examiner alternately touches body parts either on one side or on both sides at the same time. The patient identifies what body parts have been touched. Patients with inattention resulting from parietal lesions will not attend to double stimuli. If the hand is paretic, stereognosis still can be evaluated by moving the object around in the patient's palm.

MOTOR EXAMINATION

Dysfunction of the motor system can occur at any level—at the muscle, neuromuscular junction, peripheral nerve, or central nervous system. Careful and systematic examination of the motor system will give clues to the site of the dysfunction. The motor examination assesses muscle tone, bulk, and strength. It also assesses rapidity of movements, the presence of abnormal movements, and reflexes. First, the patient's muscles are observed for bulk (looking for evidence of atrophy or hypertrophy), fasciculations, and abnormal movements such as tremors. Next, tone, operationally defined as the resistance offered by the limb or other body segment when it is passively mobilized, is assessed as the examiner moves the limb through a full range of flexion and extension movements at the elbow, wrist, knee, ankle, and neck. Tone may be normal, decreased (in lower motor neuron or cerebellar lesions), or increased (in upper motor neuron and extrapyramidal disorders). The increase in tone may be perceived as a ratchety feeling of intermittent tone releases like cogwheels (cogwheel rigidity); as an increase in tone that suddenly gives way, reminiscent of a razor blade (spastic); or as a more diffuse feeling of resistance to movement without any "give" to it (lead-pipe rigidity, as seen occasionally in dystonias and akinetic rigid syndromes or the gegenhalten of the patient with dementia). To examine tone, the examiner asks the patient to relax. Then the upper extremities are examined by holding the arm above the elbow and at the hand and moving the arm through full extension and flexion. For examination of the lower extremities, the patient is placed in the supine position and again asked to relax. The leg is grasped at the level of the knee and quickly raised into the air. The heel of patients with normal or flaccid tone will stay on the bed, but it will elevate off the bed in patients with hypertonicity.

The muscle groups should be examined side to side and proximal to distal, allowing comparisons of strength to be made (Table 1.3).

TABLE 1.3. *Medical Research Council (MRC) Grading of Muscle Strength*

0/5	No movement
1/5	Flicker of movement
2/5	Moves with gravity removed but not against gravity
3/5	Moves against gravity
4/5	Provides resistance
5/5	Normal

Weakness of all muscle groups on one side would suggest a hemiparesis. Proximal muscle weakness would suggest a primary muscle problem (myopathy), whereas distal muscle weakness is suggestive of a neuropathic process. There are also patterns of weakness that suggest cervical or lumber spinal root involvement. In general, C5 innervates deltoids and biceps; C6, wrist extensions; C7, wrist flexors; C8, finger flexion; and T1, finger abduction and adduction. L1, L2, and L3 innervate the iliopsoas muscle (hip flexion); L2, L3, and L4 control knee extension; L5 controls dorsiflexion, version, and inversion of the foot; and S1 controls plantar flexion. Muscle strength is graded on a scale from 0 to 5:0 = absence of movement, 1 = a flicker of movement, 2 = movement on the horizontal plane with gravity removed, 3 = movement against gravity with resistance that can be overcome, and 5 = movement against gravity with resistance that cannot be overcome.

To test dexterity of movement (after assessing for strength), the patient is asked to open and close the hand rapidly, to alternate movements between pronation and supination, or to tap the toes. The examiner is looking for the speed, amplitude, and regularity of these movements. Impairment is suggestive of dysfunction of either the basal ganglia or cerebellum if the strength has been preserved.

Abnormal movements are observed while the patient is at rest and while he has his hands out-stretched. These abnormal movements will be discussed in Chapter 11.

REFLEXES

The deep tendon reflexes (DTRs) also known as muscle stretch reflexes are responses of muscle spindles to rapid stretch. The stretch causes rapid firing of muscle spindles. Information from the stretched muscle fibers is transmitted via afferent fibers to the spinal cord where they synapse on anterior horn cells (Table 1.4). Efferent fibers from the anterior horn cells synapse with muscle fibers at the neuromuscular junction. The muscles contract to prevent "overstretching" of the

TABLE 1.4. *Segmental Innervation of the Various Deep Tendon Reflexes*

S1, S2	Achilles reflex
L2, L3, L4	Patellar reflex
C5, C6	Biceps reflex
C6, C7, C8	Triceps reflex

muscles and hyperextension of the joints controlled by those muscles. The segmental representation of the routinely assessed DTRs can be remembered easily by simply "counting to 8," with the Achilles tendon reflex or "ankle jerk" being conveyed by fibers from the S1 and S2 nerve roots, the patellar reflexes or "knee-jerks" being conveyed by fibers from the L3 and L4 (as well as L2) nerve roots, the biceps reflex being conveyed by the C5 and C6 nerve roots, and the triceps reflex being conveyed by the C7 and C8 (as well as C6) nerve roots.

Although there are numerous DTRs, only some of them are used in a routine neurologic examination. These reflexes are the biceps, brachioradialis, and triceps reflexes of the upper extremities and the patellar and ankle responses of the lower extremities.

DTRs are elicited by using a reflex hammer to strike the tendon of interest and then palpating or visualizing a shortening of the muscle. The Achilles reflex (ankle jerk) is elicited by striking the Achilles tendon just proximal to the heel and monitoring for subsequent plantarflexion. When the patient is supine, this reflex is elicited most easily with the leg externally rotated, the knee flexed, and the ankle held in passive dorsiflexion. The patellar reflex is elicited by striking the patellar tendon just below the kneecap and monitoring for knee extension. With the patient sitting, the leg can be supported by grasping the lower leg. When the subject is supine, the reflex is elicited most easily with the patient's knee draped over the examiner's forearm. The biceps reflex is elicited by having the examiner strike his or her own finger that is pressed against the patient's biceps tendon within the antecubital fossa. The examiner then observes for flexion at the elbow. The triceps reflex is elicited by striking the triceps tendon within the olecranon fossa, just proximal to the elbow, and observing for elbow extension.

The DTRs are graded according to a standardized system, as listed in Table 1.5. Namely, absent reflexes are graded as 0, reduced reflexes as 1+, normal reflexes as 2+, and brisk reflexes as 3+. When clonus is elicited (rhythmic, oscillatory movements of the joint) a grade of 4+ is given. Unfortunately, the determination of "normal" versus "reduced" versus "brisk" is subjective. To increase reliability some authors promote the convention of using 3+ when "spread" is seen, whereby the testing of one reflex elicits responses in multiple reflex arcs (e.g., striking the biceps tendon elicits a triceps reflex). Similarly, the grade of 1+ could be reserved for instances in which "augmentation" is necessary (e.g., the patient is asked to "bite down" while the reflex is being elicited to reduce the threshold for the response). Hyperactive reflexes are considered an "upper motor neuron sign" generally seen in CNS disturbances; somewhat brisk reflexes, however, can be seen in otherwise healthy young people. Reduced reflexes can be seen in disorders of the peripheral nervous system and are considered a "lower motor neuron sign."

Asymmetric decrease or loss of a particular reflex is seen with radiculopathies, plexopathies, or mononeuropathies. Examples include ipsilateral loss of biceps and brachioradialis reflexes in pathology of the sixth cervical root and the loss of the knee reflex in femoral neuropathy. Decrease or loss of reflexes in the upper extremities with hyperflexia in the lower extremities suggests spinal cord pathology at the cervical level or amyotrophic lateral sclerosis. Bilateral decrease or absence of distal DTRs suggests peripheral neuropathy.

TABLE 1.5. *Deep Tendon Reflex Grading*

1+ Reduced
2+ Normal
3+ Increased
4+ Pathologically increased clonus

Hyperreflexia is seen in diseases affecting the upper motor neuron (motor cortex or corticospinal tract) and is associated with increase in tone (spasticity) and a positive Babinski reflex. It is seen with degenerative, neoplastic inflammatory, vascular, and posttraumatic disease affecting the brain, brainstem, or spinal cord.

The plantar response is obtained most commonly by stroking the lateral surface of the sole of the foot from heel to toe. The great toe flexes in a normal response and extends in an abnormal response (Babinski sign).

Cerebellar Function Examination

The cerebellum is an integrating way station for the control of volitional muscular movements. It integrates information from the various sensory and motor systems that results in fluid movements and postures. Dysfunction of this system is manifest in disorders of gait, abnormal speech and eye movements, hypotonia, tremors, and clumsiness of movements. Cerebellar syndromes may consist of four components, including ataxia, dysarthria, hypotonia, and nystagmus.

The clinical manifestations of these disorders can be evaluated by listening to the patient's speech; using examination techniques to demonstrate incoordination, kinetic tremor, and decomposition of movement; and observing the gait. The presence of weakness in the limbs, involuntary movements, or any other concomitant neurologic deficit will affect the cerebellar examination. In evaluating specific motor functions, the patient's ability to judge the speed, power, and distance to carry out an act should be noted. If these are faulty, dysmetria is present. If the patient has difficulty in carrying out repetitive successive acts or in stopping one motor maneuver and immediately starting an opposite motor act, dysdiadochokinesia is present.

Appendicular movements test coordination of movements of the extremities. The cerebellar hemispheres modulate these movements. The finger-to-nose-finger test and the heel-to-shin maneuver test appendicular movements.

In the former, the patient is asked to touch his finger to the examiner's finger, then to touch his finger to the examiner's finger, and then to touch his own nose. The patient's eyes are open during this testing. The examiner positions his finger at a distance such that the patient must fully extend the arm to touch it. In this way, any tremor at the extreme of arm extension can be seen. This tremor, termed a kinetic tremor, is a side-to-side pendular tremor as the patient tries to touch the examiner's finger or his own nose. An intention or kinetic tremor also can be observed in the lower extremity when the patient is asked to put his heel on his knee and then run his heel down his shin. This is performed with the patient supine.

Midline cerebellar dysfunction is characterized by ataxia of the trunk. The patient is observed sitting upright or walking to determine the ability to hold the trunk and head still. Patients with midline cerebellar lesions are unable to hold the head and trunk in position and have a swaying movement.

GAIT EXAMINATION

Like the mental examination, the gait examination starts the moment the physician greets the patient. The gait examination is best interpreted after the symptoms and signs have been gathered and diagnostic hypotheses have been framed.

The patient is asked to arise from a chair with his arms crossed. Mild difficulties are present if the patient performs this task slowly, flexing the knees while bringing the upper body forward or sliding the buttocks forward over the seating surface before trying to stand up. A measure of more difficulty in rising is the need for repeated attempts before accomplishing the task or the need to use the hands to push the body up. More severe degrees of impairment are indicated by the need for assistance. Difficulties in this area can be the result of proximal muscle weakness, basal ganglia disease, or pain in the low back or proximal lower extremities.

The patient's posture is observed. Patients with Parkinson's disease exhibit a stooping (simian) posture, which may be associated with thoracic kyphosis and additional lateral bending. Patients with progressive supranuclear palsy—another extrapyramidal disorder causing bradykinesia and rigidity—may display an erect or hypererect posture. An exaggerated lumber lordosis may be seen in patients with proximal lower-extremity weakness, as seen in muscular dystrophies and other myopathies.

The patient's ambulation is analyzed for speed, stride length, turning, and associated movements. Diseases affecting the pyramidal tract or the extrapyramidal system may shorten the stride length, slow ambulation, decrease the vertical displacement of the advancing foot, and be associated with a decrease or absence of the associated arm movement on the same side. It sometimes is impossible to distinguish, on gait examination alone, a patient who has recovered only partially from a stroke from a patient with early Parkinson's disease. Patients with a cerebellar disease, progressive supranuclear palsy, or labyrinthine disease may exhibit a cautious, wide-based stance with consequent slowing of ambulation. The festinating gait of the patient with Parkinson's disease is characterized by rapid, increasingly accelerating short steps, and the patient may have difficulty coming to an immediate halt at will.

Weakness of the tibialis anterior muscle results in inability to adequately dorsiflex the foot as the foot is being advanced and in a resultant compensatory marked elevation of the leg in what is called a step-page gait (seen in common peroneal neuropathy or L5 radiculopathy). Weakness of the same muscle may be manifested by an inability to heel walk (also seen in pyramidal tract disease). Toe-walking difficulty is indicative of gastrocnemius weakness (seen in posterior tibial neuropathy or S1-S2 radiculopathies).

Efficient turning is accomplished by an act of sequential pivoting of both legs. The leg opposite the desired direction of turn is the one making the final advance prior to the turning moment, and the posteriorly placed leg is the first to pivot. Difficulties in this area are manifested by the substitution of multiple steps or the appearance of sudden interruptions of the movement (freezing). It is at this juncture that falls are more likely to occur, and the examiner should be reasonably close to the patient to prevent this. Adequate turning or pivoting may be affected in disorders of basal ganglia, cerebellar disease, or labyrinthine disease. Freezing is viewed exclusively as an extrapyramidal (basal ganglion) dysfunction.

The patient then is asked to stand with one foot next to the other. Patients with cerebellar disease, advanced basal ganglia disease, or acute labyrinthine disease may be unable to successfully accomplish this task and may find it necessary to separate the distance between their feet. Only after a standing stance has been accomplished can the clinician proceed to perform the Romberg test. The patient is asked to close his eyes while trying to stand still. Oscillations in the lateral or anteroposterior direction may normally appear, but the feet will not move. Wider oscillations culminating in a loss of equilibrium suggest proprioceptive difficulties in the lower extremities, implying dysfunction in the posterior columns, although it also can be seen with severe sensory neuropathies.

Postural stability can be checked in the anteroposterior direction by having the clinician place him or herself behind the standing patient and firmly pushing the patient backward on the midsternal area or the anterior aspect of both shoulders. A normal response results in quick return of the displaced upper body to its preperturbation position. At times, a normal subject may have to take one or two steps back to avoid a fall. Abnormal responses are variable, ranging from the need for multiple steps to avoid the fall; the loss of generation of these multiple steps; the failure of multiple steps to avoid the fall; or the loss of generation of these multiple steps with a tendency to fall en bloc, sometimes without the compensatory forward elevation of the upper extremities. The most severely affected patients are those who need to be held while standing or walking. Basal ganglia and cerebellar disease

are the most frequent causes of problems in this area.

Postural stability is checked in the lateral direction by asking the patient to walk in tandem. Difficulties in this area include cerebellar disease, labyrinthine disease, proprioceptive difficulties in the lower extremities, and basal ganglia disease.

Neurologic Examination in Pediatric Neurology

Performing age-appropriate examinations of infants and children can be a daunting task given the amazing developmental advances that occur in early childhood. Infants and young children require adaptations of the routine adult neurologic examination including the use of more functional tasks to assess neurologic performance. A good working knowledge of normal gross motor, fine motor, and language development is essential. As with other pediatric disciplines, the child's parents can be enlisted to assist with examination. For small children and infants much of the examination can be performed on the parent's lap because the comfort and safety of the child are key. Unpleasant tests such as the testing of pain sensation (i.e., with a pin) should be avoided whenever possible.

Mental Status

The mental status examination often centers around the child's behavior with respect to the parents and surroundings. Assessment of receptive and expressive language skills can yield insight into the child's cognitive abilities even in infancy. Knowledge of normal development milestones allows the examiner to relate a child's abilities to the normal population.

Cranial Nerves

Most cranial nerves can be tested easily with creative techniques in children. Visual acuity can be assessed roughly by holding colorful or bright objects of varying size within an infant's field of vision. Similarly, one can offer a toddler a small wad of paper within one's hand. Visual fields and eye movements can be assessed by holding attractive objects in the periphery of the child's vision. Visual threat also can be used to test visual fields in infants older than 4 months of age, but this technique may be considered too threatening if not performed in a sufficiently playful manner. The funduscopic examination can be challenging but not impossible in children, especially older infants. The pupillary light reflex can be tested in standard fashion in all age groups. The corneal reflex can be reasonably elicited in young infants but may be unacceptably irksome to older children. Although not technically proper, a quick puff of air into the eye is better tolerated than a cotton swab. In any event, facial asymmetry can be assessed by observing the child's repertoire of facial expressions. Hearing can be assessed using a number of sound-producing toys held outside of the child's field of view. As with the corneal reflex, testing of the gag reflex is well tolerated by young infants but is a more sensitive issue in children. In contrast, most children relish the opportunity to protrude their tongues at an adult.

Reflexes

Testing of DTRs in children requires no special accommodations other than gentleness. Remember that an extensor plantar response (up-going toe) is normal in infants up to 1 year of age.

Motor

Assessment of muscle bulk in children is no different than in adults except that young infants may have more superficial adipose tissue. Tone can be assessed easily in older children if they are at ease or distracted. Assessment of power in infants usually is restricted to opposing their volitional movements. In young children one must rely on functional assessment of strength, observing the child perform playful tasks. Older children, how-

ever, are usually very cooperative in testing "how strong they are."

Sensory

Vibratory sensation can be tested reliably in older but not younger children. Proprioception is tested more reliably in children because the outcomes are directly observable by the examiner. Temperature sensation can be tested with a cool tuning fork. Testing of pin sensation generally should be avoided because of the inherently uncomfortable nature of the test.

Coordination

Age-appropriate testing of coordination is straightforward. Infants older than a few months can reach for colorful objects. Toddlers can be assessed for their ability to walk and reach for things. Older children can be asked to run, jump, and hop or stand on one leg.

In summary, the neurologic examination of children must be tailored to a child's age, abilities, and temperament. Gaining a child's trust is imperative.

QUESTIONS AND DISCUSSION

1. A 62-year-old man has had a feeling of generalized weakness for the preceding 3 weeks, associated with difficulty in chewing and swallowing and a change in the quality of speech. Further questioning reveals that he has been suffering from intermittent diplopia and drooping of one eyelid for the preceding year. The examination reveals ptosis of the left eyelid and impaired abduction of the left eye. There is weakness of jaw opening and nasal speech. The gag reflex is present, but the soft palate elevates poorly. Weakness is generalized, affecting both proximal and distal muscles. There are no cognitive findings (including no emotional lability) and no sensory findings. Reflexes are normal and symmetric, plantar responses are flexor, and tone is normal. The likely site of the lesion is:

A. Both cerebral hemispheres.

B. The neuromuscular junction.

C. The brainstem affecting cranial nerves III, V, VI, IX, and X.

D. The peripheral nerves in a diffuse fashion as seen in Guillain-Barré syndrome.

The answer is not (A). Bilateral hemisphere dysfunction capable of causing difficulty in chewing, swallowing, and speaking is known as a pseudobulbar state. It implies bilateral involvement of the corticobulbar fibers (i.e., a dysfunction of those connections between the cerebral hemispheres and the brainstem nuclei). This may be seen in individuals who have suffered multiple strokes. This patient had diplopia, a symptom that cannot be explained by lesions proximal to the brainstem nuclei. He also lacked cranial hyperreflexia (hyperactive jaw jerk and gag reflexes), limb hyperreflexia, Babinski responses, limb spasticity, or cognitive changes (slowness of mental function, emotional lability).

The answer is (B). Myasthenia gravis is the most commonly seen disease of the neuromuscular junction. It can affect eye movements in an asymmetric fashion, with diplopia being a frequent early complaint. This patient had difficulty in chewing because of jaw muscle weakness but no evidence of direct cranial nerve V involvement (no sensory findings over the face). The patient's difficulty in swallowing and his nasality of voice were expressive of involvement of the soft palate musculature. The fact that gag reflex and jaw jerk were not hyperactive spoke against the involvement of corticobulbar fibers. The fact that the generalized weakness was not accompanied by reflex, tone, or sensory abnormalities spoke against involvement of central (corticospinal tracts at brain, brainstem, or spinal cord level) or peripheral motor fibers.

The answer is not (C). A brainstem event may in fact be associated with diplopia by affecting cranial nerve nuclei or fibers connecting them (medial longitudinal fasciculus). Ptosis of the one eye in such a context could be the result of Horner's syndrome, but the ipsilateral pupil was not miotic. It also could be caused by involvement of cranial nerve III or its fibers before they emerge from the brainstem, but other cranial nerve III–dependent functions were not affected (no deficit of eye adduction, elevation, or depression; no pupillary dilatation). A brainstem event also could be associated with dysphagia. Dysarthria (deficit in articulation) or anarthria (absence of articulation) rather than nasality of voice is a more likely speech difficulty. An acute brainstem event (e.g., CVA) may be associated with quadriparesis but also would be associated with flaccidity of tone and hyporeflexia. As the patient recovers, spasticity and hyperreflexia will appear. Neither feature was present in this case.

The answer is not (D). An acute inflammatory polyradiculoneuropathy (Guillain-Barré syndrome) can be associated with rapid onset of generalized weakness, including bulbar dysfunction (dysphagia, difficulty with mastication, voice nasality) but is not likely to be preceded by diplopia for months, as was the case for this patient. Areflexia is a very important feature of this condition. Sensory symptoms or signs (especially distal paresthesias) also may occur.

2. A 55-year-old woman has noticed gradual loss of dexterity of her left hand and increasing difficulty with ambulation. Examination discloses an atrophied left hand and bilateral lower-extremity spasticity. The left lower extremity is weaker than the right, whereas pinprick is better perceived on that same side. The decrease in sensation to pinprick on the right side extends to the upper trunk. There are no cranial nerve findings, and cognitive functions are intact. The likely site of the lesion is:

A. An asymmetric polyneuropathy affecting the left median nerve and both sciatic nerves.

B. A cervical cord–compressive syndrome.

C. A diffuse motor neuron disorder (amyotrophic lateral sclerosis).

The answer is not (A). Polyneuropathy does not cause lower-extremity spasticity, which is a sign of upper motor neuron dysfunction.

The answer is (B). An asymmetric spasticity with the weaker lower extremity on the left and decreased sensation to pinprick on the opposite side places the site of pathology in the spinal cord, predominantly on the left side. The reason pinprick is diminished on the right is that the fibers of the spinothalamic tract cross to the opposite side shortly after entering the spinal cord. Thus, a lesion that affects the pathways for pain sensation on one side of the cord will be experienced as decreased sensation to pinprick on the opposite side of the body. The precise location of the lesion is given by the wasting of the left hand, a lower motor neuron lesion that suggests involvement of the lower motor neurons at the C8 or T1 root levels.

The answer is not (C). Motor neuron disease can present with a combination of upper and motor neuron signs such as in this case, but there is no sensory involvement.

3. A 35-year-old woman presents with complaints of painful burning feet and difficulty with ambulation. The examination discloses severe loss of position and vibratory sense in the lower extremities (distal more than proximal), lower-extremity spasticity, hyperreflexia, and abnormal Babinski responses. The upper extremities show a similar sensory deficit but to a milder degree. There are no cranial nerve or cognitive deficits. The likely site of the lesion is:

A. The posterior columns and corticospinal tracts at the level of the spinal cord.

B. The peripheral nerves, particularly the large myelinated fibers that conduct proprioceptive information.

C. The brainstem, affecting the proprioceptive fibers (medial lemnisci) and corticospinal tracts.

The answer is (A). The loss of proprioceptive information can be caused by a peripheral neuropathy affecting large myelinated fibers or to disease affecting the dorsal columns in the spinal cord. The concurrent presence of upper motor neuron signs (spasticity, hyperreflexia, and Babinski responses) points to the spinal cord as the site of pathology.

The answer is not (B). A peripheral neuropathy could be associated with selective or preferential involvement of those fibers conducting proprioceptive information, but it would not be the cause of the associated upper motor neuron findings.

The answer is not (C). The patient does not have evidence of involvement of other brainstem structures such as cranial nerves or gaze centers.

4. A 25-year-old woman with myopia presents with the complaint of blurred vision of the left eye associated with eye pain for the preceding 7 days. Past history reveals that she has been experiencing amenorrhea for the preceding 6 months. There is a very strong family history of glaucoma. The extraocular movements are intact, and there is no ptosis. The eye examination discloses no overt abnormalities of the cornea, iris, or lens. Visual acuity of the left eye is 20/80, corrected by glasses, whereas it is 20/25 in the right eye with glasses. The left pupil dilates as a light is directed from the right to the left eye. Funduscopic examination reveals blurred margins of the left disk. There are no other findings on neurologic examination. The likely site of the lesion is:

A. The optic chiasm as a result of compression by a pituitary gland tumor.

B. The right occipital lobe or right optic radiations.

C. The anterior chamber of the eye from an attack of acute glaucoma.

D. The left optic nerve

The answer is not (A). Although the patient's amenorrhea warrants investigation, it is unlikely to explain her symptoms and signs because a lesion at the level of the optic chiasm would cause loss of both temporal fields of vision and not a monocular decrease in visual acuity.

The answer is not (B). A lesion of the right occipital lobe or the optic radiations would cause a loss of vision in the nasal field of the right eye and the temporal field of the left eye (left homonymous hemianopsia).

The answer is not (C). Sudden loss of vision as a result of an acute attack of glaucoma can be associated with eye pain and even with an unreactive pupil. It is not associated with swelling of the optic disc. The patient's positive family history for glaucoma proves to be a red herring rather than a clue in this particular case.

The answer is (D). The patient's picture is very characteristic of acute optic neuritis with a decrease of central vision in one eye, associated with an afferent pupillary defect and swelling of the optic disc. Sometimes the swelling of the optic nerve may occur more posteriorly and the disc may appear normal (retrobulbar neuritis). Approximately 30% of patients who suffer optic neuritis eventually will develop multiple sclerosis.

SUGGESTED READING

Adams RD, Victor M. *Principles of neurology,* 5th ed. New York: McGraw-Hill, 1993:5–9.

De Myer WE. *Technique of the neurological examination: a programmed text,* 4th ed. New York: McGraw-Hill, 1994.

Glaser JS. *Neuro-ophthalmology,* 2nd ed. Philadelphia: JB Lippincott, 1990:37–60.

Haerer AF. *DeJong's the neurologic examination,* 5th ed. Philadelphia: JB Lippincott, 1992.

Kaplan HI, Sadock BJ. *Synopsis of psychiatry,* 5th ed. Baltimore: Williams & Wilkins, 1988.

Medical Research Council. *Aids to the examination of the peripheral nervous system.* London: HMSO, 1976.

Members of the Department of Neurology, Mayo Clinic, and Mayo Foundation for Medical Education and Research. *Clinical examinations in neurology,* 6th ed. St. Louis: Mosby Year Book, 1991:270.

2

An Approach to Neurologic Symptoms

Steven L. Lewis

In neurologic diagnosis, individual symptoms and constellations of symptoms can be of telling diagnostic importance both anatomically and etiologically. Thus, a detailed neurologic history that puts together various symptoms and their temporal development can help to define neurologic entities with significant precision; the role of the subsequent neurologic examination is to look for evidence to support, or refute, the diagnostic hypothesis generated by the symptoms elucidated by the neurologic history.

COMMON NEUROLOGIC TERMS

Before proceeding with a discussion of specific neurologic symptoms, it is worthwhile to define some terms that can be useful in characterizing neurologic symptom complexes. These words are used to indicate certain localizations of pathology (Table 2.1). Encephalopathy means disease of the brain. Although theoretically the term encephalopathy could refer to any process involving any part of the brain, it generally is used to connote dysfunction that involves the entirety of both cerebral hemispheres. Thus, the terms encephalopathy and diffuse encephalopathy are essentially synonymous. A common type of encephalopathy is metabolic encephalopa-

thy, such as that caused by hepatic, uremic, or other metabolic dysfunction.

Myelopathy means disease of the spinal cord. A patient with any symptoms or signs that are caused by spinal cord dysfunction has a myelopathy. A common type of myelopathy is a compressive myelopathy caused by a tumor or other mass lesion compressing the spinal cord, causing weakness, sensory loss, and spasticity below the level of the compression.

Radiculopathy, disease of the nerve roots (*radix* is Latin for root; a radish is a root vegetable), is the term used for any process involving single or multiple nerve roots in the cervical, thoracic, or lumbar spine. For example, a herniated lumbar disc between the fourth and fifth lumbar spine might cause an L5 radiculopathy; Guillain-Barré syndrome would cause a polyradiculopathy as a result of dysfunction of multiple nerve roots.

Neuropathy means disease of a nerve. The term connotes dysfunction of one (mononeuropathy), several (mononeuropathy multiplex), or many/diffuse (polyneuropathy) peripheral nerves. Dysfunction of a cranial nerve would be called a cranial neuropathy. Myopathy refers to any disease of muscle.

These generic terms are very helpful to the clinician in categorizing sites of pathology or dysfunction. A specific causative lesion, or causative process, is not conveyed by any of these terms. Unless there is a preceding adjective (e.g., compressive myelopathy or demyelinative polyneuropathy), a cause or mechanism is not implied. Likewise, substitution of the suffix *-itis* for *-pathy* (e.g., myositis instead of myopathy) implies, specifically, an inflammatory process, rather than an as-yet-unknown process affecting that region of the nervous system.

TABLE 2.1. *Common Terms Used to Describe Localizations of Neurologic Dysfunction*

Term	Meaning
Encephalopathy	Disease of brain (usually refers to diffuse brain dysfunction)
Myelopathy	Disease of spinal cord
Radiculopathy	Disease of nerve root
Neuropathy	Disease of nerve
Myopathy	Disease of muscle

AN APPROACH TO SPECIFIC NEUROLOGIC SYMPTOM COMPLEXES

The essential elements of the neurologic diagnostic process are an accurate and detailed history, followed by a neurologic examination. Imaging and laboratory studies follow, as appropriate. The goal is to determine where in the nervous system the problem lies, as well as how the dysfunction occurred. This section discusses the *where* part of the neurologic formulation using the history and examination. Using the temporal course of the evolution of symptoms to help determine the mechanism of dysfunction will be discussed later in this chapter. Several specific symptom complexes are discussed in the following section: mental status changes, weakness, sensory symptoms, and gait disorders.

MENTAL STATUS CHANGES

When confronted with a patient who has had a mental status change, the clinician should try to determine whether there is an alteration in the level of consciousness or an alteration of the content of consciousness. Alterations in the level of consciousness manifest in the continuum between drowsiness and coma. They result either from dysfunction of both cerebral hemispheres, dysfunction of the upper brainstem (mid pons or above), or a combination of hemispheric and upper-brainstem dysfunction. The clinical approach to the patient who presents with an alteration in level of consciousness is discussed in more detail in Chapter 5. A major goal of the neurologic examination of these patients is to determine whether there is focal brainstem dysfunction. If brainstem function is intact, the cause of the problem is unlikely to be the result of a focal structural brainstem process; it is more likely the result of a diffuse encephalopathic process (involving both cerebral hemispheres or the hemispheres and the brainstem). The actual processes that may affect the level of consciousness are vast and are discussed in more detail in Chapter 5.

Neurologic processes can affect the mental status of patients, however, by affecting the content of consciousness without necessarily altering the level of consciousness (see Chapters 15 and 16). Alterations in the content of consciousness are exemplified by psychiatric disorders or by neurologic processes that affect memory, language, awareness, or global intellectual functioning. Patients with chronic dementing illnesses (Chapter 16) usually have normal alertness despite the deterioration in cognitive functioning. Patients with aphasia—particularly those with fluent aphasias (Chapter 15)—often appear to be confused. More careful attention to the patient's speech pattern to determine the presence of paraphasic errors and neologisms often will help the clinician determine that the "confused" patient is actually aphasic; the presence of aphasia is usually a clue to focal dysfunction in the dominant (usually left) hemisphere. Patients with lesions affecting the right hemisphere also may appear to be "confused," neglectful, and unaware, whereas they actually have neglect of the left side of space and may be oblivious of their deficit (anosognosia) because of the nondominant hemisphere dysfunction.

WEAKNESS

"Weakness" as a patient complaint may have several possible meanings, besides the usually presumed meaning of a decrease in motor function in one or several extremities. The clinician should keep in mind that some patients might use the term weakness to describe generalized fatigue, malaise, or asthenia. Some patients might even describe a symptom such as the generalized bradykinesia of parkinsonism (Chapter 10) as weakness. As in all neurologic diagnosis, an accurate history and examination should suffice for clarification. Muscular fatigue, although very nonspecific, suggests the possibility of a disorder of the neuromuscular junction, such as myasthenia gravis (see Chapter 19), or a disease of muscle (myopathy), in addition to primarily non-neurologic processes causing generalized malaise and fatigue.

The following are definitions of some common terms used to describe decreases in motor function. Paresis refers to muscular weakness but not complete paralysis. Plegia is the term used to describe complete paralysis. Monoparesis and monoplegia are terms sometimes used to describe weakness or paralysis in one extremity. Hemiparesis and hemiplegia refer to weakness or paralysis in the arm and leg on one side of the body. Paraparesis and paraplegia describe weakness or paralysis in both legs, and quadriparesis and quadriplegia (sometimes alternatively called tetraplegia) denote weakness or paralysis in all four extremities.

Muscular weakness can occur as a result of dysfunction at any level of the central or peripheral nervous system. To illustrate this, it is worth considering the neuroanatomic pathway for muscle movement.

The pathway for muscle movement begins in nerve cells that are located on the precentral gyrus of each frontal lobe. The axons from these nerve cells comprise the corticospinal tract. The corticospinal tracts travel through the white matter of each cerebral hemisphere, through the internal capsule, and further downward into the brainstem, where each corticospinal tract crosses in the low medulla to the opposite side. From the medulla, the corticospinal tracts travel downward through each side of the spinal cord.

Within the spinal cord, the corticospinal tract on each side synapses with nerve cells in the anterior horns located in the spinal cord gray matter. Axons from these second-order neurons become the cervical, thoracic, and lumbosacral nerve roots. The cervical nerve roots then form the brachial plexus, and the nerves that are formed in the brachial plexus travel into the upper extremities and innervate the muscles of the upper extremities. The lumbar nerve roots travel downward within the lumbar spinal canal as the cauda equina, before exiting and forming the lumbosacral plexus and ultimately the nerves that innervate the lower-extremity musculature.

A lesion at any level of the previously mentioned pathway, from the cerebral cortex to the muscles themselves, can cause weakness. The location of this lesion causing weakness, or a history of weakness, is not always immediately obvious, even to an experienced clinician who has performed an accurate history and examination. However, there are typical, or classic, patterns of muscle weakness that lesions at various levels of the pathway for motor function usually will produce. Recognition of these typical patterns can be very helpful in attempting to decide on possible localizations of pathology in patients who present with motor weakness.

UPPER MOTOR NEURON SYNDROMES

Lesions that cause dysfunction of the corticospinal tracts are called upper motor neuron lesions; their distinctive features, in addition to weakness, include increased or pathologic reflexes and increased tone and spasticity in chronic lesions. It also should be recognized that these classic findings of upper motor neuron dysfunction might not always be evident. Upper motor neuron syndromes can result from lesions of the corticospinal tract at various levels of the central nervous system. Further clinical details—described later— help to specify whether the lesion is cortical, subcortical, or in the spinal cord. When symptoms of transient motor dysfunction occur, no abnormalities would be expected on the examination, and the site of the lesion must be inferred by the patient's description of the areas of transient weakness and associated symptoms.

Hemispheric motor cortex lesions involving the cortical motor neurons of the lateral surface of one hemisphere usually cause upper motor neuron weakness of the contralateral face (see Chapter 1) and arm, with less weakness of the leg. A lesion in this region, like all corticospinal tract lesions, often will cause predominant weakness in the extensors of the arm and flexors of the leg, with relative preservation of strength in arm flexors and leg extensors. As such, the affected arm is held mildly flexed while walking and the leg is overextended, causing it to drag stiffly, sometimes catching the toe. Hemispheric motor cortex lesions involving the medial aspect of one frontal lobe will predominantly cause contralateral leg weakness. Weakness resulting from lesions affecting cortical motor neurons often is accompanied by other signs of cortical dysfunction, giving a clue to the localization of the problem. For example, left hemisphere cortical lesions often are accompanied by abnormalities of language function (see Chapter 15). Right hemisphere cortical lesions often are accompanied by denial of the left-sided weakness or even unawareness of the presence of the left extremities (asomatognosia). Any complex behavioral change of these types suggests that the upper motor neuron lesion is cortical. Cortical lesions causing weakness often also are accompanied by some contralateral sensory disturbance because of the proximity of the cortical sensory neurons to the motor cortex.

Deep hemispheric or internal capsule lesions also will cause weakness of the contralateral body but without accompanying signs of cortical dysfunction. Lesions affecting the corticospinal tract fibers in the posterior limb of the internal capsule may produce a characteristic pure motor hemiparesis (or hemiplegia) involving the contralateral face, arm, and leg (see Chapter 6). This is characterized by significant weakness of one side of the body without sensory disturbance or signs of cortical dysfunction such as aphasia. This distinctive form of isolated weakness occurs because the corticospinal fibers from a large area of the motor cortex all lie close together in the internal capsule, segregated from the sensory fibers, and deep to the cortical structures. In contrast, a hemispheric lesion that would be large enough to cause significant weakness of an entire side of the body most likely also would involve sensory signs or symptoms and signs of cortical dysfunction.

Brainstem lesions that involve the corticospinal tract on one side also will cause weakness of the contralateral side of the body. Some unilateral ventral pontine lesions—affecting only the corticospinal tract but no other brainstem pathways—may even produce an isolated pure motor hemiparesis clinically indistinguishable from an internal capsular lesion. However, many brainstem processes producing weakness also produce brainstem signs or brainstem symptoms such as diplopia, vertigo, nausea, and vomiting, or cranial nerve palsies, which are clues to the brainstem localization of the process (see Chapter 6). One of the pillars of neurologic localization is that a brainstem lesion can cause weakness of the contralateral body (as a result of involvement of the corticospinal tract) and dysfunction of an ipsilateral cranial nerve (as a result of involvement of a cranial nerve nucleus, or the cranial nerve itself, before it exits the brainstem). An example would be a right peripheral facial palsy and left body weakness as a result of a right pontine lesion. In addition, because both the right and the left corticospinal tracts are relatively close together in the brainstem, bilateral extremity weakness can be seen in brainstem disease.

Lesions of the corticospinal tracts in the spinal cord cause weakness below the level of the spinal cord lesion. Although it is possible to have unilateral weakness resulting from a spinal cord lesion, many lesions affecting the spinal cord cause bilateral weakness because of involvement of the corticospinal tracts on both sides of the cord. The level of the spinal cord lesion causing the weakness is not always immediately obvious to the examiner, however. The corticospinal fibers destined for arm function end in the lower cervical/first thoracic portion of the spinal cord. The corticospinal tract fibers for leg function need to pass through the cervical and thoracic portions of the spinal cord before ending in the lumbosacral cord. Therefore, weakness of the upper and lower extremities, when the result of a single lesion, must be due to a lesion at least as high as the cervical spinal cord. However, weakness of the legs without weakness of the arms is not necessarily the result of a lesion below the neck. A partial or early process affecting the high (e.g., cervical) spinal cord could potentially cause clinical dysfunction primarily affecting that portion of the corticospinal tract destined for lower-extremity function, without obviously affecting those fibers involved in upper-extremity function. This has important implications in the imaging of patients with suspected spinal cord lesions.

LOWER MOTOR NEURON LESIONS

Lower motor neuron dysfunction occurs when there is dysfunction at the level of the anterior horn cell, motor nerve root, plexus, peripheral nerve, or neuromuscular junction (see Chapters 13 and 19). Lesions of the lower motor neuron may cause, in addition to weakness, decreased reflexes in the involved limb, if a clinically testable reflex is subserved by the nerve in question. In chronic lesions, lower motor neuron dysfunction may lead to clinically evident atrophy and fasciculations of muscle because of the trophic influence the lower motor neuron plays in muscle maintenance. In these cases, patients may complain that their muscles are shrinking and have small, visible twitches. Lower motor neuron weakness may be the result of either a focal or diffuse process.

Clinical localization of the source of a patient's weakness to a particular focal lower motor neuron lesion mainly rests in the finding of muscle dysfunction that appears to fit the territory of a specific nerve root (radiculopathy), region of plexus (plexopathy), or peripheral nerve distribution (neuropathy). (See Chapter 13.) In addition, when such a lesion also is affecting sensory fibers (as do most lower motor neuron lesions that are distal to the anterior horn cell), the concomitant sensory dysfunction also can be an important clue to the localization of the problem.

Examples of common diffuse lower motor neuron processes include processes that simultaneously affect multiple peripheral nerves (polyneuropathies) or multiple nerve roots (polyradiculopathies). Diffuse polyneuropathies (see Chapter 13) typically predominantly affect the most distal extremities, causing weakness that often is limited to the distal fingers and foot muscles. Distal reflexes usu-

ally are diminished or lost, fairly symmetrically. In most diffuse polyneuropathies, such as diabetic neuropathies, the sensory symptoms are more prominent than the distal motor findings, at least initially. Multifocal, rather than diffuse, polyneuropathies are characterized as a mononeuropathy multiplex. This would be seen clinically by dysfunction in the territories of two or more peripheral nerves. Polyradiculopathic processes clinically resemble (and may be difficult to initially distinguish from) the diffuse polyneuropathies but are suggested by the presence of motor dysfunction that appears to involve multiple motor nerve root territories. Concomitant sensory symptoms such as radicular pain (see later), when present, are helpful diagnostic clues to the presence of a radicular or polyradicular localization.

Disease of muscle (myopathy) is suggested when a patient presents with weakness that is predominantly proximal in distribution. However, proximal weakness is not pathognomonic for myopathy and also can be seen, for example, in some myelopathic and radiculopathic processes. It also should be noted that some myopathies cause unusual patterns of weakness (e.g., inclusion body myositis) or even predominantly distal weakness (e.g., myotonic dystrophy). (See Chapter 19.) Sometimes, myopathies cause pain and tenderness in the involved muscles, especially in inflammatory conditions.

PAIN AND SENSORY SYNDROMES

Arguably one can consider all pain to be neurologic in origin because all pain must be transmitted through sensory fibers and perceived in central nervous system structures. However, in this section, primary neurologic pain and other neurologic abnormalities of sensation are discussed and can be defined as pain and other sensory symptoms that are directly the result of dysfunction of nervous system structures. Back pain is discussed in Chapter 21 and headache is discussed in Chapter 7—these topics therefore will not be addressed specifically in this section.

Patients often report "numbness" as a neurologic symptom. However, this term has many potential meanings, including the expected sensory symptoms (also described in Chapter 13) of decreased sensation (hypoesthesia or anesthesia), a tingling/pins and needles sensation (paresthesias), or very uncomfortable/burning sensations (dysesthesias). Patients, however, sometimes use the word numbness to describe weakness or other non-sensory symptoms. A careful history, specifically asking the patient to explain the symptom of numbness in more detail, usually will suffice for clarification.

The pathways for cutaneous sensation will be summarized here. Sensation starts in the peripheral nerve endings and travels up the sensory nerves to the dorsal nerve roots and into the spinal cord. In the spinal cord, the sensory pathways ascend as the spinothalamic tract (mainly subserving pain and temperature sensation) and the posterior columns (mainly subserving vibration and proprioceptive sensation). These ascending sensory tracts in the spinal cord synapse in the thalamus. From the thalamus, thalamocortical projections send the sensory information to the cerebral cortex.

Abnormalities at any level of the sensory pathway—peripheral sensory nerve, nerve root, spinal cord, thalamus, or sensory cortex—may produce sensory symptoms. Lesions at some of these levels, particularly the sensory nerve, nerve root, or thalamus, also may produce pain.

The sensory symptoms of peripheral nerve lesions (see Chapter 13) generally consist of hypoesthesia, paresthesias, or dysesthesias conforming to the territory of the nerve. When this occurs focally, as a result of a focal peripheral nerve process, the area of numbness is usually well circumscribed, corresponding to a particular peripheral nerve distribution. When the peripheral nerve process is diffuse and symmetric, such as in a distal polyneuropathy, the area of sensory disturbance characteristically occurs in a stocking or stocking-glove pattern. The fact that these symptoms are likely the result of a neurologic process is usually evident from the history and examination.

Like peripheral neuropathic lesions, radiculopathies may cause paresthesias or hypoesthesia in the territory of a nerve root. However, these nerve root lesions often cause characteristic radiculopathic pain, characterized by sharp shooting pain, radiating proximally to distally in the distribution of the root (see Chapter 21). Radicular pain resulting from cervical or lumbar root processes can occur even in the absence of obvious neck or back pain. The possibility of a cervical or lumbar radiculopathic localization of a patient's symptoms is often apparent given the characteristic symptoms. However, thoracic radiculopathies are less common and may produce radiating pain, paresthesias, or severe dysesthesias in the territory of one or several thoracic nerve roots. Causes of thoracic radiculopathies include herpes zoster, diabetic thoracic radiculopathies, or structural lesions. Thoracic radiculopathies may mimic serious systemic processes such as intraabdominal or cardiac pathology. A clue to the primary neurologic, radicular cause of the patient's symptoms would be the presence of clear-cut cutaneous hypoesthesia or dysesthesia on the surface of the skin, conforming to a thoracic dermatomal distribution.

Spinal cord lesions (myelopathies) that affect the ascending sensory tracts cause sensory symptoms (hypoesthesia and paresthesias) below the level of the lesion. Total interruption of these sensory fibers at any level of the cord would cause complete anesthesia below that level. Myelopathies may cause Lhermitte's sign, which is an uncomfortable feeling of electricity, vibration, or tingling that radiates down the neck and/or back and sometimes into the extremities, occurring on neck flexion (see Chapter 9). Lhermitte's sign is caused by dysfunction of nerve fibers in the posterior columns. Although it can be seen in multiple sclerosis, it can occur as a result of any process affecting the cord, including compressive lesions. Therefore, when a patient reports a Lhermitte's sign, it can be a helpful clue to a spinal cord localization of pathology.

Thalamic lesions may cause decreased sensation and paresthesias over the contralateral body. This may be quite marked, and some patients with thalamic strokes, for example, may have severe sensory dysfunction over an entire half of the body up to the midline. Thalamic lesions, particularly chronic ones, sometimes also may cause severe dysesthesias (thalamic pain) in addition to the cutaneous sensory loss. Cortical lesions involving the sensory cortex will cause paresthesias or hypoesthesia in the regions of the contralateral body corresponding to the cortical territory involved. Such sensory cortical lesions also may be associated with motor abnormalities or other signs of cortical dysfunction.

GAIT DISORDERS

Disorders of gait and balance may be the result of non-neurologic or neurologic causes. Non-neurologic causes of gait dysfunction are primarily the result of orthopedic problems, such as spine, pelvic, hip, or knee problems. Gait dysfunction resulting from pain in a lower extremity is termed an antalgic gait. It is usually, although not always, evident from the history and examination that a disorder of gait is related to an orthopedic, as opposed to a primary neurologic, process.

The neurologic structures that control gait and balance include the frontal lobes, basal ganglia, cerebellum, and the pathways for motor and sensory function. Gait problems can occur as a result of dysfunction in any of these regions, which cause characteristic abnormalities evident on history and examination.

Frontal lobe disorders, as can be seen as a result of hydrocephalus or bifrontal mass lesions or as an accompaniment of aging or dementia in some patients, cause a characteristic difficulty with initiation of gait. Patients may complain that their feet are "glued" to the floor. The resulting gait disorder is very similar to a parkinsonian gait, with very short steps, although the way the feet appear to be nearly stuck to the floor and the absence of other parkinsonian features help in distinguishing this from parkinsonism. Patients with a frontal lobe gait disorder may or may

not have other symptoms of frontal lobe dysfunction, such as incontinence or dementia.

When the basal ganglia dysfunction of Parkinson's disease (see Chapter 10) affects walking, it causes a characteristic flexed posture and a slow, bradykinetic gait, with multiple steps needed for turns, which may be accompanied by impairment of postural reflexes. Patients may complain that they have a difficult time stopping their forward progress while walking, termed the festination of gait.

Disorders of the cerebellum or cerebellar pathways (e.g., in the brainstem) produce an ataxic gait. This is a wide-based, unsteady gait indistinguishable from the gait disorder of acute alcohol intoxication.

Unilateral corticospinal tract disease will produce a hemiparetic gait, often with characteristic circumduction of the stiff, overextended, hemiparetic leg, pivoting around the axis of the strong leg. Bilateral corticospinal tract disease, such as can occur as a result of myelopathies, causes both legs to be stiff, and the resulting spastic gait may include a scissoring motion of each leg around the other while moving forward.

Disorders of the lower motor neuron, or the muscles, of the lower extremities also can affect the gait. The resulting gait abnormality depends on the muscles that are weakened. When there is weakness of extension at the knee joint, the patient may lose the ability to lock the knee, and this may cause buckling and falling. This may be most bothersome in maneuvers that require the knee to lock for stabilization, and patients therefore may note buckling of a leg particularly when walking down stairs. Weakness of foot dorsiflexion may cause the patients to complain of tripping over their toes. Severe foot dorsiflexion weakness therefore will produce a steppage gait, with the leg lifted higher than normal to avoid tripping over the toes of the weak foot.

Patients with severely impaired sensation in the lower extremities also may complain of difficulty with gait, even in the absence of motor impairment. Examples include severe peripheral neuropathies or other disorders affecting proprioceptive sensory function in the legs, as can be seen as a result of vitamin B_{12} deficiency, for example. Often, these patients present to the physician because of the gait disorder; usually, they do not realize that there is an underlying disorder of extremity sensation that is the cause, especially when paresthesias or dysesthesias are not prominent. When patients have such a severe loss of proprioceptive sensation in the feet, the resulting wide-based gait disorder is a sensory ataxia. These patients need to look at their feet while walking, and they often describe a particular tendency to fall in the dark, where visual cues are lost (Romberg's sign).

ROLE OF THE TEMPORAL COURSE OF NEUROLOGIC ILLNESS IN NEUROLOGIC DIAGNOSIS

An accurate and detailed neurologic history is the cornerstone of neurologic diagnosis. In addition to learning the patient's specific symptoms, another very important aspect of the history is the elucidation of the temporal pattern of the neurologic symptomatology. This time course of neurologic symptoms can give the clinician important clues as to the probable mechanism of central nervous system dysfunction. In neurologic diagnosis, it is usually most helpful to try to decide which general mechanism of disease is most likely to be present before proceeding further diagnostically. Neurologic disease processes can be categorized as producing their dysfunction through one of these general mechanisms: compressive, degenerative, epileptic, hemorrhagic, infectious, inflammatory (including demyelinative), ischemic, migrainous, metabolic (including toxic), or traumatic. (Some congenital neurologic processes also may produce disease that results from the congenital absence of certain normal structures or tissues—whether on a subcellular or macroscopic level—thereby leading to abnormal neurologic function.)

These mechanisms of acquired neurologic disease are generic and inclusive; for example, the compressive mechanism would include such diverse disease processes as a subdural hematoma causing mass effect on the brain, a benign or malignant tumor (with or without associated edema) compressing or infiltrating brain tissue, or a cervical disc compressing the spinal cord. In addition, single pathologic processes can produce clinical symptoms via different potential mechanisms; for example, an intracerebral aneurysm may produce disease because of hemorrhage or because of compression of important structures (e.g., a posterior communicating artery aneurysm causing a compressive oculomotor nerve palsy).

Consideration of the temporal pattern of symptom development, although not specific for a single mechanism, can be most helpful in including or excluding some of these mechanisms; other clues from the history and examination then can be incorporated to narrow the choices of mechanism and specific disease process. The following discussion presents some common temporal patterns of symptomatology and the disease mechanisms they particularly suggest.

Transient focal neurologic symptoms, which may or may not be recurrent, usually are seen as a result of ischemia, migraine, or seizure. Although these three mechanisms may seem to be quite different from each other, they are not always easy to distinguish. Ischemic symptoms, when transient, can produce focal neurologic dysfunction lasting from seconds to hours. Migrainous brain dysfunction (see Chapter 7) can produce a variety of focal neurologic manifestations (even without headache). In addition to the visual scintillations of classic migraine, other neurologic symptoms can be seen as migrainous phenomena, including weakness, paresthesias, and aphasia. These migrainous symptoms typically progress and spread over a period of minutes (e.g., 15 to 30 minutes) before resolving. In contrast, the focal neurologic symptoms of seizures tend to spread somewhat more quickly (see Chapter 8). The patient's age, associated medical conditions, and other clues from the history and examination may assist in the delineation of the likely mechanism of transient focal neurologic dysfunction. It should be noted that demyelinating disease (e.g., multiple sclerosis; see Chapter 9) causes focal neurologic dysfunction that can resolve and then recur in a different region of the central nervous system. However, the symptoms of an acute attack of multiple sclerosis usually last at least days to weeks before improving, unlike the more transient symptoms of ischemia, migraine, or epilepsy. As noted in Chapter 9, some patients with multiple sclerosis do experience very brief (as short as seconds), repetitive, stereotypical paroxysmal neurologic symptoms. This is presumably because of "short circuits" (ephaptic transmission) between adjacent demyelinated axons in a multiple sclerosis plaque, and the resulting very brief paroxysmal event simply can be considered as a white matter electrical event.

Sudden-onset neurologic symptoms suggest ischemia or hemorrhage. A progressive focal neurologic symptom primarily suggests a compressive lesion, but ischemic, inflammatory, or focal infectious processes can progress gradually as well. Degenerative diseases also may produce progressive focal neurologic dysfunction, but the dysfunction is usually more diffuse, even if not symmetric. Ischemic or compressive lesions also can cause waxing and waning focal neurologic symptoms. More diffuse waxing and waning symptoms also would be expected in some toxic or metabolic processes.

Progressive diffuse neurologic symptoms are most suggestive of degenerative processes, infectious or inflammatory processes, or metabolic abnormalities. The specific time course in question can be quite helpful. For example, diffuse neurologic dysfunction that has been progressing over days would more likely be ascribed to a metabolic or infectious process, whereas the same kind of symptoms progressing over years would be more likely caused by a degenerative disease.

WHEN TO REFER THE PATIENT TO A NEUROLOGIST

It is important to know when it is appropriate to refer patients who present with neurologic symptoms to a neurologist. Table 2.2 summarizes some symptoms that should prompt evaluation by a neurologist. For more information about when to refer patients with specific symptoms, or diseases, for neurologic evaluation and treatment, please refer to the individual chapters that follow in this text.

QUESTIONS AND DISCUSSION

1. A 35-year-old man presents to the emergency room with a 3-day history of numbness and tingling from his midchest down to his

TABLE 2.2. *Ten Important Symptoms That Should be Evaluated by a Neurologist[a]*

Symptoms	Possible Causes
1. Sudden, severe headache	Subarachnoid hemorrhage, meningitis
2. Change in language function	Stroke (ischemic or hemorrhagic), encephalitis, tumor, dementia
3. Hemiparesis	Stroke (ischemic or hemorrhagic), tumor
4. Hemisensory loss	Stroke (ischemic or hemorrhagic), tumor
5. Vertigo with neurologic symptoms	Brainstem ischemia, tumor (e.g., dysarthria, diplopia, numbness, weakness)
6. Acute weakness of lower extremities	Spinal cord compression
7. Acute weakness of all extremities	Acute demyelinating polyneuropathies, spinal cord disorders
8. Sudden inability to walk (ataxic gait)	Cerebellar stroke (hemorrhage or infarction)
9. New-onset seizure	Tumor, infarct, vascular malformation
10. Poorly controlled seizures or status epilepticus	Many possible causes; requires neurologic evaluation and treatment

[a]This list is not comprehensive of all symptoms requiring neurologic attention or their causes. Further discussion of symptoms requiring neurologic referral is offered throughout this text.

legs and mild weakness in both legs. He describes an unusual sensation like an electric shock whenever he flexes his neck forward. He also has some urinary urgency. Examination shows normal mental status and cranial nerves. There is mild weakness in both legs (4/5). Sensory examination shows that pinprick is diminished below the level of the nipples, including the lower chest, abdomen, and legs. Reflexes are normal in the arms but are brisk in the legs. Toes are upgoing to plantar stimulation.

Which of the following terms best describes the localization of this patient's clinical syndrome?

A. Encephalopathy
B. Myelopathy
C. Radiculopathy
D. Neuropathy
E. Plexopathy
F. Myopathy

The answer is (B). This patient has symptoms of spinal cord (myelopathic) dysfunction. Clues to a spinal cord localization of his symptoms include the bilateral motor dysfunction in the legs as well as the bilateral sensory dysfunction with a sensory level over the trunk. There are also brisk reflexes in both legs and bilateral Babinski signs, suggestive of bilateral upper motor neuron (corticospinal tract) dysfunction. Although brainstem lesions similarly can cause bilateral motor and sensory symptoms, the absence of cranial nerve abnormalities is evidence that the lesion is below the level of the brainstem. Urinary symptoms, including urgency, are not uncommon in spinal cord processes. This patient also describes Lhermitte's sign, the electric-like sensation on neck flexion, a finding suggestive of a spinal cord process affecting the posterior columns. This patient's clinical symptoms and signs are not suggestive of pathology in the brain (encephalopathy), nerve root (radiculopathy), nerve (neuropathy), cervical or lumbosacral plexus (plexopathy), or muscle (myopathy). Although the cause of this patient's spinal cord dysfunction is not yet clear, the clinical realization that his symptoms are myelopathic is important and

will guide the clinician to the appropriate choice of imaging and other studies.

2. A 72-year-old woman with a 2-year history of diabetes mellitus presents to your office because of 4 weeks of severe pain. She describes the pain as a severe, sharp, burning sensation that begins in her medial scapula and radiates around her trunk to beneath her right breast. The pain is not worse with breathing, but she notes that the skin in this area is very uncomfortable to touch. Her only medication is an oral hypoglycemic agent. She has seen multiple physicians and has undergone extensive gastrointestinal and cardiac evaluations for the pain, which were unrevealing.

The patient's general physical examination is normal, and there is no skin rash. Neurologic examination shows normal mental status, cranial nerves, and muscle strength. Sensory testing shows that she has severe discomfort when the skin under the right breast and below the right scapula is touched with either a cotton swab or the point of a pin. This area of sensory abnormality is a strip about 2 cm in height but extending from the right mid/upper thoracic spine posteriorly to the lower sternum anteriorly. Reflexes are 1+ and symmetric, and toes are downgoing to plantar stimulation.

Which of the following terms best describes the localization of this patient's pain syndrome?

A. Encephalopathy
B. Myelopathy
C. Radiculopathy
D. Neuropathy
E. Plexopathy
F. Myopathy

The best answer is (C). This patient has characteristic symptoms and signs of a thoracic radiculopathy. (Answer (D)—neuropathy—is not entirely incorrect because it would be difficult at the bedside to be certain that her lesion is not of a thoracic nerve rather than root.) The major clue to a probable nerve root localization of her disease process is the distribution of her sensory symptoms and sensory findings to the cutaneous territory of a particular nerve root. In this case, her findings map out the territory of either the right T5 or T6 root. Another clue to this radicular localization of her symptoms is the occasional proximal-to-distal shooting pains in the territory of a right thoracic nerve root.

The generic diagnosis of a thoracic radiculopathy does not in itself give a specific clinical diagnosis for this patient. However, the clinical realization that this is the likely localization of her problem allows the physician to narrow the causative possibilities, and to reasonably exclude many possibilities, prior to further investigation. Realization that this patient's cutaneous sensory symptoms and signs are most compatible with a thoracic radicular process, and not a visceral process, probably would have saved her from some unnecessary investigation. One caveat is that visceral disease can cause referred pain syndromes suggestive of neurologic or spinal processes, such as thoracic or lumbar spine pain from deep chest, abdominal, or retroperitoneal processes.

In this patient, the most likely cause of her thoracic radicular syndrome is a diabetic thoracic radiculopathy. Herpes zoster (shingles) in this distribution would cause similar symptoms, but it is less likely given the absence of herpetic skin lesions.

3. Your office nurse tells you that your next patient is complaining of intermittent episodes of dizziness that have been occurring for the last 2 months. The patient is a 54-year-old woman who you have been following for general medical care. She has a history of hypertension but no other previous significant illnesses. Prior to coming to your office today, the patient had a few tests done by another physician, including a magnetic resonance imaging scan of the brain and a 24-hour ambulatory heart monitor test.

Which of the following choices would be the most appropriate first step in your evaluation of this patient?

A. Review the results of the previous workup.

B. Take a history from the patient.

C. Perform a general physical examination.

D. Perform a neurologic examination, including testing for positional vertigo.

The correct answer is (B). Although all of the choices are important and helpful, the first step in any neurologic evaluation should be the taking of a history. Once the neurologic history is obtained, the clinician usually should have enough clues to determine the likely locations of the lesion (the where part of the neurologic diagnostic process) and the possible disease mechanisms involved (the how part of the diagnostic process). The neurologic examination can be a very helpful adjunct to the neurologic history, and in many cases it will help exclude or include certain processes that are under consideration; it always should be performed only after the history has been obtained. The role of the neurologic history and examination in the evaluation of patients with dizziness is discussed in Chapter 14. The results of ancillary laboratory tests, although often very important in excluding or confirming specific diagnostic considerations, should be ordered and interpreted in light of the clinical history (first) and the neurologic examination (second). Clinical interpretation of a patient's diagnostic studies without regard to the findings of history and examination is fraught with potential hazard. Just as incidental abnormalities may be overinterpreted for clinical importance (red herrings), the clinician also might get false reassurance from the results of normal studies that do not answer the appropriate clinical question at hand.

4. A 25-year-old woman presents to your office because of a 5-year history of intermittent episodes of face and arm numbness and difficulty with vision and speech. The attacks are all very similar, and she has had about two attacks per year. Her symptoms begin with a visual disturbance, which she describes as difficulty seeing the right side of people's faces or the right side of a page, "as if they are obscured by heat waves." This then is followed within a few minutes by numbness and tingling in the right cheek. This numb sensation then gradually descends over the next 15 minutes to involve the right arm and hand. During

the attacks, she has difficulty with speech, which she describes as a feeling that "I know what I want to say, but I can't get the words out." The symptoms last a total of about 30 minutes then resolve and usually are followed by a moderately severe throbbing headache over the left temporal region. Although the majority of her episodes have involved her right vision and body, she recalls having had a few episodes that involved only the left side of her vision, face, and arm, but without the speech disturbance. She has no significant past medical history, except for additional occasional headaches that occur about once a month, located over either or both temples and relieved by over-the-counter analgesics. Her neurologic examination is normal when she is seen in your office.

Which of the following general mechanisms of neurologic dysfunction is the most likely cause of this patient's presenting symptoms?

A. Ischemia
B. Migraine
C. Epilepsy
D. Demyelinative

The answer is (B). This patient has recurrent episodes of transient focal neurologic dysfunction, most likely of migrainous etiology. Recurrent transient focal neurologic symptoms are usually the result of ischemia, epilepsy, or migraine. In this case, migraine is the most likely cause of her visual symptoms, which sound typical of migraine auras. Her other neurologic symptoms, which occur subsequent to the onset of her visual symptom, suggest the focal neurologic symptomatology that migraine sometimes can produce (see Chapter 7), and they progress with a typical migrainous tempo. The subsequent headache after the neurologic disturbance is also suggestive of migraine, although migrainous neurologic symptoms sometimes can occur without headache, and headache can occur with other neurologic processes, including ischemia and epilepsy. Although ischemia is possible, it is a less likely cause of this patient's symptoms because of the migrainous quality of her symptoms, the number of

episodes she has had over many years without obvious sequelae, and her age. A focal seizure is also possible, but it is less likely because of the slow tempo of progression and the fact that her symptoms have occurred on either side. Demyelinating disease is an unlikely cause of this patient's symptoms.

5. A 72-year-old right-handed woman with a 10-year history of hypertension presents to the emergency room because of right face, arm, and leg weakness. She is very alert and conversant, and she tells you that she was well until this morning, when after she awakened she realized that her right arm and leg were very weak and she was unable to move them at all. She also noted that the right side of her mouth was droopy. She called the paramedics, who brought her to the hospital. Her weakness has not improved. Although she notes that her right arm and leg are completely paralyzed, she also tells you that when the paramedics touched her on her right side, the sensation of her right arm and leg seemed normal. Her blood pressure is 140/90, and her heart rate is 68/minute and regular.

Even prior to your examination of this patient, you attempt to hypothesize the most likely location of her neurologic lesion. Of the following choices, which is the most likely localization of her lesion?

A. Cerebral cortex
B. Subcortical white matter
C. Cervical spinal cord
D. Nerve root

The answer is (B). This patient's history alone suggests that she most likely has the clinical syndrome of a pure motor hemiplegia. She describes severe weakness of her right arm and leg, without obvious sensory symptoms. In addition, her ability to give such a detailed history without obvious language impairment suggests intact left hemisphere cortical function. This combination of pure motor weakness with intact sensory and cortical function is most consistent with a subcortical stroke. The syndrome of a pure motor hemiparesis can occur as a result of a lesion in either the posterior limb of the internal capsule or on one side of the base of the pons. In either of these subcortical locations, the corticospinal fibers are segregated from sensory fibers and are deep to the cortex; therefore, a lesion in these locations will cause motor weakness without cortical or sensory dysfunction. The most likely cause of a lesion in this region would be a lacunar stroke (see Chapter 6), although a small hypertensive hemorrhage can cause lesions in the same locations and result in a similar clinical picture.

This patient's symptoms would not likely be from a cortical stroke because of the intact right hemisphere cortical function. In addition, a cortical stroke large enough to cause paralysis of an entire side of the body would be expected to cause some concomitant sensory dysfunction. A cervical spinal cord localization of her lesion would be unlikely because of the facial droop and because of the unilateral nature of her severe deficit—without the patient's description of any motor or sensory symptoms on the other side. This patient's symptoms are not suggestive of a nerve root localization.

Therefore, the most likely localizations and etiology of this patient's problem can be surmised by a simple but careful history and a little knowledge of basic neuroanatomy. The results of the subsequent neurologic examination—in particular, testing motor strength, sensory function, and assessing for left hemisphere cortical function—then would help support or refute the probable diagnosis of the syndrome of a pure motor hemiplegia. Imaging studies are then helpful in excluding a hemorrhagic, as opposed to an ischemic, lesion in the internal capsule or pons causing this patient's stroke syndrome.

SUGGESTED READING

Brazis PW, Masdeu JC, Biller J. *Localization in clinical neurology,* 4th ed. Philadelphia: Lippincott Williams & Wilkins, 2001.

Gelb DJ. *Introduction to clinical neurology,* 2nd ed. Boston: Butterworth-Heinemann, 2000.

Gilman S, Newman SW. *Manter & Gatz's essentials of clinical neuroanatomy and neurophysiology,* 10th ed. Philadelphia: FA Davis, 2002.

Haerer AF. *DeJong's the neurologic examination,* 5th ed. Philadelphia: JB Lippincott, 1992.

Patten JP. *Neurological differential diagnosis,* 2nd ed. London: Springer-Verlag, 1996.

3

Clinical Use of Neurologic Diagnostic Tests

Thomas P. Bleck

The diagnostic tests used in neurologic practice are used most effectively as adjuncts to the history and physical examination. Prior to the advent of computerized imaging studies, the noninvasive electrodiagnostic tests often were ordered as a battery to determine whether invasive radiologic studies or diagnostic cranial exploration were indicated. As computed tomography (CT) and magnetic resonance imaging (MRI) have advanced, the electrophysiologic studies are less important anatomically; however, as pathophysiologic studies they remain unchallenged. Similarly, cerebrospinal fluid (CSF) examination is indicated less often in the workup of mass lesions but is prominent in the study of neuroimmunologic disorders. Hence, diagnostic studies now can be tailored more appropriately, with a considerable decrease in risk, time, and expense. However, if these tests are used indiscriminately, rather than to include or exclude specific clinical hypotheses, they can increase costs and delay diagnosis and treatment.

CSF examination and electrodiagnostic procedures are considered in this chapter. Neuroradiologic studies, discussed in Chapter 4, are mentioned here only as an alternative means of acquiring data.

CSF Examination

Since Quincke introduced the diagnostic lumbar puncture (LP) at the end of the nineteenth century, CSF evaluation has been applied to most neurologic disorders. As other diagnostic tests have become more sophisticated, CSF examination is no longer a standard part of the analysis of all central nervous system (CNS) disorders. This procedure is indicated most commonly for the diagnosis of CNS infection, neoplastic invasion of the subarachnoid space, multiple sclerosis (MS), acute inflammatory demyelinating polyneuropathy (Guillain-Barré syndrome), other neuroimmunologic disorders, and pseudotumor cerebri.

Technique

An LP usually is performed with the patient lying on his or her side, with the knees flexed as close to the chest as possible. The patient should be informed about each stage of the procedure and should be positioned with his or her back as close to the edge of the bed as possible. The location of the intended puncture should be determined before cleansing the skin. A line connecting the posterior iliac crests crosses the L3-L4 interspace, which is usually the most rostral space used. The caudal end of the spinal cord is at L2 in most adults. After palpating the spinous processes, the examiner can mark the L4-L5 and L5-S1 interspaces with thumbnail pressure prior to gloving. The skin is cleansed with iodine followed by alcohol, and sterile drapes are positioned around the area to be punctured. The skin is anesthetized with 1% lidocaine, using a 25-gauge needle, which then is exchanged for a 22-gauge needle. This longer, stiffer needle is used to anesthetize the deeper tissue down to the epidural space. As the needle is advanced, the syringe is aspirated to avoid intravascular or subarachnoid injection. The epidural space is recognized by the sudden loss of resistance to injection.

A 20- or 22-gauge spinal needle is adequate for most LPs; smaller-caliber needles make pressure measurements difficult. The needle always should be advanced with the stylet in place (to avoid subarachnoid introduction of epidermal tissue). Although some experts replace the stylet when withdrawing the needle to avoid entrapping a spinal nerve root, the rare incidence of this complication does not appear to differ between these two techniques. The needle should be advanced with the bevel up to separate the fibers of the ligamentum flavum. The needle is angled 15 degrees cephalad to avoid the spinous processes. Dural puncture produces a "pop"; the stylet then is withdrawn. If free CSF flow does not occur, rotating the bevel toward the head is often useful. (With all movements of the needle, the stylet should be replaced.) Should it be necessary to redirect the needle, it must be withdrawn almost to the skin. Newer spinal needles, which have a conical tip and a side port rather than a beveled tip, may produce less of a dural tear and therefore fewer, less severe postprocedural headaches.

When free flow has been established, the CSF pressure is measured with a manometer attached to the needle by means of a stopcock. The patient's legs should be extended to prevent a falsely increased reading. The respiration and pulse should both fluctuate.

For accurate pressure readings, patients using ventilators (especially those receiving positive end-expiratory pressure) should, if possible, be transiently disconnected to lower the transmitted intrathoracic pressure. The Queckenstedt jugular compression test is unreliable and dangerous. Following pressure measurement, four tubes of CSF are withdrawn and processed for cell counts (at the start and end), biochemical and immunologic studies, and microbiologic analysis. The usefulness of closing pressure measurement is uncertain.

Following the withdrawal of the needle, pressure should be applied to the site of entry and the patient should be placed in the prone position. Although the evidence is inconclusive, many experts feel that 1 to 3 hours prone is the most effective method of preventing a post-LP headache, which is the major complication of the procedure.

If the physician is unable to enter the subarachnoid space with this technique, the patient should be placed in a sitting position. With the patient leaning forward on a support, the spinous processes will be palpable in the midline. When the needle is in the subarachnoid space, the patient should be returned to the recumbent position for a pressure measurement.

When lumbar spine disease or the question of an intraspinal mass prevents the lumbar approach, a lateral cervical approach can be performed by a physician trained in this technique. Newer spinal needles with a conical tip actually produce more damage to the dura, but by inciting a more robust inflammatory response they appear to result in earlier closure of the dural rent and therefore fewer postlumbar puncture headaches.

Contraindications

Prior to LP, the physician must be certain that the patient does not have an intracranial or intraspinous mass. A CSF examination is rarely useful in this situation, and the withdrawal of CSF may alter the CNS pressure dynamics sufficiently to cause herniation.

The absence of papilledema does not exclude an intracranial mass, although its presence mandates a CT scan prior to LP (as does an asymmetry on neurologic examination). It is not necessary that all patients be scanned before an LP is performed, especially if acute bacterial meningitis is suspected. If LP is delayed for CT scanning when bacterial meningitis is suspected, one should consider a single dose of empirically chosen antibiotics prior to the CT scan (after blood cultures have been obtained).

Coagulopathy is a relative contraindication to LP because epidural hematomas can arise at the puncture site. Infusions of fresh frozen plasma or platelets, as appropriate, should be given prior to the procedure if possible. If the coagulopathy is discovered after the LP, therapy still should be given because bleeding may occur for many hours. The patient should be examined frequently for signs of cauda equina dysfunction, which may necessitate surgical extirpation of the extravasated blood.

Cutaneous infection at the intended puncture site requires that a different approach (e.g., lateral cervical) be used.

Interpretation of Results

Normal lumbar CSF pressure is no more than 180 mm (of CSF) with the patient in a recumbent position. An elevated pressure suggests the presence of infection, a mass lesion, or increased CSF production or its diminished resorption. Normal pressure does not exclude an infection or a mass.

The glucose concentration in CSF is normally at least two thirds of the serum glucose; as glucose takes time to equilibrate in the subarachnoid space, the CSF value tends to lag behind the serum by about 30 minutes. Low CSF glucose concentrations are seen with meningeal inflammatory processes (e.g., infection or meningeal spread of neoplasms). The protein concentration primarily reflects albumin derived from the serum; in the lumbar space, it is usually 15 to 45 mg/dl. Elevation usually reflects an increased transudation of albumin, generally as a consequence of inflammation. The protein concentration may be low or low-normal in pseudotumor cerebri.

High-resolution electrophoretic studies of CSF proteins reveal the presence of oligoclonal antibodies in more than 90% of patients with MS. This finding also is seen in other settings in which immunoglobulins are produced in the subarachnoid space (e.g., infections) and rarely in the presence of primary brain tumors. They also frequently are present in the Guillain-Barré syndrome.

A cytologic examination of normal CSF should reveal no more than five lymphocytes per mL and no polymorphonuclear leukocytes (PMNs). The presence of PMNs indicates an acute inflammatory process; lymphocytes predominate generally in aseptic, chronic, or resolving conditions.

Cultures and stains for microbial agents should be obtained if any possibility of infection arises. These include Gram stains, India ink preparations, stains for acid-fast bacilli (AFB), routine bacterial cultures, fungal cultures, and AFB cultures. Routine viral cultures of CSF seldom reveal the etiology of aseptic meningitis or encephalitis except for human immunodeficiency virus-1 (HIV-1), but antibody titers in the CSF and serum may be helpful. Herpes simplex encephalitis is diagnosed most accurately by the detection of

TABLE 3.1. *CSF Abnormalities in Common Meningitides*

	Acute Bacterial Meningitis	Aseptic Meningitis	Tuberculous Meningitis	Cryptococcal Meningitis	Partially Treated Bacterial Meningitis	Neoplastic Meningitis	Acute HIV-1 Infection
Pressure (mm CSF)	Up to 1,000	Up to 350	300–500	300–500	Up to 500	Up to 500	Up to 350
Glucose (mg/dl)	0–40 (<35% of serum)	10–40	1–40	5–40	May be low	5–40	Usually normal
Protein (mg/dl)	Up to 1,000	Up to 200	Up to 1,000	Up to 500	May be elevated	Up to 500	Up to 200
WBCs (per mL)	500–50,000	15–200	100–500	100–500	Often elevated	20–500	Up to 500
Polys (%)	>90	May predominate early	5–15	5–15	Up to 30%	Occasional	Rare
Lymphs (%)	10	Predominate later	85–95	85–95	Predominant	Predominant	Predominant
Microbiologic studies	Gram stain culture	Culture (rarely)	AFB smear culture	India ink culture	Gram stain culture	—	Culture
Immunologic studies	CIE; limulus test	Antibodies; VDRL	—	Cryptococcal antigen	CIE; limulus test	B-2 microglobulin	Antigen, antibody studies
Other	—	—	—	—	—	Cytology	—

WBCs, white blood cell count; AFB, acid-fast bacilli; CIE, counterimmunoelectrophoresis; VDRL, Venereal Disease Research Laboratory test.

TABLE 3.2. *CSF Abnormalities in Other Disorders*

	Herpes Simplex Encephalitis	Subacute Sclerosing Panencephalitis	Acute Inflammatory Demyelinating Polyneuropathy	Cysticercosis	Acute Toxoplasmosis	Multiple Sclerosis	Subarachnoid Hemorrhage
Pressure (mm CSF)	Up to 450	Normal	Normal	Up to 250	Normal	Normal	Up to 500 (may be normal)
Glucose (mg/dl)	30–70	Normal	Normal	Normal	Normal	Normal	Usually normal
Protein (mg/dl)	Up to 200	Up to 100	Up to 100 (rarely, to 1,000)	Up to 50	Up to 100	Up to 60	Often elevated
WBCs (per mL)	Up to 1,000	6–500	0–5	Up to 300	10–50	Up to 20	Acutely, proportional to blood entry; later, elevated
Polys (%)	Up to 30	Rare	Rare	Rare	Rare	Rare	Acutely
Lymphs (%)	Predominant	Predominant	Up to 100	Predominant	Predominant	Predominant	Predominant later
Immunologic studies	Viral antibodies (late)	Measles and oligoclonal antibodies	Oligoclonal antibodies	Antibody titers	Antibody titers	Oligoclonal antibodies	—
Other	—	—	—	—	Occasional eosinophils	—	Gross blood within 1–2 hours; xanthochromia

WBCs, white blood cell count.

specific DNA by the polymerase chain reaction. This test may be falsely negative if performed at the very onset of disease or after several days of effective treatment with acyclovir. In contrast, a polymerase chain reaction (PCR) test for West Nile encephalitis is only about 50% sensitive; this latter infection is better diagnosed by the detection of specific immunoglobulin M antibody. Serologic testing for syphilis is increasingly important.

Although subarachnoid hemorrhage usually is diagnosed by CT, an LP may be necessary to confirm the diagnosis. The scan may not detect small amounts of subarachnoid blood in patients without atrophy; in this case, LP is required. The procedure also may be used to reduce CSF pressure, and thus symptoms, if there is no intraparenchymal extension of bleeding.

Tables 3.1 and 3.2 summarize the expected CSF findings associated with the more common indications for LP.

Electroencephalography

Indications for electroencephalography (EEG) have varied during the 60-year history

of this technique. Imaging studies have supplanted it as a method for localizing anatomic pathology. This has freed EEG to develop as a pathophysiologic tool, detecting abnormal cerebral function that cannot be visualized radiographically or magnetically. Thus, the use of EEG is greatest in the evaluation of transient states (e.g., seizures), evolving conditions (e.g., herpes simplex encephalitis), global disorders (e.g., dementia), and neonates. As with the other procedures considered in this chapter, the usefulness of EEG data depends on the clinical hypothesis being tested. Only a few EEG patterns are diagnostic of particular diseases, but the test is helpful in deciding among diagnostic alternatives.

Technique

The quality of EEG recording and interpretation varies dramatically among laboratories. In evaluating the standards of practice used, the physician should expect the following:

1. The technologists are trained specifically in EEG and are either eligible for, or have

obtained, certification by the American Board of Registration in Electrodiagnostic Technology.

2. The technologists participate in regular continuing education activities, both locally and nationally.
3. The electroencephalographers are neurologists certified by both the American Board of Psychiatry and Neurology and the American Board of Clinical Neurophysiology.
4. The laboratory meets the accreditation standards of the American Electroencephalographic Society.
5. The patient's head always is measured prior to the application of electrodes, according to the International 10–20 System.
6. The equipment used has at least 16 channels and is calibrated before each use.
7. Each record performed includes both wakefulness and sleep (and states this clearly).
8. Hyperventilation and photic stimulation are used routinely as activation procedures unless contraindicated.
9. Extra electrodes (e.g., sphenoidal) are used when indicated.
10. The EEG report includes both a technical description and a clinical interpretation. This interpretation attempts to correlate the EEG with the patient's history. Although it may contain suggestions for further evaluation (e.g., a sleep-deprived EEG), management recommendations beyond the scope of an EEG (e.g., the suggestion of specific medications) are inappropriate.

Topographic Mapping

Many manufacturers have adapted computer interpolation techniques to produce colorful "brain maps" of EEG (and evoked potential) data. Although these maps have a great deal of emotional appeal and eventually may be found to aid in EEG interpretation, they currently require expert technologists and electroencephalographers to be certain that the data entered are free of artifacts. The statistical analysis of these maps is in its initial stage. At present, they cannot substitute for a standard EEG.

Interpretation

The interpretation of an EEG is an attempt to answer clinical questions about the cerebrum in light of the electrophysiologic data; thus, the interpretation is most useful when the questions are well defined and are appropriate for the examination. An EEG is one of the most useful studies in the evaluation of suspected seizures, for example, but is seldom valuable in the analysis of headaches or dizziness. The most commonly encountered EEG abnormalities are epileptiform events, slowing of normal rhythms, and disorders of age-specific patterns.

Epileptiform Events

The term epileptiform is used because spikes and other sharp activity on the EEG rarely represent actual seizures. The usual EEG signature of a seizure disorder is the interictal spike. Such irritative events do occur (albeit rarely) in individuals without seizures, and their presence does not diagnose a seizure disorder (unless the actual seizure is recorded). Similarly, the absence of epileptiform abnormalities never excludes the diagnosis of a seizure disorder: this is a clinical decision.

Epileptiform activity may be divided broadly into focal, multifocal, and generalized events. In complex partial seizures of temporal lobe origin, for example, the abnormality often is localized over one anterior temporal region. In absence epilepsy, the 3-Hz discharges are typically widespread and bilaterally synchronous. This distinction is most crucial in the patient with a generalized convulsion, for whom the workup, treatment, and prognosis depend on an accurate distinction between primary generalized epilepsy and partial epilepsy with secondary generalization. Other syndromes with specific EEG patterns, such as benign Rolandic epilepsy of childhood, have predictable courses and seldom require imaging studies or further workup.

Several special EEG techniques are helpful in the diagnosis of epilepsy. Partial sleep deprivation may bring out otherwise undetected epileptiform abnormalities and should be performed whenever the routine EEG is unrevealing. Various extra electrodes have been developed and are most useful when a focal EEG abnormality is detected but is not definitely epileptiform. The most commonly used are nasopharyngeal electrodes; however, studies have shown that extra true temporal (T1 and T2) electrodes are just as valuable and are less noxious. Sphenoidal electrodes or double-density electrode arrays may be suggested by the electroencephalographer in particular clinical situations, but they are not indicated routinely. Ambulatory 24-hour EEG technology is improving and can contribute to the differential diagnosis of intermittent behavioral episodes. Prolonged inpatient recordings, sometimes using intracranial electrodes, are occasionally necessary for a definitive diagnosis.

The normal EEG contains several benign variants that may be confused with truly epileptiform activity. Small sharp spikes, positive occipital sharp transients of sleep, 14- and 6-Hz–positive spikes, "phantom" spikes, and "psychomotor variant" are embedded in the older literature but are of dubious significance. EEG reports that stress their association with epilepsy or "neurovegetative disorders" should prompt the clinician to find another electroencephalographer.

Slow Wave Abnormalities

As with epileptiform activity, the crucial distinction is among focal, multifocal, and diffuse abnormalities. A focal abnormality may result from grey or white matter dysfunction in that area; this distinction is based on other EEG characteristics. Recall here that the EEG is a physiologic test; postictal slowing from a recent seizure and the constant slowing emitted by cerebral tissue adjacent to a brain tumor may be indistinguishable on a single EEG. Imaging and electrophysiology are thus complementary, and unexplained focal slowing should prompt a radiologic or magnetic investigation.

Diffuse abnormalities are commonly a consequence of a toxic (e.g., drug), metabolic (e.g., hepatic), degenerative (e.g., Alzheimer's disease), infectious (e.g., encephalitis), or postictal condition. Pure diffuse slowing has few characteristics that distinguish among these possibilities; EEGs are most useful when acquired serially to monitor change in the patient's condition. Specific patterns, such as triphasic waves that exhibit temporospatial lags in hepatic encephalopathy, may suggest an etiology but are rarely diagnostic of a particular metabolic cause. Some forms of dementia (e.g., subacute spongiform encephalopathy) have specific EEG signatures that are usually diagnostic of that particular disorder. A paucity of EEG abnormality in an apparently demented patient raises the possibility of depressive pseudodementia.

The combination of focal and diffuse disturbances is often a useful finding. In herpes simplex encephalitis, the EEG is the earliest diagnostically useful test to become abnormal and often is used to determine the site of brain biopsy before radiologic studies are abnormal. Multifocal abnormalities, especially if intermixed with epileptiform discharges, may suggest the embolic origin of a stroke.

Electrocerebral silence ("flat EEG") is the most extreme diffuse abnormality. If hypothermia and hypnosedative drug intoxication are excluded, this finding may be used to diagnose cerebral cortical inactivity. Because the EEG does not reflect brainstem activity, the EEG is not a substitute for a physical examination in the diagnosis of "brain death." The American Electroencephalographic Society has strict published criteria for these recordings. Such a study is only supportive, however, and is subject to false-negative interpretation because of artifacts. Studies that image intracranial blood flow are more useful in this setting.

Age-Specific Patterns

Neonatal EEG recordings provide the clinician with the opportunity to assess cerebral development, as well as to detect the abnormalities previously described. The more subtle manifestations of seizures in newborns may be detected only by EEG.

A modest degree of focal slowing in the temporal regions commonly accompanies normal aging and may be overread by inexperienced interpreters.

Evoked Potentials

The role of evoked potential studies (EPs) has been in flux during the past decade. Prior to the wide availability of MR and CSF oligoclonal antibody studies, EPs were often essential in the diagnosis of MS because of their ability to detect subclinical lesions. Although they still play an ancillary role here, they are being applied increasingly to other areas.

Several sensory modalities can be investigated by EPs; the most commonly studied are the visual, auditory, and somatosensory systems. "Cognitive" potentials and the cerebral events associated with motor output are areas of current research interest that may find a clinical application in the next several years.

Technique

EPs rely on computer averaging to eliminate signals that are not related temporally to the stimulus used. Many reliable commercial systems for acquiring and displaying EP data are now available; problems arise because of variability in stimulus parameters, data manipulation, and interpretation. Standardization of techniques and interpretation is currently poor. At a minimum, the clinician should expect that the laboratory performing EPs have validated its technique and normative data by testing at least 20 normal subjects. Because the definitions of abnormality in EPs are based on numeric differences of latency and amplitude from a control population, the criteria of abnormality used must be stated clearly. The number of falsely positive and negative studies depends on how these criteria are defined, rather than on a qualitatively abnormal measurement. To reduce false-positive results, most laboratories now use three standard deviations from the control mean as the definition of abnormality.

Visual Evoked Responses

Visual evoked responses (VERs) can be elicited with various stimuli; the most commonly used are reversing checkerboard patterns, sinusoidal gratings, and repetitive flashes. The size of checks (or the spatial frequency of the grating), the luminance of the pattern, the ambient light, and the repetition rate of the stimuli are all important variables. Thus, norms derived in one laboratory may not apply to another.

The response is recorded over the occipital region. Each eye is tested separately to examine for prechiasmal lesions; stimulation of individual fields also may be performed if postchiasmal dysfunction is suspected.

Visual acuity is an important determinant of the response. If the patient wears glasses, they should be worn during pattern testing.

For pattern reversal and sinusoidal gratings, the major potential of interest is a surface positive wave occurring about 100 msec after the stimulus (termed P100). Flash responses elicit a surface negative wave approximately 80 msec after the stimulus (N3).

Brainstem Auditory Evoked Responses

Although the auditory evoked response can be followed up to the cortex, the major use of this test on brainstem auditory evoked responses (BAERs) is the evaluation of brainstem structures. The stimuli are clicks, delivered monaurally through headphones. The frequency spectra of the clicks, their intensity, their duration, and their repetition rate influence the latency and amplitude of the responses.

Five waves are recorded routinely. Wave I originates from the eighth nerve, wave II from the cochlear nucleus, wave III from the superior olivary complex, wave IV from the lateral lemniscus, and wave V from the inferior colliculus. All of these responses normally occur within 6 msec of the stimulus.

Somatosensory Evoked Responses

Upper-extremity somatosensory evoked responses (SSERs) are recorded following stimulation of the median nerve, and lower-extremity SSERs are recorded from the posterior tibial nerve. The stimulus intensity is adjusted according to the motor response. These stimuli travel in the posterior column/medial lemniscal system, so that digit movement, rather than discomfort, is used to determine the stimulation level. Repetition rate and stimulus intensity affect the latency and amplitude of the responses.

From the upper extremity, responses are recorded over the brachial plexus, at the dorsal root entry zone, and over the contralateral primary sensory cortex. Lower-extremity responses are measured at the popliteal fossa, the dorsal root entry zone, and the midline scalp over the somatosensory cortex (the foot area being located in the interhemispheric fissure).

Interpretation

The major use of EPs is in the detection of subclinical lesions. Within the visual system, asymptomatic optic neuritis is detected easily; its presence may aid in the diagnosis of MS. Abnormalities of the optic nerves are poorly visualized by MRI, making VERs an important adjunct when the diagnosis of demyelinating disease is in doubt. Similarly, BAERs and SSERs can detect physiologic lesions below the limit of resolution of imaging techniques. This is especially true for MS plaques in the spinal cord, another area where MRI has been disappointing.

In infants, VERs have been used to assess the integrity of the visual system when blindness is suspected. Paradigms to determine refractive error are under investigation.

In addition to detecting asymptomatic brainstem lesions in MS, auditory evoked responses are an excellent screening procedure when tumors of the eighth nerve are suspected. The sensitivity of BAERs in the setting is more than 90%. BAERs are often used in the operating room to help protect the eighth nerve during resection of posterior fossa lesions. The test is also useful when neuromuscular junction blockade or large doses of hypnosedative drugs have abolished the clinically testable brainstem reflexes. The presence of BAERs (beyond wave I) confirms the activity of the brainstem and also can help to localize brainstem lesions producing coma.

Analysis of BAER wave latencies as a function of intensity serves as a useful marker of auditory acuity in infants. This technique allows the early selection of hearing-impaired children for hearing aids and helps prevent their misdiagnosis as autistic or mentally retarded.

SSERs are also useful in suspected MS because they allow the documentation of unsuspected or poorly defined sensory dysfunction. As the technique evolves, dermatomal SSERs may allow better definition of nerve root compression (e.g., by a herniated disc). SSERs also have a place in the operating room, guiding the degree of tension on distracting rods during scoliosis surgery.

Electromyography and Nerve Conduction Studies

Electromyography (EMG) and nerve conduction studies are valuable primarily in the analysis of peripheral nerve and muscular disorders. They serve as adjuncts to the patient's history and physical examination and must be tailored to a specific clinical question.

Technique

EMG demands a high degree of clinical and technical skill from the physician performing the study. The laboratory should be directed by a member of the American Association of Electromyography and Electrodiagnosis. Many variables influence the interpretation of results, including anatomic variations and the cooperation of the patient.

The usual EMG study involves recording spontaneous, voluntary, and electrically stimulated muscle activity by way of small intramuscular needle electrodes. Because the voluntary contraction of muscles is crucial for some parts of the study, the procedures should be explained clearly to the patient. Some discomfort is unavoidable during the test. Patients can be premedicated with codeine or anxiolytic agents without altering the data obtained; this often results in better cooperation and tolerance.

Some conditions indicate special studies. Myasthenia gravis and the myasthenic (Eaton–Lambert) syndrome exhibit characteristic responses to repetitive stimulation; the requesting physician must communicate such suspicions to the electromyographer.

Nerve conduction velocity (NCV) studies can be performed by trained technologists under the electromyographer's supervision. These tests involve electrical stimulation of a peripheral nerve, measuring the rate of transmission and the amplitude of the response along the nerve. These results are compared to statistically derived normal ranges. Careful attention to variables such as limb temperature and length is required for a valid interpretation.

Interpretation

Abnormalities of the EMG can be produced by disease anywhere in the motor unit, from the lower motor neuron cell body to the muscle fiber. Characteristic patterns have emerged that allow the electromyographer to suspect diagnoses, but the test results are only meaningful with reference to a particular clinical problem. The analysis of the EMG and NCV data best illuminates questions of primary motor neuron or muscle disease, demyelinative versus axonal neuropathy, nerve root versus plexus disorders, and the localization of a mononeuropathy.

Motor neuron disease (e.g., amyotrophic lateral sclerosis) results in abnormal spontaneous activity of motor units and individual muscle fibers. This activity is seen throughout the body. Muscle disorders (e.g., myotonic dystrophy) produce characteristically different patterns of spontaneous activity.

Polyneuropathies cause EMG and NCV abnormalities according to their pathophysiology. Demyelinative neuropathies produce slowed conduction with preserved amplitude, whereas axonal neuropathies reduce amplitude with little effect on NCV. Chronic axonal neuropathy produces diffuse denervation responses in muscle (similar in nature to those seen focally in mononeuropathies). These tests thus can narrow the diagnostic spectrum in polyneuropathy and should be performed early to help plan the subsequent workup. In acute demyelinative neuropathies (e.g., the Guillain-Barré syndrome), special studies of conduction through the nerve roots (F responses and H reflexes) are often confirmatory when the routine NCV studies are normal.

The correct localization of a lesion along the course of a peripheral nerve (root, plexus, or at distal sites) usually is required for diagnosis and therapy. Root lesions produce denervation in paraspinal muscles in addition to distal changes; thus, a herniated disc can be separated from other pathologic lesions. Denervation changes require from 1 to 6 weeks to appear following an injury; thus, these studies rarely are indicated acutely. Such a study is important when multiple sites of pathology are detected along the course of a nerve. Some surgeons require EMG confirmation of focal lesions prior to removing a disc or transposing a peripheral nerve.

Entrapment syndromes often are diagnosed best by EMG and nerve conduction studies. The most common disorder is the carpal tunnel syndrome; this is also a situation in which clinical judgment in interpretation is crucial. Asymptomatic median nerve compression in the carpal tunnel is common; if the electrical studies are limited only to the wrist, pathology in the neck may be overlooked and the wrong therapy may be undertaken.

The routine use of EMG and NCV studies in the evaluation of neck, shoulder, or low back pain in the absence of neurologic deficits is costly and time consuming, and it seldom benefits the patient. The test is best used to confirm and define abnormalities seen on examination. Only if the clinical suspicion of a discrete lesion is high, or confirmation of equivocal imaging studies is required, should these tests be performed in such a situation.

SUMMARY

Neurodiagnostic studies can provide critical data for the evaluation of diagnostic alternatives. It is hoped that the preceding discussion has served to place these tests in their proper clinical perspective. One must use the information obtained as an extension of the history and physical examination, or incorrect diagnosis and improper therapy are likely.

The future of electrophysiologic studies is bright; improvements in automated data analysis and artificial intelligence will elicit more data from the available tests. As the power of these techniques increases, however, so does their potential for error. As the clinician becomes more dependent on other people's interpretation of data, it becomes increasingly important to be certain that the clinical laboratories used are appropriately certified.

QUESTIONS AND DISCUSSION

1. A patient presents with paraparesis and a history of optic neuritis in the left eye. An MRI study reveals no cerebral lesions and no evidence of spinal cord pathology. Which of the following tests is most likely to help confirm or refute the diagnosis of multiple sclerosis?

A. NCV studies

B. CSF evaluation for oligoclonal antibodies

C. Contrast myelography

D. BAERs

E. EEG

The answer is (B). Oligoclonal antibodies are present in more than 90% of patients with MS. NCV is not affected in MS. Contrast myelography is unnecessary if the MRI is normal. BAERs might be abnormal but would be superfluous if oligoclonal antibodies are present. The EEG is not helpful in diagnosing MS.

2. A patient with suspected complex partial seizures has a normal routine EEG. Which of these procedures would be most useful diagnostically?

A. VERs

B. LP

C. Repeat EEG with sleep deprivation and extra electrodes

D. 24-hour EEG monitoring

E. EMG studies

The answer is (C). Sleep deprivation and extra electrodes often demonstrate epileptiform activity when the routine EEG is unrevealing. Evoked response studies are not specifically abnormal in epilepsy. Twenty-four-hour EEG monitoring is helpful in special circumstances but is seldom necessary in routine practice. An EMG would not shed light on possible epilepsy.

3. Which of the following is not a contraindication to LP?

A. Papilledema, stiff neck, and fever

B. Cutaneous infection of the lower back

C. Suspected intraspinal mass

D. Posterior fossa tumor

E. Coagulopathy

The answer is (A). Papilledema is seen in states of increased intracranial pressure but does not necessarily imply a risk of herniation. In the setting of fever and stiff neck, papilledema is suggestive of meningitis so that a lumbar puncture is necessary. Patients with pseudotumor cerebri usually benefit symptomatically from an LP, and the test is necessary for the diagnosis. A CT scan, however, should precede an LP in the presence of papilledema. The other situations are all contraindications to an LP.

4. Which of the following tests is the most useful in the diagnosis of herpes simplex encephalitis?

A. EEG

B. CT scan with contrast

C. MRI

D. CSF analysis by PCR

E. Angiography

The answer is (D). Analysis of the CSF by specific PCR is the most sensitive test for herpes simplex encephalitis. The EEG frequently shows periodic lateralized epileptiform activity over one or both temporal lobes in herpes simplex encephalitis, but this finding is neither sensitive nor specific. A CT scan with contrast may or may not detect the infection. MRI is much more sensitive for herpes encephalitis, but other diseases can produce lesions in the medial temporal region, and on occasion herpes may produce encephalitis in other brain regions. Angiography may be useful in the diagnosis of herpes zoster vasculitis but would not be useful for herpes simplex encephalitis.

5. Nerve conduction studies in axonal neuropathies are characterized by:

A. Slow conduction and normal amplitude

B. No changes in either conduction velocity or amplitude

C. Loss of amplitude, with relative sparing of velocity

D. Increased conduction velocity

E. High-amplitude responses

The answer is (C). The amplitude reflects the number of nerve impulses that arrive at the neuromuscular junction; axonal neuropathies primarily reduce this number. Those impulses that are transmitted have a relatively normal conduction velocity. Demyelinative neuropathy slows conduction but does not reduce the number of fibers carrying impulses.

SUGGESTED READING

American Electroencephalographic Society. Guidelines in EEG and evoked potentials. *J Clin Neurophysiol* 1986;3 (Suppl 1).

Aminoff MJ, ed. *Electrodiagnosis in clinical neurology,* 4th ed. New York: Churchill Livingstone, 2002.

Bleck TP. Arthropod-borne virus causing central nervous system infection. In: Goldman L, Dennis Ausiello, eds. *Cecil textbook of medicine.* 22nd ed. Philadelphia: WB Saunders, 2004, 2034–2042.

Chiappa K, ed. *Evoked potentials in clinical medicine,* 3rd ed. New York: Raven Press, 1990.

Cracco RQ, Bodis-Wollner I, eds. *Evoked potentials.* New York: Alan R. Liss, 1986.

Ebersole JS, Pedley TA, eds. *Current practice of clinical electroencephalography,* 3rd ed. Philadelphia: Lippincott Williams & Wilkins, 2002.

Fishman RA. *Cerebrospinal fluid in diseases of the nervous system,* 3rd ed. Philadelphia: WB Saunders, 1992.

Liveson JA. *Peripheral neurology: case studies in electrodiagnosis,* 2nd ed. Philadelphia: FA Davis, 1991.

Niedermeyer E, Lopes da Silva F, eds. *Electroencephalography,* 3rd ed. Baltimore: Urban and Schwarzenberg, 1993.

Schaumburg HH, Spencer PS, Thomas PK. *Disorders of peripheral nerves,* 2nd ed. Philadelphia: FA Davis, 1991.

Scheld WM, Whittley RJ, Marra CM, eds. *Infections of the central nervous system,* 3rd ed. Philadelphia: Lippincott Williams & Wilkins, 2004 (in press).

4

Neuroradiology—Which Tests to Order?

M.J.B. Stallmeyer and Gregg H. Zoarski

The workup of patients with neurologic symptoms often includes multiple neuroimaging tests. At initial presentation, noninvasive imaging with computed tomography (CT) or magnetic resonance imaging (MRI) is usually the first study obtained. Depending on the disease process involved, further imaging with more advanced CT or MRI techniques, other noninvasive modalities such as positron emission tomography (PET), or invasive procedures such as angiography or myelography may be appropriate.

Stroke

Acute cerebral infarction is one of the most common clinical problems faced by neurologists, emergency medicine specialists, and neuroradiologists. With the development of effective intravenous and intraarterial thrombolytic therapy for treatment of early acute stroke, differentiating between reversibly impaired "tissue at risk" and irreversibly injured brain tissue has become critical. Thrombolysis can restore blood flow to ischemic brain; however, if blood flow is restored to large areas of irreversibly damaged brain tissue, a high risk of intracerebral hemorrhage exists. In patients with infarcts affecting greater than one-third of the middle cerebral artery territory, or with infarcts affecting significant portions of the basal ganglia, thrombolysis should not be administered. Rapid acquisition CT techniques (noncontrast CT, CT angiography [CTA], and perfusion CT), MRI, and magnetic resonance angiography (MRA) all have proved to be valuable imaging modalities in guiding which patients should undergo treatment.

The preferred initial study to be obtained in the setting of suspected stroke is noncontrast CT to determine whether stroke symptoms are caused by hemorrhage (e.g., aneurysmal subarachnoid hemorrhage, hypertensive hemorrhage, hemorrhage within a mass or vascular malformation). Noncontrast head CT obtained within a few hours of the onset of an ischemic stroke is often normal or shows only subtle changes (Fig. 4.1). Early signs of infarction that may be seen 1 to 3 hours after ictus include obscuration of grey matter–white matter differentiation, especially within the lentiform nucleus and insula; hyperdense middle cerebral artery (MCA) sign, which is specific but of limited sensitivity; and subtle effacement of sulci (Fig. 4.1). Even when trained neuroradiologists are interpreting noncontrast head CT, however, the accuracy of predicting the volume of infarct was only 76% in one study.

In perfusion CT, a bolus of contrast material is tracked as it courses through the brain vasculature while the brain is imaged using multidetector CT (Fig. 4.2). Typically this is performed prior to CT angiography to decrease background "noise" from capillary and venous contamination. In recent studies, lesion volume on perfusion CT was found to correlate well with final infarct size and clinical outcome.

In CT angiography, contrast enhancement within arteries can be visualized and displayed as a three-dimensional model. Newer scanners may be equipped with up to 16 detector rows, making scanning from the aortic arch to the intracranial vessels in 20 seconds of scan time a realistic goal. This technique can be used in rapid identification of regions of stenosis and in guiding potential endovascular intervention using intraarterial thrombolysis or mechanical disruption of clot.

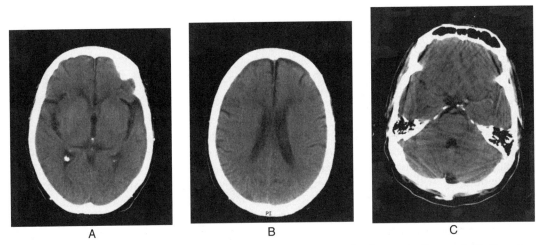

FIG. 4.1. Noncontrast computed tomography images of the brain demonstrating early findings in ischemia. **(A)** Subtle hypodensity in the anterior right insula ("insular ribbon sign"), and **(B)** loss of grey matter–white matter differentiation and effacement of sulci in the right frontal lobe, in a patient presenting 3 hours after acute onset of left-sided weakness. **C:** "Dense MCA (middle cerebral artery) sign" is demonstrated in the left middle cerebral artery in a different patient presenting 2 hours after acute onset of aphasia and right-sided weakness.

Conventional MR sequences such as T1-weighted images (T1WI) and T2-weighted images (T2WI) are limited in their ability to demonstrate acute strokes within the time window when thrombolytic treatment is likely to be effective. More recently developed techniques such as fluid-attenuated inversion recovery (FLAIR) images increase the conspicuity of developing edema within the brain but still may not show very early ischemic lesions well. Thus, diffusion-weighted imaging (DWI) sequences and perfusion-weighted MRI have become important components of the imaging workup of acute stroke.

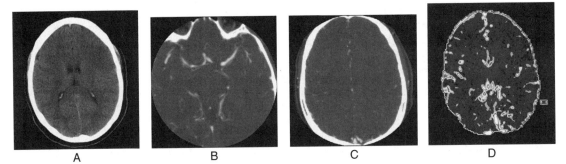

FIG. 4.2. Noncontrast computed tomography (CT) image **(A)** of a 39-year-old man presenting six hours following acute onset of aphasia and right sided weakness demonstrates well-developed focal hypodensity in the left frontal lobe, indicative of a left middle cerebral artery anterior division branch infarct. CT angiography image at the level of the circle of Willis **(B)** demonstrates gross patency of the left middle cerebral artery M1 segment; however, more superiorly **(C)** there is a relative paucity of distal left middle cerebral artery branches on the left, compared with those on the right. CT perfusion image **(D)** demonstrates mild decreased perfusion in the left frontal lobe in the region of the infarct.

DWI uses powerful imaging gradients, in conjunction with rapid spin-echo or echo-planar data acquisition to accentuate phase differences between protons of varying mobility. In regions of recent cerebral infarction (Fig. 4.3), diffusion of tissue water becomes restricted, as manifested by a decrease in its apparent diffusion coefficient (ADC). In animal models, diffusion-weighted images can reliably reveal infarcted regions within minutes of experimental vascular occlusion. Numerous clinical studies in patients have demonstrated similar results in DWI of infarcts only a few hours old.

The appearance of diffusion-weighted images changes with the age of the infarct. Diffusion-weighted images contain mixed contributions from changes in ADC and T2; this effect is called "T2 shine-through." Infarcted regions will remain abnormal on DWI for at least 14 days, and they may be abnormal for as long as 8 weeks following infarction. For the first few days, signal intensity on DWI is dominated by shortening of ADC. At 2 to 3 days, T2 effects from edema begin to dominate. Infarct volume, measured on ADC maps, may provide prognostic information for patients with acute stroke.

Perfusion-weighted MR imaging also demonstrates infarcts and ischemia within a few hours after onset of stroke symptoms.

Difference images, obtained by subtracting diffusion-weighted images from images showing disruptions in perfusion, can be used to identify an ischemic penumbra, or region of ischemic tissue at risk for infarct, to guide clinical decision making.

Indications for invasive imaging with diagnostic angiography include the preoperative workup of carotid stenosis, evaluation of stroke in the setting of suspected vasculitis and, in the setting of acute stroke, as a precursor to endovascular intervention (Fig. 4.4). Although intravenous tissue plasminogen activator (TPA) can be beneficial to some patients when given within 3 hours of stroke onset, many patients present beyond this time window. In appropriate centers and in selected cases, emergent intraarterial thrombolytic therapy, or mechanical retrieval of thrombus, may improve outcomes from an acute stroke.

Cerebral Hemorrhage: Aneurysms, Arteriovenous Malformations, and Dissections

Prior to the advent of highly sensitive cross sectional imaging modalities such as CT and MRI, cerebral angiography was the primary diagnostic tool for the indirect detection of intracranial extraaxial abnormalities such as

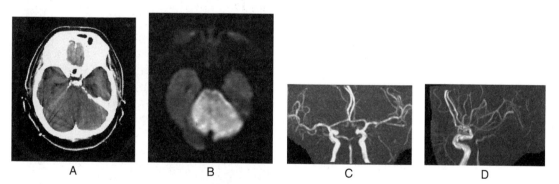

FIG. 4.3. Noncontrast computed tomography image **(A)** of a 78-year-old female patient transferred from a nursing home for obtundation demonstrates diffuse hypodensity of the cerebellum, with effacement of the fourth ventricle. Corresponding magnetic resonance diffusion image **(B)** demonstrates a large acute cerebellar infarct. Magnetic resonance angiography maximum intensity projection (MIP) images in coronal **(C)** and sagittal **(D)** planes demonstrate decreased flow signal in the distal basilar artery.

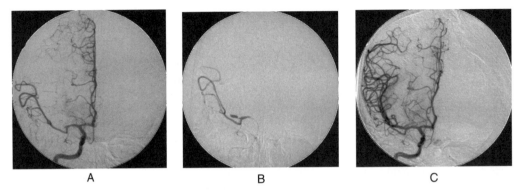

A   B   C

FIG. 4.4. Digital subtraction angiography (DSA), anterior–posterior (AP) projection, of a patient presenting 4.5 hours after acute onset of left hemiparesis demonstrates abrupt cutoff **(A)** of the right middle cerebral artery anterior division. Following passage of a microcatheter into the occluded segment **(B)**, and subsequent lysis of the clot by intraarterial infusion of r-TPA (tissue plasminogen activator), patency is restored **(C)**. The patient was neurologically intact by several hours following intraarterial thrombolysis and was discharged to home several days later.

subdural and epidural hematoma, and for intraaxial abnormalities such as brain tumors. The diagnosis was based largely upon displacement and distortion of the normal, expected vascular patterns. Conventional angiography is rarely, if ever performed now simply for the purpose of these diagnoses.

Conventional cerebral angiography remains the gold standard for the diagnosis of intracranial vascular lesions such as arteriovenous malformations, aneurysms, arteriovenous fistulas, dissection, and pseudoaneurysm formation. It is likely, however, that emerging techniques such as CTA (Fig. 4.5) and improvements in MRA will obviate the need for diagnostic cerebral angiography in many of these cases over the next several years.

Endovascular therapies for intracranial vascular lesions are becoming more frequent as research and clinical experience have advanced the technologic boundaries of this exciting specialty. A large percentage of ruptured and unruptured intracranial aneurysms now are treated with endovascular techniques instead of surgical clipping (Fig. 4.6). At some institutions, endovascular coil occlusion of cerebral aneurysms constitutes the primary mode of treatment. One large study, the International Subarachnoid Aneurysm Trial (ISAT), has documented a 26% decrease in morbidity with coiling of ruptured aneurysms when compared to traditional microsurgical clipping.

Vasospasm complicates the course of recovery in up to half of all survivors of aneurysmal subarachnoid hemorrhage. The peak onset of vasospasm typically occurs at 7 to 10 days after the ictus; the clinical presen-

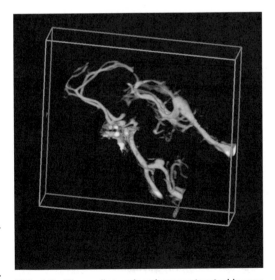

FIG. 4.5. Three-dimensional reconstructed image from a computed tomography angiogram demonstrates a distal left vertebral artery aneurysm.

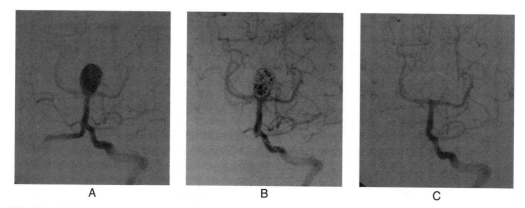

FIG. 4.6. Endovascular treatment of a basilar tip aneurysm. Anterior–posterior digital subtraction angiography (AP DSA) **(A)** demonstrates a wide-necked basilar tip aneurysm. In **(B)**, a microcatheter has been placed within the aneurysm and several coils have been placed. In **(C)**, the aneurysm lumen has been completely occluded by coils.

tation may range from a mild focal deficit such as hemiparesis to global alteration of consciousness and obtundation in the case of severe basilar artery spasm. Conventional triple-H therapy for treatment of vasospasm consists of induced hypertension, hemodilution, and hypervolemia. Calcium antagonists such as verapamil often are added to the pharmaceutical regimen. Options for endovascular intervention for vasospasm include intraarterial verapamil or papaverine infusion, or angioplasty (Fig. 4.7) which typically provides a more durable result. Because of technical limitations, angioplasty is limited to treatment of the basilar and internal carotid arteries, as well as the proximal vessels of the circle of Willis.

Extracranial carotid and vertebral stenoses, as well as intracranial stenoses, now can be treated with angioplasty alone or with angioplasty in combination with stenting (Fig. 4.8). Early data on morbidity and mortality are comparable to the results of surgical carotid endarterectomy. Antiplatelet agents such as clopidogrel may play an important role in immediate patency after angioplasty or stenting, especially in small intracranial vessels.

Arteriovenous malformations, located either within the parenchyma of the brain or on the brain surface, are thought to represent a

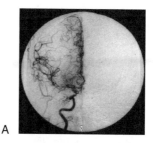

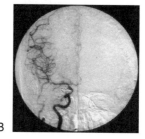

FIG. 4.7. Balloon angioplasty treatment of post-subarachnoid hemorrhage vasospasm in a patient with a ruptured right posterior communicating artery aneurysm. Anterior–posterior digital subtraction angiography (AP DSA) **(A)** demonstrates severe vasospasm in the right internal carotid artery paraclinoid segment, extending into the right middle cerebral artery M1 and M2 segments. DSA following balloon angioplasty of the right internal carotid artery and right middle cerebral artery M1 segments **(B)** demonstrates relief of spasm in the treated segments, with improved filling of middle cerebral artery branches relative to anterior cerebral artery branches. Note surgical clips obliterating the right posterior communicating artery aneurysm.

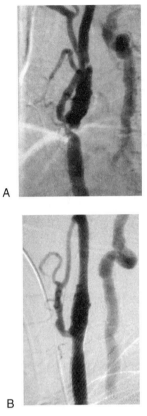

A

B

FIG. 4.8. Stenting of right internal carotid artery stenosis. Lateral digital subtraction angiography **(A)** demonstrates short-segment high-grade stenoses in the distal right common carotid artery and in the distal right internal carotid bulb. Following placement of a stent across the stenotic lesions **(B)** caliber of the artery is improved.

congenital abnormality. In the case of an arteriovenous malformation, the nidus represents a tangle of arteriovenous shunts which coalesce to drain through one or more cortical or deep cerebral veins. In the case of an arteriovenous fistula, a solitary anomaly connects a single artery to a draining vein, bypassing the normal cerebral parenchyma. In either case, an endovascular approach may be used to embolize and occlude the feeding arteries of the malformation with polyvinylalcohol particles or liquid acrylic tissue adhesive. Embolization often is performed as an adjunct to surgical excision or focused radiosurgery. Em-

bolization helps to decrease overall treatment morbidity by diminishing blood loss at surgery or decreasing the required radiation volumes.

Neoplasms

Characterization of brain tumors by imaging involves determining the location of the lesion and its enhancement characteristics. The most common primary neoplasms of the brain and spinal cord in adults are glial in origin. Astrocytomas are classified into three categories of increasing pathologic malignancy: low-grade astrocytoma, anaplastic astrocytoma, and glioblastoma multiforme (GBM). Presenting clinical symptoms include headache, seizure, and development of focal neurologic symptoms.

CT of primary brain neoplasms usually demonstrates a hypodense mass, predominantly involving the white matter. Lower grade tumors typically demonstrate somewhat less pronounced enhancement than higher grade tumors, but this is variable. On higher grade GBMs, necrosis on pathology and CT imaging is characteristic.

MRI is more sensitive than CT in detection of primary brain masses, particularly in the posterior fossa. Additionally, the multiplanar capability of MRI is often more helpful in surgical planning and in targeting of radiotherapy. Tumor infiltration along white matter tracts appears hypointense on T1WI and hyperintense on T2WI. FLAIR sequences, which increase the conspicuity of edema, are helpful in identifying smaller brain parenchymal lesions; however, distinguishing infiltrating tumor from vasogenic edema sometimes may be difficult using FLAIR.

More recently, DWI and perfusion MRI have been used to characterize primary brain tumors. DWI can aid in differentiating tumor from vasogenic edema. Regions of increased tumor perfusion may indicate regions of greatest tumor neovascularity and thus aggressiveness. The degree of contrast enhancement on MRI (Fig. 4.9), particularly in combination with more recently developed

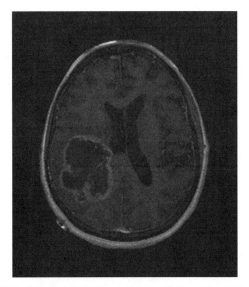

FIG. 4.9. Axial postgadolinium (Gd) contrast T1-weighted magnetic resonance image of glioblastoma multiforme (GBM), demonstrating a large, edge-enhancing necrotic mass in the right frontoparietal region.

perfusion imaging techniques, is thought to roughly correlate with the amount of vasogenic edema and tumor grade; this may not, however, correlate with gadolinium enhancement on conventional T1WI.

In brain tumor surgery, functional MRI (fMRI) data are helpful in surgical planning and guiding intraoperative brain mapping. Functional MRI maps are obtained by displaying portions of the brain activated during the performance of various tasks (e.g., motor, sensory, language, visual tasks) by the patient.

Brain tumor proton MR spectroscopy (MRS) evaluates the presence of various metabolites. N-acetylaspartate (NAA) and choline levels are often low in brain tumors; this is thought to be the result of the lack of neurons relative to glial cells in brain tumors. Choline, which is present primarily in glial cells, reflects cell membrane turnover or may reflect increased tumor cellularity. The ratio of choline-containing compounds to creatine levels, and the ratio of choline to NAA, thus may be used to distinguish tumor from nontumorous tissue. MRS is helpful in monitoring response to therapy and may be useful, at least in some cases, in differentiating recurrent tumor from radiation injury (Fig. 4.10).

PET can be used to evaluate various metabolic features of brain tumors (e.g., glucose metabolism, blood flow, and oxygen consumption). PET tumor imaging most commonly is performed using 2-[18F]-fluoro-2-deoxy-D-glucose (FDG) as a radiotracer. FDG-PET imaging of malignant brain tumors shows increased glucose metabolism in tumor cells and provides information on tumor

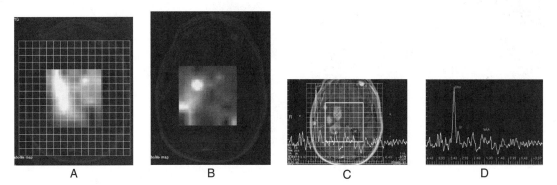

| A | B | C | D |

FIG. 4.10. Brain tumor proton magnetic resonance spectroscopy (MRS) of glioblastoma multiforme (GBM). Choline metabolite map **(A)** demonstrates multiple foci of elevated choline in GBM previously treated with radiation. The grid corresponds to that projected over a T1-weighted postgadolinium MR image in **(C)**. Creatine metabolite map **(B)** demonstrates a single focus of markedly elevated choline along the anteriomedial aspect of the tumor. Corresponding spectrum of metabolites **(D)** from a single voxel (X) demonstrates markedly elevated choline:creatine ratio, consistent with focus of viable tumor cells. (Case provided by David Lefkowitz, MD, and Katrina Read.)

grade and response to therapy, particularly when images are correlated with MRI. FDG-PET, in combination with high-resolution data from MRI, also can be used to define the most metabolically active regions of tumor for stereotactic biopsy targeting and radiosurgery and may aid in differentiating radiation necrosis from areas of high-grade tumor progression.

Metastases account for about one-third of intracranial tumors in adults. The most common appearance is that of enhancing nodular lesions in the brain parenchyma, often located at the grey matter–white matter junction (Fig. 4.11). Large brain metastases often demonstrate surrounding edema and mass effect out of proportion to the size of the enhancing lesion. In contrast, small metastases may not demonstrate appreciable mass effect. Identification of the number, location, and size of metastases is particularly crucial because this can affect treatment decisions. Solitary metastases, or a small number of metastases, may be amenable to surgical resection or focused-beam radiotherapy. With more extensive involvement, whole-brain radiotherapy or chemotherapy is indicated. In general, MRI is more sensitive than CT in evaluation of metastatic disease in the brain parenchyma. In particular, FLAIR sequences, by improving the conspicuity of edema, can be sensitive to the presence of very small lesions and lep-

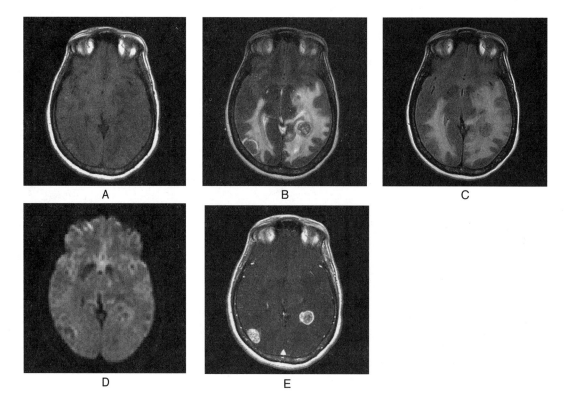

FIG. 4.11. Magnetic resonance image of metastatic disease from a breast cancer primary tumor. T1-weighted **(A)** and T2-weighted **(B)** axial images demonstrate metastatic deposits in the right and left occipital lobes, with extensive surrounding edema and signal changes suggestive of subacute to chronic hemorrhage within the tumor foci. The fluid-attenuated inversion recovery (FLAIR) image **(C)** demonstrates extensive associated edematous changes. The corresponding diffusion image **(D)** demonstrates subtle impaired diffusion immediately adjacent to the left occipital focus. Postgadolinium contrast image shows dense enhancement of the metastatic foci.

tomeningeal metastases. Double-dose gadolinium-DTPA contrast may variably improve the detection of small metastatic deposits.

Meningiomas are extraaxial benign primary brain tumors arising from arachnoid cap cells in the dura. They most commonly are located in the parafalcine regions of the convexities and occur less frequently at the skull base. On CT scan they are slightly hyperintense to grey matter because of their high cellularity. Some degree of calcification occurs frequently. On MRI, signal is usually isointense to grey matter on T1WI and slightly hypointense on T2WI. Meningiomas typically enhance prominently on both CT and MRI. Surrounding edema signal may be present and may indicate a mixed dural–pial blood supply. If the meningioma occurs in close proximity to a dural venous sinus, patency of the sinus can be evaluated with MR venogram or conventional angiography. Preoperative embolization of meningiomas may be helpful in selected patients.

Infection

Central nervous system (CNS) infections include meningitis, which predominantly affects the meninges and surface of the brain; ventriculitis, infection of the cerebral ventricular ependyma; encephalitis, with inflammation extending into the brain parenchyma; myelitis, infection in the spinal cord; brain abscess; and infections arising adjacent to the brain or spinal cord. CNS infections often require urgent diagnosis and prompt initiation of appropriate therapy to assure a good outcome. Thus, CT with and without contrast, which is more readily available than MRI in most institutions, usually will be the first study obtained. It is not uncommon, however, for initial CT studies to be normal, particularly in patients with early meningitis. Newer MRI sequences such as FLAIR and DWI are helpful in detecting subtle brain edema in early encephalitis. FLAIR sequences are also relatively sensitive and specific in detection of increased protein content in CSF within the subarachnoid space in meningitis. Additionally, postcontrast MRI offers greater sensitivity than CT for detection of meningeal enhancement.

White Matter Diseases

Multiple sclerosis (MS) is a common white matter disease that results in the demyelination of nerves of the brain and spinal cord, while sparing peripheral nerves. MS plaques are typically nodular or ovoid lesions, most often located in the periventricular white matter and corpus callosum, where they tend to be oriented perpendicular to the ventricle–white matter interface ("Dawson's fingers"). Plaques also can be located elsewhere within the white matter tracts of the brain and spinal cord.

MRI has long been established as the most sensitive imaging methodology for detections of lesions of MS. Although MS remains a clinical diagnosis, MRI is helpful in following the course of the disease and for evaluating the efficacy of treatment. T2WIs, proton density images, and FLAIR images commonly are used to detect plaques but do not distinguish between active and chronic plaques (Fig. 4.8). Magnetization transfer (MT) imaging is a relatively new technique that can be used to monitor the changes over time in the degree of demyelination and axonal loss in individual lesions. MT measurements suggest a focal increase in free water and a reduction of macromolecular material several months before the appearance of an active lesion. Gadolinium enhancement of lesions on T1-weighted sequences has been used as an indicator of active MS plaques (Fig. 4.12).

Progressive multifocal leukoencephalopathy (PML) and human immunodeficiency virus associated white matter lesions (HIV-WML) in acquired immune deficiency syndrome (AIDS) are also best evaluated with MRI. HIV-WML are nonspecific, well-defined white matter lesions, typically found in the centrum semiovale of patients with AIDS without known opportunistic infections, particularly those with advanced AIDS. They are difficult to differentiate radiographically from foci of gliosis or demyelination. FLAIR sequences and T2WI are most helpful in detection. PML, which is

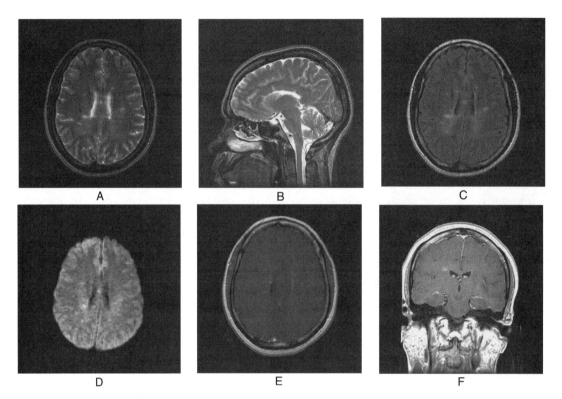

FIG. 4.12. Magnetic resonance image of multiple sclerosis. T2-weighted axial **(A)** and sagittal **(B)** images demonstrate typical hyperintense signal in periventricular and callosal plaques. Periventricular plaques are more conspicuous on fluid-attenuated inversion recovery (FLAIR) images **(C)** as a result of nulling of the cerebrospinal fluid signal and demonstrate impaired diffusion on diffusion-weighted imaging (DWI) **(D)**. Postgadolinium contrast T1-weighted axial **(E)** and coronal **(F)** images demonstrate faint enhancement in multiple plaques.

caused by infection of oligodendrocytes by the JC virus, is a demyelinating disease in patients with AIDS, affecting 2% to 7% of all AIDS patients. PML lesions are typically located in the subcortical white matter, but they also may appear in the posterior fossa. Enhancement is atypical but may occur. The larger reduction in magnetization transfer ratio for PML lesions is most likely the result of demyelination, whereas the reduction in HIV-WML may be associated primarily with gliosis. Magnetization transfer MR imaging may help distinguish these two processes. Although both PML lesions and HIV-WML cause reductions in magnetization transfer ratio, in PML, which results in demyelination, the effect is much more pronounced than in HIV-WML, which is thought to be associated primarily with gliosis.

Trauma

CT is the first-line modality for evaluation of acute injury to the brain and, with the advent of spiral and multidetector CT, is rapidly supplanting plain films in evaluation of suspected acute bony spinal injury.

Cerebral contusions may appear as foci of hyperdense blood within the brain parenchyma. Small contusions may be predominantly hypodense, with only petechial hemorrhage evident. Because many acute cerebral injuries are the result of motor vehicle collisions or falls, contusions often are located at the base of the frontal lobes or along the temporal tips. Associated subarachnoid hemorrhage may be present or may be the only finding.

Thin section CT is the methodology of choice when calvarial fracture is suspected, and it is often helpful in suspected bony spinal injury. Multiplanar reconstructed images are helpful, if not crucial, in presurgical evaluation of skull base and facial fractures and in rapid evaluation of the spinal canal in fracture-dislocations.

Subdural hematomas occur when bridging veins that traverse the subdural space are torn. On CT, acute subdural hematomas typically appear as crescent-shaped high-density collections along the cerebral convexities or tentorium. In older subdural hematomas, blood products are lower in density and may be isointense or hypodense compared with brain tissue. Large subdural hematomas may cause significant mass effect, with resultant subfalcine or transtentorial herniation.

Epidural hematomas usually occur secondary to arterial bleeding, most commonly as a result of laceration of the middle meningeal artery or laceration of a large dural venous sinus. The periosteum of the inner table of the calvarium, which is formed by the outer layer of dura, is peeled away by the hematoma, causing a characteristic lentiform shape because it is constrained at calvarial suture lines. Typically this type of hematoma enlarges rapidly and requires urgent surgical intervention.

CONCLUSION

The options for neuroradiologic investigation and imaging of disease have become increasingly sensitive, yet concurrently more complex. Consultation with colleagues in neuroradiology will help define the most efficient algorithms for patient evaluation in concert with the available imaging resources at a particular institution. Consultation regarding individual patients may be essential in unraveling the peculiarities of any one particular patient and their illness.

QUESTIONS AND DISCUSSION

1. For the evaluation of acute stroke, which of the following is (are) true?

A. T1-weighted MRI is more sensitive than CT for the diagnosis of acute subarachnoid hemorrhage (SAH).

B. A noncontrast CT (NCT) is the initial study of choice.

C. CT angiography (CTA) may be helpful in determining the location of an occluding thromboembolus.

D. Noncontrast CT often reveals infarctions earlier than does MRI.

E. Contrast-enhanced CT is more sensitive than MRI in the evaluation of the midbrain and brainstem.

The answers are (B) and (C). In general, NCT is more accurate than MRI for the evaluation of acute SAH as well as hemorrhage in other locations. Although FLAIR MRI may be sensitive in detection of small amounts of elevated protein or blood within the cerebrospinal fluid, NCT remains the preferred initial study. MRI is more useful after hemorrhage has been ruled out. MRI DWI and perfusion images are more accurate in evaluating the presence of hyperacute and acute infarctions than is CT, demonstrate ischemic changes sooner than CT, and are more sensitive in identifying additional areas of infarction. MRI is also more useful than CT in evaluation of suspected posterior fossa strokes; CT images through the posterior fossa often are degraded by streak artifacts as a result of dense bone at the skull base. CTA has been shown to be useful in determining the location of vessel occlusion in acute stroke. With the increased availability of multidetector CT scanners, CTA probably will play an increasingly important role in the imaging workup of this disease.

2. Computed tomographic angiography (CTA) (choose one or more):

A. Requires the infusion of intravenous contrast.

B. Is useful for the detection of extracranial carotid artery stenosis.

C. Has replaced cerebral angiography as the "gold standard" for detection of intracranial aneurysms.

D. Can be used to assess both the extracranial and intracranial carotid and vertebral arteries in a single scan.

E. Usually is performed prior to CT perfusion in the setting of acute stroke.

The answers are (A), (B), and (D). Infusion of intravenous contrast is necessary for CTA. CTA can be used to detect atherosclerotic lesions in the extracranial carotid and vertebral arteries, dissections, cerebral vasospasm, and brain aneurysms, but it is not yet accepted as the "gold standard" examination for detection of aneurysms. Newer generation multidetector scanners permit scanning of the major cervicocerebral carotid and vertebral arteries in a single scan. Most centers perform CT perfusion prior to CTA in the setting of suspected acute stroke to minimize "noise" from circulating contrast in the veins and capillary beds.

3. For the diagnosis of primary and secondary intracranial neoplasms, which of the following is true?

A. A contrast-enhanced study is not necessary with MRI because metastases are apparent on T2WI and FLAIR images as hyperintense (bright) areas.

B. Contrast-enhanced CT is the modality of choice.

C. Functional MRI can be helpful in planning surgical resection of tumors.

D. Noncontrast CT is more accurate than conventional MRI in the detection of osseous metastases.

E. PET imaging can help in distinguishing active tumor growth from posttreatment changes such as radiation necrosis.

The answers are (C), (D), and (E). Although many metastatic lesions will be demonstrated on T2WI and FLAIR images, contrast-enhanced T1WI always should be performed for complete evaluation. MRI is more sensitive than contrast-enhanced CT in detecting intracranial tumors, particularly small metastatic lesions and lesions in the posterior fossa. Functional MRI can be used to determine the proximity of certain eloquent areas of brain (e.g., the motor strip, visual cortex, speech areas) to tumor and has been useful in surgical planning in some patients. In general, calcification usually is seen better on noncontrast CT than on MRI. Most metastatic osseous lesions, which tend to be lytic, are better demonstrated on CT than on MRI, particularly if thin-section images and bone-technique algorithms are used; MRI, however, may be better at evaluating the extent of extraosseous spread of a metastatic lesion. PET imaging has been used to differentiate regions of active tumor growth from radiation necrosis and to define regions of active tumor growth for biopsy or radiosurgery.

4. Regarding MRI studies of white matter diseases, which of the following is or are true?

A. FLAIR images can help distinguish active MS plaques from chronic plaques.

B. Gadolinium contrast enhancement on T1WI is suggestive of active demyelination.

C. Magnetization transfer (MT) MRI imaging is a new technique that may be helpful in detection of new plaques.

D. Lesions of PML commonly enhance.

E. MRI is not helpful in detection of MS plaques in the spinal cord.

The answer is (B). FLAIR images can increase conspicuity of MS plaques, particularly those located in the periventricular white matter, but cannot distinguish areas of active demyelination from chronic plaques. Gadolinium contrast enhancement on T1WI often is used as a marker for active MS plaques. Magnetization transfer imaging has shown great promise in detection of early demyelination in MS plaques and can be helpful in following the progression of the disease or response to treatment. PML lesions do not typically enhance in most cases, but enhancement uncommonly can occur. MS plaques are uncommon in the spinal cord but may be identified by MRI as hyperintense (bright) areas on proton-density images and T2WI.

5. Regarding the use of CT and MRI in the diagnosis of various abnormalities of the brain and spine, which of the following is or are true?

A. MRI uses a slightly greater amount of ionizing radiation than does CT.

B. Contrast material such as Gd-DTPA in MRI or iodinated contrast in CT routinely localizes in the subarachnoid space.

C. The use of CTA and MRA will result in a decrease in the number of conventional catheter angiograms needed to diagnose many vascular abnormalities.

D. FLAIR MRI images can be useful in the diagnosis of meningitis.

E. Meningiomas typically enhance prominently on both CT and MRI.

The answers are (C) and (D). MRI, unlike CT, does not use ionizing radiation to produce images. Contrast material remains intravascular except in regions of blood–brain barrier breakdown or vascular rupture. CTA and MRA techniques have to some degree supplanted the routine diagnostic use of catheter angiography in evaluation of vascular diseases of the brain and spinal cord and likely will assume an increasingly important role in diagnosis and monitoring of these diseases. Catheter angiography, however, remains the "gold standard" examination for evaluation of suspected aneurysmal subarachnoid hemorrhage. FLAIR MRI can detect elevated protein within CSF, which can be useful in detection of meningitis. Meningiomas typically enhance on both CT and MRI studies; CT, however, is better at evaluating calcification within a meningioma.

SUGGESTED READING

Filippi M, Rocca MA, Comi G. The use of quantitative magnetic-resonance-based techniques to monitor the evolution of multiple sclerosis. *Lancet Neurol* 2003;2(6): 337–346.

Furlan A, Higashida R, Wechsler L, et al. Intra-arterial prourokinase for acute ischemic stroke. The PROACT II study: a randomized controlled trial. Prolyse in acute cerebral thromboembolism. *JAMA* 1999;282(21): 2003–2011.

Jackson A, Kassner A, Annesley-Williams D, et al. Abnormalities in the recirculation phase of contrast agent bolus passage in cerebral gliomas: comparison with relative blood volume and tumor grade. *AJNR Am J Neuroradiol* 2002;23(1):7–14.

Lev MH, Segal AZ, Farkas J, et al. Utility of perfusion-weighted CT imaging in acute middle cerebral artery stroke treated with intra-arterial thrombolysis: prediction of final infarct volume and clinical outcome. *Stroke* 2001;32(9):2021–2028.

Levivier M, Wikler D Jr, Massager N, et al. The integration of metabolic imaging in stereotactic procedures including radiosurgery: a review. *J Neurosurg* 2002;97(5 Suppl): 542–550.

McKnight TR, von dem Bussche MH, Vigneron DB, et al. Histopathological validation of a three-dimensional magnetic resonance spectroscopy index as a predictor of tumor presence. *J Neurosurg* 2002;97(4):794–802.

Molyneux A, Kerr R, Stratton I, et al. International Subarachnoid Aneurysm Trial (ISAT) Collaborative Group. International Subarachnoid Aneurysm Trial (ISAT) of neurosurgical clipping versus endovascular coiling in 2,143 patients with ruptured intracranial aneurysms: a randomised trial. *Lancet* 2002;360(9342):1267–1274.

Paul R, Cohen R, Navia B, et al. Relationships between cognition and structural neuroimaging findings in adults with human immunodeficiency virus type-1. *Neurosci Biobehav Rev* 2002;26(3):353–359.

Pexman JH, Barber PA, Hill MD, et al. Use of the Alberta Stroke Program Early CT Score (ASPECTS) for assessing CT scans in patients with acute stroke. *AJNR Am J Neuroradiol* 2001;22(8):1534–1542.

Roux FE, Ibarrola D, Tremoulet M, et al. Methodological and technical issues for integrating functional magnetic resonance imaging data in a neuronavigational system. *Neurosurgery* 2001;49(5):1145–1156; discussion 1156–1157.

Schaefer PW, Hunter GJ, He J, et al. Predicting cerebral ischemic infarct volume with diffusion and perfusion MR imaging. *AJNR Am J Neuroradiol* 2002;23(10): 1785–1794.

Schlemmer HP, Bachert P, Henze M, et al. Differentiation of radiation necrosis from tumor progression using proton magnetic resonance spectroscopy. *Neuroradiology* 2002;44(3):216–222.

Singer MB, Atlas SW, Drayer BP. Subarachnoid space disease: diagnosis with fluid-attenuated inversion-recovery MR imaging and comparison with gadolinium-enhanced spin-echo MR imaging—blinded reader study. *Radiology* 1998;208(2):417–422.

Smith WS, Roberts HC, Chuang NA, et al. Safety and feasibility of a CT protocol for acute stroke: combined CT, CT angiography, and CT perfusion imaging in 53 consecutive patients. *AJNR Am J Neuroradiol* 2003;24(4):688–690.

von Kummer R. Effect of training in reading CT scans on patient selection for ECASS II. *Neurology* 1998;51: 550–552.

Wintermark M, Uske A, Chalaron M, et al. Multislice computerized tomography angiography in the evaluation of intracranial aneurysms: a comparison with intraarterial digital subtraction angiography. *J Neurosurg* 2003;98(4):828–836.

Wong TZ, van der Westhuizen GJ, Coleman RE. Positron emission tomography imaging of brain tumors. *Neuroimaging Clin N Am* 2002;12(4):615–626.

5

Examination of the Comatose Patient

Jordan L. Topel and Steven L. Lewis

DEFINITIONS AND CLINICAL SYNDROMES

A discussion of the evaluation and treatment of the comatose patient requires one to define certain terms regarding different states and levels of consciousness and unconsciousness. Although the examination and diagnostic studies must be carried out in a rather organized and systematic manner, the definitions of different levels of consciousness are, by themselves, often confusing and misleading. When one physician's understanding of terms (e.g., lethargy, stupor, or obtundation) differs from that of his colleagues, he may think that a patient's condition has deteriorated, although only the terminology has changed between observers. It is better to describe specifically a patient's spontaneous movements, and reactions to external stimuli, for example, rather than to categorize the patient as being lethargic, semicomatose, or stuporous.

Consciousness is the awareness of one's self and the environment. This is a poor definition, however, because one can argue that a sleeping person is unconscious—that is, unaware of himself and his environment. Clinically, however, no one regards a sleeping person as unconscious: he can be aroused to appropriate physical and mental activity with appropriate, non-noxious stimuli.

Consciousness comprises a continuum from full alertness to deep coma, or total unresponsiveness. Drowsiness or lethargy is characterized by easy arousability with light stimuli. There may be a verbal response or appropriate limb movements to pain. Stupor reflects arousability by persistent or vigorous stimuli only, and the arousal is incomplete. There is little verbal response, but limb move-

ments still may be appropriate to the stimulus. Mental and physical activities are reduced to a minimum. Coma reflects the state in which the patient cannot be aroused to make purposeful responses. This is subgrouped into light coma, in which there may be reflex, primitive, or disorganized responses to noxious stimuli (e.g., decorticate and decerebrate responses), and deep coma, in which there is no response to painful stimuli.

Psychogenic unresponsiveness (hysterical coma) is a psychiatric phenomenon in which the patient appears unresponsive but is physiologically awake. The heart and respiratory rates are usually normal. The patient lies with the eyes closed, and the eyelids are frequently difficult to separate. Muscle tone is normal. Although there may be little resistance to passive movement, suspending the patient's hand over his face usually results in its falling to the side instead of directly downward. Pupils are equal and reactive unless certain eyedrops have been used. Ice water caloric testing produces nystagmus, a sign seen only in awake patients. The electroencephalogram (EEG) reveals a waking record.

The "locked-in" syndrome is an important condition to recognize. The patient appears to be in a coma but has essentially all higher mental activity intact. The syndrome most frequently is related to basilar pontine destruction or infarction. There is an interruption of the descending corticobulbar and corticospinal tracts, resulting in quadriplegia and paralysis of lower cranial nerves. The patient is unable to talk, breathe, or move his extremities. Because the ascending reticular activating system is spared, however, arousability and wakefulness are present. There also is sparing of fibers controlling eye blinking and vertical eye movements. Thus, the patient's only means for communication may be using eye blinks (Morse code). The ramifications of not recognizing this disturbing clinical condition are obvious. Every patient, no matter how deep in coma he appears to be, should be asked to open and close his eyes or to move them up and down.

The vegetative state is somewhat clinically opposite of the "locked-in" syndrome. The patient appears to be awake but is unable to attain higher mental functions. Simply stated, there is arousal but no awareness. Although the patient may be able to swallow or visually track the examiner, there is essentially no other appropriate response (wakeful unresponsiveness). Sleep–wake cycles may have returned, but there is no return of higher mental activity. The syndrome most frequently occurs in the setting of severe cortical dysfunction with relative brainstem sparing (e.g., patients who survive a cardiorespiratory arrest but experience significant cerebral anoxia).

It is not uncommon for patients with acute onset of global aphasia to be diagnosed initially as being in coma. The patient is indeed unable to comprehend, communicate, or carry out simple verbal commands. The diagnosis may be established by noting that he frequently appears to be awake and alert, with roving eye movements or deviation of the eyes to the left, and he most often has a right hemiplegia.

COMA

Anatomy

In the evaluation of the comatose patient, it is necessary to consider the physiologic and anatomic abnormalities that result in decreased level of consciousness. Simply stated, coma results from bilateral, diffuse cerebral hemisphere dysfunction or involvement of the brainstem (midbrain and pons) ascending reticular activating system or a combination of the two.

Coma is unusual with unilateral cerebral hemisphere disease unless there is a dysfunc-

tion of the other hemisphere or secondary pressure or destruction of brainstem structures. Most large cerebral hemisphere infarctions will result in a slightly decreased level of consciousness, but the patient still can be aroused to elicit some purposeful movements or higher mental activity. Rare exceptions may be patients with large, acute lesions affecting the dominant cerebral hemisphere. In contrast, profound coma may result from very small infarctions in the brainstem affecting the ascending reticular activating system.

A unilateral hemispheral mass lesion, such as a tumor, abscess, or expanding hemorrhage, frequently will present with unilateral focal neurologic symptoms and signs. On continued enlargement of the mass, there may be a compression of the contralateral cerebral hemisphere or a downward herniation of the ipsilateral temporal lobe, creating distortion and compression of the brainstem. At this point, coma will ensue. There is also the suggestion that horizontal displacement of the brain at the level of the pineal body may correlate more closely with levels of consciousness than downward displacement with brainstem compression.

Metabolic processes usually affect both brainstem and cerebral hemispheres to produce coma. This likely reflects a direct interference of the metabolic activity of the neurons. Initially, the patient is drowsy, but coma ensues as the metabolic process worsens.

ETIOLOGY

Coma is not an independent disease entity but a reflection of some underlying disease process. The causes of coma can be divided into two main categories: (1) those of primary central nervous system (CNS) disease and (2) those of metabolic or systemic depression (Table 5.1). The latter group contains the more common causes of a depressed level of consciousness.

Metabolic or systemic disorders generally cause depressed consciousness without focal neurologic findings. Primary CNS disorders

TABLE 5.1. *Causes of Coma*

Coma Secondary to Primary Brain Injury or Disease	
Cause	Comments
Infection	
Meningitis	Nuchal rigidity; CSF shows pleocytosis, increased protein; glucose may be decreased; meningeal enhancement on MRI
Encephalitis	May have focal findings; CSF shows mildly increased protein, increased lymphocytes, normal or slightly decreased glucose; possible focal abnormalities on MRI
Abscess	Focal findings; positive CT scan; history of ear or sinus infection or HIV or endocarditis; CSF shows mildly increased protein, increased cells, negative cultures
Tumor	
Primary or metastatic	Focal findings; progressive course; papilledema
Infarction	
Usually no coma unless bilateral or acute, large, dominant hemisphere, or involving brainstem reticular activating system	—
Hemorrhage	
Subarachnoid	Sudden onset; headache; nuchal rigidity; vomiting; positive CT scan; bloody CSF
Intracerebral	Sudden onset; headache; nuchal rigidity; vomiting; focal findings; abnormal CT scan; history of hypertension
Trauma	
Concussion, contusion	Positive history, evidence of injury on examination; uncomplicated concussion leaves no residual
Subdural hematoma	Depressed level of consciousness can occur before focal findings; may have trivial or no trauma history
Epidural hematoma	Lucid interval; skull fracture over middle meningeal artery
Seizures	
Seizure	Convulsive or nonconvulsive status epilepticus; postictal progressive improvement in level of consciousness unless other factors are involved

may or may not produce focal abnormalities on examination. A previous neurologic injury, however, may render certain neurons more susceptible to a metabolic insult. A metabolic encephalopathy thus could produce focal neurologic findings. These signs may disappear after the metabolic disturbance has been corrected.

HISTORY AND EXAMINATION

A history should be taken, but unfortunately this is often incomplete, nonexistent, or misleading. A search for "less likely" causes for coma is necessary when treatment for the "obvious" cause from the history obtained does not change the patient's clinical status. Nevertheless, aggressive management of the unconscious patient includes an aggressive pursuit of the history. For example, metabolic abnormalities most often are associated with subacute onset of coma, whereas a history of a more rapid course is suggestive of cardiac or cerebrovascular cause or drug overdose.

There should be a search for evidence of trauma. Battle's sign (purple and blue discoloration of the mastoid skin area), blood in the external auditory canal, or blood noted behind the tympanic membranes may signify a temporal bone or basal skull fracture. Raccoon eyes (purple discoloration of the eyelid and orbital regions) may signify orbital or basal skull fractures.

One should check carefully for nuchal rigidity, but several factors must be considered in doing so. If there is any suspicion of a

TABLE 5.1. *Continued*

Coma Secondary to Metabolic and Systemic Diseases

Cause	Symptoms
Exogenous Substances	
Sedatives, hypnotics, antidepressants	Positive blood or urine screens; may cause pupillary abnormalities (opiates cause miosis, and anticholinergics cause mydriasis)
Alcohol	Breath odor may not be apparent; seizures and delirium tremens on withdrawal
Methyl alcohol	Metabolic acidosis; visual symptoms
Heavy metals, cyanide, arsenic, lead, salicylates	Lead encephalopathy common in children, not in adults
Endogenous Substances	
Hepatic coma	Fetor hepaticus, jaundice, ascites, asterixis; triphasic waves on electroencephalogram
Uremic coma	Uriniferous breath; seizures; asterixis; increased BUN
CO_2 narcosis	Increased PCO_2; positive physical chest findings, electrolytes
Endocrine—pituitary, thyroid, pancreas (diabetes), adrenals	Urine and serum osmolalities; thyroid studies
Hypoxia	
Pulmonary disease, carbon monoxide intoxication, anemia	Abnormal blood gases; carboxyhemoglobin
Ischemia	
Decreased cardiac output	Congestive heart failure, myocardial infarction, arrhythmia, cardiopulmonary arrest
Hypertensive encephalopathy	Papilledema; proteinuria; headaches; seizures
Hypoglycemia	
Reversed with D_{50} unless prolonged	—
Thiamine Deficiency	
Wernicke's encephalopathy	Potentially reversible
Electrolyte Imbalance	
Inbalance	Water, sodium, acidosis, alkalosis, calcium out of balance
Temperature Regulation	
Hypothermia	Exposure; myxedema; barbiturates; circulatory failure
Hyperthermia	Heat stroke; phenothiazines (neuroleptic malignant syndrome) with muscle rigidity and elevated CK)

cervical neck fracture, there should be no manipulation of the neck. In deep coma, nuchal rigidity may be lacking despite its presence in a lighter level of consciousness. Finally, some patients with a CNS infection or subarachnoid hemorrhage may not manifest nuchal rigidity initially in the course of their illness.

The odor of the patient's breath may indicate the cause for the coma. Alcohol gives its characteristic smell, hepatic coma is often associated with a musty odor, and a fruity or acetone smell is characteristic of ketoacidosis.

After a screening general physical examination, an orderly, systemic neurologic examination is undertaken. The goal of the neuro-logic examination is essentially to determine the presence, location, and nature of the underlying process creating the decreased level of consciousness and also to give some prognosis of the patient's condition.

Respiratory patterns yield information regarding the activity of different cerebral areas. When one develops bilateral cerebral hemisphere dysfunction (essentially, functioning at the diencephalic level), Cheyne–Stokes respiration may occur. This respiratory pattern is associated with periods of hyperpnea alternating with periods of apnea. There is a regularity to the respirations: first a gradual buildup of respirations to the level of hyperpnea and then a gradual tapering off of respirations to apnea. The periods of apnea may last up to 30 seconds or more and may be accompanied by decreased responsiveness and miosis. It is believed that Cheyne–Stokes respiration relates to an abnormal response of carbon dioxide–sensitive respiratory brain centers. There is an increased ventilatory response to carbon dioxide stimulation, creating hyperpnea. After the concentration of carbon dioxide drops below the level at which the centers are stimulated, the apnea phase appears and continues until the carbon dioxide reaccumulates and the cycle repeats itself. Because sleep induces further cerebral depressing mechanisms, Cheyne–Stokes respiration may be seen in some patients during sleep, whereas they exhibit normal breathing patterns while awake.

Cheyne–Stokes respiration is, by itself, not a serious prognostic sign. Although it can be seen in focal primary CNS problems, it also can be seen early in many metabolic and systemic problems.

Central neurogenic hyperventilation appears when lower brain centers are involved; it is noted with dysfunction at the midbrain or the upper pons and often is associated with pulmonary edema. There are continuous, regular, and rapid respirations up to 40 or 50 times per minute. Arterial blood gases reveal a respiratory alkalosis with decreased PCO_2 and increased pH. The PO_2 must be greater than 70 or 80 millimeters of mercury (mm Hg). If the PO_2 is not higher than that level, it raises the possibility of an extracerebral cause (hypoxemia) for the respiratory problem. In reality, most cases of sustained hyperventilation in comatose patients are not central neurogenic hyperventilation. Cardiac, pulmonary, and metabolic (e.g., diabetes, uremia, hepatic, salicylates) problems must be ruled out as possible causes of the hyperventilation.

Apneustic respiration, noted in lower pontine lesions, consists of a prolonged inspiratory phase with a pause at full inspiration. Cluster breathing (short-cycle Cheyne–Stokes respiration), also signifying lower pontine damage, is characterized by a disorderly sequence of closely grouped respirations followed by apnea.

Ataxic respirations signify a lower pontine or medullary respiratory center problem. The breathing pattern is chaotic and haphazard with irregular pauses. It may, and usually does, lead to gasping and eventual cessation of breathing. Ataxic breathing is a forewarner of respiratory arrest, and prompt endotracheal intubation is necessary at the time of its discovery.

An examination of the pupillary responses, eye movements, and fundus must be undertaken. In a patient with a decreased level of consciousness, but who is not yet in coma, visual threat (forceful movements of the hand toward either side of the eyes) may be helpful. Blinking in response to a threat from one side, but not from the other side, suggests a hemianopsia. The abnormality thus would be in the cerebral hemisphere opposite to the side that did not blink. A funduscopic examination may reveal papilledema or retinal hemorrhages.

The pupillary response is recorded. The light reflex is mediated, in succession, through the optic nerve, the optic chiasm, the optic tract, the posterior diencephalon, and the Edinger–Westphal nuclei of the midbrain and then to the sphincter pupillae by way of the parasympathetic nerve fibers in the oculomotor nerve (cranial nerve III). Thus, it is not surprising that the most significant abnormalities of the pupils are seen with dysfunction at the level of the midbrain or oculomotor nerve.

Diencephalic pupils, the result of bilateral hemispheral dysfunction, are small and reactive. The small size likely reflects sympathetic nerve dysfunction at the level of the takeoff of the sympathetic fibers from the hypothalamus.

Midposition, unreactive (4 to 7 mm) pupils result from direct midbrain (tectal region) damage. The pupillary size likely reflects involvement of both the descending sympathetic fibers and the parasympathetic fibers of the oculomotor complex.

A widely dilated, fixed pupil usually is seen as a result of direct oculomotor nerve involvement, with unopposed dilator sympathetic tone. In addition to the pupillary abnormalities, ptosis and extraocular muscle paralysis (especially adduction of the eye) frequently are present. Because the oculomotor nerve is strategically situated at the temporal incisura, temporal lobe herniation may result in a widely dilated, fixed pupil and possibly total cranial nerve III paralysis.

Pinpoint (1 mm) pupils are seen with pontine damage but may be a transient finding for only the first 24 or 48 hours. The pupils are small and can be seen occasionally to react slightly to light if viewed through a magnifying glass. This is thought to relate to damage of the descending sympathetic tracts. Frequently, however, midposition and fixed pupils may be noted with pontine dysfunction.

Of great importance is the fact that metabolic processes do not alter pupillary re-

sponse until late in their course, if at all. For example, a deeply comatose patient with no spontaneous or reflex movements and no respirations, but with reactive pupils, must be considered to be in metabolic coma until proved otherwise.

In addition, certain drugs can alter pupillary size and response. Opiates characteristically produce pinpoint pupils (reversed with naloxone). Atropine may result in widely dilated and fixed pupils. Various eyedrops also may alter pupillary size and reaction.

The position and movements of the eyes are observed, and certain procedures are undertaken to evaluate cerebral hemisphere and brainstem integrity. The neural pathways for the control of horizontal conjugate eye movements are outlined in Fig. 5.1. Cortical control originates in the frontal gaze centers (Brodmann's area 8). Descending fibers con-

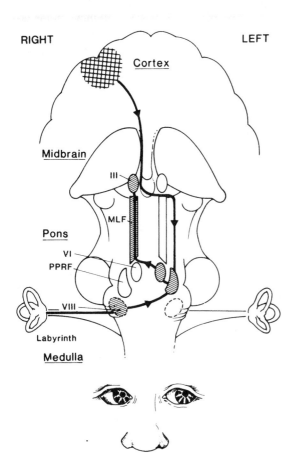

FIG. 5.1. Diagram of the conjugate vision pathways (nuclei and paths are shaded to include those important to left conjugate gaze). Fibers from the right frontal cortex descend and cross the midline, and they synapse in the left paramedian pontine reticular formation (PPRF). Fibers then travel to the nearby left cranial nerve VI nucleus (to move the left eye laterally) and then cross the midline to rise in the right medial longitudinal fasciculus (MLF) to the right cranial nerve III nucleus (to move the right eye medially). In addition to the cortical influence on the left PPRF, there is vestibular influence. With vestibular activation from the right, the left PPRF is stimulated, and the eyes conjugatively move to the left. Instillation of ice water into the right ear canal will test the integrity of this vestibular-PPRF-cranial nerve-VI-cranial nerve-III-circuit, and if the eyes move to vestibular stimulation, the brainstem from medulla to midbrain must be functioning.

trolling horizontal conjugate gaze cross the midline in the lower midbrain region and descend to the paramedian pontine reticular formation (PPRF) in the pons. The PPRF is thus the major area of confluence of pathways controlling horizontal eye movements. Neurons from the PPRF project to the nearby abducens nerve (cranial nerve VI) nucleus and thereby stimulate movement in the lateral rectus muscle of the eye ipsilateral to the PPRF and contralateral to the frontal gaze center. In addition, impulses from the abducens nerve nucleus cross the midline and ascend the median longitudinal fasciculus to the medial rectus nucleus of the oculomotor nerve (cranial nerve III) in the midbrain. This stimulates adduction of the eye ipsilateral to the frontal gaze center. Horizontal conjugate gaze thus is completed.

By following these pathways, it can be seen that stimulation of fibers from the frontal gaze center of one cerebral hemisphere results in horizontal, conjugate eye movements to the contralateral side. If one frontal gaze center or its descending fibers are damaged, the eyes will tend to "look" toward the involved cerebral hemisphere because of unopposed action of the remaining frontal gaze center. For example, a destructive lesion in the right cerebral hemisphere, involving descending motor fibers and frontal gaze fibers, will cause a left hemiplegia with head and eyes deviated to the right. In other words, the eyes "look" at a destructive hemispheral lesion and "look" away from the resulting hemiplegia.

By contrast, a destructive left pontine lesion, for example, will damage the left PPRF. The eyes, therefore, cannot go to the left and will tend to deviate to the right. Because descending pyramidal tract fibers cross the midline in the medulla, damage to the pyramidal tract fibers in the pons on the left results in a right hemiplegia. Thus, the eyes "look" away from a destructive pontine lesion but "look" toward the hemiplegia.

If the abducens nerve or nucleus is destroyed, there will be a loss of abduction of the ipsilateral eye (cranial nerve VI palsy). With destruction of the tract of the medial longitudinal fasciculus, disconjugate gaze results, with loss of adduction of the ipsilateral eye (same side as the tract of the medial longitudinal fasciculus). Abduction of the contralateral eye is preserved, but there is nystagmus. This type of disconjugate gaze abnormality also is termed internuclear ophthalmoplegia (see Chapter 23). The pathways for vertical eye movements are less well understood. Lower centers likely exist in the midbrain (pretectal and tectal) regions.

If a patient cannot follow verbal commands, two tests are used to determine brainstem integrity. An oculocephalic (doll's head) maneuver is performed by turning the patient's head rapidly in the horizontal or vertical planes and by noting the movement or position of the eyes relative to the orbits. This maneuver should not be performed if a cervical neck fracture is suspected. If the pontine (horizontal) or midbrain (vertical) gaze centers are intact, the eyes should move in the orbits in the direction opposite to the rotating head. An abnormal response (no eye movement with doll's head maneuver) implies pontine or midbrain dysfunction and is characterized by no movement of the eyes relative to the orbits or by an asymmetry of movement.

Horizontal oculocephalic maneuvers are a relatively weak stimulus for horizontal eye movements. If a doll's head maneuver is present, it is not necessary to continue with oculovestibular testing. If, however, a doll's head response is lacking, ice water calorics should be performed because it is a stronger stimulus than oculocephalic maneuvers.

Oculovestibular responses (ice water calorics) are reflex eye movements in response to irrigation of the external ear canals with cold water. The head is raised to 30 degrees relative to the horizontal plane, and the external canals are inspected for the presence of cerumen or a perforated tympanic membrane. Fifty to 100 ml of cold water is instilled into the canal (waiting 5 minutes between ears), and the resulting eye movements are noted. Ice water produces a downward current in the horizontal semicircular canal and decreases tonic vestibular input to the contralateral PPRF. Simplistically, one can think of this as an indirect means of stimulating the ipsilateral PPRF. Hence, after cold water instillation, there is a slow, tonic, conjugate deviation of the eyes toward the irrigated ear. In a waking patient, there is a correction of the eyes to the opposite side, resulting in a fast nystagmus away from the stimulated ear. In an unconscious patient, there is a loss of the fast-phase nystagmus, and only tonic deviation of the eyes is seen if appropriate pontine–midbrain areas are intact. Thus, if nystagmus is noted in a seemingly unconscious patient, the patient is either in a very light coma or psychogenic unresponsiveness.

A lack of oculovestibular responses thus suggests pontine–midbrain dysfunction. Ice water calorics can help to differentiate between the conjugate gaze weakness or paralysis caused by either cortical (cerebral hemisphere) or brainstem (pontine) damage. Oculovestibular responses should not be altered in patients with only hemispheral pathology.

Movement of the ipsilateral eye toward the irrigated ear, but no movement of the contralateral eye, suggests an abnormality of the contralateral medial longitudinal fasciculus (see Chapter 23).

Severe metabolic coma (e.g., after barbiturate overdose) may result in a lack of oculocephalic and oculovestibular responses. Reactive pupils may signify that the coma is of metabolic origin.

Ocular bobbing is characterized by a rapid downward eye movement with a slow return to the horizontal plane. This is seen most often in pontine destruction and is thought to relate to the loss of horizontal eye movements with preservation of midbrain-mediated vertical eye movement pathways. Sustained downgaze can be seen with lesions of the thalamus or pretectum or after cerebral hypoxia.

Roving eye movements signify intact brainstem mechanisms for horizontal gaze. The movements should be distinguished from those seen in patients with seizures. In the latter, the eye movements are of a jerking quality and frequently tend to lateralize to one side. Referring to Fig. 5.1, it can be seen that

an irritative cortical focus in the area of the frontal gaze center will deviate the eyes away from the side of the lesion (and possibly toward a hemiplegia). Oculovestibular responses usually will be able to overcome the eye deviations because of the strong direct input into the pons, "bypassing" the cortical effects on eye movements.

Motor movements may be spontaneous, induced, reflex, or totally absent. It is important to note not only the type of response but also the symmetry of response. An asymmetric, induced motor movement may be the only indication of an underlying focal problem.

It may be necessary to observe the patient for several minutes to note the presence or lack of spontaneous or reflex motor movements. The position of the extremities (e.g., a persistent externally rotated leg secondary to weakness of that extremity) may indicate focal pathology.

The most favorable prognostic sign related to the motor system is symmetric, spontaneous movements of all four extremities. Appropriate motor response to noxious stimuli (e.g., pain) signifies that sensory pathways are functional and there is at least partial integrity of corticospinal tracts. It is not necessary to use unusually noxious stimuli, but rather mild supraorbital pressure, pinching of the skin of the neck, or mild sternal pressure.

Reflex motor movements frequently can be elicited by light, painful stimuli or flexion of the neck or during routine care of the patient, such as tracheal suctioning. Decorticate posturing consists of flexion of the arms, wrists, and fingers and adduction of the upper extremities. In the legs, there is extension, internal rotation, and plantar flexion. Decerebrate (extensor) posturing consists of extension of the arms as well as adduction and hyperpronation of the arms. There may be opisthotonic posturing of the neck. The movement of the lower extremities is similar to that seen in decorticate posturing. Although not completely anatomically specific, bilateral decerebrate posturing often is seen in lesions of the midbrain and pons, whereas decorticate posturing often implies a higher corticospinal tract lesion. Decerebrate posturing is generally a poorer prognostic sign than decorticate posturing. However, decerebrate posturing also occasionally can be seen in the setting of severe, although potentially reversible, metabolic encephalopathies.

A common mistake regarding the interpretation of motor responses is that of relating a withdrawal response in the legs as representing an appropriate cortical response. When the bottom of the foot is stroked, or a noxious stimuli is applied to the leg, there may be hip flexion, knee flexion, and dorsiflexion of the foot (triple flexor response). This signifies spinal cord reflex integrity and does not signify an intact cerebral response.

Asymmetric extensor toe signs (i.e., flexion on one side, extensor response on the other) are of moderate value in localizing a focal cerebral lesion. Bilateral extensor toe signs can be seen in any form or at any level of coma and are, by themselves, neither prognostic nor localizing. For example, transient extensor toe signs are common in hypertensive encephalopathy.

The Glasgow Coma Scale (Table 5.2) is the most widely used clinical scale for assessment of comatose patients. Although it initially was designed for trauma cases, it is used now for all causes of coma. It measures the "best responses" of eye opening, motor response, and verbal response. A lower score usually signifies a more serious neurologic problem and possibly a poorer prognosis. However, there can be falsely low scores such as in patients who cannot speak because of mechanical ventilation or aphasia.

LABORATORY EVALUATION AND TREATMENT

Initial emergency treatment for a comatose patient is essentially the same as for all other medical emergencies. An adequate airway should be established. Endotracheal intubation and artificial ventilation may be necessary. The cardiovascular status must be evaluated promptly, and shock and blood pressure should be controlled. The temperature should be noted because hypothermia or hyperthermia may play a prominent role in the identification of the underlying problem.

Following the establishment of an airway, assisting of respirations, and maintenance of circulation, certain laboratory tests (Table 5.3) and therapeutic measures (Table 5.4) are undertaken, often occurring simultaneously

TABLE 5.2. *Glasgow Coma Scale*

Eye Opening	
Spontaneous	4
To speech	3
To pain	2
None	1
Motor Response	
Obeys	6
Localizes	5
Withdraws (flexion)	4
Abnormal reflex (flexion)	3
Extension	2
None	1
Verbal Response	
Oriented	5
Confused	4
Inappropriate	3
Incomprehensible	2
None	1

Adapted from Jennett B, Teasdale G, Braakman R, et al. Prognosis of patients with severe head injury. *Neurosurgery* 1979;4:283.

TABLE 5.3. *Tests in the Evaluation of the Comatose Patient*

Blood Tests
  Complete blood count
  Glucose, electrolytes, calcium, blood urea nitrogen, and creatinine
  Liver function studies and serum ammonia
  Coagulation studies
  Arterial blood gases
  Drug/toxin screen
  Thyroid function studies[a]
  Magnesium[a]
  Serum osmolality[a]
  Blood cultures[a]
Urine Tests
  Urinalysis
  Drug/toxin screen
  Urine osmolality[a]
  Urine culture[a]
Imaging Studies
  Electrocardiogram
  Chest x-ray
  Computed tomography brain scan[a]
  Magnetic resonance imaging scan of the brain[a]
Lumbar Puncture[a]

[a]If indicated.

TABLE 5.4. *Treatment of the Comatose Patient*

Problem	Comment
Respiration	Immediately obtain an airway and consider intubation. Early intubation prevents aspiration, decreases risk of transferring patient to other hospital areas, and allows for more aggressive treatment of seizures.
Blood Pressure	
Hypotension	Treat with fluids, volume expanders, or pressors.
Hypertension	Aggressiveness of treatment depends on etiology and level of elevation. Hypertensive encephalopathy suggested by papilledema, history of headaches, seizures, and marked elevation in blood pressure.
Arrhythmias	May point to etiology of coma or can be a secondary factor: continuous cardiac monitoring is necessary.
Hypoglycemia	50 mL of 50% dextrose in water. Risk of worsening hyperglycemia outweighed by benefits of treating hypoglycemia.
Thiamine deficiency	To be considered in alcoholic patients or patients who are chronically malnourished. Glucose load may precipitate Wernicke's encephalopathy. Give thiamine (100 mg) intravenously and add to intravenous solutions.
Drug overdose	Obtain urine and blood toxicology screens. For suspected narcotic overdose, give naloxone intravenously (see text for details). Use of other specific antidotes depends on history, clinical examination, and results of toxin screens.
Increased intracranial pressure	Worsening level of coma, focal abnormalities, change in respiratory pattern, pupillary dilation.
	Intubation, hyperventilation, and mannitol infusion.
	Possible use of intracranial pressure monitor. Consider need for surgical intervention.
Seizures	Correct any underlying metabolic or systemic problem.
	Treat status epilepticus with lorazepam or diazepam.
	Infuse loading dose of phenytoin or fosphenytoin for long-term anticonvulsant effect. Barbiturates may be needed if seizures are not initially controlled.
	Midazolam or propofol for refractory status epilepticus. (See Chapter 25 for doses.)
General medical and nursing care	Fluids and acid–base balance, continued observation of metabolic status. Watch and treat changes in temperature (hyperthermia or hypothermia), agitation, and infections; prevent corneal abrasions and decubiti.

Modified from Weiner WJ, Shulman LM, eds. *Emergent and urgent neurology,* 2nd ed. Philadelphia: Lippincott Williams & Wilkins, 1999.

with obtaining a history and performing a neurologic examination.

Blood is drawn for a complete blood count (CBC); electrolyte, glucose, calcium, blood urea nitrogen (BUN), and creatinine determinations; liver function tests; arterial blood gas determinations; and a drug/toxin screen. Urinalysis and urine drug screening are performed. An electrocardiogram and chest roentgenograms are obtained. If hypoglycemia is suspected, or if the cause of the coma is uncertain, 25 to 50 ml of 50% dextrose in water is given intravenously (IV). Hypoglycemia is an extremely important, potentially reversible cause of coma that, if not treated promptly, will lead to irreversible cerebral damage. For suspected opiate overdose, naloxone 0.4 mg IV is given and is repeated every 5 to 15 minutes as needed. Repeated infusions should be instituted if the

response to glucose or naloxone is incomplete. Other medications can be given for specific drug overdoses when appropriate, such as intravenous flumazenil for benzodiazepine overdose. If chronic or acute ingestion of alcohol is suspected, thiamine should be given IV to treat or prevent the Wernicke–Korsakoff syndrome. Correction of any other underlying metabolic process (e.g., hyponatremia) must be undertaken. If there is significant evidence for increased intracranial pressure, intubation with hyperventilation and the use of mannitol must be considered. Corticosteroids may be beneficial to reduce vasogenic edema related to neoplasms, but their effect is not immediate. Neurosurgical intervention may be considered for insertion of an intracranial pressure monitor or possibly surgical decompression. Hypothermia has been shown to improve neurologic outcome and decrease mortality in postcardiac arrest patients.

Seizure activity may be generalized or focal and necessitates prompt treatment and a search for a cause. Myoclonic jerks (symmetric or asymmetric rapid, brief movements of the extremities) frequently are seen in metabolic encephalopathies and are common following anoxia (e.g., after cardiac arrest). Unfortunately, myoclonic jerks in the setting of severe anoxic coma are often difficult to treat, and their appearance following anoxia is a poor prognostic sign.

It may be necessary to proceed with further neurologic studies if the cause of the coma remains unclear. Computed tomography (CT) will demonstrate intracerebral or extracerebral blood, mass lesions, infarctions, and abscesses as well as skull fractures. Magnetic resonance imaging (MRI) will show the brain in greater detail and may reveal abnormalities earlier than a CT scan, but it is often difficult to obtain an MRI on a comatose patient. Patients will need to be left unattended for a longer scanning time. Unconscious patients are often on ventilators, which usually cannot be placed near the MRI scanner. If a CNS infection or subarachnoid hemorrhage is suspected, a lumbar puncture is indicated, although a CT scan will identify most subarachnoid hemorrhages sufficient to cause coma. A CT scan usually should be obtained prior to the lumbar puncture to rule out a focal mass lesion or increased intracranial pressure.

The EEG may be helpful in the diagnosis of an overdose from sedatives (excessive fast activity), hepatic or uremic encephalopathy (triphasic waves), or psychogenic unresponsiveness (normal EEG) or in differentiating focal from diffuse disease. It can be used to rule out subclinical seizure activity as a cause for prolonged, unexplained coma. An EEG with no evidence of cerebral activity can be reversibly noted secondary to barbiturate intoxication (and occasionally other drugs) and also with hypothermia.

PROGNOSIS

Several studies that have dealt with postanoxic coma have revealed that the prog-

nosis is generally better for the patient with spontaneous motor movements or appropriate movements in response to noxious stimuli and those with pupillary reactions and oculocephalic or oculovestibular responses. Patients studied after cardiopulmonary arrest reveal that depth and duration of postarrest coma correlated significantly with poor neurologic outcome. Motor unresponsiveness, lack of pupillary responses, and lack of oculocephalic and oculovestibular responses were associated with a poor prognosis for neurologic functional recovery. In addition, the prediction of survival and outcome could be based on a loss of consciousness alone within 3 days after cardiopulmonary arrest. Those patients not awakening within 72 hours had the worst prognosis.

Prognosis for patients with metabolic encephalopathies or drug overdose cannot be based solely on the level of consciousness. For example, patients with barbiturate overdose in deep coma may have no spontaneous respiration, absent oculovestibular responses, and absent cerebral activity on the EEG, yet have a complete neurologic recovery. No alternative interventions can be recommended in the acute management of neurologic conditions causing coma. In patients who survive and remain comatose (persistent vegetative state), passive range of motion and other physical therapies may help in the presentation of contractures and decubiti that can complicate hygienic maintenance care.

WHEN TO REFER THE PATIENT TO A NEUROLOGIST

A neurologist should be consulted for almost all comatose patients, especially when the etiology of the coma is uncertain. The neurologist will aid in arriving at a diagnosis, localize the abnormalities, and assist in the treatment of the underlying cause of coma and the secondary medical problems. In addition, the neurologist will be able to provide in most cases a prognosis for survival and functional recovery (e.g., ability to function independently). This information also will enable the family and all treating physicians to make important further decisions regarding the patient's medical care.

QUESTIONS AND DISCUSSION

1. A 24-year-old man is brought to the emergency room with a decreased level of consciousness. On arrival, he suffers a respiratory arrest and is intubated. An examination reveals small, reactive pupils (2 mm), a lack of oculocephalic and oculovestibular responses, and no response to painful stimuli. Which of the following is correct?

A. The most likely diagnosis is a pontine hemorrhage.

B. A CT scan should be obtained immediately.

C. The pupils should be pharmacologically dilated to obtain a good funduscopic examination.

D. Neurosurgical consultation should be sought immediately to evacuate a subdural hematoma.

E. Drug screen and other blood tests should be obtained immediately, and glucose and naloxone should be given IV.

The answer is (E). Metabolic encephalopathies can result in a lack of oculocephalic and oculovestibular responses, with preserved pupillary responses. Any comatose patient with preserved pupillary responses should be considered as having a metabolic cause of the coma.

2. Cheyne–Stokes respiration:

A. Is associated with irreversible brain disease

B. Is pathognomonic of midbrain dysfunction

C. Is characterized by sustained inspirations

D. May occur in noncomatose patients while they are asleep

E. Is associated with decerebrate posturing

The answer is (D). Cheyne–Stokes respirations are related to bilateral hemispheral dysfunction. During sleep, increased inhibitory influences may create this pattern of respiration. Cheyne–Stokes respirations are reversible and are not a poor prognostic sign.

3. A right hemispheral destructive lesion may produce:

A. Lack of caloric responses, eyes conjugately deviated to the left, and left hemiplegia

B. Right eye deviated to the right, left eye midline, and left hemiplegia

C. Eyes conjugately deviated to the right, left hemiplegia, and present caloric responses

D. Ocular bobbing and left hemiplegia

E. Present caloric responses, eyes conjugately deviated to the left, and left hemiplegia

The answer is (C). Eyes "look toward" a destructive hemispheral lesion. Caloric responses are preserved because the pathway for the oculovestibular responses does not involve hemispheral connections. Eyes "look away" from the side of a destructive pontine lesion.

4. Lack of caloric (oculovestibular) responses bilaterally:

A. Signifies marked suppression of both cerebral hemispheres

B. Is pathognomonic of pontine hemorrhage

C. Frequently is associated with Cheyne–Stokes respiration

D. Can be seen in metabolic encephalopathy

E. Is always reversible

The answer is (D). Oculovestibular responses are mediated by brainstem (i.e., pontine) pathways. The responses are reversible if a metabolic encephalopathy is corrected in appropriate time.

5. Decerebrate posturing:

A. May be associated with central neurogenic hyperventilation

B. Is seen in patients with bilateral frontal lobe dysfunction

C. Consists of flexion of the arms and wrists

D. Signifies integrity of spinal cord and occipital lobe synapses

E. Is a good prognostic sign

The answer is (A). Decerebrate posturing, which partially consists of extension and hyperpronation of the upper extremities, often is associated with midbrain dysfunction (as is central neurogenic hyperventilation). It usually is considered a poor prognostic sign.

SUGGESTED READING

Bates D. Predicting recovery from medical coma. *Br J Hosp Med* 1985;33:276.

Bernard SA, Gray TW, Buist MD, et al. Treatment of comatose survivors of out-of-hospital cardiac arrest with induced hypothermia. *N Engl J Med* 2002;346:557.

Buettner WW, Zee DS. Vestibular testing in comatose patients. *Arch Neurol* 1989;46:561.

Fisher CM. The neurological examination of the comatose patient. *Acta Neurol Scand* 1969;45(suppl 36):1.

Hamel MB, Goldman L, Teno J, et al. Identification of comatose patients at high risk for death or severe disability. *JAMA* 1995;273:1842.

Hoffman RS, Goldfrank LR. The poisoned patient with altered consciousness: controversies in the use of a "coma cocktail." *JAMA* 1995;274:562.

Jennett B, Teasdale G, Braakman R, et al. Prognosis of patients with severe head injury. *Neurosurgery* 1979;4:283.

Levy DE, Caronna JJ, Singer BH, et al. Predicting outcome from hypoxic-ischemic coma. *JAMA* 1985;253:1420.

Lewis SL, Topel JL. Coma. In: Weiner WJ, Shulman LM, eds. *Emergent and urgent neurology,* 2nd ed. Philadelphia: Lippincott Williams & Wilkins, 1999.

Plum F, Posner JB. *The diagnosis of stupor and coma,* 3rd ed. Philadelphia: FA Davis, 1980.

Rabinstein AA, Atkinson JL, Wijdicks EF. Emergency craniotomy in patients worsening due to expanded cerebral hematoma: to what purpose? *Neurology* 2002;58(9):1367.

Wijdicks EFM, Parisi JE, Sharbrough FW. Prognostic value of myoclonus status in comatose survivors of cardiac arrest. *Ann Neurol* 1994;35:239.

Young GB, Ropper AH, Bolton CF. *Coma and impaired consciousness.* New York: McGraw-Hill, 1998.

6

Cerebrovascular Disease

Roger E. Kelley and Alireza Minagar

Cerebrovascular disease includes both ischemic stroke (large artery thrombotic, small artery thrombotic = lacunar, embolic, vasculitis-induced infarction, vascular dissection-induced infarction, sinovenous thrombotic infarction) and hemorrhagic stroke (primary intracerebral hemorrhage and subarachnoid hemorrhage). Stroke is a common presentation in the emergency department, and most strokes are readily diagnosed on the basis of a sudden constellation of neurologic deficit in a patient with well-recognized risk factors for cerebrovascular disease. The frequency of stroke type varies depending on the patient population being assessed. For example, a retirement community is more likely to have patients of advanced age with a relatively high incidence of atherosclerotic disease seen in tandem with hypertension, diabetes mellitus, hyperlipidemia, and coronary artery disease. A hospital in a community of young and middle-aged people will tend to see more esoteric causes of stroke such as lupus vasculitis, hypercoagulable states, sinovenous occlusive disease as a complication of pregnancy, stroke related to oral contraceptive use, paradoxical cerebral embolism related to an atrial septal defect, and vascular dissection (which often has trauma as an initiating factor).

Roughly 80% to 85% of all stroke is primary ischemic and 15% to 20% is primary hemorrhagic. Of the ischemic strokes, approximately 50% to 60% are large artery thrombotic; 20% are small artery thrombotic (lacunar); 15% to 20% are cardiogenic or artery-to-artery emboli; and 5% to 10% are less common etiologies such as vasculitis, dissection, septic or non-septic emboli, or sinovenous occlusive disease. Approximately 5% to 6% of all strokes are subarachnoid hemorrhage (SAH), usually related to rupture of

a cerebral aneurysm or bleeding from an arteriovenous malformation (AVM), whereas 10% to 15 % are primary intracerebral hemorrhage (ICH). Of particular note, primary ischemic stroke can undergo hemorrhagic transformation (Fig. 6.1), and this secondary bleeding can be dramatic enough to look like a primary ICH. The major stroke etiologies are listed in Table 6.1.

It has become increasingly important to recognize the risk factors for stroke (Table 6.2) because there is an increasing armamentarium of potential therapies to reduce stroke risk. Conversely, the interventional therapies for acute stroke remain quite limited. For example, transient ischemic attack (TIA) is a warning of ischemic stroke and it can precede up to 15% of all stroke. It represents an opportunity to identify a patient who is at particular risk for ischemic stroke in an effort to institute effective prevention. In a recent study of patients with TIA presenting to the emergency room (ER), 10.5% of patients returned to the ER within 90 days with a stroke and half of these events occurred within 2 days of the TIA.

EPIDEMIOLOGY

It is estimated that there are 750,000 first-ever or recurrent strokes in the United States. This is approximately 250 per 100,000 population. The risk of stroke increases exponentially with age, and the risk is higher for males. African Americans are at greater risk than whites and tend to have a higher mortality rate. The overall 30-day mortality rate of stroke is 20%, and stroke remains the third leading cause of death in the United States and the leading cause of neurologic disability in adults. Roughly 15% of first-ever stroke

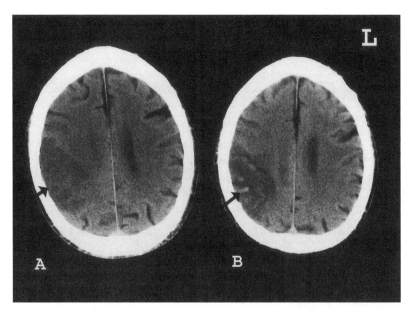

FIG. 6.1. A: Non-contrast computed tomography brain scan that reveals an acute ischemic stroke in the distribution of the right middle cerebral artery *(arrow).* **B:** Follow-up scan several days later that reveals hemorrhagic transformation of the infarct *(arrow).*

survivors suffer a recurrent stroke over the next 5 years, and the mortality rate for this second stroke is 25% within 28 days. A population-based study of survival and recurrence after the first cerebral infarction, from 1975 through 1989, found a risk of recurrent stroke of 2% at 7 days, 4% at 30 days, 12% at 1 year, and 29% at 5 years. Predictors of recurrent stroke were age and diabetes mellitus. The

risk of death after the first cerebral infarction was 7% at 7 days, 14% at 30 days, 27% at 1 year, and 53% at 5 years. Predictors of early recurrent ischemic stroke include major hemispheric stroke syndrome, atherothrombotic stroke mechanism, and atrial fibrillation.

TABLE 6.1. *Major Etiologies of Stroke*

Primary Ischemic	Primary Hemorrhagic
Thrombotic	Spontaneous
Large artery	intracerebral
Small artery	hemorrhage
(lacunar)	Aneurysmal rupture
Sinovenous	Bleeding from
thrombosis	arteriovenous
Vascular dissection	malformation
with propagation	
of thrombus	
Hemodynamic	
Mechanical obstruction	
Embolic	
Cardiogenic	
Aortic arch atheromata	
Artery-to-artery	
Arteritis	

TABLE 6.2. *Risk Factors for Stroke*

Major Risk Factors	Minor Risk Factors
Age	Hypercholesterolemia
Sex	Oral contraceptives
Race	Migraine
Genetic predisposition	Obesity
Hypertension	Physical inactivity
Diabetes mellitus	Mitral valve prolapse
Acute myocardial	Patent foramen ovale
infarction with thrombus	Bacterial endocarditis
Peripheral vascular disease	Marantic endocarditis
Cigarette smoking	Sick sinus syndrome
Valvular heart disease	Polycythemia
Hyperhomocysteinemia	Thrombocytosis
Atrial fibrillation	Bleeding diathesis
Dilated cardiomyopathy	Sympathomimetic
Aortic arch atheromata	agents
Hypercoagulable state	
Transient ischemic attack	
and prior stroke	

Studies of recurrent stroke provide conflicting information. In one study, recurrent stroke most commonly was associated with a history of TIA, atrial fibrillation, male gender, and hypertension. However, recurrence did not correlate with age, alcohol consumption, smoking, diabetes, ischemic heart disease, serum cholesterol, or hematocrit. In another study of the potential protective effect of optimal blood pressure control on stroke recurrence, the risk ratio for stroke recurrence for diastolic blood pressure 80 mm Hg or more compared to less than 80 mm Hg was 2.4. The risk ratio for systolic blood pressure 140 mm Hg or more compared to less than 140 mm Hg was also 2.4. Thus, optimal blood pressure control is effective not only for primary prevention of stroke but also for protection against recurrence. This is especially important in primary ICH where the most common mechanism remains longstanding poor blood pressure control resulting in hyaline degeneration of smaller cerebral vessels, the formation of Charcot–Bouchard microaneurysms, and a predisposition toward bleeding within the basal ganglionic and thalamic regions.

DIAGNOSTIC EVALUATION

The history is an important part of the diagnostic assessment of patients presenting with strokelike symptoms. It is even more important with the advent of thrombolytic therapy (recombinant tissue plasminogen activator, or rt-PA), which must be administered within 3 hours of symptom onset. This is the only agent presently available for acute ischemic stroke interventional therapy. To be eligible for rt-PA, patients need to be assessed, have certain blood tests performed, and have a non-contrast computed tomography (CT) brain scan performed within the 3-hour time window before the agent can be started by intravenous infusion. There are important parts of the history with special emphasis on determining the exact time that the symptoms began and any other factors in the history, such as prior bleeding, recent surgery, or trauma that might enhance the bleeding complication

rate with rt-PA. It is important to note that patients that wake up with their deficits have to have the onset assigned to the time that they were last neurologically unaffected. For example, if they woke up with a stroke at 6 AM and were last awake at 11 PM the evening before, then it has to be assumed that the stroke occurred just after 11 PM. However, if the patient had gone to the bathroom at 5 AM, and they were perfectly fine at this time, and then went back to bed and awakened at 6 AM with the stroke, then it can be assumed that the stroke occurred just after 5 AM. This would translate into a 2-hour window of opportunity for treatment with rt-PA (i.e., 6 AM to 8 AM).

The use of rt-PA mandates a more standardized approach to the neurologic evaluation for a patient with acute stroke, and this, fortunately, has been extended to most stroke patients even if they are not candidates for the medication. For example, it is important to obtain a CT brain scan at the time of presentation to readily distinguish a primary ischemic stroke from a primary hemorrhagic stroke. Generally, contrast is not necessary unless there are clinical concerns that the patient might have a tumor or abscess instead of a stroke. It is important to recognize that the CT brain scan has a sensitivity of the order of 90% to 95% for the detection of subarachnoid hemorrhage (11). Therefore, clinical suspicion for SAH, even with a negative CT brain scan, mandates the performance of a lumbar puncture unless there are contraindications to the performance of this procedure. In addition to the CT brain scan, routine immediate blood work includes a complete blood count (CBC), platelet count, metabolic profile, prothrombin time (PT)/ international normalization ratio (INR), and partial thromboplastin time (PTT).

Furthermore, a more standardized approach to the neurologic examination has been adopted to quantitate the degree of deficit in a more objective and reproducible pattern. This is especially pertinent for patients who are potentially eligible for rt-PA. The National Institutes of Health (NIH) Stroke Scale is being used to provide such standardization. This is in recognition of the fact that rt-PA should only be considered for patients with a significant neurologic deficit at the time of presentation, rt-PA should not be used if the patient is rapidly improving on their own, and there are potentially greater risks of complications of rt-PA and a reduced chance of benefit from therapy when the patient has a high score on their NIH Stroke Scale. This scale correlates with a severe neurologic deficit.

Table 6.3 outlines the first-, second-, and third-tier diagnostic studies that are part of the stroke evaluation. The first tier represents the routine studies that are performed on any patient presenting with symptoms of TIA or stroke. Obviously the clinical picture will affect the choice and speed with which the study is performed. For example, a patient presenting with new-onset TIA should undergo immediate evaluation of the potential

TABLE 6.3. *Hierarchy of Studies in Acute Ischemic Stroke*

First Tier
    Non-contrast CT brain scan
    CBC, platelet count, PT, INR, PTT
    Serum chemistry profile
    EKG
Second Tier (If clinically indicated)
    Contrast-enhanced CT brain scan
    MRI brain scan
    Carotid/vertebral duplex scan
    Transcranial Doppler ultrasonography
    Echocardiogram
    Holter monitor
    Magnetic resonance angiography and/or venography
    Blood cultures
    Lumbar puncture
Third Tier (If clinically indicated)
    ESR
    Syphilis serology
    HIV testing
    Stress EKG
    Bleeding time
    Platelet function studies
    Special clotting factor studies
    Fasting lipid profile
    Fasting homocysteine level
    Protein C and S levels
    Antiphospholipid antibodies
    Antithrombin III level
    Cerebral arteriography
    Spiral CT angiography
    Sickle cell prep

EKG, electrocardiogram; ESR, erythrocyte sedimentation rate.

ischemic mechanism in an effort to intervene before a stroke occurs. The same is true for relatively minor stroke associated with resolution of signs and symptoms within days to weeks (Fig. 6.2). However, there is usually little to offer the patient who is moribund from a stroke. In such a circumstance, once it has been established by examination and neuroimaging that the prognosis for meaningful recovery is nil, then tests that will have no impact on management should be avoided.

The CT brain scan is often the only neuroimaging study that is necessary for acute stroke evaluation. Contrast is usually not necessary, and this represents a practical and cost-effective approach for most patients. However, there are certain patients in whom a magnetic resonance imaging (MRI) brain scan may provide worthwhile information that may affect patient management—for example, in the patient with an atypical or fluctuating clinical picture with evidence of brainstem or cerebellar involvement, an MRI typically provides a much better image of this area and can help to confirm or refute the clinical impression (Fig. 6.3). Other potential advantages of MRI include the greater safety of using contrast-enhanced MRI, as opposed to contrast-enhanced CT scan. In addition, magnetic resonance angiography (MRA) and venography (MRV) have the ability to provide a reasonably accurate view of the extracranial and intracranial circulation, which often allows information complimentary to the MRI. However, MRA and MRV can vary considerably in quality between institutions and it does not have the accuracy of the "gold standard" for the evaluation of the cerebral circulation, which remains intraarterial cerebral arteriography.

The MRI brain scan has been the subject of a number of reports with perfusion and diffusion-weighted imaging (DWI) in acute ischemic stroke. DWI allows detection of cellular injury and cytotoxic edema, whereas MR perfusion imaging can identify brain tissue that is susceptible to infarction but that is in a potentially reversible stage of tissue injury. Thus, a so-called "perfusion–diffusion mis-

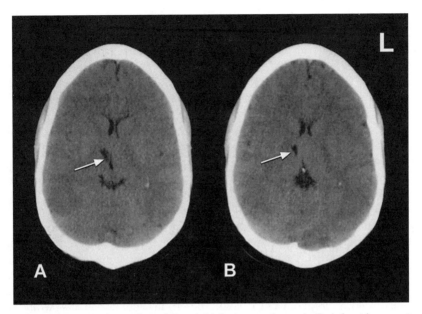

FIG. 6.2. A: Small infarct in the region of the right thalamus *(arrow).* **B:** Infarct is seen to extend in a rostral-caudal pattern *(arrow)* in this 23-year-old woman who had a postpartum stroke that resolved over several weeks.

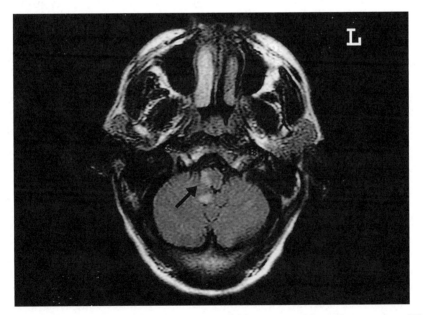

FIG. 6.3. Magnetic resonance imaging brain scan (fluid-attenuated inversion recovery [FLAIR] image) that demonstrates a right lateral medullary infarct *(arrow)* with the computed tomography brain scan normal on repeated study. There is also some involvement of the cerebellum manifested by increased signal intensity.

match" might be of value in identifying acute ischemic stroke patients who are most likely to respond to rt-PA. However, such an approach requires ready availability of these newer MRI techniques and immediate reading of the images. Any delay associated with obtaining these studies further prolongs the initiation of rt-PA, which limits the usefulness of perfusion–diffusion images.

Cardiac evaluation is of value in the assessment of potential cardiogenic sources of embolism. This can include imaging of the aortic arch where atheromata have the potential to break off and enter the brain circulation. However, one must factor in the costs versus benefits of extensive cardiac evaluation unless the results are going to definitely affect management of the patient. Specifically, transesophageal echocardiography (TEE) and long-term cardiac monitoring are reserved for patients with a reasonable chance of having a potential cardiogenic source of embolism and who should be considered for anticoagulant therapy. One also must address the potential coexistence of coronary artery disease in patients with ischemic stroke because this association is not at all uncommon. Cardiac stress testing might be appropriate in some patients with cerebral events.

Well-documented cardiac disease in a patient presenting with symptoms of stroke warrants the performance of transthoracic echocardiography and consideration of heart monitoring to assess for structural cardiac disease, with the former study, and the possibility of a paroxysmal cardiac arrhythmia (e.g., atrial fibrillation [AF]) with the latter. TEE usually is restricted to patients who have unexplained stroke (i.e., with no risk factors for stroke). TEE is useful when there is concern about a possible patent foramen ovale in a patient with the possibility of paradoxical cerebral embolus. TEE is useful to assess the left atrium and left atrial appendage and to more effectively assess the aortic arch for atheromata. Vegetations, either septic or nonseptic, as well as thrombus formation tend to be better detected with TEE. Concern about possible bacterial endocarditis mandates blood cultures. An erythrocyte sedimentation rate can be useful for the detection of endocarditis, atrial myxoma, or a vasculitic process. Syphilis serology and human immunodeficiency virus testing also can be important in susceptible individuals presenting with strokelike symptoms.

Evaluation for a hypercoagulable state is predicated on the clinical picture of prior thromboembolic events, a positive family history, a history of spontaneous abortions, and unexplained ischemic stroke in a young person. Antiphospholipid antibody titers are particularly important when there is a well-documented hypercoagulable state or in patients with systemic lupus erythematosus in association with ischemic stroke. Protein C, protein S, and antithrombin III deficiencies are ordered in young patients with unexplained stroke, but the yield tends to be quite low unless there is a history of thromboembolic events and/or a positive family history. Thrombocythemia, with a platelet count greater than 1,000,000/uL, polycythemia, and sickle cell disease are additional hematologic factors associated with ischemic stroke. Conversely, a low platelet count or factor deficiency can result in a bleeding diathesis with secondary ICH.

Noninvasive vascular imaging now includes carotid and vertebral duplex ultrasound, which combines the anatomic information of B-mode scanning with the physiologic information of Doppler and transcranial Doppler ultrasonography (TCD), which allows assessment of the flow velocities of the intracranial major arteries, as well as MRA and CT angiography. However, routine intraarterial cerebral arteriography remains the "gold standard" for the most accurate information about the extracranial and intracranial circulation. This is useful for the detection of intracranial or extracranial vascular stenosis, possible vasculitis, vascular dissection, the presence of an aneurysm, or the presence of an AVM. Moyamoya disease, with progressive occlusion of the intracranial vasculature, is another entity that requires assessment with angiography.

Second- and third-tier studies primarily are performed in an effort to prevent a subsequent event. These can include a fasting lipid profile. This is in recognition of the fact that statin therapy has been demonstrated to be of some efficacy for stroke prevention in certain patients. The plasma homocysteine level and C-reactive protein (CRP) level also can help to identify individuals with an enhanced risk of ischemic stroke. Both elevated levels of homocysteine and CRP have been implicated. The finding of a relationship between CRP levels and stroke risk raise the possibility that inflammation is a potential mechanism for ischemic events.

ISCHEMIC STROKE AND TRANSIENT ISCHEMIC ATTACK

Presentation and Localization

Thrombotic stroke and embolic stroke can look very much alike in terms of presentation. However, there are certain features that may help distinguish one from the other. Features supportive of a thrombotic versus embolic mechanism are outlined in Table 6.4. A subcategory of thrombotic stroke (small vessel) is known as lacunar-type. Major lacunar syndromes include pure motor hemiparesis, pure

TABLE 6.4. *Features of a Thrombotic Versus Embolic Stroke*

Thrombotic	Embolic
Premonitory transient ischemic attack(s)	Sudden onset of maximal deficit
Stepwise progression	Cardiogenic source of embolus
Evidence of atherosclerotic disease	Multiple vascular territory involvement
Large artery or small artery territory infarction pattern	Potential association with syncope at onset
	Potential association with seizure at onset
	Greater likelihood of hemorrhagic infarct
	Branch occlusion infarct pattern
	Embolic involvement of other organs
	Severe deficit at onset followed by rapid resolution

TABLE 6.5. *Carotid Versus Vertebrobasilar Distribution of Stroke/TIA Symptoms*

Carotid Distribution	Vertebrobasilar Distribution
Aphasia	Bilateral visual loss
Transient monocular blindness (amaurosis fugax)	Ataxia
	Quadriparesis
	Perioral numbness
Hemiparesis	"Crossed" sensory or motor deficits
Hemisensory deficit	
Homonymous hemianopsia in combination with motor or sensory deficit	Two or more of the following: Vertigo Syncope Dysarthria Diplopia Nausea Dysphagia Drop attack, especially when seen in association with a motor or sensory deficit

sensory stroke, sensorimotor, clumsy hand dysarthria, and hemiataxia–hemiparesis.

Of particular importance is the distinction between carotid distribution versus vertebrobasilar distribution ischemia. Carotid endarterectomy is of value for stroke prevention in symptomatic patients when carotid stenosis ipsilateral to the involved cerebral hemisphere is demonstrated. However, it is not expected that prophylactic carotid endarterectomy would be of any value for a patient presenting with vertebrobasilar distribution symptoms who also was found to have moderate or severe carotid stenosis. The features that help to distinguish carotid distribution symptoms of stroke or TIA from vertebrobasilar distribution are outlined in Table 6.5.

Treatment

Atherosclerosis is a primary factor in the pathogenesis of ischemic stroke. It has been clearly established that the formation of atherosclerotic plaque correlates with stroke risk. Measures that interfere with the deposition of plaque material are presently the most effective means for reducing the incidence of stroke and TIA. Lipohyalinosis of the small penetrating arteries, with secondary occlusion, is the most common mechanism of lacunar-type stroke. Effective blood pressure control is of particular importance for both primary and secondary stroke prevention. Two agents that have been identified for their potential in preventing secondary stroke are ramipril and perindopril plus a diuretic.

Statin agents are established for the primary prevention of stroke in certain high-risk patients. Statin agents have been associated with a 25% relative risk reduction in fatal and non-fatal stroke. Studies are under way to look at the potential efficacy of statin agents in the secondary prevention of stroke. Additional measures that may reduce stroke risk include the intake of supplemental folic acid, vitamin B6, and vitamin B12 to reduce the homocysteine level and enhanced consumption of omega-3 polyunsaturated fatty acids and whole grains. Optimal glucose control in patients with diabetes mellitus is associated with a reduced risk of vascular complications including stroke. Smoking cessation is of utmost importance.

Antithrombotic agents can be of benefit in stroke prevention, as well as in acute ischemic stroke treatment, but one must weigh risks versus benefit in terms of choice of therapy. For example, aspirin was not found to be of benefit in the primary prevention of stroke in middle-aged healthy men. Warfarin now is identified as the agent of choice in the primary prevention of stroke in patients with atrial fibrillation who are at relatively high risk for stroke as well as for other cardiac conditions that are associated with a significant risk of cardioembolic events. Warfarin also has a place in the management of certain conditions associated with a hypercoagulable state. However, warfarin was not found to be superior to aspirin in symptomatic stroke patients who did not have a cardiogenic source of embolism.

Presently available antiplatelet agents include aspirin and low-dose aspirin combined with high-dose timed-release dipyridamole, clopidogrel, and ticlopidine. There has been considerable debate over the optimal aspirin dose for stroke prevention. It has been demonstrated that aspirin at a dose of either 81 mg or 325 mg per day is superior to doses of either 650 mg or 1300 mg per day in preventing vascular events around the time of carotid endarterectomy. Aspirin is the first line of antiplatelet therapy for protection against ischemic stroke in patients with symptoms of stroke. This is in recognition of its efficacy—roughly a 20% relative risk reduction in vascular events compared to placebo—its safety profile, and its limited cost.

For patients who are symptomatic on aspirin ("aspirin failures"), alternative antiplatelet agents either are substituted or added to the aspirin. In one analysis, ticlopidine was associated with a relative risk reduction of stroke of roughly 33.5%, clopidogrel 27.2%, and the combination of low-dose aspirin–high-dose dipyridamole (25/200 mg twice a day) 37%. The decision about substituting an antiplatelet agent, and which agent to use, often is based on several factors including cost; the risk of side effects; concerns about the low dose of aspirin in cardiac patients with the aspirin–dipyridamole combination; and the easy bruising seen with these agents, which tends to cause the patients considerable concern. Table 6.6 outlines the potential prophylactic medications available.

TABLE 6.6. *Pharmacologic Treatment Approaches for Stroke Prevention*

Antihypertensives
Ramipril
Perindopril with diuretic
Alternative antihypertensives
Statin Agents
Pravastatin
Simvastatin
Alternative statin drugs
Agents to Lower Homocysteine Level
Folic acid
Vitamin B6
Vitamin B12
Antiplatelet Agents
Aspirin 81 mg to 325 mg/day
Clopidogrel 75 mg/day
Ticlopidine 250 mg with meals bid
Aspirin/dipyridamole 25/200 mg bid
Anticoagulants

Warfarin at a dose to achieve an INR of 2.0 to 3.0 for nonvalvular atrial fibrillation, although higher dosing may be necessary for other conditions.

Carotid endarterectomy is the most effective means of preventing stroke in patients with symptomatic high-grade carotid stenosis (Fig. 6.4). There is possibly some potential benefit for patients with 50% to 69% symptomatic stenosis, but the greatest benefit is in those with 70% to 99% stenosis. Careful patient selection and risk versus benefit analysis is required. Carotid angioplasty is an option for patients who have unacceptable surgical risk but who clearly may benefit from correction of their stenosis. This is an evolving procedure, but it may be particularly attractive for certain patients with asymptomatic carotid stenosis where the potential benefits of endarterectomy do not clearly justify the risks.

rt-PA is approved for acute ischemic stroke in patients who fulfill the criteria for its use and in whom there are no contraindications (Table 6.7). It is associated with roughly a 30% increased chance of full neurologic recovery at 3 months and 12 months compared to placebo. It is most effective when given early on, and the more normal the CT brain scan, the more likely is one to see some benefit. Conversely, the greater the evolution of

TABLE 6.7. *Indications and Contraindications to the Use of Recombinant Tissue Plasminogen Activator for Acute Ischemic Stroke*

Indications	Contraindications
Acute ischemic stroke presentation and treatment possible within 3 hours	Hemorrhage on CT brain scan
Persistent significant neurologic deficit on repeat examination	Uncontrolled hypertension with SBP >185 mm Hg and/or DBP >110 mm Hg over time
Absence of significant improvement on serial examination	History of intracranial hemorrhage
Absence of marked anemia, severely abnormal blood glucose level, or other severe metabolic disturbance or bleeding diathesis by admission or laboratory testing	Thrombocytopenia with platelet count <100,000 µL Active anticoagulant therapy Active internal bleeding Recent serious head trauma, recent prior ischemic stroke, or recent intracranial surgery
No associated seizure activity at onset	Clinical suspicion for SAH
No recent arterial or lumbar puncture	

SBP, systolic blood pressure; DBP, diastolic blood pressure; SAH, subarachnoid hemorrhagic stroke.

the infarct by CT brain scan, the less the likelihood of a good response and the greater the chance of intracerebral hemorrhage as a complication. This is seen in approximately 6.4% of patients treated with rt-PA for acute ischemic stroke, but this figure can be considerably higher in certain medical centers, which is, perhaps, related to less experience with this agent. Theoretically, ischemic stroke associated with clot within a cerebral vessel (Fig. 6.5) should be most responsive to thrombolytic therapy.

Aspirin therapy (160–300 mg/day) in acute ischemic stroke now appears to be indicated as long as there is no medical contraindication to the use of aspirin. The primary benefit is to reduce the risk of early recurrent stroke. Of note, aspirin should not be given within 24 hours of the use of rt-PA nor should anticoagulant therapy.

Anticoagulant therapy for acute ischemic stroke continues to be a controversial subject. However, there is increasing evidence indicat-

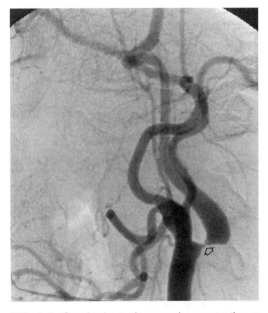

FIG. 6.4. Cerebral arteriogram demonstrating a high-grade internal carotid artery stenosis at the origin *(arrow).*

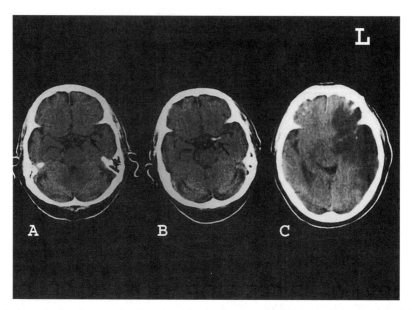

FIG. 6.5. A: Non-contrast computed tomography brain scan that demonstrated a patent left middle cerebral artery *(arrow)* in a patient with transient ischemic attack. **B:** Follow-up study, the next day, after the patient develops symptoms of evolving stroke and there is now hyperdensity of the left middle cerebral artery *(arrow)* representing a fresh clot within the vessel. **C:** Subsequent evolution of a large left middle cerebral artery infarct.

ing that anticoagulant therapy is of no benefit for acute ischemic stroke, whereas aspirin therapy is of some benefit. The accumulated evidence of a number of trials has led to published guidelines of the American Academy of Neurology and American Stroke Association in reference to anticoagulants and antiplatelet agents in acute ischemic stroke. These guidelines conclude "there is no convincing evidence that anticoagulants are effective for any particular stroke subtype." Anticoagulants do reduce the frequency of deep venous thrombosis in acute stroke, and antiplatelet agents do not.

There are certain standard measures for acute stroke management, which are outlined in Table 6.8. These include protection of the airway with aspiration precautions, careful monitoring of the vital signs, and early mobilization if at all possible. In acute ischemic stroke, it is important not to be overly aggressive with blood pressure control, and systolic blood pressures of 160 ± 20 mm Hg and diastolic blood pressure of 100 ± 10 mm Hg gen-

erally are not treated in the first several days to weeks of the acute event. This is in recognition of the potential for sudden drops in blood pressure to reduce cerebral perfusion and cause extension of the infarction related

TABLE 6.8. *Guidelines for the General Management of the Patient with Acute Stroke*

1. Stability of vital signs
2. Avoidance of aggressive blood pressure control in acute ischemic stroke
3. Avoidance of glucose- or dextrose-containing intravenous fluids in acute ischemic stroke
4. Initiation of aspirin therapy in acute ischemic stroke if no contraindication
5. Protection of airway with aspiration precautions
6. Assessment of swallowing capacity
7. Early mobilization as clinically indicated
8. Bowel program
9. Prevention of pressure sores
10. Antiembolus measures
11. Rehabilitation therapy evaluation as indicated by the deficit
12. Social Service evaluation
13. Assessment for evidence of poststroke depression
14. Long-term management of risk factors for stroke

to disruption of cerebral autoregulation in acute stroke. It is also now well recognized that elevated blood glucose can have a deleterious effect on stroke outcome and enhances the risk of complications with rt-PA.

INTRACEREBRAL HEMORRHAGE

Clinical Approach

The most common causes of ICH are listed in Table 6.9. Hypertensive ICH most commonly affects the basal ganglionic–thalamic region; pontine hemorrhage and cerebellar hemorrhage are other uncommon locations. The patient typically presents with maximal deficit at onset, and a patient who complains of sudden severe headache followed by obtundation and focal neurologic deficit, in association with a markedly elevated blood pressure, usually is found to have ICH rather than ischemic stroke. However, relatively small hematomas can present with minor deficit; this is why it is important to obtain a CT brain scan immediately at the time of presentation because this readily distinguishes an intracerebral hematoma from an evolving infarct (Fig. 6.6). It is important to recognize that acute bleeding shows up immediately on the CT brain scan, whereas it generally takes 3 to 6 hours or longer for an acute ischemic stroke to evolve on the CT brain scan.

Lobar hematomas are less likely associated with a hypertensive mechanism; other etiolo-

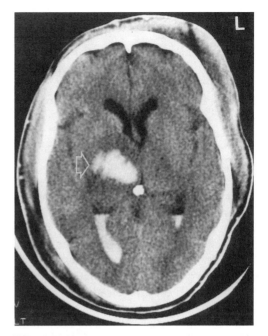

FIG. 6.6. Non-contrast computed tomography brain scan that demonstrates a right thalamic intracerebral hematoma *(arrow)* with intraventricular extension of the bleed.

gies need to be considered. Roughly one-half of all lobar hematomas are not attributable to hypertension. Alternative explanations can include cerebral amyloid angiopathy. This typically is seen in patients in their 60s or older, and it is characterized by lobar hematoma, dementia, and congophilic (amyloid) angiopathy on pathologic specimen. This entity is important to recognize clinically because surgical evacuation should be avoided. The involved vessels tend to be quite friable, and this can be associated with an unexpected challenge in terms of control of bleeding. Vascular anomalies such as AVMs and aneurysms are also in the differential diagnosis of lobar hemorrhage.

A severely low platelet count, generally below 30,000/uL, can be associated with brain hemorrhage as can factor VIII and factor IX deficiency, with the latter two entities being familial in nature. Routinely, a PT and PTT are obtained in patients with ICH, and a bleeding time can be useful to assess for

TABLE 6.9. *Causes of Spontaneous Intracerebral Hemorrhage*

---

1. Hypertension
2. Intracranial aneurysm
3. Arteriovenous malformation
4. Bleeding diathesis
5. Complication of anticoagulant therapy
6. Illicit drug use (e.g., cocaine)
7. Mycotic aneurysm
8. Hemorrhagic metastasis
9. Bleeding into a primary brain tumor
10. Bleeding into a brain abscess
11. Arteritis (primary, connective tissue disorder, syphilitic, etc.)
12. Amyloid angiopathy
13. Hemorrhagic leukoencephalopathy
14. Idiopathic ? cryptic arteriovenous malformation

platelet dysfunction. Hypofibrinogenemia is another potential hematologic explanation for ICH. In addition, the presence of fibrinogen degradation products with fragmented erythrocytes suggests disseminated intravascular coagulation as an explanation. Acquired immune deficiency syndrome can have a multitude of effects that can promote ICH; one of them is severe thrombocytopenia. Meningovascular syphilis also remains in the differential diagnosis of ICH.

The increasing use of anticoagulant therapy to protect against cardiogenic embolism in susceptible individuals will translate into an increased incidence of ICH. This can be prevented, in most circumstances, with an extremely rigorous approach toward monitoring of the patient, their medications, and their INR. A good general rule is to have only one physician taking responsibility for prescribing all medications; over-the-counter preparations should be discouraged if at all possible.

Certain drugs can promote ICH, including cocaine and amphetamines. Agents with a sympathomimetic effect can cause a sudden increase in blood pressure that can "unmask" a preexisting cerebrovascular anomaly such as an AVM or aneurysm. There also can be a vasculitic effect with so-called "beading" of the cerebral blood vessels similar to what one can see with a connective tissue disorder such as systemic lupus erythematosus and polyarteritis nodosa. Phenylpropanolamine, a sympathomimetic agent, which, until recently, commonly was found in cough and cold over-the-counter preparations and in appetite suppressants, has been implicated as a factor in certain patients with ICH who have no other discernible etiology.

Bleeding into a primary CNS neoplasm or metastatic disease are other etiologies. The most likely metastatic lesions to be associated with ICH include lung, breast, thyroid, renal cell, and melanoma. One also can see bleeding related to septic embolism from bacterial endocarditis as well as non-septic embolism from marantic endocarditis, and it is possible to have bleeding into a brain abscess.

Treatment

With hypertensive ICH, bleeding can persist for up to 6 hours, which can produce major deleterious effect on outcome. There has been some controversy about what degree of blood pressure control is desirable in the acute setting. There has been concern that aggressive reduction of a markedly elevated blood pressure can lead to secondary hypoperfusion of brain tissue surrounding the hematoma and can lead to worsening of the outcome. However, this has not been demonstrated. It is recognized that expansion of the hematoma to a critical level, related to persistent intracranial bleeding, can accurately identify those patients with no hope for meaningful recovery. It appears that aggressive blood pressure management, with agents such as sodium nitroprusside or labetalol, have some potential to reduce expansion of the hematoma and to limit end-organ damage to other areas such as the heart and kidneys. Surgical evacuation of primary ICH remains controversial with insufficient evidence of risks versus benefits.

ICH related to the use of unfractionated heparin requires immediate discontinuation of the heparin infusion and infusion of protamine sulfate. Warfarin-related ICH is managed most effectively with fresh frozen plasma. It can take vitamin K up to 8 to 24 hours to correct a prolonged prothrombin time, which is far too long in such an emergency setting.

A lobar hematoma has the potential to be removed surgically if it does not involve a vital part of the brain such as the motor strip or speech area. Surgical evacuation usually is considered when there is significant mass effect associated with the hematoma and the patient is demonstrating clinical deterioration. This is of utmost importance for a cerebellar hematoma, especially if the patient is beginning to show long tract signs or other evidence of brainstem compression. Acute obstructive hydrocephalus associated with intraventricular extension of the bleed often is treated with a ventricular shunt. However, the effectiveness of such an approach is questionable.

SUBARACHNOID HEMORRHAGE

Intracranial Aneurysm

Aneurysmal subarachnoid hemorrhage has an annual incidence in the United States of roughly 1 in 10,000 people. It is estimated that 0.5% to1% of adults have an incidental aneurysm. Each year, new aneurysms may develop in up to 2% of patients with previously ruptured aneurysms, and the rupture rate is up to 6 per 10,000 per year. The risk of aneurysmal rupture is associated with female sex, age, amount of cigarettes smoked, hypertension, moderate to heavy alcohol consumption, and ingestion of sympathomimetic agents. Genetic factors include Marfan's syndrome, autosomal dominant polycystic kidney disease, Ehlers–Danlos syndrome Type IV, and neurofibromatosis type 1.

Aneurysmal rupture has a mortality rate that approaches 50%. It is extremely important to recognize that a "warning leak" can precede a major rupture in up to 25% of patients and that recognition of this premonitory syndrome can be life saving. Patients presenting with an atypical or particularly severe headache, especially when there is clinical evidence of meningeal irritation, are most worrisome. The CT brain scan has a sensitivity of roughly 90% to 95% during the initial 24 hours of the bleed, whereas the lumbar puncture has essentially 100% sensitivity. Thus, the lumbar puncture is indicated even if the CT brain scan appears to be completely negative, but there is clinical suspicion for an aneurysmal bleed. On occasion, one actually can see the aneurysm on the CT brain scan, but this can be a subtle finding (Fig. 6.7). Cerebral arteriography remains the definitive study for documentation of an aneurysm or aneurysms because they can be in multiple locations, and they typically are seen at branching points of the major cerebral arteries. MRA and spiral CT angiography have some value for noninvasive "screening" purposes. Roughly 80% to 85% of cerebral aneurysms are seen in the anterior circulation, with the most common locations at the junction of the internal carotid artery and the posterior communicating artery, in the region of the anterior communicating artery, and at the trifurcation of the middle cerebral artery. Posterior circulation aneurysms most commonly are found at the tip of the basilar artery or at the junction of a vertebral artery with the posterior inferior cerebellar artery. The clinical manifestations

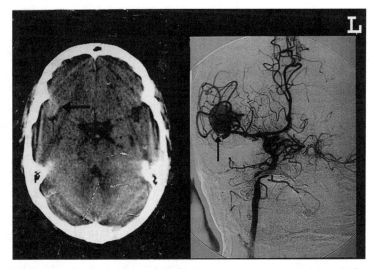

FIG. 6.7. A (left): Demonstration of the subtle finding of an unruptured right middle cerebral artery aneurysm *(arrow)* on non-contrast computed tomography brain scan. **B (right):** Cerebral arteriogram demonstrates the large right middle cerebral artery aneurysm *(arrow)* following rupture.

of a ruptured cerebral aneurysm typically reflect its location. Most patients have a severe headache with clinical evidence of meningeal irritation (i.e., neck stiffness and pain), which is aggravated by neck motion. Some patients have syncope as the primary manifestation, with headache as a more minor component of the presentation. Subhyaloid hemorrhage on funduscopic examination can be an important clue. So-called "classic" presentations include the patient stating they are experiencing the "worst headache" of their life with no localizing neurologic features or having a severe headache with a third cranial nerve palsy. The third nerve palsy lateral to the ruptured aneurysm identifies the location of the aneurysm at the junction of the internal carotid artery with the posterior communicating artery in the vicinity where the third cranial nerve is traversing from the midbrain toward the eye.

The major therapeutic approach is to have early surgical clipping of the ruptured aneurysm as soon as possible in an effort to prevent further bleeding. There are a number of potential complications of the initial rupture (Table 6.10), and rebleeding is the most worrisome. Up to 10% to 20% of patients will suffer rebleeding if early surgery, within the first 48 to 72 hours of presentation, cannot be performed. Another not infrequent complication is vasospasm. This tends to correlate with the amount of subarachnoid blood present, and it is most commonly seen 3 to 15 days after the initial rupture. The agent nimodipine, a calcium channel blocker, is available to help prevent aneurysmal rupture-induced vasospasm. Some centers now are using endovascular balloon angioplasty. These latter therapeutic approaches require effective obliteration of the aneurysm. An alternative approach to such obliteration is the placement of endovascular coils within the aneurysms that induce electrothrombosis of the aneurysmal sac. There is some evidence that outcome following aneurysmal rupture was better with endovascular coiling than with surgical clipping.

Arteriovenous Malformation

An AVM represents an anomaly of embryonal development in which there is a conglomeration of arteries and veins with no intervening capillaries. The prevalence of AVM in the general population is estimated at 0.14%, and most remain clinically silent throughout life. They are reported to be twice as common in men as in women. Although present at birth, they tend to become clinically evident most commonly between the ages of 10 and 40 years.

Approximately 50% of people who become symptomatic from an AVM present with either ICH, SAH, or both. It is the second most common cause of spontaneous SAH after aneurysmal rupture. Approximately 30% of patients with AVM present with seizures; the remaining 20% present with headache, focal neurologic deficit, or cognitive impairment. Roughly 25% of patients with ICH secondary to AVM will suffer serious morbidity or death. Overall, the first bleed is fatal in 4.6% of patients. In a population-based long-term follow-up study, the risk of first hemorrhage is lifelong and increases with age. The recurrence rate for brain hemorrhage is roughly 7% for the first year following the initial bleed. Of the patients with AVM who present with seizure, 1% will suffer ICH within 1 year. The headache that is associated with AVM can be very difficult to distinguish from migraine, and there is always the possibility that the two coexist.

Fortunately, the risk of rebleeding from an AVM is not analogous to that of aneurysmal rupture. This gives the clinician time to carefully plan optimal management once the patient is stable. The most effective course is to surgi-

TABLE 6.10. *Complications of Aneurysmal Rupture*

---
1. Rebleeding
2. Vasospasm with secondary ischemia
3. Hydrocephalus
   a. Obstructive
   b. Communicating
4. Diffuse cerebral edema
5. Chemical meningitis
6. Subdural hematoma
7. Intracerebral hematoma

---

cally remove the AVM, if this is feasible. However, not all AVMs can be resected because of the extent of the vascular supply, the location, or both. AVMs located within the deep brain structures or those involving vital brain function areas are the most challenging from a surgical approach. In an effort to reduce the vascular supply of the AVM, endovascular occlusion has been used. With the use of superselective vascular catheterization, one can insert a permanent balloon, sclerosing drugs, quick-acting glues, or thrombosing coils to interrupt the vascular supply. In certain instances, these endovascular procedures can obliterate the AVM. However, the usual purpose is to allow the AVM to be more effectively, and safely, managed from a surgical standpoint. This is in recognition of the proposed surgical risk of extirpation based on size of the lesion, type of venous drainage, and location.

Radiotherapy is an alternative to more invasive approaches. It can involve the use of gamma knife, proton beam, or linear accelerator. The purpose is to focus the radiotherapy at the vascular supply of the AVM in an effort to promote occlusive vascular injury, over multiple courses of therapy, in an effort to thrombose the involved vessels. Theoretically, radiotherapy, also known as radiosurgery, can obliterate the AVM in a best-case scenario and remove its risk of ever bleeding or rebleeding. It is important to point out that both radiotherapy and endovascular occlusion are in the developmental stages and it is expected that outcome will improve as these techniques are perfected.

WHEN TO REFER TO A NEUROLOGIST

Acute stroke management is usually the most pressing within the first several hours. It is important to obtain the opinion of the neurologist in regard to the possible use of rt-PA, if this is feasible and does not result in an unnecessary delay in treatment. In addition, patients who require a more sophisticated opinion in reference to recurrent symptoms of stroke or TIA should have access to a neurologic opinion. Issues such as choice of an-

tiplatelet therapy, indications for the use of anticoagulant therapy, decision making in reference to carotid endarterectomy, and informed opinions about the evaluation of the patient with unexplained ICH as well as the approach to the patient with aneurysmal rupture and the management of AVM are potentially helped with the input of a neurologist.

SPECIAL CHALLENGES FOR HOSPITALIZED PATIENTS

It is important to recognize that patients presenting with acute stroke or new-onset TIA require immediate evaluation and management; hospitalization is the preferred approach for this. Within several days of admission, the mechanism of the cerebral ischemia or hemorrhage should be identified in the majority of patients; this allows institution of effective management sooner rather than later. Patients who are neurologically unstable should be admitted to an intensive care unit. This is particularly important for monitoring purposes after they have received rt-PA. Cardiac monitoring can be especially important for patients who are at significant risk for cardiac arrhythmia as an explanation for their symptoms. Many medical centers now have stroke units available, which allow a multidisciplinary approach toward the various special needs of the patient with acute stroke. These include nursing staff with special expertise in neurologic monitoring of patients with stroke; supervision by neurologists with special expertise in stroke; and a dedicated stroke rehabilitative staff to address communication disorders secondary to stroke, cognitive dysfunction, psychologic sequelae including depression, swallowing and/or respiratory impairment. The staff also can assess and treat motor dysfunction, incoordination, and gait impairment.

QUESTIONS AND DISCUSSION

1. A 32-year old right-handed woman presents to your ER complaining of right-sided head and neck pain. She also has a mild right hemiataxia, loss of sensation over the right

side of her face, a right Horner's syndrome, and left arm and leg sensory loss. Her complaints date back to a motor vehicle accident a week before in which she sustained a whiplash-type injury. Her CT brain scan is negative, and her estranged husband reports that she has had recent severe emotional problems. What do you believe is the most likely explanation for her presentation?

A. Conversion reaction

B. Spinal contusion

C. AVM of the midbrain

D. Right lateral medullary (Wallenberg's) syndrome

E. None of the above

Answer (D). This patient has obvious objective findings on examination despite the normal CT brain scan and the history of recent emotional difficulty. Her findings could reflect cervical spinal cord contusion, but the selective involvement makes it much more likely that the location of involvement is the lateral tegmentum of the right medulla. The normal CT brain scan most likely reflects the fact that this is a lesion of the posterior fossa where the CT brain scan is less sensitive for detecting small ischemic lesions. This is where the MRI brain scan tends to be far superior to the CT brain scan. However, the negative CT brain, along with the clinical presentation, makes it unlikely that this patient is presenting with a midbrain AVM. Her clinical picture is most compatible with a dissection of the right vertebral artery, secondary to the recent motor vehicle accident, with secondary infarction of the lateral medulla of the brainstem. Wallenberg's syndrome consists of ipsilateral cranial nerve V, IX, X, XI involvement with ipsilateral Horner's syndrome, cerebellar ataxia, and contralateral loss of pain and temperature sense.

2. A 54-year old right-handed male presents to your ER with the sudden onset of aphasia, right homonymous hemianopsia, and right hemiparesis. He developed the symptoms at 7 AM, and it is now 9 AM. Measures necessary to determine if he is a potential candidate for rt-PA include all of the following *except:*

A. CT brain scan, which reveals no evidence of intracerebral hemorrhage

B. Routine blood work, which reveals no significant metabolic disturbance such as severe hypoglycemia or hyperglycemia

C. The exclusion of the presence of a so-called hyperdense middle cerebral artery sign on CT brain scan reflective of a clot within the involved middle cerebral artery

D. Blood work to rule out significant thrombocytopenia

E. Blood work to rule out the possibility of him being on anticoagulant therapy in a therapeutic range

Answer (C). This patient is a potential candidate for rt-PA if he presents with an ischemic stroke within 3 hours of onset and with enough time to exclude contraindications to the use of this drug. A CT brain scan is mandatory to exclude intracerebral hemorrhage or evolution of the infarct to the point that there is already significant tissue damage present, which would raise serious questions about the exact onset of the ischemic insult and would increase the likelihood of hemorrhagic transformation as a complication of the therapy. Patients also must have enough of a deficit to warrant the use of this agent, and they should not be demonstrating significant spontaneous resolution of their signs and symptoms during the evaluation period because this contraindicates the need for this potentially dangerous agent. One must exclude a severe metabolic derangement, such as a very low or very high blood glucose, which can produce focal neurologic deficit. It is also important to exclude focal seizure activity as part of the presentation because this can contribute to the neurologic deficit. The hyperdense middle cerebral artery sign identifies patients with a clot within the affected vessel, which makes them, theoretically, most appropriate for treatment with this "clot-busting" agent. Contraindications include a clinically significant bleeding diathesis or anticoagulant therapy that is in a therapeutic range.

3. A 67-year-old right-handed woman presents to your office with recurrent episodes of speech disturbance and right-sided weakness. Her neurologic examination is normal as is her CT brain scan and electroencephalogram

(EEG). Appropriate evaluation of this patient should include which of the following?

A. Auscultation for carotid bruits, for cardiac murmur, and for cardiac rhythm disturbance

B. Performance of a carotid and vertebral duplex scan

C. Performance of an electrocardiogram

D. Routine blood work including CBC, PT, PTT, INR, and platelet count

E. All of the above

Answer (E). This patient is at risk for stroke, and evaluation for possible contributing factors to her transient ischemic attacks is very much in order. She requires evaluation for carotid stenosis, valvular heart disease, or a clinically significant cardiac rhythm disturbance such as atrial fibrillation. It is also important to determine whether she is anemic, which raises concerns about the possible use of antithrombotic therapy; this issue also is addressed with assessment of her clotting status. It is generally a good idea to admit patients immediately for the new onset of TIA so that the mechanism can be potentially determined as quickly as possible and appropriate therapy can be instituted.

4. A 34-year-old woman presents to your ER with severe headache and is found to have some pain on motion of her neck. Her husband reports a longstanding history of migraine and that she "overdid it" with red wine the night before. She reports to you that this headache is similar in severity to previous "bad migraines," but she also states that it is not a "typical" migraine for her. She is afebrile with normal vital signs. You elect to obtain a non-contrast CT brain scan, and it is officially read as normal. Before you send her home, you should seriously consider which diagnostic test?

A. An MRI brain scan

B. An EEG

C. A serum protein electrophoresis

D. A lumbar puncture

E. A Lyme titer

Answer (D). A patient presenting to the ER with a severe headache is always a cause for concern, especially if it is called "the worst headache of my life." Atypical headaches also should raise particular concern so that one does not miss the so-called "warning leak" of subarachnoid hemorrhage or an early meningitis or encephalitis. The CT brain scan has a sensitivity of the order of 90% to 95% within the first day of an aneurysmal subarachnoid hemorrhage, and, thus, it does not fully exclude the possibility of such a life-threatening bleed. To completely exclude this possibility, when there is any clinical suspicion, one must perform a lumbar puncture.

SUGGESTED READING

Barnett HJM, Taylor DW, Eliasziw M, et al. Benefit of carotid endarterectomy in patients with symptomatic moderate or severe stenosis. *N Engl J Med* 1998;339: 1415.

Friday G, Alter M, Lai S-M. Control of hypertension and risk of stroke recurrence. *Stroke* 2002;33:2652.

Gorelick PB. Stroke prevention therapy beyond antithrombotics: unifying mechanisms in ischemic stroke pathogenesis and implications for therapy—an invited review. *Stroke* 2002;33:862.

The Homocysteine Studies Collaboration. Homocysteine and risk of ischemic heart disease and stroke. *JAMA* 2002;288:2015–2022.

Johnson SC, Gress DR, Browner WS, et al. Short term prognosis after emergency department diagnosis of TIA. *JAMA* 2000;284:2901.

Mohr JP, Thompson JLP, Lazar RM, et al. A comparison of warfarin and aspirin for the prevention of recurrent ischemic stroke. *N Engl J Med* 2001;345:1444.

The National Institute of Neurological Disorders and Stroke rt-PA Stroke Study Group. Tissue plasminogen activator for acute ischemic stroke. *N Engl J Med* 1995;333:1581.

Report on the Joint Stroke Guideline Development Committee of the American Academy of Neurology and the American Stroke Association (a Division of the American Heart Association). Anticoagulants and antiplatelet agents in acute ischemic stroke. *Neurology* 2002;59:13.

Strauss SE, Majumdar SR, McAlister FA. New evidence for stroke prevention: scientific review. *JAMA* 2002;288: 1388.

Van Walraven C, Hart RG, Singer DE, et al. Oral anticoagulants vs. aspirin in nonvalvular atrial fibrillation: an individual patient meta-analysis. *JAMA* 2002;288:2441.

7

Headache Disorders

Joel R. Saper and Todd D. Rozen

EPIDEMIOLOGY

Primary headache disorders are highly prevalent conditions affecting tens of millions of U.S. citizens and hundreds of millions of individuals worldwide. The lifetime prevalence of common headache disorders can be more than 78%, with migraine prevalence greater than 20% in adult females. The economic and quality-of-life burden of migraine alone is substantial, with the most disabled half of migraine sufferers accounting for more than 90% of migraine-related work loss. Barriers to successful care include failure to properly diagnose, underestimation by both the professional and public domains of the morbidity of these conditions, and denied access to appropriate treatment.

PRIMARY AND SECONDARY HEADACHES

Primary headaches include those in which intrinsic dysfunction of the nervous system, often genetic in origin, predisposes to increased vulnerability to headache attacks. Examples include cluster headache and migraine. Secondary headaches are those in which the headache is secondary to an organic or physiologic process, intracranially or extracranially.

Table 7.1 is a short overview version of the International Headache Society's (IHS) classification of primary headaches. Table 7.2 lists some of the more frequently occurring categories of illnesses that produce secondary headaches.

MIGRAINE

Migraine is a complex neurophysiologic disorder characterized by episodic and progressive forms of head pain in association with numerous neurologic and non-neurologic (autonomic, psychophysiologic) accompaniments. These can precede, accompany, or follow the headache itself.

Migraine is classified into three major subtypes:

1. Migraine with aura—characterized by heralding neurologic events lasting 30 minutes to 1 hour and preceding the head pain attacks (only 20% of migraine attacks). A migraine aura should last longer than 5 minutes and less than 60 minutes. If an aura is consistently less than 5 minutes in duration, then a "secondary aura" should be suspected (arteriovenous malformation, epileptic aura). If an aura lasts longer than 60 minutes in duration, it is termed a "prolonged aura," and an underlying pathology should be ruled out.

TABLE 7.1. *IHS Classification of Primary Headaches*

Episodic migraine
   With aura (including basilar [brainstem] migraine)
   Without aura
Chronic migraine (new IHS criteria)
Cluster headache (episodic/chronic)
Tension-type headache (episodic/chronic)

IHS, International Headache Society.

TABLE 7.2. *Secondary Headache Conditions*

More than 300 conditions can produce secondary headaches. Among the conditions are the following:
   Cerebrovascular/cardiovascular ischemia
   Metabolic disorders
   Intracranial mass lesions
   CSF hypotension/hypertension
   Infectious disorders (systemic, intracranial)
   Endocrine dysfunction
   Cervical (neck) disorders
   Temporomandibular/dental disorders

2. Migraine without aura—in which attacks of migraine and accompaniments occur without clearcut preheadache neurologic symptomatology. This is the most common form of migraine (80%–85%).

3. Chronic migraine—a progressive form of migraine in which intermittent attacks occur at increasing frequency, eventually reaching 15 or more days per month. By definition, chronic migraine occurs on a backdrop of episodic migraine without aura, often accompanied by comorbid neuropsychiatric phenomena. Chronic migraine frequently is associated with medication overuse and "rebound." Comorbid conditions associated with migraine, particularly chronic migraine, include depression, anxiety and panic disorders, bipolar disorder, obsessive-compulsive disorder, character disorders, and perhaps fibromyalgia.

Migraine—Clinical Symptoms

Between 80% and 90% of patients with migraine have a family history. In childhood there is a ratio of 1:1, males to females, but in adulthood a 3:1 female-to-male gender ratio occurs. This is primarily thought to result from the adverse influence on the headache mechanism by estrogen. At older ages, the gender ratio again declines to almost 1:1, suggesting that estrogen is likely to be influential.

Each attack generally lasts between 4 and 72 hours and can be accompanied by a wide range of autonomic and cognitive symptoms. In complex cases, particularly in chronic migraine, a likely association with several neuropsychiatric comorbid disorders, including depression, panic/anxiety syndromes, sleep disturbance, obsessive-compulsive disorder, and others. Predisposed individuals are particularly vulnerable to provocation (triggering) by certain extrinsic and intrinsic events, including hormonal fluctuation, weather changes, certain foods, delayed meals and fasting, extra sleeping time, stress, and others.

TABLE 7.3. *Key Concepts in Migraine Pathogenesis*

Trigeminal-mediated perivascular (neurogenic) inflammation resulting in painful vascular and meningeal tissue

The perivascular release of vasoactive neuropeptides, particularly calcitonin-gene-related-peptide (CGRP)

The development of allodynia and central sensitization as attacks progress

The presence of an active "modulator zone" in the dorsal raphe nucleus of the midbrain during migraine attacks

Activation and threshold reduction of neurons in the descending trigeminal system following C2-C3 cervical stimulation

The deposition of non-heme iron in the brainstem, roughly correlated to increasingly frequent attacks

A yet-to-be-defined relationship to nitrous oxide

Pathophysiology of Migraine

Migraine is a brain disorder that renders the brain "hypersensitive" and overresponsive to a variety of internal and external stimuli. Trigeminal/cervical connections and cervical activation may be important phenomena in the clinical manifestations, pathogenesis, and treatment. The key features of current pathophysiologic understanding are identified in Table 7.3.

TENSION-TYPE HEADACHE

This controversial disorder is classified into both episodic and chronic forms. Episodic forms have certain features that overlap with migraine without aura, although there is a general absence of throbbing pain and autonomic accompaniments. Chronic tension-type headache overlaps in clinical features with chronic migraine. Both forms of tension-type headache may be present in patients who have otherwise typical migraine headaches. Some authorities believe that these disorders are variant forms of migraine.

CHRONIC DAILY HEADACHE

Chronic daily headache is a frequency-based descriptive term that embodies four overlapping clinical subtypes. These include the following:

TABLE 7.4. *Features of Rebound Headache*

Weeks to months of excessive use of abortive
　agents, with usage exceeding 2–3 days per week
Insidious increase of headache frequency
Dependable and predictable headache,
　corresponding to an irresistible escalating use of
　offending agents at regular, predictable intervals
Evidence of psychologic and/or physiologic
　dependency
Failure of alternate acute or preventive medications
　to control headache attacks
Reliable onset of headache within hours to days
following the last dose of symptomatic treatment

1. Chronic migraine, with or without medication overuse
2. Chronic tension-type headache, with or without medication overuse
3. New daily persistent headache—the onset of daily, persistent head pain without the progressive features of chronic migraine but that often is associated with comorbid and medication misuse features
4. Hemicrania continua—unilateral, generally persistent hemicranial discomfort with some features of migraine and cluster headache and that in 20% of cases appears to arise as a consequence of head trauma

REBOUND HEADACHE

Rebound headache (or medication misuse headache) is a self-sustaining headache condition characterized by persisting and recurring headache (usually migraine forms) against a background of chronic, regular use of centrally acting analgesics, ergotamine tartrate, or triptans. The key features of this condition are noted in Table 7.4.

CLUSTER HEADACHE AND ITS VARIANTS

Cluster headache is a relatively rare disorder that affects more men than women in a ratio of 3:1. Current concepts of pathophysiology suggest disturbances within the hypothalamus with relevant involvement of autonomic systems and alterations in melatonin function. Melatonin "fine tunes" endogenous cerebral rhythms and homeostasis.

The clinical features of cluster headache include the presence of headache cycles or bouts (clusters) lasting weeks to months and occurring one or more times per year or less. During these periods, repetitive attacks of short-lasting headache attacks occur daily. Individual attacks of headache last 1 to 3 hours (averaging 45 minutes). The attacks are associated with focal orbital or temporal pain, which is always unilateral; of extremely severe intensity; and accompanied by lacrimation, nasal drainage, pupillary changes, and conjunctival injection. Attacks of headache

TABLE 7.5. *Clinical Features Distinguishing Between Cluster and Migraine Headaches*

Feature	Cluster	Migraine
Location of pain	Always unilateral, periorbital; sometimes occipital referral	Unilateral and bilateral
Age at onset (typical)	Onset 20 years or older	10–50 years (can be younger or older)
Gender difference	Majority male	Majority female in adulthood
Time of day	Frequently at night, often same time each day	Any time
Frequency of attacks	1–6 per day	1–10 per month in episodic form
Duration of pain	30–120 min	4–72 hours
Prodromes	None	Often present
Nausea and vomiting	20%	85%
Blurring of vision	Infrequent	Frequent
Lacrimation	Frequent	Infrequent
Nasal congestion/drainage	70%	Uncommon
Ptosis	30%	1–2%
Polyuria	2%	40%
Family history of similar headaches	7%	90%
Miosis	50%	Absent
Behavior during attack	Pacing and agitation	Resting in quiet, dark room

TABLE 7.6. *Trigeminal Autonomic Cephalgias*

Cluster headache
Chronic and episodic paroxysmal hemicrania
SUNCT syndrome (short-lasting unilateral
neuralgiaform pain with conjunctival injection and
tearing)
Cluster-tic syndrome (the association of cluster head
ache with trigeminal neuralgia symptomatology)

commonly occur during sleeping times or napping and can be provoked by ingestion of alcohol or nitroglycerin. It is interesting that a high likelihood of blue or hazel-colored eyes; ruddy, rugged, lionized facial features; and a long history of smoking and excessive alcohol intake characterize the majority of men with cluster headache. Table 7.5 lists the clinical distinctions between cluster headache and migraine.

Cluster headache may occur in its episodic form (bouts or cycles of recurring headaches followed by a period of no headache [remission], lasting weeks to years) or in a chronic form without an interim period, with headache attacks daily for years without interruption. Treatment differences may exist.

In addition to cluster headache, several short-lasting headache entities are recognized and currently are classified with cluster headache in a category referred to as the trigeminal autonomic cephalgias. These disorders are characterized primarily by the presence of short-lasting headaches of variable duration—seconds (short-lasting unilateral neuralgiform headaches with conjunctival injection and tearing [SUNCT]) to 3 hours (cluster headache). The attacks are associated with autonomic features. Table 7.6 lists the current members of the trigeminal autonomic cephalgia group.

TREATMENT OF PRIMARY HEADACHES AND RELATED PHENOMENA

The following represent the key principles in the approach to treatment of headaches and related phenomena. These key treatment principles include the following:

- Diagnosing the specific primary headache entity
- Determining attack frequency and severity
- Establishing the presence or absence of comorbid illnesses (e.g., psychiatric, neurologic, medical)
- Identifying confounding factors, including external or internal phenomena, such as the following:
  Rebound
  Psychologic, comorbid illnesses, and medication factors (e.g., estrogen replacement, nitroglycerin)
  Hormonal disturbances
  Use of or exposure to toxic substances
  Other
- Identifying previous treatment successes and failures

Treatment Modalities

Numerous treatment modalities are available (Table 7.7). Nonpharmacologic treatments can be very helpful, particularly when combined with pharmacologic therapy. Behavioral modification, biofeedback, exercise, and dietary manipulation add a dimension of help beyond the administration of medications and also provide patients with a method of helping themselves. Pharmacologic therapy provides the essential treatment for the majority of patients with primary headache. Increasing attention has focused on the important contribution that interventional treatment may provide patients with primary headache. Occipital nerve blocks, although not reversing the primary problem, can be particularly useful for symptomatic treatment.

TABLE 7.7. *Therapeutic Categories of Treatment for Primary Headache*

Nonpharmacologic treatment
Pharmacologic treatment (acute and preventive)
Interventional procedures, including the following:
Neuroblockade (nerve, facet, epidural space)
Radiofrequency and cryolysis procedures
Implantations and stimulation
Others
Hospital/rehabilitational programs

Nonpharmacologic Treatments for Primary Headaches

A variety of factors related to health, habits, and education can assist patients with headache. Education on headache triggers and eliminating headache-producing behaviors can be essential. Reduction of medication use and the treatment of rebound provide a fundamental and critical element to the treatment of patients with chronic headache when medication overuse phenomena exist. Discontinuing smoking, establishing regular eating and sleeping patterns, and getting regular exercise are reported as helpful by many patients with headache. Biofeedback and behavioral treatment, together with cognitive behavioral therapy, may be of value in many cases. Formal psychotherapy is helpful in individual cases.

Treatment of Rebound

Rebound headache (or medication overuse headache) requires treatment because continued use of the medication renders patients refractory to effective treatment. Outpatient and inpatient strategies are available, depending on the intensity of medication usage and the characteristics of the case. Table 7.8 identifies important principles in the approach to the treatment of rebound or medication overuse headache.

Rebound headaches, which most likely result from chronic changes to receptors, must be distinguished from headaches resulting from toxic substances or other exposure to

TABLE 7.8. *Principles in Treating Rebound Headache*

Discontinuation of offending agent (taper if contain opioid or barbiturate)
Aggressive treatment of resulting severe "withdrawal" headache
Hydration, including intravenous fluids and support in severe cases (treat nausea)
The development of pharmacologic prophylaxis
Implementation of behavioral therapies
Use of outpatient infusion or hospitalization techniques for advanced and severe conditions

agents or drugs. These have a direct provocative influence.

Pharmacologic Treatment of Migraine

The pharmacologic treatment of headache involves the use of abortive (acute) and preventive medications. Abortive treatments are used to terminate evolving or existing attacks. Preventive treatment is implemented to reduce the frequency of attacks and prevent overuse of acute medications. Most patients require combination treatment. Preemptive treatment is a short-term preventive course of therapy used in anticipation of a predictable event, such as a menstrual period, or vacation-related headache. The wide variety of pharmacologic agents used in headache management and clinical information regarding their use are listed in Table 7.9.

Acute Treatment of Migraine

There are numerous agents used for the acute treatment of migraine. Some agents, such as analgesics, are of general value for pain, whereas others, such as the ergots and triptan medications, are specific and influence receptor and transmitter systems thought to be relevant to migraine pathogenesis. Table 7.10 lists the various categories of abortive agents.

The triptans represent narrow-spectrum, receptor-specific (serotonin [5-HT$_1$]) agonists that stimulate the 5-HT$_1$ receptors to reduce neurogenic inflammation. The ergot derivatives are broader spectrum agents, affecting the serotoninergic receptors and also alpha-adrenergic and dopamine receptors (and others). Whereas many patients respond well to the triptans, others appear to require the broader influence of ergot derivatives. Experienced clinicians are adept at administering several of the triptans as well as the ergots. Short-acting, rapidly effective triptans include almotriptan, sumatriptan, rizatriptan, zolmitriptan, and eletriptan, whereas naratriptan and frovatriptan have the longest half-lives. Several delivery formats are available in addi-

TABLE 7.9. *Selected Drugs Used in the Pharmacotherapy of Head, Neck, and Face Pain*[a]

Drug Name	Mg/Dose	Standard Daily Admin.	Notes
SYMPTOMATIC DRUGS			
ANALGESICS			
**Excedrin	—	Varies	Avoid more than 2 days/wk of use
NSAIDs			
**Naproxen sodium (p.o.)	275–550	bid–tid	Avoid extended, daily use
Indomethacin (p.o.)	25–50	bid–tid	"
Indocin SR (p.o.)	75	1 q day or bid	"
Indomethacin (p.r.)	50	bid–tid	"
Meclofenamate (p.o.)	50–200	bid	"
**Ibuprofen (p.o.)	600–800	bid–tid	"
Ketorolac (p.o.)	10	qid	"
Ketorolac (IM)	30	tid	" Appears particularly valuable when ergot derivatives & narcotics must be avoided and parenteral therapy is necessary. No more than occasional, short-term use is advisable because of renal toxicity, most likely in predisposed patients
SPECIAL MIGRAINE DRUGS			
**Isometheptene combinations (Midrin, etc.)	—	2 caps at onset, 1–2 q 30–60 min	Max 5–6 caps/day; 2 days/wk
**Ergotamine tartrate (ET) Oral (Cafergot, Wigraine, etc.)	1 mg ET, 100 mg caffeine	2 tabs at onset, 1–2 q 30–60 min	Max 4–6/day; 2 days/wk
Suppositories (Cafergot, Wigraine)	2 mg ET, 100 mg caffeine	½–1 at onset; may repeat in 60 min	Max 2/day; 2 days/wk
Sublingual (Ergomar, Ergostat)	2 mg ET	1 at onset; may repeat after 15 min	Max 2/day; 2 days/wk
**Dihydroergotamine (DHE) IM/IV	0.25–1.0	0.25–1 mg SC, IM, IV tid 0.25–1 mg SC, IM, IV tid	Can be used 2–3 ×/day in conjunction with antinauseant, analgesic, etc. IM more effective than SC
**DHE Nasal Spray	1	1 spray each nostril (½ mg/spray). Repeat in 15 min (4 sprays=2 mg)	Use no more than 2–3 ×/wk, on separate days
**Sumatriptan (parenteral)	6 SC	May repeat in 1 hr	Cannot be used within 24 hrs of ergotamine-related meds or other triptans; should not be used in presence of cardiovascular and/or cerebrovascular, severe hypertension, Prinzmetal angina, or peripheral vascular disorders. No more than 2 doses in 24 hrs. Limit 2 days/wk usage. Do not take within 2 weeks of MAOI discontinuation
**Sumatriptan (oral)	25–100	Take at HA onset; may repeat at 2 hrs; max 100 mg/day	"
**Sumatriptan (nasal spray)	5 or 20	1 spray in 1 nostril only; may repeat in 2 hrs; max 40 mg/24 hrs	"

Continued

TABLE 7.9. *Continued*

Drug Name	Mg/Dose	Standard Daily Admin.	Notes
**Zolmitriptan (oral)	2.5–5	1 at onset; may repeat in 2 hrs; max 10 mg/24 hrs	"
**Zolmitriptan (ZMT)	"	"	"
**Naratriptan (oral)	2.5	1 at onset; may repeat in 4 hrs; max 5 mg/24 hrs	"
**Rizatriptan (oral)	5–10	1 at onset; may repeat in 2 hrs; max 30 mg/24 hrs	"
**Rizatriptan (MLT)	"	"	"
**Almotriptan	12.5	1 at onset; may repeat; max 25 mg/24 hrs	"
**Frovatriptan	2.5	1 at onset; may repeat after 6–8 hrs; max 7.5 mg/24 hrs	"
**Eletriptan	20–40	1 at onset of HA; may repeat if necessary after 2 hrs	The above & because metabolized by the cytochrome P-450 hepatic enzyme 3A4, it should not be used with cimetidine, diltiazam, nicardipine, verapamil, or fluoxetine
**Valproic acid intravenously	250–750	1 to 3 dosages/day IV	See valproic acid discussion in Prevention section of this table
ANTINAUSEANTS/NEUROLEPTICS			
Chlorpromazine (p.o.)	25–100	bid–tid	Limit 3 days/wk, except for persistent nausea; avoid extended use. Monitor for hypotension & cardiac rhythm effects (QT interval)
(supp)	25–100	bid–tid	"
(IM)	25–100	bid–tid	"
(IV)	2.5–10	bid–tid	"
Metoclopramide (p.o.—tablet & syrup)	10–20	tid	"
(parenteral)	10	tid	"
Promethazine (p.o.)	25–75	tid	Limit 3 days/wk, except for persistent nausea; avoid extended use. Monitor for hypotension & cardiac rhythm effects (QT interval)
(IM)	25–75	tid	"
Perphenazine (p.o.)	4–8	bid–tid	"
(IM)	5	bid	"
ANTIHISTAMINES			
Hydroxyzine (p.o., IM)	25–75	bid–tid or at hs	Can be used as a symptomatic or preventive treatment
Cyproheptadine (p.o.)	2–4	tid–qid	"
Diphenhydramine (IM, IV)	25–50	1 to 3 dosages per day	Used essentially as acute, abortive agent
STEROIDS			
Prednisone (p.o.)	40–60	In 1 or divided doses	4–10 day program. Avoid repeated use
PREVENTIVE DRUGS (avoid sustained use for more than 6 mo w/o trial reduction)			
TRICYCLIC ANTIDEPRESSANTS			
Amitriptyline	10–150	Divided doses or hs	Bedtime dose aids sleep disturbance
Nortriptyline	10–100	"	"

Drug	Dose	Frequency	Notes
Doxepin	10–150		"
OTHER ANTIDEPRESSANTS			
Fluoxetine	20	20–80 mg/day in divided dose	Actual efficacy for HA uncertain. Administer with care to pts using lipophilic beta blockers (propranolol, metoprolol, etc.) or switch to hydrophilic beta blockers such as nadolol. Value for HA of numerous other antidepressants under investigation
Others (SSRIs, etc.)			
MAO INHIBITORS			
Phenelzine	15–30	15–90 mg/day in divided dose	Dietary & medication restrictions mandatory
BETA-ADRENERGIC BLOCKERS			
**Propranolol	20–50	tid–qid (standard dose)	Monitor cardiac function, BP, pulse, lipids
Atenolol	50–100	bid	"
**Timolol	10–20	bid	"
Metoprolol	50–100	bid	"
Nadolol	20–120	bid	"
CALCIUM CHANNEL ANTAGONISTS			
Verapamil	80–160	tid–qid	Monitor cardiac function, BP, pulse, lipids; eliminated by kidneys
Nimodipine	30–60	tid	Monitor cardiac function, BP, pulse
Diltiazem	30–90	tid	"
ERGOTAMINE DERIVATIVES			
**Methysergide	1–2	tid–5 ×/day	After 6 months of tx, review cardiac, pulmonary, & retroperitoneal regions for fibrotic changes. Carefully observe contraindications
Methylergonovine	0.2–0.4	tid–qid	"
ANTICONVULSANTS			
**Valproic acid	125–500	1–2 g/day in divided doses	Monitor hepatic, metabolic (platelets), & metabolic parameters carefully. Consider dose reduction when used w/antidepressants, lithium, verapamil, phenothiazines, benzodiazepines, other anticonvulsants. Observe warnings carefully; avoid using with barbiturates and perhaps benzodiazepines.
**Valproic acid (ER)	250–1000	500 mg–1 g/day, once per day dosing	"
Valproic acid (IV)	250–750	1 to 3 dosages/day IV	"
Carbamazepine	100–200	300–1200 mg/day in divided doses	Monitor hepatic & metabolic parameters carefully. Consider dose reduction when used w/anticonvulsants, lithium, verapamil, phenothiazines. Observe warnings carefully. Reduces oral contraceptive efficacy.
Gabapentin	100–400	1800–3600 mg/day	May cause agitation & other CNS AEs
Topiramate	25–50	25 mg bid, tapered slowly to 100–200 mg/day	Sedation, cognitive impairment, tingling, abdominal cramps, & risk for renal stones are limiting features. Liver function disturbances, acute myopia, and closed angle glaucoma (in 1st month) require careful monitoring & immediate discontinuation. Weight loss may occur.
OTHERS			
Baclofen	10–20	tid–qid	Increase & decrease dose slowly & allow tolerance to develop; taper when discontinuing.

Continued

95

TABLE 7.9. *Continued*

Drug Name	Mg/Dose	Standard Daily Admin.	Notes
Tizanidine	2–8	2–8 mg tid or prn; max dose 32–36 mg/day	May be used as abortive or preventive agent. Sedation, hypotension, liver function disturbances must be considered & monitored. Careful use with other alpha-adrenergic agonist agents, such as clonidine and with hepatotoxic agents is recommended. Max dose is 36 mg/day.
Lithium	150–300	bid–tid	Reduce dose in conjunction with verapamil, other calcium channel antagonists, & NSAIDs; monitor metabolic parameters
Oxygen inhalation	100% O$_2$ w/mask	7 liters/min for 10–15 min	Must be used at onset of attack of cluster HA; avoid around extreme heat or flame, such as cigarettes
**Stadol Nasal Spray (butorphanol)	1 mg/spray; max use 2 dose days/wk		Useful for acute migraine but important side effects. Dependency & addictive potential significant. Avoid in pts with addictive or obsessive drug-taking patterns or hx of drug overdose. Avoid in pts with daily or almost daily HA. Withdrawal symptoms can be severe
Botulinum toxin	Uncertain	Uncertain	At this time controlled studies have not firmly established efficacy in headache
Melatonin	3–15	Usually at h.s.	Its value in cluster headache is currently tentative but promising; risks in asthma & vasoconstrictive diseases remain to be defined

^{a}Few of the medications listed in this table are either approved specifically for headache or have been shown by controlled studies to be effective for headache. Their inclusion reflects that they have been recommended from various sources as possibly useful for the treatment of some cases of headache. Those drugs that have been approved by the FDA for the treatment of migraine, cluster headache, or tension-type headache are designated by **.

Modified with permission from Saper, et al., *Handbook of Headache Management*, Lippincott Williams & Wilkins, 1999.

TABLE 7.10. *Categories of Medications Used in the Treatment of Migraine*

Simple and combined analgesics (acetaminophen, Excedrin, nonsteroidal antiinflammatory drugs, and others)

Mixed analgesics (barbiturate and simple analgesics, such as aspirin ± acetaminophen, ± caffeine)—often avoided because of the likelihood of dependency and misuse

Ergot derivatives, including dihydroergotamine

Triptan medications, including the following:
  Sumatriptan
  Naratriptan
  Almotriptan
  Rizatriptan
  Zolmitriptan
  Frovatriptan
  Eletriptan

tion to tablets: injection (sumatriptan), nasal spray (sumatriptan and zolmitriptan), and rapidly dissolving forms (zolmitriptan and rizatriptan).

Patients who have not responded to less potent medications require triptans or ergots for maximum benefit. It is imperative that the triptans, and probably the ergot derivatives as well, be administered to patients in the early phases of an ensuing headache attack to bring about maximum benefit and reduce the possibility of recurrence (the return of headache within the same 24-hour period). It is important that clinicians encourage patients to take these medications early, unless patients have a history of medication overuse or would unreasonably anticipate an attack, thus increasing the potential for medication misuse.

Acute medications are used in conjunction with antinauseants and in combination with each other for maximum efficiency (do not combine ergots and triptans). Clinicians must be familiar with important contraindications and safety warnings of each of these medication groups as well as adverse effects and influence on hepatic metabolism, particularly when these drugs are used in combination with others.

Finally, for reasons that are not fully understood but perhaps related to the cervical/trigeminal connections, occipital nerve blocks may relieve acute migraine attacks in some

individuals. This method has been used historically by anesthesiologists but is increasingly used by neurologists and others treating headache. Long-term value is rare, but short-term relief frequently is seen.

Preventive Treatment of Migraine

Many agents are available for the prevention of migraine. However, the clinician must determine when preventive pharmacotherapy should be introduced. Table 7.11 lists certain clinical guidelines that can be used to make this determination.

The categories of medications useful in prevention are listed in Table 7.12. A wide range of therapies is available, and increasingly useful are those that appear to work on specific neurotransmitter systems. The reader will note that several of these categories do not relate to vasculature or blood flow, suggesting that the primary pathogenesis of migraine seems more likely to involve neuronal rather than vascular dynamics.

Tricyclic antidepressants and beta blockers are well-established, firstline medications for preventive treatment of migraine in those patients who do not have contraindications or restrictions to either medication. Calcium channel blockers are generally not as effective. The anticonvulsants have considerable value and are particularly useful in the presence of neuropsychiatric comorbidities or other conditions, such as seizures or bipolar disorders, which might accompany migraine.

TABLE 7.11. *Guidelines for Determining the Need for Preventive Treatment*

1. Disability from migraine headaches (loss of time at work or at home)
2. Migraine headaches occur two or more days per week
3. Patient is overusing acute medication (analgesic rebound headache)
4. Risk of permanent neurologic dysfunction because of the headache condition (hemiplegic migraine, migraine with prolonged aura)
5. Acute medications are contraindicated or ineffective
6. Patient preference, provided clinical justification exists

TABLE 7.12. *Categories of Preventive Medications*

Tricyclic antidepressants (particularly amitriptyline, nortriptyline, and doxepin)
Beta-adrenergic blockers (particularly propranolol and nadolol)
Calcium channel blockers (verapamil)
Anticonvulsants (valproic acid, gabapentin, topiramate)
Ergot derivatives (methylergonovine and methysergide)
Monoamine oxidase inhibitors (for refractory cases)
Others
   Selective serotonin reuptake inhibitors
   Neuroleptics
   Tizanidine
   Botulinum toxin?
   Riboflavin

The selective serotonin reuptake inhibitors are helpful for neuropsychiatric comorbidities, such as depression and panic and anxiety disorders, but generally do not have a strong antimigraine influence. Some patients with migraine-related headaches benefit from the antidopaminergic influence of the new neuroleptics, although the potential for adverse effects limits their widespread use. Tizanidine, an alpha-adrenergic agonist, has been shown to be effective in an adjunctive, preventive role. Botulinum toxin is increasingly administered for the prevention of migraine. Numerous uncontrolled studies support efficacy, but there is a paucity of controlled data at this time. If botulinum toxin is shown to work for migraine, it is likely to work through a central mechanism and not through a primary muscular influence.

The treatment of chronic migraine is similar to that of episodic migraine. Treatment is directed at both the daily or almost daily pain and periodic attacks. Because of the likely presence of a progressive course, medication overuse, and neuropsychiatric comorbidities in this population, a more comprehensive approach beyond medications alone is required. This includes cognitive behavioral therapy and other forms of psychotherapy and family therapy. Organic illness must be ruled out with appropriate testing in patients with frequent or daily headache and in those with neurologic findings.

TABLE 7.13. *Acute Treatment of Cluster Headache*

Oxygen inhalation (8–10 L/min 100% oxygen via non-rebreather face mask)
Triptans/ergot (avoid more than 2 usage days per week)—best efficacy is with sumatriptan injectable
Indomethacin, which is occasionally useful

Treatment of Cluster Headache

Cluster headache responds and is treated differently than migraine. Because cluster headache attacks generally occur numerous times daily (1–8), the use of abortive medications is limited to only a few agents that are safe for such frequent use. Unlike migraine, preventive therapy is necessary for cluster headache unless the typical cluster cycle is 2 weeks in duration or less.

Acute Treatment of Cluster Headache

Table 7.9 describes in detail agents used in the acute and preventive treatment of cluster headache. Table 7.13 lists the agents useful in the acute management of cluster headache, which is limited by the need to use medications up to several times a day when effective preventive treatment is not available or has not yet become effective.

Preventive Treatment of Cluster Headache

Table 7.14 lists the available preventive agents for cluster headache. The most reliable agents for prevention are the steroids, but because of their inherent risks with long-term usage, they are inappropriate except in transi-

TABLE 7.14. *Preventive Treatment of Cluster Headache*

Verapamil (120–160 mg tid–qid)
Lithium
Divalproex/topiramate
Melatonin 6–15 mg h.s.
7-day prednisone burst (steroids generally are effective for cluster headache prevention, and short-term trials can be dramatically effective, but risks limit utility)
Ergot derivatives (methylergonovine/methysergide)

TABLE 7.15. *Recommended 7-Day Prednisone Program (5 mg. Tablets—Dispense 60 Tablets)*

Day	Breakfast		Lunch	Dinner
	(mg)	(mg)	(mg)	(mg)
1	20 (4 pills)		20	20
2	20	20	20	
3	20		15 (3 pills)	15
4	15	15	10 (2 pills)	
5	10	10	10	
6	10		5 (1 pill)	5
7	5	5		

TABLE 7.16. *Diagnostic Testing*

Physical examination
Metabolic evaluation
  Hematologic
  ESR/CRP
  Endocrinologic
  Chemistry
  Toxicology (drug screens)
Standard x-rays
Neuroimaging
  CT
  MRI/MRA/MRV
  Arteriography
Dental and otologic examination
Lumbar puncture
Diagnostic blockades
Cardiac ultrasound (PFO, etc.)

ESR, erythrocyte sedimentation rate; CRP, C-reactive protein; MRV, magnetic resonance venography.

tional regimens. Steroids can be used, for example, at the onset of treatment while other preventive agents are being titrated upward; during particularly vulnerable times, such as when traveling; or when other medications are in transition. Table 7.15 lists a recommended prednisone protocol.

For intractable cases, hospitalization is recommended. In some cases surgical intervention is required, but surgical treatment is limited because of the likelihood of postsurgical painful sequelae. Occipital nerve injection is effective in treating some acute attacks, and subcutaneous occipital stimulation has been reported as anecdotally effective.

Treatment of Other Primary Headache Disorders

Chronic paroxysmal hemicrania (CPH) and episodic paroxysmal hemicrania (EPH), as well as hemicrania continua, are characteristically sensitive to treatment with indomethacin at a dose of 25 to 50 mg three times a day. SUNCT syndrome may respond to lamotrigine, topiramate, or gabapentin.

DIAGNOSTIC TESTING AND SECONDARY HEADACHE DISORDERS

More than 300 entities may produce symptoms of headache, many of which mimic the primary headache disorders. The clinician has the burden of ruling in and ruling out potentially relevant conditions in patients with re-curring or persistent headache. Diagnostic testing includes a wide range of studies, including the investigation of metabolic, endocrinologic, toxic, dental, traumatic, cervical, and infectious disorders and space-occupying lesions. Disturbances of cerebrospinal fluid (CSF) pressure, ischemic disease, and allergic conditions must be considered. Table 7.16 lists diagnostic tests that are among those that should be considered in intractable or variant cases.

Important specific conditions to consider include those of the temporomandibular or dental structures, sphenoid sinuses (must specifically image and evaluate for sphenoid sinus disease), carotid and vertebral dissection syndromes, cerebral venous occlusion, and cardiac abnormalities (PFO, etc.).

Because of the relevance of the cervical spine to the descending trigeminal system and headache physiology (trigeminal cervical connection), disturbances at the level of the upper cervical spine and its nerves and joints have become important targets for the treatment of otherwise pharmacologically resistant headaches. Premature or excessive use of interventional procedures is unwarranted, but when selective and expertly administered, they clearly have a role in the overall spectrum of diagnosis and treatment for headache conditions. Treatments such as implantable stimulators are on the horizon.

REFERRAL AND HOSPITALIZATION

It is advisable to refer patients with intractable headache to specialists, specialized clinics, and tertiary centers. Hospitalization is required for many complex patients whose medication misuse or the presence of intractable pain and behavioral/neuropsychiatric symptomatology has reached an intensity and complexity that makes outpatient therapy no longer appropriate. Aggressive and thorough diagnostic assessment is mandatory either to rule out organic, toxic, or physiologic illness or to define unrecognized provocative factors.

Hospitalization

Patients with intractable headache can respond to the more aggressive therapeutic environment and milieu in specialty inpatient programs when outpatient therapy has failed to establish efficacy. Table 7.17 lists the criteria that can be used when hospitalization is considered.

The principles of hospitalization include hospitalization for acute and prolonged headache is a complex undertaking because it must address not only the refractoriness of the symptoms, the often-present confounding influence of medication overuse headache (rebound), but the behavioral and psychological factors that often influence these dilemmas. Discontinuation of medication and the weaning process bring with them a predictable escalation of headache and the emotional factors that are characteristic to that patient. The principles of hospitalization are listed in Table 7.18.

TABLE 7.18. *Principles of Inpatient Care*

Interrupt daily/intractable headache pain with parenteral protocols
Discontinue offending analgesic medications if rebound is present
Implement preventive pharmacotherapy
Identify effective abortive therapy
Treat behavioral and neuropsychiatric comorbidities
Use interventional modalities when indicated
Educate
Discharge and perform outpatient planning

Hospitalization length of stay varies, depending on the intensity and type of medication that is overused and that requires discontinuation, the amount of pain and its duration during this weaning process, the behavioral issues that emerge, and the confounding factors that often are present in patients with these symptoms. Developing a preventive treatment during this time is difficult because it takes time for medications to work and because generally patients are in a refractory period that may last up to weeks to months after discontinuation of the offending agents. Readers are encouraged to refer patients with complex and intense headache problems to specialists and/or referral centers, which can address more effectively the many issues that arise and have experience in using multiple medication and behavioral regimens simultaneously.

A variety of parenteral agents can be used during hospitalization to control attacks, particularly during rebound withdrawal (Table 7.19). These protocols also can be used for emergency department treatment of acute episodic migraine.

TABLE 7.17. *Criteria for Hospitalization*

Symptoms are severe and refractory to outpatient treatment.
Symptoms are accompanied by drug overuse (dependency) or toxicity not treatable as an outpatient.
Intensity of neuropsychiatric and behavioral comorbidity renders outpatient treatment ineffective.
Confounding medical illness is present.
Treatment urgency in a desperate patient is present.

TABLE 7.19. *Parenteral Regimens to Treat Intractable Headaches*

Dihydroergotamine (0.25–1.0 mg IV or IM, tid)
Diphenhydramine (25–50 mg IV or IM, tid)
Various neuroleptics (i.e., chlorpromazine 2.5–10 mg IV, tid)
Ketorolac (10 mg IV, tid; 30 mg IM tid)
Valproic acid (250–1,000 mg IV, tid)
Magnesium sulfate (1 g IV, bid)

IV, intravenous; IM, intramuscular.

When to Use Opioids

Experience and evidence support the avoidance of sustained opioid administration in the chronic headache population. Use in acute situations when other treatments are contraindicated remains appropriate, but dose and amounts of prescriptions should be limited and monitored carefully to avoid misuse. Sustained opioid administration can be considered in the following limited circumstances:

When all else fails, following a full range of advanced services, including detoxification
When standard agents are contraindicated
In the elderly or during pregnancy

Experience suggests that, although some patients with difficult headache problems respond to sustained opioid therapy, there is significant risk for untoward reactions and confounding of the already complex problem. It is my belief that sustained opioid therapy for intractable headache should not be started on a primary care level but that patients who do not respond to standard treatment should be referred to specialists and/or centers where more complex regimens of treatment can be imposed, where rebound can be treated most effectively, and where psychological influences on headache refractoriness can be most effectively addressed.

Except in the elderly or during pregnancy, patients should be refractory to aggressive and creative therapies before opioids are administered regularly. Nearly 75% of refractory patients placed on daily opioids fail to gain effective control. Approximately one-half of those maintained on opioids demonstrated noncompliant drug-related behavior. Despite reports of pain reduction, a major improvement in function was not noted in a significant percentage of patients.

SUGGESTED READING

Argoff CE. A focused review of the use of botulinum toxins for neuropathic pain. *Clin J Pain* 2002;18:S177–S181.

Bartsch T, Goadsby PJ. Stimulation of the greater occipital nerve (GON) enhances responses of dural responsive convergent neurons in the trigeminal cervical complex in the rat. *Cephalalgia* 2001;21:401–402.

Boes CJ, Dodick DW. Refining the clinical spectrum of chronic paroxysmal hemicrania: a review of 74 patients. *Headache* 2002;42:699–708.

Burstein RH, Cutrer FM, Yarnitsky D. The development of cutaneous allodynia during a migraine attack. *Brain* 2000;123:1703–1709.

Ferrari MD, Roon KL, Lipton RB, et al. Oral triptans (serotonin 5-HT[1b/1d] agonist) in acute migraine treatment: a meta-analysis of 53 trials. *Lancet* 2001;358:1668–1675.

Goadsby PJ, Lipton RB, Ferrari MD. Migraine—current understanding and treatment. *N Engl J Med* 2002;246:257–270.

Goadsby PJ. Short-lasting primary headaches: Focus on trigeminal autonomic cephalgias and indomethacin-sensitive headaches. *Curr Opin Neurol* 1999;12:273–277.

Lake AE III, Saper JR, Madden SF, et al. Comprehensive inpatient treatment for intractable migraine: a prospective long-term outcome study. *Headache* 1993;33:55–62.

Limmroth V, Katsarav AZ, Fritsche G, et al. Features in medication overuse headache following overuse of different acute headache drugs. *Neurol* 2002;59:1011–1014.

Nixdorf DR, Heo G, Major PW. Randomized control trial of botulism toxin A for chronic myogenous orofacial pain. *Pain* 2002;99:465–473.

Olesen J. Classification and diagnostic criteria for headache disorders, cranial neuralgias, and headache pain. *Cephalalgia* 1988;8(supp)7:1–96.

Olesen J, Tfelt-Hansen P, Welch KMA, eds. *The headaches,* 2nd ed. Philadelphia: Lippincott Williams & Wilkins, 2000.

Peres MF, Rozen TD. Melatonin in the preventive treatment of chronic cluster headache. *Cephalalgia* 2001;21:993–995.

Saper JR. Chronic daily headache: a clinician's perspective. *Headache* 2002;42:538.

Saper JR. What matters is not the differences between triptans, but the differences between patients. *Arch Neurol* 2001;58(9):1481–1482.

Saper JR, Lake AE III. Borderline personality disorder and the chronic headache patient: review and management recommendations. *Headache* 2002;42:663–674.

Saper JR, Lake AE III, Hamel RL, et al. Long-term scheduled opioid treatment for intractable headache: 3-year outcome report. *Cephalalgia* 2000;20:380.

Saper JR, Lake AE III, Madden SF, et al. Comprehensive/tertiary care for headache: a 6-month outcome study. *Headache* 1999;39:249–263.

Saper JR, Silberstein SD, et al. *Handbook of headache management,* 2nd ed. Philadelphia: Lippincott Williams & Wilkins, 1999.

Silberstein SD. Practice parameter: Evidenced-based guidelines for migraine headache (an evidence-based review): Report of the Quality Standards Subcommittee of the American Academy of Neurology. *Neurol* 2000;55:754–762.

Silberstein SD, Lipton RB, Dalessio DJ, eds. *Wolff's headache and other head pain,* 7th ed. New York: Oxford University Press, 2001.

Weiller CA, May A, Limmroth V, et al. Brainstem activation and spontaneous human migraine attacks. *Nat Med* 1995;1:658–660.

Welch KM, et al. Periaqueductal gray matter dysfunction in migraine: cause or the burden of illness. *Headache* 2001;41:629–637.

8

Epilepsy

Donna C. Bergen

A tonic–clonic or grand mal seizure may occur singly and acutely at any time of life as a result of trauma, metabolic disturbances, stroke, alcohol withdrawal, substance abuse, or other causes. Approximately 6% of the population have an afebrile seizure at some point in their lives. The recurring seizures of the chronic disorder called epilepsy also may begin at any time of life and include various other types of attacks. The prevalence of epilepsy in the United States is about 0.5%, making it one of the most common neurologic disorders. Incidence across the lifespan is a U-shaped curve, with the first year of life and old age being the most common times for epilepsy to start.

Epilepsy is a disorder primarily of the cerebral cortex, with seizures occurring when populations of neurons discharge in abnormal patterns. The pathophysiology of epileptic disorders is not well understood and no doubt varies depending on seizure type and epilepsy syndrome (see later in this chapter). Some of the genetically determined epilepsies, for example, have been shown to be the result of channelopathies or structural abnormalities of neurotransmitter receptors. Animal models of focal epilepsies, however, suggest that glial proliferation, loss of inhibitory neuronal activity, cortical remodeling, excessive excitatory activity, and other chronic cortical changes all may play a part in producing an epileptogenic focus.

TYPES OF SEIZURES

The diagnosis of epilepsy is made on the basis of the clinical history of the seizures taken from the patient and often from a witness. The prototypical seizure, the tonic–clonic seizure (previously called grand mal seizure), often starts with sudden loss of consciousness, with the patient falling stiffly (the tonic phase); this is followed by rhythmic jerking of the limbs and torso (the clonic phase), which slows and then stops abruptly. Such seizures usually last only 60 to 90 seconds. The patient awakens after a period of postictal stupor, which usually lasts less than 15 minutes, but confusion may persist considerably longer. Such seizures coincide with very rapid, abnormal cortical and subcortical neuronal activity, which is recruited so rapidly that it appears synchronously in all brain areas when recorded on an electroencephalogram (EEG).

Obvious physical stresses and physiologic abnormalities may accompany these attacks, including apnea, hypoxemia, acidosis, and autonomic disruptions such as cardiac arrhythmias and hypertension. Pulmonary edema may occur and may play a role in the syndrome of sudden death that occurs occasionally even in young, otherwise healthy patients with epilepsy. Other physical complications may include dislocation of the shoulder, vertebral collapse, and aspiration pneumonia.

Focal or partial seizures begin in a localized cortical area, with the ictal phenomena being determined by the brain region involved. For example, seizures beginning with abnormal neuronal activity in primary motor cortex may cause initial twitching of the face or limb, depending on the exact site of onset. The patient with an occipital focus may report flashing lights or globes, often in the visual field contralateral to the focus. The more common temporal lobe focus produces autonomic symptoms such as nausea or complex experiences such as intense feelings of familiarity (déjà vu) or feelings of strangeness. Such recalled seizure onsets commonly are called auras; they are not the warnings of seizures but the beginnings of the seizures themselves. Focal seizures that end without impairment of consciousness are termed simple partial seizures. The duration of such attacks is generally 30 to 60 seconds.

Whether they begin with an aura or with sudden loss of awareness, focal seizures that impair consciousness are called complex partial seizures. A witness typically reports that the patient stares and becomes unreactive. Falls are uncommon, and the patient may carry out simple motor activities such as picking at the clothes, walking about, or most typically smacking the lips. Complex partial seizures also last about a minute and may or may not be followed by postictal confusion. Either the simple or the complex partial seizure may spread throughout the brain, developing into a typical tonic–clonic seizure.

There are also less dramatic seizure types, many occurring more commonly in children than in adults.

An *absence seizure* (previously called petit mal seizure) refers to a brief episode of loss of awareness. It occurs without warning, lasts for a few seconds, and ends with immediate resumption of consciousness. The patient usually stops what he is doing; the eyes remain open or may blink rapidly, but the patient does not fall. Absences may occur many times per day. Patients often are unaware of them, and they commonly are noted first by family members or teachers.

Another brief seizure type is the *myoclonic seizure*, which consists of sudden single or repetitive jerks of the limbs without warning. The myoclonic seizure occurs without warning and generally lasts only a few seconds. Consciousness sometimes is impaired, but like the absence seizure, the myoclonic seizure is followed by immediate return to full awareness without a postictal state.

Less common are the brief *atonic* or *akinetic seizures*, which consist of sudden falls without warning, sometimes with loss of consciousness. Although brief, these seizures can be very dangerous, with patients often suffering injuries to the face or skull.

Epilepsy Syndromes

The primary generalized epilepsies are a group of disorders that usually present in childhood, respond well to treatment, and may have high rates of remission. They generally are considered genetic in origin, most having obscure inheritance patterns but family clustering, suggesting polygenetic etiologies. The types of seizure seen in these syndromes vary and may include generalized tonic–clonic seizures, absence seizures, and myoclonic seizures.

Patients with primary generalized epilepsies usually have normal neurologic examinations, are of normal intelligence, and give no history suggesting prior brain injury. The EEG shows normal background activity, often interrupted by bursts of generalized spike-and-wave discharges. Primary generalized epilepsies make up 30% to 40% of childhood epilepsies.

Virtually all of the primary generalized epilepsies are age-related, beginning and often remitting at specific times of life. The most common syndrome is *febrile seizures*, which occur in nearly 5% of children, generally between the ages of 1 and 3 years. Uncomplicated febrile seizures stop by the age of 5 years and are not associated with an increased risk of seizures in later life. When the seizures are prolonged (30 minutes or more), repeated, or followed by postictal hemiparesis (Todd's paralysis), children have an increased risk of developing a chronic seizure disorder, sometimes appearing years later in the form of complex partial seizures. Such syndromes are called complicated febrile seizures.

Childhood absence epilepsy usually begins between the ages of 4 and 10 years with absence seizures. In some cases, tonic–clonic seizures appear around the time of puberty. Seizures usually respond easily to medical treatment, and the remission rate by young adulthood may reach 80% to 90%. Before treatment, the EEG usually shows normally developed background activity interrupted by hyperventilation-induced three per second spike-and-wave activity (see later in this chapter), which is characteristic and helpful for diagnosis.

Juvenile myoclonic epilepsy is one of the most common genetically based epilepsies, with onset between the ages of 10 and 20 years. Patients usually present with a tonic–clonic seizure occurring without warning, often in the early morning. If specifically asked, they also give a history of recent involuntary jerks of the limbs or dropping of objects from the hands. These myoclonic jerks occur most commonly in the morning and often immediately precede the "big" seizure that brings them to medical attention. Sleep deprivation or alcohol use may trigger seizures. The EEG shows characteristic polyspike-and-wave discharges elicited by strobe lights. The seizures themselves, however, are not sensitive to flashing lights. This type of epilepsy persists for decades or may be lifelong.

In contrast to the previously mentioned seizure types, almost all adult epilepsies, as well as the majority beginning in childhood, are *focal or localization-related epilepsies*, and the seizures are focal or partial seizures. The occurrence of focal seizures implies the existence of focal brain pathology. An almost unlimited variety of focal seizure phenomena may occur, depending on the site of brain injury. In the diagnosis of all forms of epilepsy, taking a meticulous history from the patient as well as from witnesses to the seizures is essential. The precise sequence of events making up the attacks reveals the site of seizure onset in the brain and the route and extent of seizure propagation through the brain.

For example, a patient with a meningioma growing over the right cerebral hemisphere may present with focal motor seizures of the left leg resulting from irritation of nearby cerebral motor cortex by the tumor. Such an attack may spread down along the precentral (motor) gyrus, involving the cortex controlling the left arm before stopping in 1 or 2 minutes. If the patient remains conscious throughout the seizure, the episode is called a *simple partial seizure*. Commonly, however,

intrinsic cerebral inhibitory mechanisms fail to keep the seizure localized, and the electrical discharge may spread suddenly into thalamic and other brain structures with strong, widespread cortical projections. In this case, a generalized tonic–clonic seizure ensues. Unless the clinician obtains the history of focal onset of such an attack, a mistaken diagnosis of primary generalized epilepsy may be made, and a search for localized brain disease may be left undone.

A completely different symptom complex may be reported by the patient with temporal lobe injury, such as that following encephalitis, anoxia, or complicated febrile convulsions. A *complex partial seizure* often begins with a subjective experience such as a sudden feeling of strangeness or an abrupt sensation of nausea moving upward from the epigastrium. If the seizure discharges remain confined to a small area of the temporal lobe, the attack may not proceed further and may end in 30 to 60 seconds. If, however, it spreads throughout both sides of the limbic system, consciousness may be altered or lost. The patient may stare vacantly or may appear to look about, becoming unresponsive and often making simple movements (automatisms) such as lip smacking, grimacing, or hand wringing. He or she may stand or sit still or may walk about aimlessly. Because of the intimate relationship between limbic cortical structures and the hypothalamus, autonomic signs and symptoms such as piloerection, change in skin color, borborygmus, or an urge to urinate are common in complex partial seizures. If the seizure stops at that point, the altered behavior also stops abruptly, but the patient may remain confused for several minutes or longer. If the seizure has started in the speech-dominant hemisphere, language function may be temporarily impaired postictally. If the ictal activity spreads further to affect both cerebral hemispheres, however, a full-fledged tonic–clonic seizure occurs. Patients may be able to describe vividly the onset or aura of such attacks, but many subjects with temporal lobe seizures have no recall of events before loss of consciousness, and the physician must rely on witnesses for a full description of the episodes.

Focal epilepsy, with or without secondary generalization of the attacks, is by far the most common form of seizure disorder seen by the primary care physician and by most neurologists. Within that category, complex partial seizures are the most prevalent type. Many patients with partial seizures find complete relief from attacks with medication, but about 30% continue to have some seizures even with competent medical advice and optimal therapy.

The clinical picture becomes even more complex in the patient with multifocal or diffuse brain injury. Such a person may be subject to two or sometimes three seizure types. Generalized motor convulsions, focal seizures of any type, or absence attacks all may occur chronically. Additional patterns also may be present, often as fragments (tonic seizures) or distinctive types of episodes such as sudden losses of muscle tone with falling (akinetic seizures). Patients with these multiple seizure types nearly always bear other stigmata of serious cerebral injury such as mental retardation or cerebral palsy. In such cases, seizures are usually difficult if not impossible to control with drugs, are almost always lifelong, and are best handled with the help of a neurologist or epileptologist.

Epilepsy takes a heavy toll on many aspects of patients' lives. Although prejudicial attitudes are softening gradually, epilepsy is still a condition often hidden from those outside the family. Social stigmatization is still surprisingly high, often affecting employment, insurability, and self esteem. When the condition is poorly controlled, it can dominate and define relationships between parents, children, spouses, and siblings. Children may be sheltered excessively by parents and teachers, which may cause social maturation to be delayed or prevented. Depression is very common and underdiagnosed in those with epilepsy, and suicide rates are above average.

Details of state regulations vary, but usually the patient with epilepsy who cannot demonstrate complete, long-term control of the attacks is prohibited from driving. Public transportation and car pools are often inadequate solutions for day-to-day autonomy. Because a diagnosis of epilepsy has far-reaching implications for the life of the patient it is essential that the diagnosis be neither missed nor misapplied.

DIAGNOSING EPILEPSY

Epilepsy is diagnosed through the patient's history—not by head scans, EEGs, or the neurologic examination. In cases when a seizure disorder is suspected, the physician must spend adequate time with the patient and often with witnesses to the attacks to make a reliable diagnosis.

In most cases, asking the patient for a detailed account of the last episode, or of the last one the patient recalls well, often evokes precise details and a coherent impression. Physicians should ask what the patient was doing when the attack began. They should inquire about the first thing that occurred when the attack started and what happened next. They also should ask how the patient felt after the episode ended and if any focal weakness or speech difficulty was present.

The stereotypy of the attacks is an important diagnostic point because for the individual patient, seizures are highly consistent events. Even when there is more than one seizure type, each type has its own stereotypy. Significant variation in the pattern of attacks argues against epilepsy.

The duration of seizures is generally invariant. Except for brief absence or myoclonic seizures, which generally last 5 to 15 seconds, most focal or tonic–clonic seizures last 30 to 90 seconds. The postictal recovery period depends on the type of seizure, but actual seizurelike episodes that last many minutes to hours are usually not epileptic.

Finally, a brief history from a witness is often crucial. What does the witness see and how does the attack begin? Patients with clear auras at the start of a seizure ("Oh, I'm going to have a seizure") sometimes may have postictal amnesia for a focal onset that was obvious to onlookers. The physician should inquire if the patient was fully or partially responsive during an attack.

Discriminating between absence and complex partial seizures sometimes may be a diagnostic hurdle but one that is easily cleared. The latter is much more common than the former, especially in adults. Making the correct diagnosis is important because only complex partial seizures imply the presence of focal brain disease and the therapies for the two types are different. If a reliable witness can be found, the two seizure types can be distinguished accurately by the duration of the attack. Almost all absence seizures last less than 15 seconds, and many are shorter. However, most complex partial seizures continue for more than 30 seconds, with many lasting 1 to 1.5 minutes. Auras, automatisms, and postictal confusion are common with complex partial seizures but are not characteristic of absence seizures. Postictal language difficulty or other focal neurologic signs may be reported after a complex partial seizure.

The EEG almost always demonstrates abnormal neuronal discharges (spikes) during a seizure. When seizures are not occurring, many EEGs show single spikes that often are reported as "epileptiform discharges" on EEG reports. Such discharges may be focal or diffuse ("generalized"), depending on the type of epilepsy. Some are so characteristic of specific epilepsy syndromes that an expert electroencephalographer may be able to corroborate the likely clinical diagnosis very specifically, given an adequate history. This rule is particularly true in patients with childhood absence epilepsy where the EEG shows characteristic three per second discharges and in subjects with complex partial seizures associated with focal spikes over the temporal lobe.

Epilepsy cannot be diagnosed by the EEG alone, however. Although the typical abnormality is seen in more than 80% of untreated patients with absence seizures, there is a dismaying 50% false-negative rate in a single EEG in patients with focal seizures. In addition, the EEG may be falsely positive in up to

5% to 10% of children, especially those with a family history of epilepsy. Focal epileptiform discharges in adults are more specific, occurring in only 2% to 3% of those without epilepsy.

Magnetic resonance scanning of the head with infusion is indicated, unless a specific genetically determined, nonfocal epilepsy syndrome is identified with some assurance. Most patients, even those with focal epilepsy, have normal scans, but up to 30% demonstrate focal pathology such as cortical migrational abnormalities, mesial temporal sclerosis, vascular malformations, infarctions, or neoplasms.

DIFFERENTIAL DIAGNOSIS

Neurocardiogenic (vasovagal) syncope should not be missed because the typical prodrome almost always is remembered vividly by the patient. Giddiness, weakness, sweating, nausea, and fading or graying-out of vision are highly suggestive of true syncope. Urinary incontinence is not rare in syncope; tongue biting is rare, however, and usually implies a convulsion.

Witnesses report the victim of syncope as crumpling or sliding to the ground, whereas the patient with convulsions usually falls stiffly. Consciousness is regained very quickly after syncope, whereas confusion or somnolence is common after seizures. The diagnosis of neurocardiogenic syncope may be made more difficult by the occurrence of a few myoclonic jerks during the syncope, which may be reported by witnesses as seizure activity (so-called convulsive syncope). A history of the typical prodrome and syncopal triggers (dehydration, overheating, prolonged standing, micturition) will prevent confusion.

Cardiogenic or Stokes–Adams attacks also must be differentiated from seizures. Most patients with this syndrome are late middle aged or elderly. The patient usually loses consciousness without warning or after brief palpitations. The patient usually falls suddenly and limply to the ground. Syncope from cardiac arrhythmias rarely causes incontinence or tongue biting. The attacks are usually short, and consciousness is regained quickly and completely.

Panic attacks sometimes are mistaken for seizures, particularly if they include an element of dissociation reported as altered consciousness. The typical symptom complex of fear, chest pain, dyspnea, numbness (especially in the fingertips and lips as a result of hyperventilation), and weakness are not typical of seizures.

Pseudoseizures or psychogenic seizures usually present as seizurelike attacks that do not respond to antiepileptic drug (AED) treatment. Like true seizures, pseudoseizures vary from convulsivelike episodes to transient alterations in consciousness or sensation, but the astute clinician may note incongruous or atypical elements in the history. For example, the person with pseudoseizures resembling tonic–clonic seizures may report continuing awareness of surroundings during the throes of an attack. Urinary incontinence and even bodily injury occur with surprising frequency in pseudoseizures and do not rule out the diagnosis. A firm diagnosis can be made only with the help of the EEG (see later in this chapter). Pseudoseizures and true epileptic seizures can occur in the same patients, making diagnosis and treatment particularly difficult.

MANAGEMENT OF EPILEPSY

Medical therapy is begun once a diagnosis of epilepsy has been firmly established. The goal of treatment should be complete control of seizures, and the ideal therapy is a single drug without side effects. This goal is initially achievable in 70% of patients. Eventually a substantial minority of patients (10% to 30%) will demonstrate refractoriness to drug therapy, however (see later).

Epilepsy is a fearsome diagnosis for most patients or parents, so the physician should be prepared to spend some time dispensing information about the disorder, its prognosis, expectations of therapy, problems relating to

pregnancy, and safety measures. Informational pamphlets can be acquired from a local or regional Epilepsy Foundation office; the phone number for the national office is 800-332-1000, and the Web site is www.epilepsy-foundation.org.

The choice of initial treatment depends on an accurate diagnosis of seizure type(s). Absences and myoclonic seizures, for example, respond to valproate, lamotrigine, and zonisamide, and these drugs also prevent tonic–clonic and focal seizures. Ethosuximide, however, will stop absence seizures but not other seizure types. Most other AEDs are effective against the most common seizure types (i.e., focal seizures and tonic–clonic seizures) (Table 8.1). Treatment of the patient with mental retardation, cerebral palsy, or structural cerebral pathology who has multiple seizure types or akinetic seizures is particularly challenging and usually requires the assistance of a neurologist or epileptologist.

Because many AEDs cause side effects if introduced too quickly, standard practice is to start the chosen AED strictly according to instructions on the package insert. This practice involves starting with a low dosage and building to a recommended effective dose or serum level. An exception is phenytoin, which gen-

TABLE 8.1. *Treatment of Common Seizure Types*

A. Partial (focal)	Phenytoin (Dilantin, Phenytek)
Simple partial	Carbamazepine (Tegretol, Carbatrol)
Complex partial	Valproate (Depakote)
Tonic–clonic	Primidone (Mysoline)
	Phenobarbital
	Gabapentin (Neurontin)
	Lamotrigine (Lamotrigine)
	Topiramate (Topamax)
	Tiagabine (Gabitril)
	Oxcarbazepine (Tripleptal)
	Zonisamide (Zonegran)
	Levetiracetam (Keppra)
B. Absence seizures	Valproate
	Lamotrigine
	Zonisamide
	Ethosuximide (Zarontin)
Myoclonic seizures	Valproate
Lamotrigine	
Zonisamide	

TABLE 8.2. *Properties of AEDs*

AED	Plasma Half-Life	% Protein Bound	Target Levels (mcg/ml)
Ethosuximide	30–60	<10	40–100
Gabapentin	5–9	0	4–16
Lamotrigine	15–24[a]	55	2–20
Levetiracetam	7	<10	20–60
Oxcarbazepine	10–15	40	5–50
Phenobarbital	65–110	45	10–30
Phenytoin	10–24	90	10–20
Primidone	8–15	<20	10–30[b]
Tiagabine	2–9	96	5–70
Topiramate	12–30	15	2–25
Valproate	5–15	70–90	50–150
Zonisamide	50–70	55	10–40

[a]60 hours when used with valproate.
[b]Reported as phenobarbital.

erally is started at a full, usually well-tolerated, adult daily dosage of 300 mg/day.

The effective dose of many AEDs is often very close to the dose that causes side effects, and interactions among AEDs themselves and between some AEDs and other drugs are common. Careful attention to the pharmacokinetics of the AED is essential, and the physician managing epilepsy must be aware of all drugs that the patient chronically or intermittently ingests (Table 8.2).

Serum Antiepileptic Drug Levels

Recommended "therapeutic" serum levels of AEDs are simply values below which patients have been observed to be at risk for seizures and above which many patients complain of dose-related side effects. It is prudent to titrate doses of carbamazepine, phenytoin, valproate, and the barbiturates to within the usual therapeutic levels. Optimal therapeutic levels for the newer AEDs have not been well established, although clinical laboratories provide estimates, and these AEDs usually are increased to a therapeutic dose (Table 8.2). If seizures or side effects occur, an AED may be increased or decreased carefully within or even outside normal levels or dosages. If the first AED fails to control the seizures, a second drug is added; when the dosage is stable, the first, ineffective drug then is withdrawn slowly.

Serum AED levels also can aid decision making when a patient taking more than one drug becomes toxic. Drug levels also may be helpful if patient compliance is questionable. When drawn at the same time of day at the same laboratory, and without interference from other medications or illness, AED levels are remarkably stable from sample to sample.

Individual Antiepileptic Drugs

Although some general principles govern their use, individual AEDs vary enough in their metabolism, side effects, and interactions with other drugs that they require separate comment. Carbamazepine, especially in one of its long-acting forms, is probably the AED most frequently chosen by neurologists for treatment of new-onset focal or tonic–clonic seizures. A readily reversible rash occurs in about 3% to 5% of patients, but serious hypersensitivity reactions are rare. Early, mild leucopenia may be seen but is generally reversible and its importance is overrated. Predictable, reversible, dose-related side effects are blurred vision, diplopia, and nausea. Chronic side effects include macrocytosis, low-normal serum levels of folate, and occasionally hyponatremia.

Partly because it is available in a parenteral form and a loading dose is well tolerated, phenytoin is prescribed more commonly by primary care physicians. Nystagmus may be seen at therapeutic doses that are well tolerated by the patient. High serum levels of phenytoin are associated with cerebellotoxic effects such as ataxia and tremor. Elevated serum alkaline phosphatase, macrocytosis, and low T4 (but normal thyroid-stimulating hormone) are common and require no action. Metabolism of phenytoin is saturable, so that small increases in dosage in the therapeutic range may cause large increases in serum levels; incremental daily doses larger than 300 mg should be no more than 25 to 50 mg. The common long-term cosmetic effects of phenytoin (acne, hirsutism, gingival hyperplasia, possibly coarsening of facial features) may be significant, especially in children.

Both carbamazepine and phenytoin are powerful inducers of some P450 hepatic enzymes, and phenytoin is strongly protein-bound, so physicians prescribing these drugs must always be aware of possible interactions with other drugs (e.g., Coumadin [warfarin], certain antimicrobials). Both drugs reduce the serum levels of valproate, lamotrigine, topiramate, tiagabine, zonisamide, oxcarbazepine, and each other.

The barbiturates, phenobarbital and primidone, share these interactive properties. These highly sedating drugs are little used by neurologists, and should be drugs of last resort, because other AEDs have become available.

Valproate is generally tolerated well, but side effects such as weight gain, reversible alopecia, and tremor can present a problem. Fatal toxic hepatitis has been reported, mainly in young children on polytherapy during the first 6 months of use; the drug is not recommended for children younger than 2 years of age. Blood levels tend to vary more than they do with other anticonvulsants, so they are less useful. Drug interactions with valproate may be significant: it is an inhibitor of certain liver metabolic pathways, but its own metabolism may be enhanced by other drugs. Valproate dramatically raises the serum level of lamotrigine.

Newer Antiepileptic Drugs

Since 1993 many new AEDs, most of them pharmacologically unrelated to older AEDs, have become available for treatment of seizure disorders. All are U.S. Food and Drug Administration-approved for treatment of focal (partial) and tonic–clonic seizures, most as add-on drugs. All are used by most epileptologists as monotherapy. "Therapeutic" blood levels of the newer AEDs may be underestimated by many laboratories and in some cases are not known; doses generally may be increased carefully as tolerated, without frequent monitoring of blood levels. Many of these drugs offer some advantages in terms of fewer drug interactions. All are considerably more costly than the older AEDs.

Gabapentin is a derivative of gamma-amino-butyric acid (GABA), the main inhibitory neurotransmitter of the brain. Because gabapentin is not metabolized or protein-bound, it demonstrates no interactions with other drugs; it is therefore very useful in the elderly, who are often taking a variety of other pharmaceuticals. It is a relatively safe drug; no safety monitoring is necessary. The most common dose-related side effect is drowsiness. Patients starting gabapentin should be warned that weight gain is common with chronic use.

Lamotrigine is a powerful AED that must be introduced very slowly to reduce the incidence of skin rash to a tolerable 3% to 4%. Titration must be even slower, beginning at lower doses, when valproate also is used, because of pharmacokinetic interactions. Blood levels may not be helpful; reasonable initial target doses are 400 mg/day without valproate or 200 mg/day with valproate. Lamotrigine is not recommended for children because of a higher incidence of life-threatening rashes. Adding lamotrigine to carbamazepine usually requires lowering the dose of the latter to avoid diplopia and dizziness—toxic effects of both drugs. Insomnia also may limit its use.

Topiramate is a sulfonamide derivative with some evidence of efficacy in absence seizures as well as other seizure types. Slow introduction of the drug (25 mg per week at first) is essential to minimize cognitive and behavioral side effects. Weight loss with chronic use may be considerable. The concomitant use of hepatic enzyme-inducing drugs such as phenytoin or carbamazepine significantly lowers the blood level of topiramate, a fact that must be considered when adding or subtracting these drugs. A reasonable initial target dose of topiramate is 300 to 400 mg/day.

Tiagabine is another GABA agonist, whose metabolism is briskly enhanced by enzyme-inducing drugs, and its dose must be managed accordingly. Twice-a-day dosing has been shown to be effective. Confusion and difficulty thinking are common during dose escalation and can be minimized by slow titration of the drug.

Oxcarbazepine is a derivative of carbamazepine, with the advantage of fewer drug interactions and with a similar side effect profile and cost. Oxcarbazepine may increase serum levels of phenytoin.

Zonisamide is another sulfonamide derivative that is useful not only for focal seizures and tonic–clonic seizures but also for absences and myoclonic seizures. Cognitive or behavioral changes may occur during titration or with the use of higher doses. Some cases of nephrolithiasis have been reported.

Levetiracetam has a very good safety profile but also must be introduced slowly to avoid cognitive side effects. Once a stable dose is established, it is very well tolerated. Efficacy has been demonstrated taking as little as 1,000 mg/day.

For "rescue" therapy in patients with clusters of seizures, prepackaged syringes of diazepam for rectal use are safe for home use and are very effective.

Surgical Therapies

A novel treatment for drug-resistant epilepsy is vagus nerve stimulation, shown to be effective in treating partial and tonic–clonic seizures. This pacemakerlike device is implanted subcutaneously, and it operates both by programmed, intermittent stimulation and by being switched on when a seizure is felt or seen to begin. Although about 30% of patients improve with vagus nerve stimulation, it is always used with concomitant AEDs, and complete cessation of seizures is unusual.

If three appropriate AEDs at therapeutic dosages fail to control epilepsy in adults or children, the possibility of definitive surgical therapy should be considered. The most common procedure is temporal lobectomy, which has a low morbidity and a high probability of complete cessation of seizures, particularly in patients with mesial temporal sclerosis.

Stopping Antiepileptic Drugs

Many epilepsies, particularly those beginning in childhood, eventually go into remission. The point at which AEDs may be safely stopped in a well-controlled patient is debatable. A seizure-free period of 2 years in children and 3 years in adults is considered a reasonable time at which to consider a trial without drugs. Unfortunately, the outcome of AED withdrawal in an individual case cannot be predicted.

Dietary and Alternative or Rehabilitative Treatments

The ketogenic diet is an extreme, high-fat diet sometimes used for short periods in children with intractable epilepsy. It customarily is initiated and supervised by a pediatric neurologist, usually with the assistance of a dietitian experienced in its use. No other dietary changes, herbs, or supplements have been found to help in the treatment of epilepsy.

Hypnosis has been successful in isolated cases but is not customarily used. In the absence of complication, no specific physical or occupational rehabilitation is necessary in treating epilepsy.

Women and Epilepsy

Phenytoin, carbamazepine, the barbiturates, and topiramate all enhance the metabolism of oral contraceptive hormones; high-dose preparations with 50 mcg of estradiol are recommended. Folate metabolism also is enhanced by phenytoin, carbamazepine, and the barbiturates. Because inadequate maternal folate has been associated with spina bifida, 1 mg/day of supplemental folic acid should be given to all women of reproductive capacity taking these drugs.

All of the AEDs that have been studied have been shown to increase the rate of fetal malformations by a factor of two, and all AEDs are Category C drugs in pregnancy. Valproate has been associated with a significant increased risk of midline neural tube defects. Because of the serious risks of seizures during pregnancy, however, most women with epilepsy continue to use an AED when pregnant. Stopping or changing an AED after pregnancy is discovered generally is not advised.

Special Challenges for Managing Hospitalized Patients

Patients with epilepsy who are admitted to hospital for other conditions should have their routine AEDs continued. Currently the only chronically used AEDs available in parenteral form are phenytoin, valproate, and phenobarbital. If patients cannot take their usual AED by mouth for more than 24 hours, a parenteral AED should be used, preferably with the help of a neurologist. Many surgical procedures will interrupt oral AED therapy by less than a day, and the usual drug simply may be resumed as soon as the patient is able to take it.

WHEN TO REFER THE PATIENT TO A NEUROLOGIST

Although most patients with epilepsy are helped to achieve substantial control of seizures, many patients on optimal drug therapy continue to have seizures serious or frequent enough to cause major disruptions to life. If seizures have not been completely controlled after 2 years, or if the patient has failed to respond to two AEDs, such patients should be referred to a neurologist or epilepsy center. Some of these patients turn out to have disorders other than epilepsy; some have types of seizures responsive to more appropriate AEDs; others are appropriate for surgical therapy. Surgical cure rates for some types of intractable seizures are high with low morbidity.

QUESTIONS AND DISCUSSION

1. Patients with primary generalized epilepsy may have which of the following types of seizures?
A. Absence
B. Myoclonic
C. Grand mal
D. All of the above
E. None of the above

The answer is (D). Patients may have any combination of these seizures. Sometimes grand mal attacks are preceded or led into by clusters of absence or myoclonic spells.

2. The physiologic substrate of clinical seizure activity is:
A. Abnormal neuronal discharge
B. Hyperactive glial potentials
C. Repeated disturbances in cerebral blood flow
D. Autoimmune mechanisms

The answer is (A). In focal epilepsy, groups of hyperirritable neurons, perhaps affected by loss of inhibitory input, excessive excitatory activity, and anatomic distortions, overact and are able to hypersynchronize the activity of other neuronal populations. This activity spreads and causes focal or even generalized seizures.

3. Some cause(s) of new epilepsy after adolescence is/are:
A. Brain tumor
B. Penetrating head injury
C. Cerebral infection
D. B and C
E. A, B, and C

The answer is (E). New onset of seizure disorder in adulthood demands a full investigation into the cause. Epilepsy is thus better regarded as a symptom rather than as a disease.

4. High blood levels of phenytoin usually are accompanied by:
A. Somnolence
B. Hair loss
C. Ataxia
D. Pulmonary edema
E. Weakness

The answer is (C). Ataxia is much more common than somnolence. Sedation is caused by phenytoin only at extremely high levels, as would be caused by deliberate overdosing. Hair loss may occur with valproate but not with phenytoin. Neither pulmonary edema nor muscle weakness is typical of phenytoin effect. Ataxia is seen in most patients with blood levels higher than 30 mg/dl.

SUGGESTED READING

Annegers JF, Shirts SB, Hauser WA, et al. Risk of recurrence after an initial unprovoked seizure. *Epilepsia* 1986; 27:43.

Brodie MJ, French JA. Management of epilepsy in adolescents and adults. *Lancet* 2000;356;323–329.

Browne TR, Holmes GL. Epilepsy. *N Engl J Med* 2001;344; 1145–1151.

Dodrill C, Batzel LW. Interictal behavioral features of patients with epilepsy. *Epilepsia* 1986;27(Suppl 2):564.

Fish DR, Smith SJ, Quesney LF, et al. Surgical treatment of children with medically intractable frontal or temporal lobe epilepsy: results and highlights of 40 years' experience. *Epilepsia* 1993;34:244.

Leppik IE, Goldensohn ES, Hauser WA, et al. Epilepsy through life: recent advances in understanding and treating epilepsy during pregnancy, childhood, adulthood, and old age. *Epilepsia* 1992;33(Suppl 4):S1.

Lowenstein DH, Alldredge BK. Status epilepticus. *N Engl J Med* 1998;338;970–976.

Schachter SC, Saper CB. Vagus nerve stimulation. *Epilepsia* 1998;39:677–686.

Schachter SC, Schomer DL, eds. *The comprehensive evaluation and treatment of epilepsy.* San Diego: Academic Press, 1997.

Scheuer ML. Seizures and epilepsy in the elderly. In: Pedley TA, Meldrum BS, eds. *Recent advances in epilepsy,* No. 6. Edinburgh: Churchill Livingstone, 1995.

Sirven JI. Acute and chronic seizures in patients older than 60 years. *Mayo Clin Proc* 2001;76:175–183.

Theodore WH, Porter RJ, Penry JK. Complex partial seizures: clinical characteristics and differential diagnosis. *Neurology* 1983;33:1115.

Wyllie E. *The treatment of epilepsy: principles and practice,* 3rd ed. Philadelphia: Lea & Febiger, 2001.

9

Multiple Sclerosis

Peter A. Calabresi

Multiple sclerosis (MS) is an inflammatory disease of the central nervous system (CNS) of unknown etiology. The disease is characterized pathologically by inflammatory infiltrates and demyelination followed by varying degrees of secondary axonal degeneration. It is the most common non-traumatic cause of neurologic disability in young adults and affects between 250,000 and 400,000 people in the United States. MS affects women two to three times more commonly than men. Most patients start with a period of unpredictable relapses and remissions, which in the majority is followed by an accumulation of neurologic dysfunction and a chronic progressive course. The life expectancy has been shown to be only 6 to 7 years less than that for a control population without MS, but the emotional and economic cost to society as a result of the disability is enormous.

HISTORY

The earliest account of a disease that appears likely to have been MS is found in writings from the 14th century describing the illness of a Dutch nun, "Blessed Lidwina of Schiedam." The earliest pathologic descriptions by Carswell and Cruveilher date to between 1838 and 1845. Charcot generally is credited with the first comprehensive account of the clinical and pathologic features of MS, which was published in 1868.

Epidemiology

Epidemiologic studies have shown that MS has an unequal geographic distribution with large regional and ethnic variations in the prevalence of disease (Fig. 9.1). MS is rare in the tropics and increases in frequency at higher latitudes north and south of the equator. The prevalence in the United States is reported at 57.8 per 100,000 and is almost twice as common in the Northern as compared to the Southern United States. The prevalence rate has been increasing, probably because of better recognition of MS and improved treatment of complications with a correspondingly increased longevity of those affected. Prevalence rates of less than 5 per 100,000 are found in Asia, Africa (except English-speaking whites in South Africa), and northern South America. MS also is said to be much less common among Eskimos, Gypsies, and African Americans. However, these patterns may be changing with increased travel; cases of MS have been reported in native Africans who have not traveled out of the country, and the prevalence of African Americans with MS has not been reexamined adequately in the magnetic resonance imaging (MRI) era of diagnosis.

Migration studies suggest that the risk of acquiring MS is related to the location in which one has lived before puberty. Individuals migrating from high- to low-risk areas decreased their expected risk of developing MS, as determined from their area of birth. Conversely, migration from low- to high-risk areas increased the risk of acquiring MS. The reliability of migration studies has been questioned, and no definite conclusions can be made from these data.

Numerous instances of MS clusters have been reported. Several clusters have been related to exposure to heavy metals and canine distemper virus, but no conclusive link has been established. Genetic studies strongly suggest that the disease is polygenic and that genetic factors may have a stronger influence in determining susceptibility to MS than environmental factors.

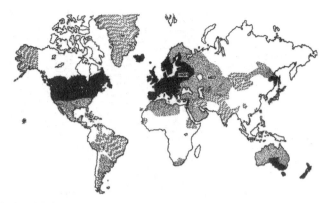

FIG. 9.1. Map of the world depicting areas of high (prevalence 30+/100,000, *solid*), medium (prevalence 5–29/100,000, *dotted*), and low (prevalence 0–4/100,000, *dashed*). *White* areas are regions without data or people. (From Kurtzke. Epidemiology. Burks JS, Johnson KP, eds. *Multiple sclerosis: diagnosis, medical management, and rehabilitation.* New York: Demos Medical Publishing, 2000. Reproduced with permission from Demos Medical Publishing.)

Pathology of Multiple Sclerosis

Pathology

Classic descriptions of the MS lesion as predominantly demyelinating with relative sparing of axons still hold true today. Modern tools have afforded more detailed descriptions of the immunologic and structural events occurring within lesions and have reemphasized the secondary axonal degenerative stage of the lesion. Major advances in the classification of MS pathology have been made from biopsy and rapid autopsy material. Clinicopathologic correlations using MRI and spectroscopy provide hope that advances in our understanding of the pathologic state will allow guided therapeutic interventions.

The MS plaque appears to begin with migration of lymphocytes and macrophages across the blood–brain barrier into the perivenular space (Fig. 9.2). This is followed by diffuse parenchymal infiltration by inflam-

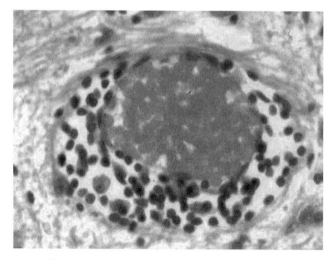

FIG. 9.2. Perivenular infiltrate typical of the early acute inflammatory event in an active lesion.

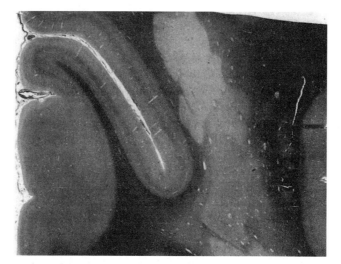

FIG. 9.3. Luxol fast blue stain revealing loss of myelin in several irregular geographic lesions.

matory cells, edema, and active stripping of myelin from axons by macrophages leading to multifocal areas of demyelination (Fig. 9.3). Subsequently, astrocytic hyperplasia and the accumulation of lipid-laden macrophages ensue. As plaques enlarge and coalesce, the initial perivenular distribution of the lesions becomes less apparent. The inflammatory reaction usually is less pronounced in grey matter, probably because of the smaller amount of myelin in these areas. The extent of axonal loss in the demyelinated areas is highly variable. The sparing of axons is relative, and some axonal loss occurs in almost all lesions and can become substantial in severe cases.

Plaquelike areas of pale myelin staining are called shadow plaques and generally are regarded as evidence of partial remyelination. Several studies have confirmed a remarkable potential for oligodendrocyte proliferation and partial remyelination, which seems to be impeded by as-yet-unknown local factors.

Myelin and Nerve Conduction

Proteolipid protein (PLP), myelin basic protein (MBP), and their isoforms make up 80% to 90% of the protein with 2', 3' cyclic nucleotide 3' phosphohydrolase (CNPase), myelin-associated glycoprotein (MAG), myelin oligodendrocyte protein (MOG), and other minor proteins making up the rest. Both PLP and CNPase are restricted to CNS myelin, whereas MBP constitutes about 10% of the protein in PNS myelin. Lipids constitute 80% of the dry weight of myelin. Cultured oligodendroglial cells contain a family of gangliosides of which GM_3 and GM_1 are the principal components.

One oligodendrocyte usually forms internodal segments of myelin on several different nerve fibers. This differs from the peripheral nervous system, where one Schwann cell contributes myelin to only one internodal segment. This difference may account, in part, for the much greater efficiency of regeneration in peripheral myelin. The nodes of Ranvier have a high concentration of sodium channels concentrated in the nodal membrane, which are required for saltatory conduction. During an episode of inflammatory demyelination, conduction may be transiently impaired as a result of edema, loss of myelin, and some degree of metabolic dysfunction of the nerve axon. Conduction can recover acutely on resolution of edema, subacutely with redistribution of sodium channels along the internodal membrane, or chronically after partial remyelination.

Pathologic Correlations with Magnetic Resonance Imaging

The profound impact of modern imaging technologies is evident from its expanding role in the diagnosis and prognosis of MS. High signal (bright) T2-weighted lesions correlate well with the presence of lesions on gross pathology. However, T2 lesions lack specificity for microscopic tissue pathology and seem to represent a composite of factors including edema, demyelination, remyelination, gliosis, and axonal loss. Therefore, the T2 lesion burden does not correlate strongly with clinical disability even in clinically eloquent areas of the CNS (brainstem and spinal cord) because not all T2 lesions purport the destructive axonal pathology. Indeed, this is exactly what the T2-weighted lesion volume studies show—a weak but significant correlation with clinical disability (Expanded Disability Status Scale, or EDSS, and cognitive dysfunction). Because of the imprecise specificity of T2 images, more emphasis is being placed on T1-weighted images in which persistent low signal (black holes) seems to correlate better with axonal dropout and clinical disability. However, one must be cautious because during the acute enhancing phase of a lesion, and perhaps for several months thereafter, low signal T1 lesions may represent extracellular edema that can resolve.

Another misunderstood aspect of imaging is that there is a temporal sequence of lesion pathology such that acute contrast-enhanced lesions correlate well with the perivenular infiltrate and the likelihood of a clinical exacerbation but also predict future formation of black holes and brain atrophy. Indeed in a clinical trial of interferon beta (IFNβ), the drug suppressed inflammation on the MRI in the first year of treatment but did not slow brain atrophy until the second year. This suggests that those axons that were already demyelinated prior to treatment may follow an inexorable course of degeneration during the first year of treatment, but the axons that were salvaged from demyelination by suppression of the inflammatory attack in the first year are spared degeneration in the second year. This also would explain why in two recent short-term trials of potent immunosuppressive drugs used for 12 months or one dose, contrast-enhancing lesions were reduced, but there was no effect on progression of disability or brain atrophy. Newer methods such as magnetization transfer imaging and proton magnetic resonance spectroscopy (^{1}H-MRS) may be more sensitive measures of underlying structural pathology.

Etiology and Immunopathogenesis

Although the cause of MS remains uncertain, our understanding of the underlying mechanisms and pathology has grown enormously. The best formulation of the pathogenesis of MS is that the disease is an autoimmune process that occurs in a genetically susceptible individual after an environmental exposure. This hypothesis is supported by an extensive and diverse literature but is based on three seminal discoveries. The recognition by Rivers that the acute paralytic encephalitis that occasionally followed rabies and small pox vaccination was an autoimmune reaction to contaminating self-proteins, led him to the discovery of experimental allergic encephalomyelitis (EAE), which has since been studied extensively as an animal model for MS. The discoveries that genes influence disease susceptibility and specifically that the human leukocyte antigen (HLA) class II region on the short arm of chromosome 6 is associated with the risk of developing MS has led to a multitude of studies suggesting that polygenetic influences predispose certain individuals to acquiring MS. Finally, the observations made regarding latitudinal gradient, migration, and disease clustering have strongly suggested an environmental role in the disease. Although no specific microbial agent has stood the test of time, modern molecular immunology has provided numerous potential mechanisms through which numerous infections could mediate autoimmunity.

Genetics

Genetic susceptibility to MS has long been suspected, based on widely differing prevalence in different ethnic populations. Family studies have found that first-degree relatives of patients are at 20-fold increased risk of developing MS. Furthermore, monozygotic twins are more likely to be concordant for MS (20%–40%) than dizygotic twins (3%–4%). Nonbiologic first-degree (adopted) relatives are no more likely to develop MS than the population at large, which further supports the notion that familial clustering for MS is largely genetic in origin. However, unless one invokes incomplete penetrance of genes, the twin studies also suggest a strong environmental component because no more than 40% of monozygotic twins are concordant for MS. Widely different MS prevalence among similar high-susceptibility genetic groups that inhabit different environments (such as Anglo-Saxons in England versus in South Africa) presumably must be tied to this second, environmental, element of disease etiology. Studies of candidate genes and whole-genome screens suggest that multiple weakly acting genes interact epistatically to determine risk toward MS as suspected from epidemiologic studies.

Immunology of Multiple Sclerosis

The inflammatory reaction in MS is of unknown origin. Although no infectious agent has been proved to be the cause of MS, it is hypothesized that many common viruses can trigger autoimmune-mediated demyelination in susceptible individuals through molecular mimicry (cross reactivity between microbial proteins and myelin). In addition, there is evidence that quiescent autoreactive T cells that are present in healthy individuals may be activated through bystander activation by cytokine or polyclonal T-cell activation mediated by bacteria or viruses.

It remains uncertain how tissue injury (to myelin, oligodendroglia, axons, and neurons) occurs in MS, but the inflammatory events surrounding the vast majority of acute MS lesions seem to suggest a direct immune-mediated pathology. The MS lesion resembles a delayed type hypersensitivity (DTH) reaction, containing activated T cells, B cells, numerous mononuclear phagocytes, inflammatory cytokines, and adhesion molecules. Electron microscopy studies suggest the macrophage may play a major role in the direct stripping of myelin from axons, although this could be a secondary phagocytic response to excitotoxic injury of oligodendrocytes or neurons.

Disease Course and Clinical Patterns

The clinical course of MS is divided into categories according to neurologic symptoms as they develop over time. A new classification for MS categories was developed by consensus among MS experts (Table 9.1).

TABLE 9.1. *Multiple Sclerosis Clinical Categories*

Disease Category	Explanation
Relapsing-remitting (RR-MS)	Episodes of acute worsening with recovery and a stable course between relapses
Secondary progressive MS (SP-MS)	Gradual neurologic deterioration with or without superimposed acute relapses in a patient who previously had RR-MS
Primary progressive MS (PP-MS)	Gradual, nearly continuous neurologic deterioration from onset of symptoms
Progressive-relapsing MS (PR-MS)	Gradual neurologic deterioration from onset but with subsequent superimposed relapses

Lublin FD, Reingold SC. Defining the clinical course of multiple sclerosis: results of an international survey. *Neurology* 1996;46:907–911.

Relapsing-remitting Multiple Sclerosis

Relapsing-remitting MS (RR-MS) is the most common form in patients younger than age 40 years. Patients may develop focal neurologic symptoms and signs acutely or over a few days. These exacerbations or attacks are remarkably unpredictable and heterogenous in character, probably because they result from varying degrees of inflammation that can occur in any part of the brain or spinal cord. Common presentations include blurred/double vision, sensory symptoms (numbness, tingling, or pain), weakness, vertigo, or impaired balance. A new symptom commonly will present over 24 to 72 hours, stabilize for a few days or weeks, and then improve spontaneously over 4 to 12 weeks. Subsequent new focal symptoms or signs typically follow the initial attack months or years later and again remit partially or completely. It is very common for old symptoms to persist or reoccur, especially in response to periods of stress such as infections or prolonged elevations of core body temperature. Over time it becomes difficult to determine whether the symptom flare represents a new exacerbation or worsening symptoms referable to past disease. Recovery from relapses is often incomplete, and permanent disability can accumulate in a stepwise fashion at this stage of the disease.

Secondary Progressive Multiple Sclerosis

Secondary progressive MS (SP-MS) refers to the patient with an initial RR-MS course who then progressively worsens over months (at least 6) to years. Natural history studies have shown that with time most patients with RR-MS convert to SP-MS. This usually occurs after 10 to 20 years from onset or after the age of 40. A patient with SP-MS still may experience relapses but does not stabilize between relapses. The predominant clinical pattern is one of continued clinical worsening. As time passes, relapses become less discrete, and the pattern becomes one of continued worsening without relapses. Conversion to SP-MS is considered a poor prognostic sign because this stage of the disease is much more refractory to the presently available immunomodulatory therapies. Some patients with SP-MS spontaneously stabilize for considerable periods, although they only rarely recover after deficits have persisted for 6 months. The pathogenic mechanisms underlying conversion from RR-MS to SP-MS may relate to failure of remyelination and progressive axonal injury.

Primary Progressive Multiple Sclerosis

In approximately 10% to 15% of patients, primary progressive MS (PP-MS) is characterized by progressive worsening from the onset of symptoms without interposed relapses. Patients with PP-MS are more likely to be men and older than 40 years of age at symptom onset. This form of the disease often presents with progressive gait disorder as a result of leg weakness, spasticity, and impaired coordination. In cases of progressive neurologic dysfunction, it is extremely important to rule out structural pathology, infections, and hereditary and other neurodegenerative diseases. Patients with PP-MS have fewer gadolinium-enhancing brain lesions on MRI, less tissue inflammation on histopathologic assessment, and less cerebrospinal fluid (CSF) inflammation than typical for SP-MS; pathologic studies have suggested this form of the disease may represent a primary problem with the oligodendrocyte.

Progressive-relapsing Multiple Sclerosis

According to the new classification, progressive-relapsing MS (PR-MS) refers to the rare patient with progressive disease from symptom onset who subsequently experiences one or more relapses. In all likelihood, this is another form of SP-MS without clinically apparent relapses in the early stages of disease, and if considered separately this group comprises only 6% or fewer of all patients with MS.

Disease patterns change over time, and it may be difficult at a given time to clearly categorize a patient's disease. The problem is particularly difficult when a patient is converting from a purely relapsing remitting to a purely progressive disease course. This has been termed relapsing progressive MS by some and transitional MS by others, but these disease categories cannot be defined precisely by current methods. Observation for as long as 1 year may be required to categorize such a patient with confidence.

Other Variants of Multiple Sclerosis

Several other variants of MS have been described and are important to recognize. An acute rapidly progressive form of MS often called Marburg's disease is characterized by a person who develops acute or subacute progressive neurologic deterioration leading to severe disability within days to months. The disease may progress steadily to a quadriplegic obtunded state with death as a result of intercurrent infection, aspiration, or respiratory failure from brainstem involvement. Postmortem studies have documented inflammation in the optic nerves, optic chiasm, cerebral hemispheres, and spinal cord. The pathology reveals a pronounced mononuclear cell infiltrate with severe axonal damage and tissue necrosis. Neuromyelitis optica (Devic's disease) refers to the patient who presents with both optic neuritis and transverse myelitis, occurring either simultaneously or separated by only a few months. Several features differentiate this disease from classical MS, including the absence of white matter lesions on a brain MRI, multilevel spinal cord lesions, and severe disability and death as a result of respiratory failure in one-third of all patients. Pathologically, the syndrome is variable with some lesions characterized by inflammation and demyelination, but it is invariable with severe necrosis and many patients having cavitary lesions in the spinal cord. Those patients who survive the acute attack commonly follow a course with features indistinguishable from RR-MS but have a worse prognosis. Acute disseminated encephalomyelitis (ADEM) and its hyperacute form, acute necrotizing hemorrhagic encephalopathy (ANHE), are thought to be forms of immune-mediated inflammatory demyelination. They differ from MS in that they are typically monophasic, whereas MS is by definition multiphasic or chronically progressive. Patients with ADEM or ANHE usually present with fever, headache, meningeal signs, and altered consciousness, which are exceedingly rare in MS. Multiple reports of clinical and pathologic overlap have been published. Some authors have suggested that the MRI can be used to differentiate MS from ADEM, but no reliable clinical criteria to differentiate the two processes exist.

Clinically Isolated Syndromes and Prognosis

In the era of partially effective prophylactic MS therapies, there has been increased emphasis on making a diagnosis early in the course of the disease to initiate appropriate preventative treatment. The use of MRI as a diagnostic tool is discussed later. T2-lesion burden at the time of first MS symptoms not only determines the likelihood of converting to clinically definite MS but also is predictive of future disability. The frequency of gadolinium-enhancing lesions correlates with the likelihood of having a clinical exacerbation and predicts future brain atrophy. However, because T2-weighted lesions lack specificity for tissue pathology and gadolinium enhancement is transient (2 to 8 weeks), T1 hypointense lesions ("black holes") and brain atrophy may be a better measure of axonal loss and have been shown to correlate more strongly with both present and future disability. The presence of mild atrophy or persistent T1 black holes early in the course of MS should alert the physician to a potentially aggressive form of the disease.

Precipitating Factors

Exposure to viruses and bacteria has been associated with precipitating disease exacerbations. The risk of an exacerbation decreases

TABLE 9.2. *Initial Symptoms in Patients with Multiple Sclerosis*

Symptom	Percentage
Sensory disturbance in one or more limbs	33
Disturbance of balance and gait	18
Vision loss in one eye	17
Diplopia	13
Progressive weakness	10
Acute myelitis	6
Lhermitte's symptom	3
Sensory disturbance in face	3
Pain	2

Paty DW, Poser CM. Clinical symptoms and signs of multiple sclerosis. In: Poser CM ed. *The diagnosis of multiple sclerosis.* New York: Thieme & Stratton, 1984:27.

during pregnancy, with the rate being decreased by approximately two-thirds in the third trimester. The risk of an acute attack in the first 3 months postpartum is increased and has been estimated that 20% to 40% of postpartum patients with MS will have an exacerbation. The decreased relapse rate during pregnancy probably is related to a family of immunosuppressive hormones and T_H2 cytokines. Overall, pregnancy probably has little overall effect on the course of the disease and therefore remains a realistic possibility for woman with MS.

Symptoms and Signs

See Tables 9.2 and 9.3.

Optic Neuritis

Multiple sclerosis commonly affects the optic nerves and chiasm, and approximately 30% of patients present with visual symptoms. In acute optic neuritis, the patient experiences monocular loss of central vision and often has eye or brow pain, which worsens on lateral eye movement. The symptoms may present over a few hours to 7 days, with a few cases progressing over several weeks. Loss of

TABLE 9.3. *Common Symptoms and Signs in Patients with Multiple Sclerosis*

Symptom	Sign	Comment
Visual blurring, central visual loss, eye pain	Diminished acuity, central scotoma, deafferented pupil	Syndrome of optic neuritis, usually seen early in the disease
Diplopia, oscillopsia	INO, more rarely other oculomotor weakness, ocular dysmetria, or flutter	May be associated with nausea, vertigo, or other brainstem signs
Loss of dexterity, weakness, tightness, pain	Upper motor neuronal signs affecting legs	Develops in most patients with MS over time early in disease, arms later
Shaking, imbalance	Intention tremor, dysmetria, dysarthria, truncal or head titubation	Occurs in about 30% of patients; may be predominant manifestation in certain patients
Paresthesias, loss of sensation	Decreased vibration and position sense in legs more than arms; decreased fine sensation in hands	Sensory symptoms often painful and distressing
Inability to concentrate or learn; distractibility	Diminished concentration, processing speed, or verbal learning on neuropsychologic testing	May be subtle or inapparent clinically, but may have severe impact on patient and family; severe dementia in <10% of patients
Emotional lability or pathologic laughing and weeping	Episodic crying or laughing	Distressing to patient; generally not related to the patients' actual emotions
Depression	—	Commonly unrecognized or underestimated
Fatigue	—	Disabling in many patients with MS; does not correlate with severity of motor signs
Pain		Numerous etiologies (see text)
Urinary urgency, hesitancy, incontinence	Requires urodynamic testing to characterize	Often complicated by intercurrent UTI

INO, internuclear ophthalmoplegia; MS, multiple sclerosis; UTI, urinary tract infection.

visual acuity and color perception often are considerable. Most patients will recover significantly after 2 to 3 months, although continued improvement can occur as long as a year later; however, some patients sustain permanent damage and can become blind. Acuity is variably diminished in the affected eye. A central or centrocecal scotoma (marked enlargement of the blind spot to involve central vision) can be documented at the bedside with an Amsler grid, and red desaturation can be demonstrated with color plates or with a red-tipped hat pin. Using the swinging flashlight test in a darkened room, one can demonstrate a defect in the afferent pathway such that pupillary constriction in the affected eye is greater with contralateral than with direct light stimulus. A positive test reveals a relative afferent pupillary defect, sometimes called a Marcus Gunn pupil. Funduscopic examination is usually normal in acute retrobulbar neuritis. When the optic nerve is affected anteriorly, the disk may be congested and swollen, thus resembling papilledema. Several months after an optic neuritis, the disc often appears pale, especially at the temporal border, and this can provide evidence of a previous attack. Occasionally, optic nerve demyelination and axonal damage can manifest silently and is noticed only in the setting of other symptoms suggestive of MS.

Oculomotor Syndromes

Eye movement abnormalities are also extremely common in MS and include broken (saccadic) smooth pursuits, nystagmus, ocular dysmetria (over-shooting target), and the classical internuclear ophthalmoplegia (INO). An INO results from damage to the medial longitudinal fasciculus, and its presence in a young adult is highly suggestive of MS. In its complete form, one eye is unable to adduct and the other has abducting nystagmus. More commonly one observes varying degrees of adduction lag with dysconjugate nystagmus. The patient is asked to make a rapid saccade from midline to a laterally situated target, and the examiner focuses on whether the eyes move in a conjugate manner. The condition is frequently bilateral, with one eye being more involved than the other. Quantitative infrared oculography has demonstrated that the frequency of subtle INOs is probably much greater than can be clinically appreciated.

Weakness

Weakness, spasticity, hyperreflexia, and Babinski's sign (upgoing toe) are common manifestations of damage to the pyramidal tracts in patients with MS. This most commonly presents in the legs (spastic paraparesis) because of the relative length that these fibers have to travel, which makes them more susceptible to numerous areas of demyelination and noticeable conduction delays. It is not uncommon for cervical lesions to manifest first in the lower extremities. Concomitant symptoms include stiffness, spasms, and pain. Extreme hyperreflexia causes clonus, which usually is described by the patient as a shaking or tremor.

Cerebellar Signs

End-point tremor (dysmetria) on finger to nose testing is most noticeable in the upper extremities probably because of their important role in fine movement tasks. Lower extremity and midline truncal ataxia result in gait impairment, and some patients with MS are mistaken for being intoxicated. Head or truncal titubation or scanning dysarthria (impaired prosody) can become disabling aspects of the disease.

Sensory Symptoms

Approximately one-third of patients with MS present initially with sensory disturbance involving the limbs, and the majority of patients will have paresthesias as the disease progresses. Symptoms usually are described as "pins and needles" and less commonly as a loss of sensation. Paresthesias can be painful burning or electrical sensations. The sensory symptoms follow a spinal cord pattern often with an incomplete loss of sensation to either vibration (posterior columns) or pinprick (spinothalamic) pathways. It is important to distinguish the spinal pattern from peripheral or root lesions, which follow cutaneous or dermatomal patterns of sensory loss. Occasionally, patients will describe patches of numbness or symptoms in an apparently non-anatomic distribution, which presumably could relate to multifocal areas of demyelination or may be a manifestation of psychiatric disease.

Lhermitte's phenomenon refers to an electric tingling sensation that is precipitated by neck flexion, usually into the arms or down the back. Lhermitte's phenomenon suggests cervical spinal cord disease. It is very common in patients with MS with cervical spinal cord involvement but is not specific for MS.

Pain

Pain is very common in MS and may be caused directly by abnormal firing of sensory nerves, as a result of severe spasticity, or because of secondary orthopedic injuries. Trigeminal neuralgia or atypical facial pain are common causes of severe pain in MS.

Cognitive and Memory Symptoms

Approximately 50% of patients with MS exhibit significant short-term memory loss or difficulty with concentration, attention, and processing speed. Cortical deficits relating to language and visual spatial function are much less common. In only a minority of patients is dementia an incapacitating aspect of the disease. Correlations between the severity of cognitive impairment and the extent of MRI changes have been found.

Psychiatric Manifestations

Inappropriate laughing and weeping, often in response to minor provocation, occurs in more than 10% of patients with MS. Approximately 50% of patients with MS will have an episode of major depression during the course of their illness, and many patients will have chronic low-level depressive symptoms. MRI studies have confirmed an association with lesion load or atrophy, especially in the frontal and temporal lobes, and depression in MS. The health care provider should have a heightened awareness of the risk of suicide in patients with MS. Depression also may be part of a bipolar illness, which is more common in patients with MS than in control populations.

Fatigue

Fatigue may be the most common single complaint of patients with MS and can be disabling. Fatigue usually comes on late in the afternoon or may occur with strenuous activity or with exposure to heat. Short rest periods usually restore function. A less specific and more generalized fatigue also is seen and may take the form of overwhelming lassitude, which can be disabling. Episodic fatigue may herald clinical disease exacerbation. The mechanisms underlying MS fatigue are unknown.

Bladder, Bowel, and Sexual Dysfunction

Bladder dysfunction is common and can be divided into two categories. Patients may fail to empty urine adequately, causing urinary hesitancy, postvoid fullness or dribbling, or frank inability to initiate urination despite a feeling of fullness. Alternatively, patients may fail to properly store urine, causing urgency, urge incontinence, dysuria, frequency, and nocturia. The correlation between bladder symptoms and the underlying pathophysiology is often imperfect; therefore objective testing by cystometrogram is often necessary to characterize the problem and to guide management.

Constipation is also common in MS and should be managed aggressively to prevent complications. Fortunately, fecal incontinence is relatively rare but when present is socially devastating.

Sexual dysfunction is reported by 50% to 75% of patients with MS and is exacerbated by a variety of problems including fatigue, decreased sensation, decreased libido, erectile dysfunction, spasticity, impaired lubrication, body image disorder, and depression.

TABLE 9.4. *McDonald Diagnostic Criteria*

Clinical Presentation	Paraclinical Tests Needed	
	Space	Time
Two attacks; 2 locations	No	No
Two attacks; 1 location	MRI abnormal or 2 MRI lesions + CSF	No
One attack; 2 locations or	No	MRI ≥ 3 months or second attack
One attack; 1 location (CIS)	MRI abnormal or 2 MRI lesions + CSF	MRI ≥ 3 months or second attack
PP–MS[a]	9 MRI brain or 2 MRI cord or 4–8 MRI brain + VEP or <4 MRI brain + 1 MRI cord	MRI ≥3 months or clinical presentation for 1 year

CIS, clinically isolated syndromes; PP-MS, primary progressive multiple sclerosis; VEP, visual-evoked potential.

[a]Must have positive CSF.

Modified from McDonald WI, Compston A, Edan G, et al. Recommended MRI diagnostic criteria. *Ann Neurol* 2001;50:121–127.

Other Manifestations

Paroxysmal disorders in MS include dystonic spasms, tic douloureux, episodic paresthesias, seizures, ataxia, and dysarthria. Various other disease manifestations occur more rarely, including hearing loss, spasms, aphasia, homonymous hemianopsia, gait apraxia, movement disorders (myoclonus and chorea), and autonomic dysfunction (sweating, feeling hot and cold, edema, and postural hypotension).

Diagnosis of Multiple Sclerosis

MS is diagnosed clinically through the demonstration of CNS lesions disseminated in time and space and with no better explanation for the disease process. There is no single diagnostic test, and several other diseases can mimic MS. Therefore, diagnostic criteria based on clinical features supplemented by laboratory tests have been used. The new McDonald criteria were developed by a panel of MS experts and were based on review of extensive supportive scientific studies focusing on the sensitivity and specificity of MRI diagnostic criteria (Table 9.4). The major change associated with the latest criteria is that a diagnosis of MS can be made early after a clinically isolated syndrome if a follow up MRI performed 3 months later demonstrates the formation of a new lesion (Table 9.5). These

TABLE 9.5a. *MRI Criteria for Brain Abnormality*

Three of four of the following:[a]
  One Gd-enhancing lesion or nine T2-hyperintense lesions if there is no Gd-enhancing lesion
  At least one infratentorial lesion
  At least one juxtacortical lesion
  At least three periventricular lesions

Gd, gadolinium.
[a]One spinal cord lesion can be substituted for one brain lesion.
McDonald WI, Compston A, Edan G, et al. Recommended MRI diagnostic criteria. *Ann Neurol* 2001;50:121–127.

TABLE 9.5b. *Dissemination in Time*

First scan ≥3 months after clinical event
  Gd-positive lesion: dissemination in time
    If not same site
  Gd-negative lesion: follow-up MRI at ≥3 months
    New T2W or Gd+ lesion: dissemination in time

Gd, gadolinium; T2W, T2-weighted.
McDonald WI, Compston A, Edan G, et al. Recommended MRI diagnostic criteria. *Ann Neurol* 2001;50:121–127.

criteria also define MRI lesion characteristics that increase the likelihood of MS: number (>9), abutting the ventricles, juxtacortical, infratentorial, spinal, and contrast enhancing. As with all the criteria, the clause that "there must be no better explanation" remains a critical part of the definition of MS. Critics of these criteria have complained they are too restrictive, whereas purists remain unconvinced of the utility of MRI for diagnosis. The lack of specificity for MS of white matter lesions seen on MRI also must be remembered, and overreliance on imaging to the exclusion of the clinical picture can lead to diagnostic errors. Ultimately, how one defines the clinical syndrome of MS, within the recognized spectrum of multifocal demyelination discovered at au-

topsy to hyperacute demyelinating syndromes, remains an ongoing debate. The recent McDonald criteria provide an important update and have been adopted for the incorporation of patients in research studies.

Laboratory Features

MRI

MRI is the single most useful test in confirming the diagnosis of MS. A brain MRI performed on a high field (≥1.5 Tesla) magnet is abnormal in 95% of patients with clinically definite MS, and the absence of high signal abnormalities in either the brain or spinal cord is strong evidence against the diagnosis of MS. MS lesions appear as areas of high signal

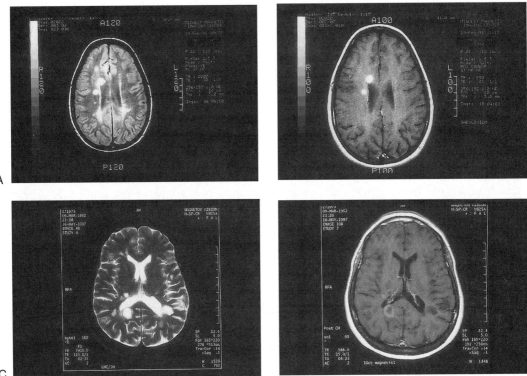

FIG. 9.4. Magnetic resonance imaging scans of the brain of a patient with multiple sclerosis. **A:** Fluid-attenuated inversion recovery (FLAIR) sequence demonstrating typical periventricular white matter lesions. **B:** On T1-weighted image with contrast only two of these lesions appear active. **C:** In a separate patient, T2-weighted scan demonstrating two demyelinating lesions of apparent equal intensity. **D:** The T1-weighted images with contrast reveals one lesion is active and the other is hypointense, suggesting formation of a T1 black hole. Persistence of T1 holes correlates with axonal dropout.

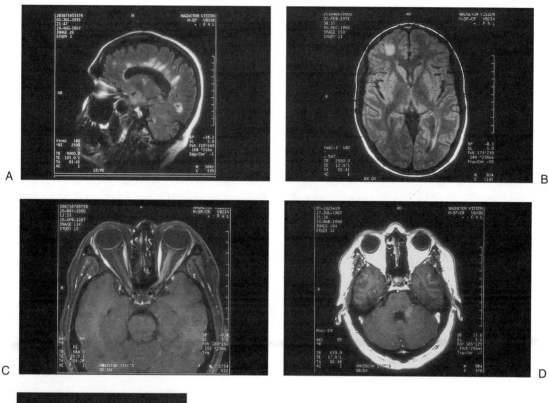

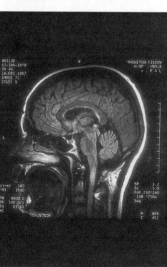

FIG. 9.5. Magnetic resonance imaging scans of the brain of a patient with multiple sclerosis demonstrating typical lesion locations. **A:** Periventricular lesions extending perpendicularly from the ventricles (Dawson's fingers). **B:** Juxtacortical lesion. **C:** Edematous enhancing optic nerve. **D:** Enhancing lesion on the cerebellar peduncle. **E:** Lesions in the corpus callosum and high cervical cord.

usually in the cerebral white matter on T2-weighted images (Figs. 9.4 and 9.5). They are typically round or ovoid but may appear as fingerlike projections extending perpendicularly from the ventricular wall (Dawson's fingers). Typical locations include the corpus cal-losum, abutting the walls of the ventricles, in the juxtacortical lesions (grey–white junction), in the posterior fossa (pons and cerebellar peduncles), and in the spinal cord (cervical twice as commonly as thoracic). Fluid-attenuated inversion recovery (FLAIR) is more sensitive than conventional T2-weighted imaging for cerebral lesions but is less useful in the posterior fossa or spinal cord. Short tau inversion recovery (STIR) images have the highest sensitivity for detecting demyelination in the spinal cord. All MRIs performed in suspected or definite patients with MS should be done before and after intravenous administration of the paramagnetic agent gadolinium diethylenetriaminepentaacetic acid (GdDTPA). Lesions that enhance after GdDTPA have been shown to represent acute inflammatory lesions and as such increase the likelihood that a lesion is related to MS as opposed to a non-specific small-vessel disease process. Enhancing lesions also are used as a measure of disease activity in clinical trials. Enhancing lesions only last for 2 to 8 weeks and therefore can be missed easily, so FLAIR is a more reliable measure of the total burden of disease or for infrequent serial scanning. MRI is also useful for ruling out non-MS related structural lesions such as spinal tumors, syrinxes, Chiari malformations, and herniated disc material.

CSF Analysis

CSF studies to rule out infectious and neoplastic etiologies and to look for the presence of intrathecal immunoglobulin (Ig) synthesis are an important part of laboratory testing in cases in which the clinical picture and MRI are not diagnostic. The presence of more than 50 mononuclear cells/mm^3, any neutrophils, or a CSF protein of greater than 100 mg/dl should raise concern about a diagnosis of MS. Depending on the laboratory and technique, approximately 80% to 90% of patients with clinically definite MS will have two or more IgG bands present on a CSF gel electrophoresis and not in a matched serum sample (oligoclonal bands). Quantitative increases in the CSF IgG index provide similar information but do not always correlate with the presence of oligoclonal bands and should therefore also be ordered as part of CSF analysis. The sensitivity of these tests in clinically isolated syndromes is lower. In addition, oligoclonal bands are not specific for MS and have been

observed in 50% of patients with infectious diseases of the nervous system and in about 15% of patients with non-inflammatory diseases such as tumors and infarctions. MBP is released after CNS tissue injury from many processes, and other than documenting an organic etiology to the clinical presentation, the test is not helpful.

Evoked Potentials

Sensory evoked potentials are used in MS to provide objective evidence to supplement subjective sensory symptoms or occasionally to reveal clinically silent lesions. This can be particularly valuable if a psychiatric basis for the symptoms is being considered or in early cases in which MRIs are inconclusive. Of the three types of evoked potentials, brainstem auditory evoked response (BAER), somatosensory evoked potential (SSEP), and visual evoked response (VER), the latter is the most useful because remote optic nerve disease is common and not well visualized on MRI.

Serologic Testing

As part of excluding other disease processes it is often prudent to obtain peripheral blood to test: vitamin B12, thyroid stimulating hormone, erythrocyte sedimentation rate, antinuclear antibodies, Lyme titer, and rapid plasma reagin. In unusual cases, more extensive testing may include antineutrophil cytoplasmic antibodies, antiphospholipid antibodies, Sjögren's syndrome A and B, hepatitis profile, and angiotensin-converting enzyme. Rarely, human immunodeficiency virus and opportunistic infection can mimic MS. Some risk exists of obtaining false-positive tests, and some experts have questioned the cost effectiveness of extensive serologic testing.

Errors in Diagnosing Multiple Sclerosis

Conditions commonly misdiagnosed for MS are listed in Table 9.6. The rules of dissemination in time and space are critical to

TABLE 9.6a. *Conditions Commonly Mistaken for Multiple Sclerosis*

Vascular diseases	Small-vessel cerebrovascular disease
	Vasculitis
Structural lesions	Malformation, or base-of-skull anomaly or tumor
	Posterior fossa tumor or AVM
	Spinal cord tumor or cervical spondylosis
Degenerative diseases	Motor system disease
	Spinocerebellar degeneration
Infections	HTLV-1 infection
	HIV myelopathy or HIV-related cerebritis
	Lyme disease
Other conditions	Cobalamin deficiency
	Sjögren's syndrome
	Sarcoidosis
	Nonspecific abnormalities visible on MRI

AVM, arteriovenous malformation; HTLV-1, human T-cell lymphotrophic virus type-1.

TABLE 9.6b. *Diseases That Mimic Multiple Sclerosis on MRI*

ADEM	Histiocytosis
HTN/small vessel disease	HTLV-1
CADASIL	Lyme disease
Sarcoidosis	Leukodystrophies
Vasculitis	Mitochondrial disease
Migraine	Lupus
Aging-related changes	Behçet's disease
Organic aciduria	HIV

ADEM, acute disseminated encephalomyelitis; HTN, hypertension; HTLV-1, human T-cell lymphotrophic virus type-1; CADASIL, cerebral autosomal-dominant arteriopathy with subcortical infarcts and leukoencephalopathy.

making an accurate diagnosis of MS. ADEM can appear clinically and radiographically like MS but is usually a monophasic disease process. Similarly, the presence of a cervicomedullary lesion such as with a Chiari malformation can cause multiple symptoms emanating from one location in the nervous system, so careful attention to documenting a clear second location is critical. In both situations, MRI has proved extremely useful; however, T2-weighted lesions are not specific for MS, and therefore vascular, infectious, and neoplastic etiologies of multifocal disease must be considered. The extent of exclusionary testing usually is dictated by the clinical presentation. In a case of RR-MS with typical findings and confirmatory brain MRI, little other testing is necessary. In atypical presentations with unusual historical features (fever, exposures, no relapses), strong family history, no eye findings, or purely progressive disease, more extensive testing is mandatory. Finally,

psychiatric disease must be considered in the patient with numerous symptoms and little objective evidence for disease. The experienced clinician, however, recognizes that early in the course of MS, objective evidence may be lacking and comorbid psychiatric disease can be the primary symptom. The level of confidence in the diagnosis of MS increases with time, and the physician always should be alert to alternative or coexistent disease processes even in patients who carry a diagnosis of MS.

When to Refer a Patient to a Neurologist

MS is a complicated neurologic disease, and the approaches to diagnosis and treatment are changing rapidly. It is therefore appropriate to refer any patient suspected of having MS to a neurologist with MS experience. Symptoms that are suspicious for MS include unexplained numbness/tingling, fatigue, urinary urgency, loss of vision in one eye, or impaired coordination. Although many of these symptoms occur commonly in healthy people, it is the persistence of a symptom or multiple symptoms that should provoke further evaluation. The non-neurologist should not be dissuaded by concomitant emotionality or psychiatric disease because this can be part of the presentation of MS. A brain MRI is a good first step in screening for MS. The presence of any high signal lesions in a young person warrants neurologic consultation.

Therapy of Multiple Sclerosis

Symptomatic Therapy

Despite the recent advances in immunomodulating therapies to decrease new disease activity, many patients continue to suffer from ongoing symptoms related to preestablished lesions. Appropriate recognition and treatment of ongoing symptoms can greatly improve quality of life in patients with MS (Table 9.7).

Spasticity

Mild spasticity may be managed by stretching and exercise programs such as aqua ther-

apy and yoga. Drug therapy is indicated when stiffness, spasms, or clonus interfere with function or sleep. Baclofen is a good first choice for monotherapy. It exerts an antispastic effect by stimulating receptors for the inhibitory neurotransmitter, GABA. The initial dosage is 5 to 10 mg three times a day with intermittent upward dosage adjustments to achieve a therapeutic response or maximum tolerated dose, which may exceed 100 mg in some patients. Some patients may only require bedtime dosing to control nocturnal spasms. The principal limiting side effects of baclofen are confusion, sedation, or increased muscle weakness, and careful attention must be given to not overmedicate patients who are dependent on their muscle tone to ambulate. Baclofen may also unpredictably improve or worsen bladder function. Patients should never abruptly discontinue baclofen from doses greater than 30 mg/day because a withdrawal syndrome can occur consisting of confusion, seizures, or both. Tizanidine is an alpha-adrenergic agonist that exerts an antispastic effect by stimulating central pathways that provide descending inhibitory input to the spinal cord. Tizanidine is best initiated very slowly, starting with 2 mg at bedtime, with gradual dosage adjustment by 2 to 4 mg increments to a maximum of 12 mg three

TABLE 9.7. *Pharmacologic Treatments: Symptomatic*

Drug	Indication	Starting Dose	Stable Dose	Comments
Baclofen	Spasticity	5 mg tid	10–40 mg tid/qid	Severe withdrawal reaction
Tizanidine	Spasticity	2 mg qhs	4–8 mg tid	—
Diazepam	Spasticity, anxiety, insomnia, vertigo	2–5 mg qhs	5–10 mg tid	—
Meclizine	Vertigo	12.5 mg tid	25 mg tid	—
Oxybutynin	Urinary urgency	5 mg qd	5–10 mg bid	Anticholinergic effects may be contraindicated with glaucoma
Tolterodine	Urinary urgency	1 mg qd	1–2 mg bid	Anticholinergic effects may be contraindicated with glaucoma
Sildenafil	Erectile dysfunction	50 mg 0.5–4 hrs prior to intercourse	25–100 mg	Contraindicated in macular degeneration and with nitrates
Modafinil	Fatigue	200 mg qam	100–200 mg qd/bid	Contraindicated with certain heart conditions
Amantadine	Fatigue	100 mg bid	100 mg bid	—
Gabapentin	Pain, dystonic spasms	300 mg qhs	300–900 mg tid/qid	—
Carbamazepine	Pain, dystonic spasms	100 mg qd	100–600 mg tid/qid	Contraindicated in patients with preexisting cytopenias

times a day. The principal side effects are sleepiness, orthostatic hypotension, and dry mouth. Tizanidine is said to be less likely to cause motor weakness than baclofen, but its efficacy often is limited by somnolence. It can be used alone but is often successful in low doses combined with baclofen. Gabapentin and benzodiazepines also have muscle-relaxant properties. In cases of extreme spasticity, continuous intrathecal baclofen can be delivered through an implantable infusion pump placed in an abdominal subcutaneous pocket and connected to a plastic catheter that is tethered in the lumbar subarachnoid space.

Pain and Spasms

Patients with disagreeable paresthesias, atypical facial pain, or tic douloureux often respond to antiepileptic drugs such as carbamazepine, phenytoin, or gabapentin. Occasionally amitriptyline can be helpful. Narcotic analgesics are rarely the solution for chronic pain in MS. For refractory trigeminal neuralgia, intravenous phenytoin may provide rapid relief. Baclofen, mexiletine, misoprostol, valproic acid, topiramate, and lidocaine also have been suggested but have shown variable success. Surgical procedures to relieve medically intractable pain include rhizotomy, injection of anesthetics, and gamma knife. Paroxysmal dystonic spasms can be seen in MS and respond well in most instances to low doses of the same antiepileptic drugs.

Bladder, Bowel, and Sexual Dysfunction

The first step in managing a neurogenic bladder is to determine whether the problem is one of failure to empty, failure to store, or a combination of both called detrusor external sphincter dyssynergia. A thorough history and urinalysis to rule out infection is appropriate. Immediate treatment of bacteruria with antibiotics, even in the absence of typical dysuria, is necessary in MS because of the known propensity for infection to cause disease exacerbation. A postvoid residual urinary volume is the best means to determine if

there is retention. Anticholinergic drugs are the initial drugs of choice for irritative bladder symptoms in the absence of infection. Oxybutynin, 5 mg, is increased gradually until symptom relief or distressing side effects, such as dry mouth, blurred vision, or worsening constipation, occur. Oxybutynin is also available in a long-acting formulation with reduced peak side effects and enhanced efficacy compared with other agents. Tolterodine, 1 to 2 mg twice a day, is a useful alternative with fewer anticholinergic side effects. Propantheline bromide and hyoscyamine sulfate are older alternative anticholinergic agents. Anticholinergic drugs can be used intermittently if bladder symptoms are distressing at particular times, such as at bedtime or before a long automobile ride. The patient should be made aware of possible urinary retention with anticholinergics. Urinary residual volume should be checked after initiating therapy or should concerns arise about retention. In cases of concomitant retention and urgency, anticholinergics can be used in combination with intermittent bladder self-catheterization. Patients failing to achieve urinary continence with anticholinergic pharmacotherapy, with or without self-catheterization, need formal urologic evaluation for consideration of diversion procedures.

Drug treatment of urinary retention is usually ineffective, but some patients may benefit from attempts at decreasing bladder neck tone using alpha-1 adrenergic receptor antagonists such as terazosin, doxazosin, and tamsulosin. Desmopressin, a vasopressin analogue, can be used at a dose of 20 mg by intranasal administration nightly to treat nocturnal incontinence by temporarily suppressing urine production. This approach should be used with caution in patients with hypertension.

Constipation is very common in MS and should be managed aggressively to avoid long-term complications. For fecal incontinence, the addition of fiber in the form of a bulk fiber laxative (e.g., Metamucil) twice a day can provide enough bulk to the stool to allow a partially incompetent sphincter to hold in the bowel movement long enough to allow the patient to reach a bathroom. The use of anticholinergics or antidiarrheal agents may be effective for short periods to combat incontinence associated with diarrhea.

A careful sexual history to determine the problem(s) is a good first step in treating sexual dysfunction. Counseling the patient regarding avoiding the ill effects of elevated body temperature can be critical in managing problems that worsen with sexual intimacy. Erectile dysfunction in MS can be managed with sildenafil effectively initiated at 50 mg 60 minutes before intercourse (higher doses may be necessary). Sildenafil should be used with caution in older patients or in those with a history of heart disease and is contraindicated in patients with macular degeneration. Discontinuation of medications known to decrease libido (selective serotonin reuptake inhibitors (SSRI) or impotence (beta blockers) should be considered if possible.

Neurobehavioral Manifestations

The most common neurobehavioral manifestation amenable to drug therapy is depression, which occurs in more than 50% of patients with MS. Moderate or severe depression should be treated with one of the SSRIs. For patients with psychomotor retardation and depression, fluoxetine, 20 to 80 mg daily, or sertraline, 50 to 200 mg daily, may be particularly effective. Paroxetine, 100 to 200 mg daily, is often useful for patients who are anxious and depressed. These drugs increase the levels of tricyclic antidepressants, so care should be exercised in combining SSRIs with tricyclic antidepressants (TCAs). Amitriptyline, 50 to 200 mg at bedtime, can be useful in depressed patients who are also having difficulty sleeping, headaches, or other pain. Treatment should be instituted gradually to minimize anticholinergic or CNS side effects. The patient and family should be warned of the delay between initiating therapy and observing a benefit. The pseudobulbar syndrome of pathologic laughing or weeping may respond to amitriptyline in low doses. Several

newer antidepressants may be useful when the anticholinergic side effects of TCAs or the sexual side effects of SSRIs (decreased libido and orgasm) become intolerable. Bupropion, citalopram, and venlafaxine all may be better tolerated.

Alprazolam, a benzodiazepine analogue, has been useful for anxiety in some patients. A dose of 0.25 to 0.50 mg two or three times a day is usually sufficient. Diazepam can be used as an alternative drug. As with other symptomatic therapies, the need for pharmacotherapy over time should be assessed intermittently, and the drug should be tapered if appropriate.

Fatigue

Some types of MS fatigue may respond to short periods of rest, but if this is not possible, or in cases of severe fatigue, medication should be considered. Amantadine, 100 mg twice a day, may be effective in treating about one-third of the cases of fatigue. Modafinil, a new narcolepsy drug that acts as a CNS stimulant, was found to be effective in patients with MS at a dose of 200 mg in the morning. Occasionally, treatment with an SSRI (fluoxetine and sertraline) can have a positive effect on fatigue even in the absence of overt depression.

Corticosteroids

Corticosteroids are the mainstay of acute relapse treatment and are discussed as a symptomatic therapy because at this time no conclusive evidence exists that they have any effect on the natural history or long-term outcome of a disease exacerbation. There is evidence that corticosteroids shorten the duration and severity of an exacerbation. Intravenous methylprednisolone (IVMP), 1,000 mg, is administered daily for 3 to 5 days in the office or at home by a visiting nurse. On completion of the IVMP, prednisone may be started, 60 mg orally in the morning and reduced by 10 mg every other day until tapered off. The prednisone taper is not necessary but helps reduce withdrawal symptoms in some patients. An H_2 blocker or proton pump inhibitor may be coadministered in patients with a history of ulcer or heartburn. Metoclopramide may be useful in patients who develop singultus (hiccups). The effects of steroids appear to diminish with repeated usage, and many patients reach a stage of unresponsiveness to steroids. It is unclear whether that stage can be delayed or prevented by restricting the use of steroids, but this appears to be a wise approach. Patients who become refractory to a short course of IVMP may respond to higher doses (2 g/day) or longer courses (10 days).

The most common side effects of treatment are irritability, difficulty sleeping, and fluid retention. Additional well-recognized risks include hypokalemia, gastrointestinal side effects, and osteoporosis. Fluid retention can be minimized by salt restriction during the therapy, and diuretic use is discouraged because of the exaggerated risk of hypokalemia. Ankle edema can be minimized by wearing elastic stockings and elevating the leg. Hypokalemia is usually not a problem in the absence of concurrent potassium wasting, such as with diuretic therapy, but in the presence of heart disease or with concurrent diuretic therapy, oral potassium replacement should be administered and electrolyte levels should be monitored during therapy. Anxiety and difficulty sleeping are usually minor problems. Patients may on rare occasions develop significant depression or mania during corticosteroid therapy.

In the Optic Neuritis Treatment Trial (ONTT) the rate of visual recovery was significantly faster in the IVMP group than in patients treated with placebo or oral prednisone, but no significant differences in visual outcome were found between groups at 6 months. Prednisone therapy alone increased the risk of new episodes of optic neuritis in either eye. The ONTT results have led to widespread use of IVMP for patients with optic neuritis and an abnormal brain MRI and have discouraged the use of oral prednisone alone for MS relapses. Hints of a neuroprotective effect of steroids in other studies await confirmation.

Disease-Modifying Therapies

Four partially effective disease-modifying therapies for the initial management of MS are available in the United States: IFNβ-1a (Avonex), IFNβ-1a (Rebif), IFNβ-1b (Betaseron), and glatiramer acetate (Copaxone). A fifth agent, mitoxantrone (Novantrone), was approved in the United States for treatment of worsening forms of RR-MS and SP-MS. Table 9.8 lists these immunomodulating pharmacologic treatments.

TABLE 9.8. *Pharmacologic Treatments: Immunomodulating*

Drug	Indication	Starting Dose	Stable Dose	Comments
Avonex (Interferon beta 1a)	Relapsing MS, clinically isolated syndromes	30 mcg IM qd	30 mcg IM qd	Flulike side effects
Betaseron (Interferon beta 1b)	Relapsing MS	2–4 MIU SC qod	8 MIU SC qod	Flulike side effects
Rebif (Interferon beta 1a)	Relapsing MS	22 mcg SC tiw	22–44 mcg tiw	Flulike side effects
Glatiramer acetate	Relapsing MS	20 mg SC qd	20 mg SC qd	Harmless idiosyncratic reaction of chest pain and palpitations lasts 10–20 min.
Methylprednisolone	Acute exacerbation	1000 mg IV qam	1000 mg IV qam for 3–5 days	Contraindicated in avascular necrosis
Mitoxantrone	Worsening forms of relapsing MS and SPMS	5–12 mg/m^2 IV	5–12 mg/m^2 IV Q3 months for 2–3 years	Maximum dose 140 mg/m^2; cardiotoxicity and leukemia reported

MS, multiple sclerosis; IM, intramuscularly; MIU, million international units; SC, subcutaneous; SPMS, secondary progressive multiple sclerosis; IV, intravenous.

Beta Interferons

Beta interferons are naturally occurring cytokines with a variety of immunomodulating and antiviral activities that may account for their therapeutic utility. IFNs may act through several mechanisms including modulation major histocompatibility complex (MHC) expression, suppressor T-cell function, adhesion molecules, and matrix metalloproteinases. All three IFNβ drugs have been shown to reduce relapses by about one-third in double-blind placebo-controlled trials and are recommended either as firstline therapies or for glatiramer acetate intolerant patients with RR-MS. In addition, in each of these trials, IFNβ resulted in a 50% to 80% reduction of the inflammatory lesions visualized on brain MRI. Evidence also exists that these drugs improve quality of life and cognitive function.

The major difference between the IFNβ drugs is that Avonex is given weekly intramuscularly (IM) and Rebif and Betaseron are given three times a week subcutaneously (SC). The adequacy of IFNβ-1a weekly dosing has been questioned. Studies appear to support a modest dose-response effect for IFNβ; however, one study of double dose (60 μg IM) Avonex, once a week, found no benefit over the single-dose regimen. Whether the benefit of more frequent dosing is sustained for periods longer than 2 years remains unclear, and the increased incidence of neutralizing antibodies with the more frequent SC dosing also must be considered.

Flulike symptoms, including fever, chills, malaise, muscle aches, and fatigue, occur in approximately 60% of patients treated with either IFNβ-1a or IFNβ-1b and usually dissipate with continued use and premedication with non-steroidal antiinflammatory drugs (NSAIDS). Other side effects include injection-site reactions, worsening of preexisting spasticity, depression, mild anemia, thrombocytopenia, and elevations in transaminases, which are usually not severe and rarely lead to treatment discontinuation.

Development of neutralizing antibodies (NAbs) can occur with any of the IFNβ products. Although the results are variable, IFNβ-1a weekly IM (Avonex) is reported to have the lowest incidence. The effect of NAbs on long-term efficacy remains to be fully defined. Some experts recommend that the results of a NAb assay in patients who exhibit insufficient treatment response may guide decisions for alternative therapy.

Glatiramer Acetate

Glatiramer acetate (Copaxone) is a polypeptide mixture that originally was designed to mimic MBP. The mechanism of action of glatiramer acetate is distinct from that of IFNβ; therefore patients may respond differently to this drug. Glatiramer acetate (20 mg SC QD) has also been shown to reduce the frequency of relapses by approximately one-third and therefore is also recommended as a firstline treatment for RR-MS or for patients who are IFNβ intolerant. Glatiramer acetate results in a one-third reduction in the inflammatory activity seen on MRI.

Glatiramer acetate is generally well tolerated and unassociated with flulike symptoms. Immediate postinjection reactions associated with administration of glatiramer acetate include a local inflammatory reaction and an uncommon idiosyncratic reaction consisting of flushing, chest tightness with palpitations, anxiety, or dyspnea, which resolves spontaneously without sequelae. Routine laboratory monitoring is not considered necessary in patients treated with glatiramer acetate, and the development of binding antibodies does not interfere with the therapeutic efficacy of glatiramer acetate.

Mitoxantrone

Mitoxantrone is an anthracenedione antineoplastic agent that was shown in a phase III, randomized, placebo-controlled, multicenter trial to reduce the number of treated relapses by 67% and slowed progression on EDSS, ambulation index, and MRI measures of disease activity. It therefore is recommended for worsening forms of MS. Acute side effects of mitoxantrone include nausea and alopecia. The lifetime use of this drug is limited to 2 to 3 years (or a cumulative dose of 120 to 140 mg/m^2) because of its cumulative cardiotoxicity, and more rapid cardiotoxicity can occur. There is also some concern about treatment-related leukemias with this drug. Mitoxantrone is a chemotherapeutic agent that should be prescribed and administered only by experienced physicians.

Other Drugs Used in Multiple Sclerosis

Several other drugs are commonly used in MS despite the lack of U.S. Food and Drug Administration approval and definitive evidence of efficacy. Numerous small clinical trials support the modest effect of intravenous immunoglobulin G (IVIg), azathioprine, methotrexate, and cyclophosphamide.

Initiation of Early Therapy

Evidence is accumulating that the best time to initiate disease-modifying treatment is early in the course of the disease. Data indicate that irreversible axon damage may occur early in the course of RRMS and that available therapies appear to be most effective at preventing new lesion formation but do not repair old lesions. With disease progression, the autoimmune response of MS may become more difficult to suppress. Weekly IM IFNβ-1a (Avonex) has been proved to reduce the cumulative probability of developing clinically definite MS in patients who present with a first clinical demyelinating episode and have two or more brain lesions on MRI. Based on these data, the National Multiple Sclerosis Society recommends initiation of immunomodulating treatment at the time of diagnosis. The clinician must weigh these considerations against the practical concerns of young patients, for whom the prospect of starting a therapy that requires self-injection may be frightening and burdensome. There are also few long-term (more than 10 years) data regarding the safety and sustained efficacy of disease-modifying drugs. Some patients will opt to defer therapy, hoping to be among the minority of patients with benign MS, but certain MRI and clinical features should prompt the physician and patient to reconsider this approach. An MRI with contrast-enhancing lesions, large burden of white matter disease, or presence of any T1 low signal lesions (black holes) suggests a relatively poor prognosis. It may be useful to repeat the brain MRI in 6 months or 1 year to determine how quickly the disease process is evolving. The presence of spinal cord lesions or atrophy also suggests a poor prognosis (Figs. 9.6 and 9.7). Clinical features may be less useful for assessing prognosis, and once definite disability develops it may be too late to treat that component of the disease.

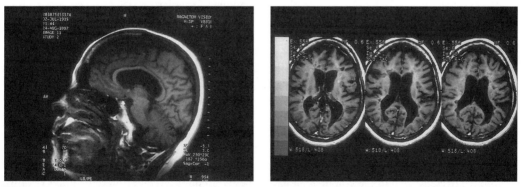

FIG. 9.6. T1-weighted magnetic resonance imaging scans of the brain of a patient with multiple sclerosis demonstrating atrophy. **A:** Sagittal image revealing thinned corpus callosum and ventriculomegaly. **B:** Axial image with extensive ventriculomegaly and T1 black hole formation.

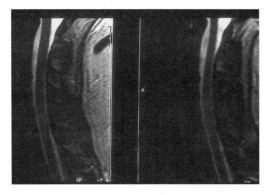

FIG. 9.7. Magnetic resonance imaging scans of the spinal cord of a patient with multiple sclerosis revealing multiple high signal lesions best seen using the short tau inversion recovery (STIR) sequence.

Combination Therapy

Several trials are studying the addition of oral immunosuppressive drugs, IVIg, or glatiramer acetate to IFNβ in patients who continue to have disease activity. The rationale for this approach is based on experience with other diseases, but further testing is required both to ensure its safety and to ensure that the mechanism of action of one drug does not interfere with that of the other drug. Two 6-month trials of Avonex administered along with either glatiramer acetate or oral methotrexate suggested that the combinations were safe, and longer-term trials to assess clinical effects are planned.

Special Challenges for Hospitalized Patients

Patients with MS may be hospitalized either during severe exacerbations or for other medical problems. In the case of an MS exacerbation, the patient should be screened for sources of infection and treated with antibiotics as appropriate. Rapid control of fever is also important to prevent worsening of symptoms. Exacerbations that warrant hospitalization usually are related to acute inability to ambulate or loss of self-care in the more advanced patient, and IV corticosteroids usually are instituted. Physical and occupational therapy should be initi-

ated immediately, and a rehabilitation plan should be put in place with attention to adaptive devices for the home and orthotics or ambulation aids. For non–MS-related hospitalization it is equally important to be vigilant about infections to prevent exacerbation. MS rarely causes respiratory compromise, and there are no absolute contraindications to anesthesia. Cosmetic surgery is discouraged, but necessary operations are usually well tolerated. Patients with MS do not have any impairment in wound healing. Postpartum exacerbations usually do not occur for several weeks after delivery and thus are not a major obstetric complication. Counseling, social work, and attention to severe depression should be considered during periods of stress such as may occur during hospitalization.

Alternative Therapies Used by Patients with Multiple Sclerosis

Numerous alternative therapies have been advocated for MS but rarely are they tested in a placebo-controlled manner and, therefore, they cannot be recommended. Because MS is an unpredictable disease characterized early by relapses and spontaneous recovery, patients are very susceptible to placebo effects and misguided judgments about the efficacy of alternative therapies. Bee stings have been used for many years, and for those who are not allergic, about half of patients report a temporary boost in energy perhaps related to endogenous corticosteroid release in response to cutaneous inflammation. Procarin is a patch used by some patients with MS and contains vitamin B12, histamine, caffeine, and a proprietary substance. Several diets for MS, such as the Swank diet, have been popular. Acupuncture is used to relieve pain and sometimes boost energy. Naltrexone is advertised on the Internet for MS. None of these approaches has been tested adequately. Complementary medicine advocates recommend yoga, meditation, aqua therapy, body cooling devices, and stress reduction, all of which are reasonable and safe approaches to dealing with MS.

Physical Therapy

Physical therapy has an important role in managing MS. Regular exercise and stretching decrease MS symptoms of stiffness, weakness, and pain and improve overall well being. Physical therapy has been shown to improve disability from MS independent of drug interventions and should be continued on a regular basis as part of a maintenance regimen.

Novel Experimental Immunomodulatory Approaches

Several treatments are being tested in preliminary trials, including antibodies to various critical immune molecules (IL-12 [interleukin-12], VLA-4 [very late antigen-4], and IL-2 receptor), phosphodiesterase inhibitors, novel NSAIDs, beta-adrenergic agonists, and immunosuppressive regimens used during organ transplantation and malignancies. Of these therapies, a monoclonal antibody directed against the adhesion molecule VLA-4 (natalizumab) had promising results in a phase II trial, and phase III clinical trials are in progress. Immunoablative protocols using extremely high doses of chemotherapies, followed by autologous stem-cell rescue, have been used in particularly aggressive forms of MS. This approach has afforded disease stabilization, both clinically and by MRI, but has an unacceptably high morbidity and mortality at present.

Remyelination and Neuroprotection

Theoretic approaches to remyelination include enhancing existing oligodendrocyte precursors or neural stem cells by using growth factors or direct transplantation of oligodendrocytes or autologous Schwann cells. Growth factors such as insulinlike growth factor carry the inherent risk of non-specifically activating the immune system. Schwann cell transplantation has been done in three patients with MS to determine viability and proof of concept, but no data are available at this time.

QUESTIONS AND DISCUSSION

1. A 24-year-old nursing school student presents to her primary care physician (PCP) with complaints of numbness and tingling in her hands for 1 month. On questioning, she responds that she has had recent fatigue and mild depression, which she attributed to stress. She denies any other past medical history and is only taking birth control pills. Her entire physical examination is normal. The next appropriate step is to:

A. Tell her she probably has carpal tunnel syndrome and recommend splinting.

B. Tell her that because she has no abnormal signs on examination that the symptoms are probably from stress and not to worry.

C. Order blood tests and then a brain MRI.

D. Treat her for depression.

The answer is (C). This woman could have early signs of MS, and because there is strong evidence to support early initiation of therapy it is important to make a diagnosis. Blood testing is indicated to exclude thyroid disease, vitamin B12 deficiency, other inflammatory neurologic disorders, and infections. A brain MRI is the single best screening tool for MS. Depression may be a symptom of MS and should not be considered an adequate explanation for ill-defined somatic symptoms. Carpal tunnel syndrome is common but usually unilateral and is detectable on examination by eliciting symptoms through tapping or compression of the median nerve or detection of sensory and/or motor loss in a median nerve distribution.

2. Blood tests are normal on this patient and the brain MRI is reported to show two periventricular lesions, which are suspicious for demyelination. The woman is referred to a neurologist for further evaluation. The neurologist also finds no sensory loss in the hands to pinprick but thinks there may be some loss of vibratory perception in both the hands and feet. In addition, there is a partial loss of vibratory perception below C4 level in the neck bilaterally. The next appropriate step is to:

A. Tell her she probably has a herniated disk in her neck, and get C-spine x-rays.

B. Tell her she has evidence for spinal cord disease and that a C-spine MRI is the most sensitive test for evaluating the spinal cord.

C. Tell her she has clinically definite MS and should be treated immediately.

D. Tell her to wait and see if the symptoms resolve spontaneously.

The answer is (B). Vibratory loss in all four extremities with a partial cervical level is highly suggestive of a dorsal column lesion in the spinal cord, and direct imaging of this area is indicated to exclude compressive and neoplastic processes. Although the absence of pain and the brain MRI are more consistent with a demyelinating process, she does not have evidence for "lesions separated in both time and space," which is critical to the diagnosis of MS.

3. The C-spine MRI reveals a high signal lesion in the dorsal spinal cord at C3-C4, which does not enhance with contrast or cause swelling of the cord. The neurologist explains to her that it is highly likely that she has the beginnings of MS, and there is scientific evidence that initiation of therapy in "clinically isolated demyelinating syndromes" prolongs the time to a second attack and a clinically definite diagnosis. She declines immunomodulating therapy and prefers to "wait and see." The patient is treated for her depression with an SSRI and notices improvement in both her depression and fatigue. Three months later a repeat MRI is obtained and reveals a new gadolinium-enhancing lesion. The neurologist should tell her:

A. She has clinically definite MS according to McDonald criteria but that treatment is not indicated because this is probably a benign case.

B. She has clinically definite MS according to McDonald criteria and that treatment with either IFNβ or glatiramer acetate is appropriate.

C. She has PP-MS and there is no treatment.

D. She has clinically definite MS according to McDonald criteria and that because of the spinal cord involvement and active MRI she should be treated with mitoxantrone.

The correct answer is (B). The demonstration of a new lesion on MRI more than 3 months later provides evidence for dissemination in time and now fulfills criteria for a definite diagnosis of MS. The National Multiple Sclerosis Society and many MS experts now favor early initiation of therapy. Benign MS is defined as no disability after at least 10 years and only can be diagnosed retrospectively. Progressive MS is defined as 6 months of unabated worsening without exacerbations. The presence of oligoclonal bands in the CSF also is required to make a diagnosis of PPMS. Mitoxantrone is a chemotherapeutic agent, which is indicated for worsening forms of RR-MS or SP-MS but is usually not a firstline agent.

4. A 36-year-old woman with RR-MS presents for routine follow-up. She is being treated with IFNβ injections and although she has had no exacerbations since being on treatment she complains of increased stiffness in her legs, and on questioning she also admits to urinary urgency with occasional episodes of incontinence. On examination she is more spastic and hyperreflexic in her legs than 6 months ago, but there is no clear sensory level over her spine or weakness. You tell her:

A. There is nothing you can offer her because she now has secondary progressive disease.

B. It is likely that she has failed IFNβ and she should switch to another immunomodulating drug.

C. She should have a urinalysis to look for infection and if negative, offer her symptomatic treatment with Baclofen (for spasticity) and oxybutynin (anticholinergic for bladder).

D. These are likely side effects of her IFNβ and she should stop taking the medication.

The correct answer is (C). Minor changes in neurologic function do not constitute progressive disease, and it is likely that the reduction in relapses suggests that the IFNβ is effective. Although exacerbation of spasticity can be a side effect of IFNβ, bladder frequency is part of underlying MS and is often a sign of urinary tract infection. Antibiotic treatment of bacteruria often alleviates the bladder symptoms and sometimes other new symptoms as well.

5. Two years later the patient presents with blurred vision in her left eye and is treated with a 3-day course of IV methylprednisolone for optic neuritis by her ophthalmologist. Three months after this event she presents to the office with dizziness, diplopia, and trouble walking straight. There has been no obvious precipitating factor (infection, heat, stress), and she has been taking her medications on a regular basis. On examination she is noted to have several new findings including bilateral INO, finger to nose dysmetria, severe gait ataxia, and facial asymmetry. You recommend the following:

A. A 3- to 5-day course of iv methylprednisolone.

B. Physical therapy evaluation and treatment for gait stability.

C. A brain MRI 30 days after the steroids.

D. Discussion of alternative or combination therapies and/or referral to an MS clinical trials center.

E. All of the above

The answer is (E). The patient is having an acute disabling exacerbation and should be retreated with IV methylprednisolone. Physical therapy is very important in improving functional outcome, and therapists can make recommendations of appropriate aids such as canes, crutches, and walkers. A brain MRI is a useful means of assessing disease activity (gadolinium-enhancing lesions and new T2 lesions) and determining the extent of breakthrough disease activity. Steroids may mask enhancement for 30 days; therefore the MRI should be delayed if possible. Given that the patient has had two rapid exacerbations, and/or if there are numerous new lesions on a follow-up MRI, it is appropriate to consider alternative therapies. The options include switching drugs, adding an immunosuppressive drug, or referring for enrollment in an investigational drug trial.

SUGGESTED READING

Arnold DL, Matthews PM. MRI in the diagnosis and management of multiple sclerosis. *Neurology* 2002;58: S23–S31.

Brex PA, Ciccarelli O, O'Riordan JI, et al. A longitudinal study of abnormalities on MRI and disability from multiple sclerosis. *N Engl J Med* 2002;346:158–164.

Brex PA, Miszkiel KA, O'Riordan JI, et al. Assessing the risk of early multiple sclerosis in patients with clinically isolated syndromes: the role of a follow up MRI. *J Neurol Neurosurg Psychiatry* 2001;70:390–393.

Comi G. Why treat early multiple sclerosis patients? *Curr Opin Neurol* 2000;13:235–240.

Dhib-Jalbut S. Mechanisms of action of interferons and glatiramer acetate in multiple sclerosis. *Neurology* 2002;58:S3–S9.

Frohman EM, Zhang H, Kramer PD, et al. MRI characteristics of the MLF in MS patients with chronic internuclear ophthalmoparesis. *Neurology* 2001;57:762—768.

Grudzinski AN, Hakim Z, Cox ER, et al. The economics of multiple sclerosis: distribution of costs and relationship to disease severity. *Pharmacoeconomics* 1999;15:229–240.

Hemmer B, Archelos JJ, Hartung HP. New concepts in the immunopathogenesis of multiple sclerosis. *Nat Rev Neurosci* 2002;3:291–301.

Krupp LB, Rizvi SA. Symptomatic therapy for underrecognized manifestations of multiple sclerosis. *Neurology* 2002;58:S32–S39.

Lucchinetti C, Bruck W, Parisi J, et al. Heterogeneity of multiple sclerosis lesions: implications for the pathogenesis of demyelination. *Ann Neurol* 2000;47:707–717.

McDonald WI, Compston A, Edan G, et al. Recommended diagnostic criteria for multiple sclerosis: guidelines from the International Panel on the diagnosis of multiple sclerosis. *Ann Neurol* 2001;50:121–127.

Trapp BD, Peterson J, Ransohoff RM, et al. Axonal transection in the lesions of multiple sclerosis. *N Engl J Med* 1998;338:278–285.

10

Parkinson's Disease

William J. Weiner and Lisa M. Shulman

Parkinson's disease is the most common akinetic rigid syndrome and the most frequently
encountered extrapyramidal movement disorder. It is a neurodegenerative disease of unknown etiology that most often begins at 58 to
60 years of age. Approximately 10% to 15% of
patients will have disease onset before age 50.
As the population of the United States ages, the
number of people at risk for the development of
Parkinson's disease increases. Diagnostic and
therapeutic knowledge is important not only because of the prevalence of the disorder but also
because the pharmacology of Parkinson's disease has led to fundamental changes in the way
investigators and physicians view central nervous system neurotransmitter function.

CLINICAL FEATURES

Parkinson's disease is characterized by a
typical history of progressive neurologic disability and the following four major neurologic
signs: resting tremor, cogwheel rigidity,
bradykinesia, and impaired postural reflexes. It
is often observed that by the time a patient presents to a physician for evaluation of early
symptoms, the syndrome has been present for
1 to 2 years. Unilateral tremor involving a single limb is the most common presenting symptom and sign. However, careful history taking
often reveals that difficulty buttoning shirts or
blouses, fastening snaps, and cutting food with
the proper utensils; alterations in handwriting
(Fig. 10.1); a feeling of stiffness; or a general
feeling of overall slowness may have been
noted up to 12 to 24 months earlier and that
these symptoms have gradually become worse.
In addition, a patient may note that his voice
fluctuates and seems to intermittently lose volume. Inquiring whether the patient has difficulty rising from low, soft chairs or sofas; dif-

ficulty entering and leaving an automobile, difficulty turning in bed; or difficulty walking
and maintaining balance in a crowd highlight
the functional impact of bradykinesia, rigidity,
gait impairment, and impaired postural reflexes. The patient may notice that occasionally
he or she is unable to stop walking forward
(propulsion) or backward (retropulsion). Family members also may report that the patient's
facial expression has changed and that he or
she does not smile as much (masked faces; Fig.
10.2), that he or she seems to stare all the time
(reptilian stare), that her or his posture has become stooped and flexed (simian posture; Fig.
10.3), and that he or she has become exasper-
atingly slow. It may take 30 to 90 minutes to
dress in the morning and even longer to disrobe
in the evening.

The elucidation of this history may make
the diagnosis of parkinsonism evident. Not all
patients will present with all of these symptoms, and a patient occasionally will present
with only a single symptom and yet will have
parkinsonism. Inquiring whether the onset of
symptoms was abrupt or insidious; whether
there has been a gradual progression of symptoms; whether there is a family history of neurologic syndromes; and whether there is concurrent drug use, past history of encephalitis,
or exposure to various toxins including the
use of street drugs may help determine the etiology of the syndrome.

Resting tremor is the most frequent presenting sign in these patients. The appearance of
this tremor often precipitates the patient's visit
to the doctor. The tremor is highly characteristic and consists of a low-to-medium-amplitude
with four to five cycles per second alternating
movement. Tremor is defined as the involuntary rhythmic oscillatory sinusoidal movement
that results from the alternating or synchro-

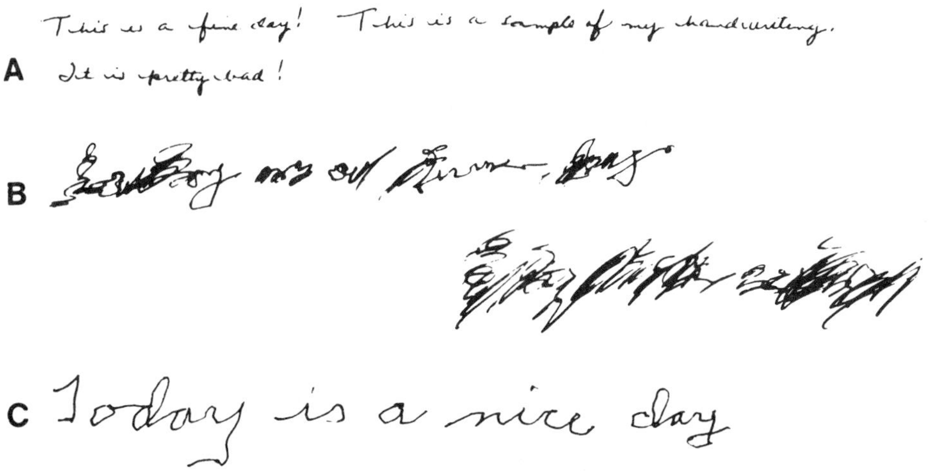

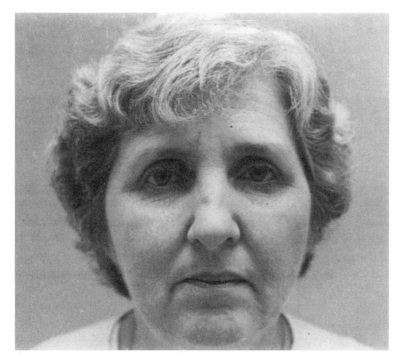

FIG. 10.1. A: This handwriting sample from a 55-year-old patient with untreated Parkinson's disease is a good example of the typical micrographic handwriting that is often characteristic of this condition. The handwriting samples shown in *B* and *C* are from a patient with essential tremor. **B:** Prior to treatment, the sample shows the typical large, sloppy script. **C:** This sample, taken from the same patient with essential tremor while being treated with propranolol (160 mg/day), shows obvious improvement. Changes in written script can provide excellent clues to the type of movement disorder that is present (see Chapter 11).

FIG. 10.2. Typical masked faces in a patient with Parkinson's disease.

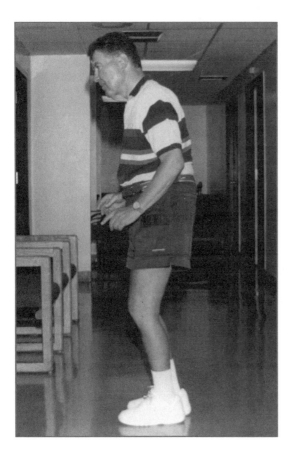

FIG. 10.3. Moderate simian posture in a patient with Parkinson's disease. Note the flexion of the upper extremities, upper trunk, and head. Facial masking is also apparent.

nous contractions of reciprocally innervated antagonistic muscles. Resting tremor has been described as "pill rolling" because of the movement of the fingers and thumb. Its appearance resembles the activity of an "old time" pharmacist preparing a pill. The tremor, however, may begin in the hands, legs, or face and most often appears unilaterally in a single limb. It often will progress to involve the second limb of the same side before becoming bilateral. Tremor is the initial presenting symptom in 75% of patients. With the exception of impaired postural reflexes, the major signs of parkinsonism usually appear unilaterally. Careful observation of the tremor will reveal that it is a resting tremor that is ameliorated with purposeful movement. A simple way of assessing whether a tremor is primarily resting, postural, or kinetic is to have the patient perform the finger-to-finger and finger-to-nose maneuver and to observe the affected limb at rest, with outstretched posture and with movement. The patient with a resting tremor will have a marked amelioration of tremor when the arm springs into action. The patient with kinetic tremor will have no tremor at rest but typically will develop increased tremor as the hand approaches the target. When the resting limb is raised to an outstretched position, the tremor of Parkinson's disease will diminish, although with maintained posture, the tremor may reappear until movement is initiated again. When the limb is totally supported and at rest, the patient with resting tremor will be seen to have the tremor, whereas those patients with kinetic tremor will not.

Cogwheel rigidity is a sign that can be present either unilaterally or bilaterally depending on the stage of illness. The patient does not complain of "cogwheeling." This sign is elicited by passive movement of the limb or neck through a full range of motion. When present, this sign is best elicited by slow flexion and extension of the wrist or neck. In addition to increased tone, a characteristic ratchetlike sensation is sensed by the examiner with passive movement. There are some patients in whom the initial symptomatology is cervical or low back discomfort, and the question of whether increased muscle tone is responsible for this symptom has been raised.

Bradykinesia is responsible for much of the disability associated with parkinsonism. Slowness of voluntary movement contributes to increasing difficulty with the activities of daily living such as getting in and out of a car, rising from chairs, cutting meat, preparing food, dressing, and walking. Some of these difficulties can be observed easily during an examination by watching the patient rise from a chair, walk to the examining room, and undress. Postural reflexes refer to the ability of the patient to right himself and to keep from losing balance when sustaining postural perturbations (e.g., being jostled in a crowd). In addition, these reflexes are also important when turning around and changing direction while walking without losing balance. These reflexes can be evaluated simply and effectively by observing the patient walk 10 to 15 steps and turn around. A patient with normal postural reflexes should be able to pivot and turn without taking extra steps. In parkinsonism, one often will observe that the patient takes three to five steps to change direction. Another test of postural reflexes during the office visit is a firm backward pull on the shoulders or chest with the admonition to the patient that he should attempt to stop his backward motion in one to two steps. The examiner must be positioned behind the patient during this maneuver and prepared to stop the retropulsive movement or prevent a fall if necessary (Fig. 10.4). Impaired postural re-

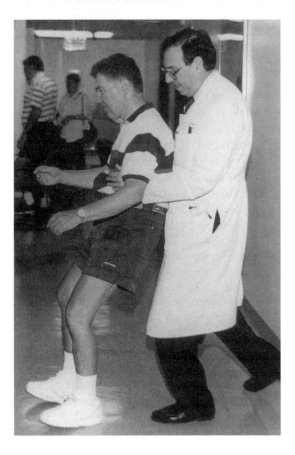

FIG. 10.4. A loss of postural reflexes often is seen in patients with Parkinson's disease. After instructing the patient to maintain his or her posture, the examiner has administered a backward thrust to the patient's chest. The postural response is quite poor: rather than maintaining a fixed postural response to the thrust or taking one or two steps backward, the patient has lost balance entirely and requires the assistance of the examiner to prevent him or her from falling to the ground.

flexes with frequent falls are a source of severe disability and injury in advanced parkinsonism (e.g., subdural hematoma, fractures of the hip or wrist). It should be noted that when postural reflex impairment is a prominent early sign of parkinsonism, the diagnosis more often than not is not true Parkinson's disease but instead one of the other neurodegenerative disorders that produces parkinsonism, such as progressive supranuclear palsy (PSP) or multiple system atrophy (MSA).

There is no single pathognomonic sign of Parkinson's disease; instead, the informed and experienced clinician uses a constellation of symptoms and signs to make the diagnosis. There is also no known biologic marker of Parkinson's disease, and there is no definitive laboratory or imaging study to confirm the diagnosis. Furthermore, identifying parkinsonism by history and clinical examination does not imply that the diagnosis is Parkinson's disease, which is characterized by a specific neuropathology. The substantia nigra (a pigmented midbrain nucleus) bears the brunt of the pathologic changes in Parkinson's disease, with depigmentation, neuronal loss, and the presence of intracytoplasmic inclusion bodies (Lewy bodies) that stain for alpha-synuclein. Patients with a minimum of two of the four cardinal symptoms (tremor, rigidity, bradykinesia, and impaired postural reflexes) in the absence of this specific neuropathology are diagnosed as having an akinetic rigid syndrome or parkinsonism, but not Parkinson's disease. The most common cause of parkinsonism is Parkinson's disease. Clinical features that help distinguish Parkinson's disease from parkinsonism include unilateral presentation of symptoms and signs, slow progression, resting tremor, and responsiveness to dopaminergic agents.

MECHANISMS OF DISEASE

Parkinson's disease is defined pathologically by the loss of dopaminergic neurons in the substantia nigra pars compacta and the presence of intracytoplasmic Lewy bodies, which stain for alpha-synuclein. The idiopathic degeneration of these neurons leads to loss of dopaminergic input to the corpus striatum. The progressive failure of the nigrostriatal pathway results in the symptoms of Parkinson's disease. Neuropathologic examination of the brain of a patient with a history of Parkinson's disease reveals loss of the pigmented neurons in the substantia nigra and loss of dopamine in the striatum where the nigrostriatal fibers project.

The etiology of Parkinson's disease remains elusive. Although numerous epidemiologic studies have investigated Parkinson's disease, definitive environmental factors have not been identified. Nevertheless, there are many leads, and the presence of significant environmental toxin exposure in genetically predisposed individuals remains a strong possibility. In a relatively small number of families, dominant (alpha-synuclein) and recessive (Parkin associated) inheritance has been identified. However, surveys of large numbers of patients seen in movement disorder centers do not reveal a family history of Parkinson's disease in the majority of patients with Parkinson's disease. Nonetheless, identifying the alpha-synuclein and Parkin mutations has led to the discovery that the Lewy body is partly composed of alpha-synuclein and to the potential role of the proteosome in the pathogenesis of Parkinson's disease.

The demonstration in 1967 that orally administered levodopa could produce dramatic improvement in the symptoms of Parkinson's disease was a remarkable therapeutic advance. For levodopa to have a therapeutic effect, it must cross the blood–brain barrier and be decarboxylated to dopamine. The enzyme that decarboxylates dopa to dopamine is ubiquitous and also decarboxylates several other aromatic amino acids. This enzyme, termed aromatic amino acid decarboxylase or dopa decarboxylase, is found in several extracerebral locations, including the gastrointestinal tract, liver, and kidney. When orally administered, levodopa is absorbed; acted on by the extracerebral decarboxylase; and converted to dopamine, which cannot cross the blood–brain barrier. If levodopa is administered alone, enormous quantities are required to overcome the peripheral decarboxylase systems and achieve a therapeutic benefit. The use of a peripheral decarboxylase inhibitor (carbidopa) with levodopa results in a marked reduction in the dose of levodopa necessary to achieve a central effect.

Another enzyme that plays a role in determining how much levodopa circulating in the blood reaches the brain is catechol-O-methyltransferase (COMT). COMT methylates levodopa and also reduces the concentration of levodopa that is available for transport across the blood–brain barrier. Peripheral COMT inhibition is another therapeutic maneuver to enhance levodopa bioavailability in the brain to increase central dopamine activity.

Because increasing the concentration of dopamine in the striatum results in dramatic clinical improvement in patients with Parkinson's disease, the neural substrate that dopamine acts on (the striatal dopamine receptors) are obviously relatively intact. The dopamine receptor sites are divided into five different subtypes, but there are two main families: the D_1 and D_5 group and the D_2, D_3, and D_4 group. Drugs acting as dopamine receptor agonists must have D_2 activity to be effective in the treatment of Parkinson's disease. The dopamine receptor agonists that are available to treat Parkinson's disease include ergot-derived (bromocriptine and pergolide) and non–ergot-derived (pramipexole and ropinirole) compounds. Pramipexole and ropinirole, the most recently marketed, were both introduced for the treatment of Parkinson's disease in 1997. Although all of the dopamine receptor agonists have D_2 activity, they have somewhat different profiles of activation for the various dopamine receptors. Although all agonists have similar efficacy and adverse event profiles, there are variations among individual patients in regard to which agonist is the most efficacious. Although the number of antiparkinsonian medications grows steadily, levodopa remains the gold standard of therapy, the most potent drug for the symptomatic treatment of Parkinson's disease.

TREATMENT

All medications currently used to treat Parkinson's disease only provide symptomatic relief and do not alter the underlying pathogenesis of the disorder; in other words, the natural progression of Parkinson's disease continues despite current treatment. The treatment of each patient with Parkinson's disease should be highly individualized to provide functional improvement. If a patient's symptoms are very mild and causing no impairment in the activities of daily living, delay of treatment may be the appropriate choice. If a patient's symptoms are mildly troublesome, with tremor as the predominant feature, low-dose anticholinergics (e.g., trihexyphenidyl, benztropine) may be all that is required. The anticholinergics, the oldest drugs available to treat Parkinson's disease, remain useful because the striatum contains high levels of both dopamine and acetylcholine, and the dopamine deficiency state in the striatum of patients with Parkinson's disease results in a relatively elevated cholinergic tone. Anticholinergics exert their beneficial effect by partially correcting this relative cholinergic excess. Anticholinergics must be used with caution in older patients because they can induce memory dysfunction and confusion. In older men, anticholinergics also can lead to urinary hesitancy and retention.

Amantadine is also useful in the treatment of early Parkinson's disease and can be helpful for early bradykinesia. Amantadine has anticholinergic activity, mild dopaminergic activity, and antiglutaminergic activity. Amantadine is also useful in treatment of drug-related dyskinesia in more advanced Parkinson's disease. Other options for patients with early troublesome symptoms include monotherapy with the dopamine receptor agonists (pramipexole or ropinirole), or low-dose carbidopa–levodopa with or without a COMT inhibitor (tolcapone or entacapone). The progression of the disease process eventually will result in the need for more powerful dopaminergic stimulation.

The use of levodopa as a precursor loading strategy to increase central dopamine and to ameliorate Parkinson's disease has been one of the major therapeutic advances in neurology. However, high-dose levodopa administration without the addition of a peripheral dopa decarboxylase inhibitor, such as carbidopa, produces anorexia, nausea, and vomiting. These symptoms occur because of the high levels of circulating peripheral dopamine that are present as a result of extensive extracerebral decarboxylation and result in the stimulation of the area postrema (emesis center) of the brain. The development of peripheral dopa decarboxylase inhibitors in large part ameliorated these problems and led to the development of combination therapy with carbidopa and levodopa. This drug is available in fixed rations of 10:100, 25:250, and 25:100, with the numerator indicating the milligram dose of carbidopa and the denominator indicating the milligram dose of levodopa. The most important advantage of this drug is the ability to administer less levodopa to obtain the same central effect with a marked reduction in nausea and vomiting. In fact, the ease of administration of carbidopa–levodopa therapy both for patient and the treating physician has resulted in it being used almost exclusively in the treatment of patients with Parkinson's disease who require levodopa. Carbidopa–levodopa in a controlled-release (CR) formulation (CR 25/100, CR 50/200) provides a slower and longer-lasting effect of levodopa. CR preparations may be useful to treat motor fluctuations, night-time bradykinesia resulting in sleep disruption, early morning painful dystonic cramps, and early morning severe bradykinesia. There is now a triple combination (levodopa/carbidopa/entacapone) tablet to treat Parkinson's disease, which will allow some patients to take fewer pills daily.

There are four direct-acting dopamine receptor agonists available in the United States that have been demonstrated to be effective in the treatment of Parkinson's disease (Table 10.1). Because dopamine receptor agonists exert their effect on the striatal dopamine re-

TABLE 10.1. *Dopamine Receptor Agonists for the Treatment of Parkinson's Disease*

Generic	Trade Name
Bromocriptine	Parlodel[a]
Pergolide	Permax[a]
Pramipexole	Mirapex[b]
Ropinirole	Requip[b]

[a]Ergot derived.
[b]Nonergot.

ceptors (which presumably are not involved in the substantia nigra degenerative process), it was felt that they might be an effective substitute for levodopa. Although dopamine agonists have assumed an important role in Parkinson's therapy, none of the agonists are as potent as levodopa for relief of symptoms of Parkinson's disease. Clinical experience with all four has shown that they are effective not only in the treatment of Parkinson's disease but also in ameliorating motor fluctuations in patients treated with carbidopa–levodopa. Bromocriptine, the first dopamine agonist introduced, is rarely used today both because of its cost and because the new agonists are generally more potent and effective. Pergolide, although effective, has been tentatively linked to valvular heart disease (fibrotic changes associated with ergot-derived preparations). The use of pergolide is likely to decline until the prevalence of the problem is more clearly understood. Pramipexole and ropinirole have been approved for use in both early and late Parkinson's disease. These nonergot dopamine agonists are effective and well tolerated in early Parkinson's disease. The use of these drugs instead of levodopa as initial therapy has been shown to delay the onset of drug-induced dyskinesia. They are also very helpful in managing motor fluctuations and dyskinesias in more advanced Parkinson's disease.

Because there are no known neuroprotective agents that modify disease progression in Parkinson's disease, treatment is directed at symptomatic improvement. If the diagnosis of Parkinson's disease is made, there is no need to start treatment with any anti-Parkinsonian medications unless the patient is experiencing functional disability in activities of daily living, on the job, or in recreational activities.

There is continuing controversy about whether to start treatment with levodopa or a dopamine agonist when functional impairment begins. A number of clinical trials of pramipexole, ropinirole, and levodopa in early untreated patients with Parkinson's disease have demonstrated that levodopa is more effective than the dopamine agonists in relieving motor symptoms and that dopamine agonists induce less motor fluctuations and dyskinesias in the early years (2–5) of Parkinson's disease. The American Academy of Neurology issued a practice parameter examining this issue and concluded that initial symptomatic treatment of Parkinson's disease could begin with either levodopa or a dopamine agonist. When choosing initial treatment, many factors including age, degree of disability, cognitive status, and cost all need to be considered.

Selegiline, a monoamine oxidase type B (MAO B) inhibitor also know as l-deprenyl, inhibits the catabolism of dopamine and promotes dopaminergic activity. Selegiline has been used in early Parkinson's disease and has been shown to delay the need for levodopa. There has been considerable discussion as to whether this effect in early Parkinson's disease is "neuroprotective" or simply symptomatic. The evidence strongly suggests that the effect of selegiline is symptomatic

Rasagiline, another MAO B inhibitor that is not metabolized to amphetamine byproducts, has been demonstrated to be effective in early Parkinson's disease and in managing motor fluctuations in advanced Parkinson's disease. Rasagiline is likely to be studied as a potential neuroprotective agent in the future. Rasagiline is under review by the Food and Drug Administration (FDA) and is likely to be approved for use in Parkinson's disease in 2004.

Entacapone and tolcapone are COMT inhibitors approved for the treatment of Parkinson's disease. COMT inhibitors must be administered in combination with levodopa, resulting in increased bioavailability of levodopa to the brain. COMT inhibitors may enhance dopaminergic side effects; therefore downward titration of carbidopa–levodopa may be required, particularly in patients who already have dyskinesia. Tolcapone and entacapone have been shown to be effective in patients experiencing motor fluctuations. Both drugs are easy to administer, and their therapeutic efficacy can be ascertained quickly. The FDA determined that hepatotoxicity associated with tolcapone necessitates stringent liver function monitoring and informed consent when prescribing this drug. Entacapone is not associated with liver toxicity. Entacapone has been combined with levodopa and carbidopa in one tablet.

It should be noted that all of the anti-Parkinson's medications may be used in combination, particularly in the advanced patient with complex symptoms.

COMPLICATIONS

Although there is no question that carbidopa–levodopa is the mainstay of therapy in this disorder, numerous problems are associated with its use (Table 10.2). However, it should be recognized that several long-term follow-up studies of patients with Parkinson's disease who were treated with levodopa demonstrated that at the end of 5 years of treatment, most patients' motor function was no worse than prior to treatment or, in many cases, still better than before they were treated. This finding is extraordinary because prior to levodopa therapy, the prognosis in Parkinson's disease was dismal.

TABLE 10.2. *Toxicity Associated with Chronic Levodopa Therapy*

Central toxicity	Dyskinesias
	Motor fluctuations
	"On-off" phenomenon
	Sleep disturbances
	Psychiatric disturbances
Peripheral toxicity	Nausea and vomiting
Mixed central and ?	
Peripheral toxicity	Orthostatic hypotension

Several major side effects are associated with the use of carbidopa–levodopa, including drug-induced dyskinesias, drug-induced psychiatric problems, and motor fluctuations. Levodopa-induced dyskinesias are a striking long-term complication of this therapy. The dyskinesias are most often choreic. Chorea consists of irregular, unpredictable, brief, jerky movements that flit from one body part to another in a continuous random sequence. Occasionally, levodopa-induced dyskinesias are dystonic. Dystonia describes movements that are dominated by sustained muscle contraction, frequently resulting in twisting repetitive movements and abnormal postures. The dyskinesia may involve the lingual, facial, and buccal regions; the limbs; and the axial musculature. It is particularly striking to see patients with this drug-related movement disorder because patients with Parkinson's disease previously were characterized by slowness and poverty of movement. The chorea seen in this setting may resemble the chorea seen in Huntington's disease or tardive dyskinesia.

Levodopa-induced dyskinesias are common and may be seen in more than half the patients at the end of 5 years of carbidopa–levodopa treatment. However, patients with onset of dyskinesias during the first 5 years of levodopa treatment will experience very mild abnormal movements that do not interfere with function. The severity of the chorea may increase with continued treatment, and the dose of levodopa required to elicit chorea may decrease with time. A reduction in levodopa dosage invariably will ameliorate this drug-induced movement disorder. Although the chorea may be severe, the parkinsonian patient often does not find the movement troubling; it is usually the family or the physician who first notices the chorea. This is probably best explained by the fact that while a patient is choreic they are still able to move voluntarily with relative ease. Given a choice, most parkinsonian patients prefer excess movement to bradykinesia. However, severe levodopa-induced dyskinesia can be as disabling as bradykinesia.

The psychiatric side effects of long-term dopaminergic therapy include altered sleep patterns, vivid nightmares, auditory and visual hallucinations, paranoia, and psychosis. Although there may be a continuum of increasing severity of psychiatric symptomology with increasing dopaminergic medication dose and duration, in some patients these symptoms develop insidiously, whereas in others they begin acutely. These drug-related complications can be ameliorated by reduction of dopaminergic medications.

The simplest approach to drug-induced psychosis in Parkinson's disease is to reduce the dosage of antiparkinsonian medications and particularly to reduce the administration of other medications that depress the nervous system, including sedatives, hypnotics, anxiolytics, anticholinergics, opiates, and muscle relaxants. When this is not sufficient to relieve hallucinations and delusions, the use of antipsychotic medications is indicated to be able to continue dopaminergic medications at a level to maintain the patient's motor function. There are several atypical neuroleptic drugs available that can reduce or abolish psychosis with less potential for extrapyramidal side effects. Clozapine is the only neuroleptic medication that does not produce adverse motor effects, whereas olanzapine (Zyprexa) and quetiapine (Seroquel) have reduced extrapyramidal side effects as compared to the traditional neuroleptics, which should be avoided in parkinsonian patients. All of the atypical neuroleptics are used in much lower dosage in Parkinson's disease than when indicated for schizophrenia.

Fluctuation in motor performance is an additional complication associated with chronic dopaminergic therapy. After a variable period of treatment, patients note that the beneficial effects of the drug begin to wear off before they are due to take their next dose ("wearing off" or end-of-dose akinesia) and that they may be very akinetic in the morning before the first dose of medication (morning akinesia). One or more doses often do not seem to work. Later, particularly in patients on multiple overlapping doses of carbidopa–levodopa, the fluctuations from a mobile state or "on" to "off" with obvious parkinsonism may appear random with no obvious relation to dosage timing. The transition between relatively normal functions to complete reemergence of the parkinsonian state can occur in several minutes, and it can persist for up to 3 to 4 hours. Sudden, rapid, unpredictable fluctuations between these two extremes also can occur. Clinically, these fluctuations can be striking, and the dramatic nature of these transitions occasionally can be observed during an office evaluation. A patient may be seen in a severely parkinsonian state ("off") with marked cogwheel rigidity, resting tremor, and severe akinesia to the degree that the patient is unable to rise from a chair and have impaired postural reflexes to the point of falling or being unable to stand. During 5 to 6 minutes, the same patient may turn "on" and be observed to be able to stand and sit without difficulty, to have no tremor, and to be able to walk relatively normally and not look at all parkinsonian. The observer who is unfamiliar with these rapid transitions is astounded by these fluctuations, and the uninformed observer may even believe that the severe parkinsonian state, or "off," may reflect a functional or nonorganic problem.

This perplexing problem seems to be related to alterations in central dopamine receptor-site responsiveness and to fluctuating levels of available dopamine. There are many therapeutic maneuvers to use in a patient with motor fluctuations, including increasing the antiparkinsonian medication dose or dosing frequency, adding the controlled-release formulation of carbidopa–levodopa, adding a dopamine receptor agonist, adding a COMT inhibitor, or implementing a restricted-protein diet. New medications should be added one at a time. Both levodopa and the dopamine receptor agonists (bromocriptine, pergolide, pramipexole, ropinirole) must be initiated at a low dose and gradually titrated upward to the therapeutic range, whereas the COMT inhibitors (tolcapone or entacapone) are initiated at an effective dose. The restricted-protein diet is mainly helpful in patients who report a significant effect of diet on their response to carbidopa–levodopa. Levodopa shares the same gastrointestinal transport system with aromatic amino acids, and high-protein meals result in greater competition for the uptake system, reducing the amount of levodopa available to the brain. In patients who note loss of efficacy of carbidopa–levodopa when it is administered with a protein meal, the restricted-protein diet may provide smoother motor response throughout the day. This is not a low-protein diet; it restricts daytime protein intake to enhance motor performance during the day and shifts a greater proportion of the daily protein to the evening meal.

The symptoms of Parkinson's disease remain responsive to the effects of levodopa throughout the duration of the illness; however, as the disease advances, the degree of symptom relief is less satisfying as the complications of motor fluctuations, dyskinesia, and hallucinosis emerge. The administration of levodopa or a dopamine agonist should begin when the patient's ability to carry out daily functions is impaired. The precise timing is individualized based on many issues including lifestyle and individual response to symptomatology. There is no benefit to withholding treatment until advanced disability ensues.

Management of advanced Parkinson's disease is challenging because the clinician often confronts a double bind; the patient requires increased levodopa to improve his or her parkinsonism but needs decreased levodopa to reduce dopaminergic adverse events. The introduction of dopamine receptor agonists often can be useful for problems with motor fluctuations and drug-related dyskinesia. Dopamine receptor agonist administration provides dopaminergic stimulation of the postsynaptic striatal dopamine receptors and also often allows a reduction in carbidopa–levodopa dose. In some patients the combination of dopamine agonist with levodopa will result in more consistent motor improvement with less dyskinesia.

SURGERY

The history of surgical treatment of Parkinson's disease goes back more than 60 years. In

1968–1969 when levodopa treatment became widely available, surgical procedures for Parkinson's disease dropped precipitously and almost disappeared. However, in the last 15 years there has been a resurgence of interest in surgical treatment. This has developed because pharmacologic treatment has limitations, greater insight into basal ganglia function was achieved, and improved surgical techniques and technologies became available. Pallidotomy utilizing updated stereotactic techniques has been reintroduced to treat advanced Parkinson's disease. In this procedure, a small lesion is made by the neurosurgeon in the globus pallidus in an attempt to disrupt the physiologic outflow of the basal ganglia and relieve the symptoms of Parkinson's disease. Some centers report a 20% to 30% improvement in the motor symptoms of Parkinson's disease and resolution of dyskinesia in selected patients. Neurosurgical complications include intraparenchymal hemorrhage, cerebral vascular accident, and altered mental status. Patients with severe intractable drug-related dyskinesia are generally the best candidates for this procedure.

Another surgical procedure increasingly used for the symptoms of Parkinson's disease is deep brain stimulation (DBS). DBS is a neurosurgical stereotactic procedure in which a stimulating electrode is placed in a selected brain region (target) and wires are subcutaneously passed from the target to an electronic stimulator that is implanted in the chest wall (analogous to a cardiac pacemaker). The stimulator can be turned off and on by the patient with the use of a magnetic "wand." DBS for Parkinson's symptoms has been targeted at the Vim nucleus of the thalamus, the globus pallidus, or the subthalamic nucleus. When the target is the Vim nucleus of the thalamus, relief of tremor is most likely to be achieved; however, the other symptoms of Parkinson's disease (bradykinesia, rigidity, loss of balance) are not relieved by this procedure. When the target is the globus pallidus or the subthalamic nucleus, more pervasive symptomatic relief including tremor, rigidity, bradykinesia, and dyskinesia may be

achieved. Currently, the most common target for DBS is the subthalamic nucleus, although there have been no formal trials comparing pallidotomy to DBS procedures for Parkinson's disease.

There has been considerable interest in the role of fetal tissue (mesencephalon) implants in the treatment of Parkinson's disease. This concept involves the transplantation of the dopamine-producing mesencephalon cells from an aborted fetal brain into the brain of the patient with Parkinson's disease. Unfortunately, two well-controlled, blinded trials of human fetal tissue transplants in Parkinson's disease failed to demonstrate therapeutic benefit and provoked uncontrollable dyskinesias in a number of study subjects.

DRUG-INDUCED PARKINSONISM

Drug-induced parkinsonism can be precipitated by any drug that reduces central dopaminergic activity. Drugs that block the dopamine receptor (e.g., neuroleptics, metoclopramide) or deplete central dopamine (e.g., reserpine, tetrabenazine) often result in parkinsonian symptomatology. Parkinsonism induced by drugs can mimic all of the features seen in idiopathic Parkinson's disease. Akinesia and rigidity are generally the most common signs, and resting tremor is seen less often. Other features that may help distinguish drug-induced parkinsonism from Parkinson's disease include a clear history of ingestion of a compound known to interfere with central dopamine activity, a relatively short time from onset of parkinsonian symptoms to significant disability (about 1 to 2 months as opposed to 12 to 24 months), bilateral presentation instead of unilateral presentation of symptoms and signs, and the presence of other drug-related motor abnormalities (e.g., tardive dyskinesia; see Chapter 11).

The diagnosis of drug-induced parkinsonism requires a high index of suspicion. Once the diagnosis is made, treatment should be directed at stopping the offending drug. In almost all patients with this syndrome, the parkinsonism will resolve over time. If active treatment is required, anticholinergics, amantadine, and levodopa–carbidopa have been used successfully. When drug-induced parkinsonism does not resolve, idiopathic Parkinson's disease may have been unmasked.

FURTHER CONSIDERATIONS

Although the etiology of Parkinson's disease remains unknown, there have been recent attempts to modify the natural history of this disorder and delay progression. This approach to treatment, sometimes referred to as "neuroprotective" or "disease-modifying therapy," has been based on a wide variety of theoretic and preclinical models. Attempts to modify disease progression using vitamin E (2,000 units/day) and selegiline (5 mg bid) failed. Vitamin C in doses of 1,500 to 3,000 mg/day has been proposed as an additional antioxidant treatment, but vitamin C never has been tested adequately. At present, there is no "neuroprotective" therapy for Parkinson's disease; however, there is mounting interest in disease-modifying therapies and a number of new trials are in progress.

The levodopa treatment era in Parkinson's disease with improved function and life expectancy led to broadening the scope of what is considered to be the central nervous system dysfunction seen in this disorder. Although James Parkinson did not originally describe cognitive dysfunction as part of the illness, it is apparent that cognitive improvement and dementia often is associated with Parkinson's disease. There is evidence from the pre-levodopa era to suggest that 25% to 30% of patients with Parkinson's disease eventually were institutionalized because of dementia and not because of incapacitating motor performance. However, the increased longevity and maintenance of communicative abilities in patients with Parkinson's disease led to further understanding of cognitive dysfunction in Parkinson's disease. Studies confirm earlier observations that as many as 25% of patients with Parkinson's disease may develop dementia. Dementia must be differentiated from drug-induced altered mental states because

the former is not amenable to treatment but the latter is.

There is considerable interest in other nonmotor symptoms of Parkinson's disease including depression, apathy, fatigue, anxiety, and sleep disruption. Studies indicate that all of these non-motor symptoms are much more frequent than previously understood.

Any drug or degenerative process that interferes with central dopaminergic activity can lead to parkinsonism. The dysfunction of the dopamine system may involve the nigral (presynaptic) neuron or the striatal dopamine receptor (postsynaptic). Drugs or degenerative processes that affect not the presynaptic nigrostriatal dopaminergic pathway but the striatal dopamine receptors may result in the same clinical signs. The latter situation sometimes is referred to as postsynaptic parkinsonism. Examples of postsynaptic parkinsonism include some drug-induced states and metabolic disturbances that result in calcification of the basal ganglia and familial striatonigral degeneration. Because the pathology in these syndromes is located primarily within the striatum and involves the dopamine receptors, it should not be surprising that carbidopa–levodopa therapy is less effective in these disorders. Other neurodegenerative disorders have elements of both presynaptic and postsynaptic dopaminergic dysfunction including the spinocerebellar atrophies (SCA), PSP, and MSA. Clinical clues to identify these syndromes include variable response to levodopa, the presence of a kinetic tremor (SCA), the failure of voluntary conjugate gaze (PSP), and the presence of severe orthostatic hypotension and other autonomic signs (MSA).

When to Refer to a Neurologist

Parkinson's disease is a common disorder, and it is believed that there may be 1 million people in the United States with this illness. Because there is no specific imaging study or biomarkers to confirm the diagnosis, Parkinson's disease is a clinical diagnosis. Physicians making this diagnosis should be comfortable in determining that a patient has

Parkinson's disease based on the patient's history and examination. Parkinson's disease is a chronic progressive illness that ultimately results in significant disability; the diagnosis is a serious one.

Although the diagnosis of Parkinson's disease certainly can be made by a non-neurologist, many patients and families will ask for referral for confirmation. There is great interest in clinical research trials for neuroprotective agents for Parkinson's disease, and most of these trials seek to enroll early patients. Referral of patients for possible participation in studies can be of great value for the patient because there currently are no drugs that slow the progression of Parkinson's disease and it may give the patient a sense of being more proactive about dealing with this diagnosis.

The early years of symptomatic treatment are often uneventful and the patient can be cared for by the non-neurologist. If patients develop motor fluctuations, dyskinesias, or hallucinations and psychosis, referral to a neurologist is indicated for further treatment.

Complementary Therapies

Some people say that there are no alternative therapies in medicine—only therapies that work and those that don't. This applies to Parkinson's disease. Few alternative therapies in Parkinson's disease have been tested. High-dose vitamin E (2,000 units/day) was demonstrated to have no effect in modifying disease progression. Early studies of coenzyme Q10 were promising, but it is premature to conclude that it is "neuroprotective."

A small study of acupuncture was conducted in Parkinson's disease. Acupuncture was ineffective for all motor and non-motor symptoms with the exception of some benefit for sleep and rest.

There is no special diet for most patients with Parkinson's disease. In some patients with motor fluctuations that are sensitive to protein intake (after a protein meal medications may not work as well), a protein redistribution diet may be of value. A wide variety of additional treatments are marketed as possible therapeutic agents for Parkinson's disease. These include over-the-counter antioxidants, food supplements, ginkgo biloba, ginseng, herbal preparations, massive doses of vitamins, spa treatments, NADH (reduced form of nicotinamide adenine dinucleotide) preparations, and chelation therapy. None of these have been shown to be effective.

Special Challenges for Hospitalized Patients

When patients with Parkinson's disease enter the hospital for medical or surgical conditions unrelated to Parkinson's disease, special precautions are indicated. Most patients with moderate Parkinson's disease have specific requirements for the timing of their medications to maintain optimum motor function. Hospital routines often do not accommodate well to complicated time-specific oral medication schedules. One way to address this problem is to have patients and families remain in control of administering the antiparkinsonian medications. The staff must remain fully informed about the medications being administered.

If hospitalized patients with Parkinson's disease become agitated, with delirium or psychotic ideation, care must be taken to avoid agents that interfere with the efficacy of Parkinson's disease medications. The use of traditional neuroleptics, and certain antiemetics, or gastrointestinal agents (metoclopramide) can interfere with dopamine neurotransmission and result in motor worsening.

The dramatic changes in motor function of the patient with Parkinson's disease with motor fluctuations may result in confusion on the part of the hospital staff. Staff may observe a patient "on" who is able to perform all activities of daily living without assistance and later observe the same patient "off" and immobile. During "off periods" the patient may require assistance and the staff mistakenly may believe the patient's request for assistance is not necessary. Staff education about the changeable nature of symptoms in fluctuating patients is important.

All medical and surgical services caring for patients with Parkinson's disease should be proactive in instituting preventative measures to avoid deep-vein thrombosis and aspiration pneumonia in patients with Parkinson's related immobility.

QUESTIONS AND DISCUSSION

1. A 62-year-old right-handed man presented to his physician with the following problems. He has noticed for the last 6 months that his handwriting has changed and that it appears small and cramped. In addition, he has the feeling that his right hand is not as strong as it used to be, and he often has to struggle to button his shirt. The week prior to his visit, his wife noticed that his right hand appeared to be shaking when he was resting quietly in an easy chair.

The most likely diagnosis in this patient based on history alone is:

A. Parkinson's disease

B. Wilson's disease

C. Huntington's disease

D. Dystonia

Neurologic signs present on examination might include which of the following?

A. Bilateral limb chorea, linguofaciobuccal dyskinesias

B. Resting tremor of the right hand, cogwheel rigidity of the right upper extremity

C. Fixed dystonic posturing of the right hand

D. Kinetic tremor of the right hand

E. Three-step retropulsion, two to three extra steps in turning maneuvers

The answer to the first part of the question is (A) and the answer to the second part is (B). This is a typical history of Parkinson's disease characterized by slow progression and a predominantly unilateral presentation of the symptoms and signs. In addition, the handwriting is described as cramped and small (micrographic). The feeling of weakness in an involved extremity is a common complaint, although there is usually no objective sign of weakness. The presence of unilateral signs of tremor and cogwheel rigidity is typical. If postural reflexes are impaired (retropulsion and increased steps on turning maneuvers) early in the presentation the diagnosis of Parkinson's disease is questionable. However, postural reflex impairment is a common sign in advanced Parkinson's disease.

2. A 59-year-old right-handed woman has an 8-year history of left upper extremity resting tremor. She has been treated with carbidopa–levodopa for the last 7 years. Although she states that originally her tremor was much improved, she has been having difficulty with increasing involuntary "dancelike" gyrating, non-purposeful movements of the left upper and lower extremities. In addition, her husband reports that occasionally his wife sees visitors in the house when they are alone. Questioning the patient reveals that she often sees people who are not really there. She speaks lucidly about this and recognizes that they are not real. The correct diagnosis in this patient would be:

A. Dystonic posturing of the left upper extremities

B. Tardive dyskinesia

C. Parkinson's disease with dopaminergic adverse events

D. Wilson's disease and dopaminergic adverse events

The answer is (C). The patient's initial presenting complaint is the spontaneous appearance of a unilateral resting tremor that is relieved by dopaminergic agents. This is a characteristic early presentation of unilateral Parkinson's disease, and the additional information that dopaminergic therapy ameliorated the symptoms suggests the diagnosis of Parkinson's disease. The patient's present complaints are adverse events associated with chronic dopaminergic therapy, specifically levodopa-induced chorea and hallucinations. Choreiform movements that are induced by dopaminergic therapy in patients with Parkinson's disease are not phenomenologically distinguishable from the chorea seen in many other choreatic states. The hallucinations reported by this patient are typical, non-threatening visual hallucinations.

Answer (A) is incorrect because dystonic postures and movements are not "dancelike" and gyrating. (B) is incorrect because there is no drug history of neuroleptic medication and tardive dyskinesia is by definition secondary to chronic dopamine receptor blockade. (D) is incorrect because Wilson's disease does not present so late in life. The average age of onset of Wilson's disease presenting with neurologic symptomatology is 19 years.

The most appropriate therapy in this patient would be:

A. Raising the dose of carbidopa–levodopa

B. Adding an anticholinergic

C. Reducing the dose of carbidopa–levodopa

D. Administering an atypical neuroleptic if levodopa reduction is not possible

The correct answers are (C) and (D). The patient's current problem of dyskinesias and hallucinations are secondary to chronic dopaminergic stimulation, and the appropriate therapy is to reduce the dose of dopaminergic therapy if possible. These drug-induced effects will be ameliorated when dopaminergic agents are reduced. When the dose of the dopaminergic is reduced or discontinued, the patient's parkinsonian symptoms will become worse.

If reduction in levodopa dosage results in excessive motor dysfunction with functional impairment, the addition of an atypical neuroleptic may be necessary. First, confirm that the patient is not taking other types of medications that may significantly contribute to confusion and psychotic ideation, such as sedatives, tranquilizers, and anticholinergics. If the drug regimen is simplified but the psychotic symptoms persist, choose either clozapine or quetiapine for their antipsychotic effects. Use the lowest effective dosage to avoid adverse effects. If drug-induced dyskinesia persists and is very troublesome despite maximal reduction of antiparkinsonian medications, surgical intervention may be considered.

Answer (A) is incorrect because this is a drug-induced syndrome and raising the dose of the drug will not ameliorate the problem—it will exacerbate it. (B) is incorrect because anticholinergics will not improve chorea and are likely to increase the psychotic symptoms.

3. A 65-year-old right-handed man presents with generalized slowing of mobility and difficulty seeing the food on his plate. His family says that his problem has been getting worse for the last 12 months and that the patient also has difficulty walking up stairs. In addition, he describes that he is having difficulty buttoning his shirt, rising from a chair, and turning over in bed. The family also reports that his facial expression has changed (he does not smile as much) and that a tremor of this left hand occasionally is noted. Examination reveals that there is a resting tremor of the left hand, cogwheel rigidity in the left upper extremity is present, and postural reflexes are mildly impaired. Additional findings include increased extensor tone in the neck and marked impairment of voluntary conjugate gaze. The patient is unable to look down voluntarily, and there is also moderate impairment of upward gaze. In addition, right and left lateral gaze are not normal. The correct diagnosis in this patient would be:

A. Wilson's disease

B. Huntington's disease

C. Parkinson's disease

D. Progressive supranuclear palsy

E. Multiple system atrophy

The answer is (D). PSP is an idiopathic midbrain and brainstem degenerative disorder that is characterized by parkinsonian features and progressively impaired voluntary conjugate gaze. This patient is described as having parkinsonian features (resting tremor, cogwheel rigidity, impaired postural reflexes, and mild bradykinesia) and has markedly impaired conjugate gaze. A useful office maneuver to determine whether the gaze dysfunction is supranuclear or nuclear is the doll's head procedure. In this maneuver, the head is passively flexed and extended, and in a separate maneuver it is rotated to the right and to the left while the passive motion of the eyes is observed. In a patient with supranuclear gaze dysfunction, the eyes will move reflexly and conjugately in an appropriate direction. This maneuver and its physiology are discussed in greater detail in Chapter 5.

Answer (A) is incorrect because of the late onset of neurologic symptoms and the type of eye movements observed. (B) is incorrect because of the late onset of neurologic symptoms and because the movement disorder is not that seen in adult-onset Huntington's disease. Although definite parkinsonian features are present, (C) is incorrect because of the additional findings of disturbed volitional gaze. (E) is incorrect because of the pronounced oculomotor dysfunction.

4. The degenerative cellular pathology seen in Parkinson's disease is localized primarily in the:

A. Cerebral cortex

B. Thalamus

C. Cerebellum

D. Substantia nigra

E. Corpus striatum

The loss of cell bodies and their projection systems in the correct answer to the first part of this question results in what biochemical lesion?

A. Loss of acetylcholine in the striatum

B. Loss of dopamine in the striatum

C. Loss of dopamine in the cerebral cortex

D. Loss of acetylcholine in the cerebellum

The answer to the first part of the question is (D), and the answer to the second part of the question is (B). Parkinson's disease is pathologically characterized by depigmentation, Lewy bodies, and cell loss in the substantia nigra. The destruction of the nigral striatal projection system results in the loss of dopamine in the striatum. Dopamine is the neurotransmitter used by this system, and the dopamine within the striatum is contained primarily within the axonal terminations of the nigral neurons.

5. A 65-year-old woman was diagnosed with Parkinson's disease 9 years ago when she developed a resting tremor of the left hand. When levodopa–carbidopa treatment was started she had a positive response and her tremor, clumsiness of the left hand, and gait improved. She is now taking levodopa–carbidopa 25/100 2 tablets qid, pramipexole 1 mg tid, and entacapone 200 mg qid. On this schedule she experiences end-of-dose wearing off and moderate dyskinesias. She has no hallucinations or delusions, is not depressed,

and is otherwise in good health. The motor fluctuations and dyskinesias have become troublesome to her.

Management of her motor fluctuations and dyskinesia may include:

A. Reduce levodopa–carbidopa dosage and frequency.

B. Reduce pramipexole dosage.

C. Introduce amantadine 100 mg bid.

D. Perform surgical procedures (DBS or pallidotomy).

E. All of the above.

All answers are correct (E). This patient has a complex problem that reflects advancing parkinsonism and drug-associated problems. Decreasing the dosage of pramipexole, entacapone, or levodopa will ameliorate her dyskinesia. However, her parkinsonism may worsen to an unacceptable degree. Introducing amantadine may reduce dyskinesia. DBS is a possible therapeutic choice because, when successful, it can alleviate both motor fluctuations and dyskinesias.

Which of the following excludes a patient from DBS surgery for Parkinson's disease?

A. Unstable medical conditions

B. Cognitive impairment

C. No response to levodopa

D. Neurobehavioral problems

E. Unrealistic expectations

F. Atypical Parkinsonism

G. All of the above

All answers are correct (G). The best DBS candidates with the best chance of a successful outcome are relatively healthy, have no cognitive impairment or significant behavioral problems (depression, anxiety), still have some good response to levodopa administration, have idiopathic Parkinson's disease, and understand that DBS or ablative surgery for Parkinson's disease is not a cure.

SUGGESTED READING

Cotzias GC, Van Woert MH, Schiffer LM. Aromatic amino acids and modifications of Parkinsonism. *N Engl J Med* 1967;276:374.

Factor SA, Weiner WJ, eds. *Parkinson's disease: diagnosis and clinical management.* New York: Demos Press, 2002.

Havemann J. *A life shaken—my encounter with Parkinson's*

disease. Baltimore: Johns Hopkins University Press, 2002.

Jankovic J, Marsden CD. Therapeutic strategies in Parkinson's disease. In: Jankovic J, Tolosa E, eds. *Parkinson's disease and movement disorders,* 3rd ed. Baltimore: Williams & Wilkins, 1998:191.

The Parkinson Study Group. Effect of deprenyl on the progression of disability in early Parkinson's disease. *N Engl J Med* 1989;321:1364.

Weiner WJ, Shulman LM, Lang AE. *Parkinson's disease: a complete guide for patients and families.* Baltimore: Johns Hopkins University Press, 2001.

11

Hyperkinetic Movement Disorders

Stewart A. Factor and William J. Weiner

Abnormal involuntary movements are the hallmarks of a number of neurologic diseases; they collectively are termed hyperkinetic movement disorders (also referred to as dyskinesias). In such conditions, the movements are easily visible, and intelligent observation allows the clinician, in most instances, to suggest the proper diagnosis or class of disorders. The characteristic tremor of Parkinson's disease, which is present at rest but lacking during volitional movements, is such an example (see Chapter 10). In this chapter, six other neurologic diseases will be described. All are dramatic visually because bizarre and abnormal involuntary movements are their major descriptive neurologic feature. The non-neurologist certainly will encounter these patients in an office practice and will identify them in public (e.g., in parks, trains, shopping centers). The disorders discussed are dystonia, essential tremor (ET), Huntington's disease (HD), Wilson's disease (WD), Gilles de la Tourette's syndrome (GTS), and tardive dyskinesia (TD).

DEFINITIONS

Dystonia: Involuntary sustained muscle contractions producing twisting or squeezing movements and abnormal postures. Dystonia can have stereotyped, repetitive movements that vary in speed from rapid to slow and that may result in fixed postures from the sustained muscle contractions.

Tremor: Involuntary rhythmic oscillating movement that results from the alternating or synchronous contraction of reciprocally innervated antagonist muscles. Tremor may be classified according to its prominence during activity or at rest.

Chorea: Excessive, spontaneous movements that are irregularly timed, nonrepetitive, randomly distributed, and often have a flowing "dancelike" quality that involves multiple body parts.

Tics: Repetitive, brief, rapid, involuntary, purposeless, stereotyped movements that involve single or multiple muscle groups. The tic can be a patterned sequence of coordinated movements that may be complex or simple.

Myoclonus: Rapid, shocklike, arrhythmic (usually), and often repetitive involuntary movements. Myoclonus can be classified by location (focal, multifocal, or generalized) and by etiology.

DYSTONIA

Dystonia is divided into primary (idiopathic) and secondary forms. Several types of primary dystonia have been identified but they share the characteristic that dystonia is the sole clinical feature. The prevalence of primary dystonia is estimated to be 33 per 100,000. Dystonia of primary origin has a number of unusual but characteristic features. At onset, the movements may occur in relation to specific voluntary actions by the involved muscle groups (such as in writer's cramp) or with varied movements, so-called action-induced dystonia. It may occur in one body part with movement of another (overflow dystonia). Later, with progression of disease, dystonia becomes present at rest. Dystonic movements typically worsen with anxiety, heightened emotions, and fatigue, whereas they decrease with relaxation and disappear during sleep. There may be diurnal fluctuations in dystonia, which manifest as little or no involuntary movements in the morning followed by severe disabling dystonia in the afternoon and evening. Whereas morning improvement is seen with several types of dystonia, one particular form of childhood-onset dystonia is characterized by this feature (dopa-responsive dystonia [DRD] or Segawa's dystonia).

Dystonia may occur in nearly any muscle group. The following terms are used to describe dystonia in varied distributions. When the upper face and eyelids are involved and the eyes are involuntarily kept closed the patient is said to have blepharospasm. When the lower face, lips, and jaw are involved and the patient presents with involuntary opening or closing of the jaw, retraction or puckering of the lips, and repetitive contractions of the platysma, he is experiencing oromandibular dystonia. Pharyngeal dystonia is associated with dysphagia, dysphonia, or dysarthria and is typically action induced. Lingual dystonia may occur at rest, presenting as sustained or repetitive protrusion of the tongue or upward deflection of the tongue against the hard palate, or it may be action induced via speaking or eating. Laryngeal dystonia (involving the vocal cords) causes spasmodic dysphonia in which the speech is tight, constricted, and forced, or it may be more whispery, depending on whether the adductor or abductor muscle groups are involved. The smooth flow of speech is lost, and certain sounds are held longer and overemphasized. Spasmodic dysphonia is typically action induced by speech, and it most commonly involves the adductor muscles of the larynx. Abductor dysphonia resulting in a soft whispery voice is less common. Some patients have a mixed form.

Dystonic contractions of the neck muscles, referred to as spasmodic torticollis or cervical dystonia, result in torticollis, retrocollis, anterocollis, or laterocollis. In spasmodic torticollis, rapid jerking and twisting neck movements along with tremor may accompany sustained posturing of the neck. Some patients may appear to have a fixed abnormal neck posture without the spasmodic movements. The shoulder on the side of the head tilt typically is elevated. Dystonic movements

of the arms (brachial dystonia) most commonly present with pronation of the arm, often behind the back. With hand dystonia, the movements are often action induced as in writing (writer's cramp), manipulating a musical instrument (musician's cramp), and other occupational maneuvers. Truncal or axial dystonia manifests as lordosis, scoliosis, kyphosis, tortipelvis, or opisthotonus. Dystonic movements of the legs (crural dystonia) may occur with action or at rest and present most commonly with equinovarus posturing of the foot while walking, twisting of the foot, or increased elevation of the leg when walking. The knee usually maintains a hyperextended position with crural dystonia. It is interesting that some patients are able to walk backward or run without incident, but when they attempt to walk normally, the dystonia recurs. Certain combinations are fairly common and make up specific syndromes.

Patients with dystonic disorders often discover ways to suppress or hide the movements using an interesting array of "tricks." These usually consist of postural alterations or counterpressure maneuvers that are primarily sensory in nature. Examples include touching an eyebrow in blepharospasm, which leads to eye opening, or the classical geste antagonistique, where a finger placed lightly on the chin will neutralize neck-turning in spasmodic torticollis. There are also motor tasks that may deactivate dystonia, including singing or whistling by patients with blepharospasm or oromandibular dystonia and dancing by patients with cervical or truncal dystonia. Typically, these tricks lose their effectiveness as the disease progresses.

The pathophysiology of dystonic movements and tricks remain a mystery. However, in recent times some clues have emerged, although it is beyond the scope of this chapter to describe them in detail. Briefly, it is believed that dystonia is the result of basal ganglia dysfunction. This is primarily based on work involving cases of secondary dystonia. There appears to be decreased output from the primary output nucleus of the basal ganglia, the medial globus pallidus. There are two pathways from putamen to medial globus pallidus that control this output—the direct and indirect pathways—and they have opposite effects. Overactivity of the direct pathway, or underactivity of the indirect pathway, can lead to dystonia. Microelectrode recordings from the globus pallidus in patients undergoing surgery have demonstrated irregular, intermittent group discharges leading to irregular output from that region to the thalamus and cortex. This supports the notion that the basal ganglia are the source of the problem. The altered output somehow leads to a loss of reciprocal inhibition mechanisms for muscle contraction controlled at the brainstem or spinal levels. This allows antagonist muscle groups to contract simultaneously, resulting in dystonia. There also appears to be sensory and motor cortical involvement. Sensory involvement is suggested by the usefulness of sensory tricks and studies demonstrating abnormalities in sensory fields in thalamus and cerebral cortex in patients with dystonia. Physiologic studies also have demonstrated that motor cortex is hyperexcitable and that there is decreased activation of these regions. It is possible that certain patterned or learned tasks (tricks), both sensory and motor, interrupt the production of dystonia through alterations in cortical activity, which in turn changes input of direct or indirect pathways to medial globus pallidus.

Dystonia often is misdiagnosed as hysterical or psychiatric in origin. The basis for this arises from its typical features, including the varied, often bizarre, movements and postures; the fact that they are often action induced; the worsening of dystonia with stress and improvement with relaxation; the diurnal fluctuations; and the effectiveness of various sensory tricks. Knowledge of the unusual characteristics of dystonic disorders will be helpful in avoiding a misdiagnosis.

CLASSIFICATION

Classification of dystonia has been based on (a) age of onset, (b) distribution of movements, and (c) etiology. Clinical and genetic studies have demonstrated that they are all connected. Use of the first two items in the patient's initial assessment can lead to consideration of etiology. The age-of-onset classification separates patients into early onset (younger than age 26 years) and late onset (older than age 26 years). Early onset typically begins with limb involvement and carries a worse prognosis than the older group because of the more likely possibility of generalization of the movement disorder. Early patients are more likely to have hereditary disease, most commonly DYT1. The late onset cases have focal or segmental dystonia that primarily involves the craniocervical region and does not generalize.

The distribution of dystonia is categorized as focal, multifocal, hemidystonia, or generalized. Focal dystonia refers to dystonia in a single body part. Multifocal dystonia includes dystonic movements in more than one body part yet not fulfilling the criteria for generalized dystonia; segmental dystonia is a form of multifocal dystonia in which contiguous body parts are affected. In hemidystonia, an arm and a leg on the same side are involved. Finally, generalized dystonia refers to the presence of dystonia in at least one leg, the trunk, and an additional body part (cranial, cervical, or brachial) or in both legs and the trunk. This classification is also important in formulating a proper diagnosis. For example, hemidystonia is usually the result of an infarction or space-occupying lesion, whereas generalized dystonia is most likely primary early-onset disease and has a worse prognosis than focal dystonia or hemidystonia.

Classification by etiology has undergone substantial change in the last few years, primarily because of the linkage (or non-linkage) of many types of dystonia to a variety of genes. Table 11.1 demonstrates the latest scheme, first introduced at the Third International Dystonia Symposium in 1996. The primary dystonias (also known as idiopathic torsion dystonias [ITD]) are defined as syndromes in which the sole manifestation is dystonia, with the exception that tremor may be present as well. It is considered to be neurochemical in origin rather than degenerative.

TABLE 11.1. *Classification of Dystonia*

Primary Dystonia
  Early-onset dystonia (Oppenheim's dystonia):
    chromosome 9q–DYT1
  Non DYT1 autosomal-dominant early-onset
    dystonia with whispering dysphonia—DYT4
  Autosomal recessive dystonia: DYT2
  Adult-onset familial torticollis
  Adult-onset familial cervicocranial dystonia:
    chromosome 18p–DYT7
  Mixed adult and childhood-onset dystonia:
    chromosome 8p–DYT6
  Mixed but predominantly adult-onset segmental
    dystonia (occasionally childhood onset and
    generalized): chromosome 1p36—DYT13
  Adult-onset sporadic focal dystonia
Dystonia—Plus Syndromes
  Dopa-responsive (Segawa's) dystonia:
    chromosome 14q22 & 11p–DYT5
  Myoclonus dystonia: chromosome 7q21—DYT11
  Rapid-onset dystonia, parkinsonism: chromosome
    19q—DYT12
Secondary Dystonia (See Table 11.2)
  Hereditary and degenerative diseases
Degenerative Disorders
  Parkinson's disease
  Huntington's disease
  Progressive supranuclear palsy
  Corticobasal degeneration
  Hallervorden-Spatz disease
  Olivopontocerebellar atrophies
  Lubag (Filipino X-linked dystonia parkinsonism):
    chromosome Xq13–DYT3
Hereditary metabolic disorders
  Wilson's disease
  Leigh's disease
  GM 1 and 2 gangliosidoses
  Hexosaminidase deficiency
  Leber's optic neuropathy with dystonia

TABLE 11.2. *Secondary Forms of Dystonia*

Drugs
  Dopamine antagonists (i.e., haloperidol, thoridizine,
    compazine, metoclopramide)
  Dopamine agonists (i.e., levodopa, bromocriptine)
  Antidepressants (tricyclics, SSRIs, lithium)
  Antihistamines
  Calcium channel blockers
  Stimulants (cocaine)
  Buspirone
Vascular Disease
  Basal ganglia infarction
  Basal ganglia hemorrhage
  Arteriovenous malformation
Neoplasms
  Astrocytoma or glioma of the basal ganglia
  Metastatic neoplasm
  Cervical spinal cord tumor
Others
  Head trauma
  Thalamotomy
  Anoxia (in adulthood or perinatal)
  Meningitis (fungal or tuberculosis)
  Syringomyelia
  Colloid cyst of the third ventricle
  Münchhausen syndrome
  AIDS (toxoplasmosis abscess of basal ganglia,
    PML)

SSRIs, selective serotonin reuptake inhibitors; PML, progressive multifocal leukoencephalopathy.

Primary dystonia is genetically and clinically heterogeneous, which leads to the various categories. Dystonia genes are depicted by the symbol DYT (followed by a number) by the Human Genome Organization/Genome Database. DYT designations have been assigned to a variety of dystonic syndromes clinically defined and unmapped, linked primary dystonias, or others not classified as primary but with dystonia as a predominating feature (Table 11.1). Eleven genes causing dystonia have been mapped to human chromosomes, and four are for primary dystonias; these will be discussed in more detail.

The second category comprises the dystonia-plus syndromes. These also are considered to be neurochemical in origin, but they have features other than dystonia (e.g., patients with DRD have parkinsonian features). The third category is secondary dystonia, which develops as the result of a wide variety of known etiologies (Table 11.2). The fourth category includes hereditary and degenerative syndromes that have dystonia as part of the clinical spectrum. Examples include Parkinson's disease, WD, HD, and X-linked dystonia parkinsonism (Lubag).

PRIMARY INHERITED DYSTONIAS

Dystonia is typically the only neurologic abnormality in patients with primary dystonia (although many also may have tremor), and any distribution of abnormal involuntary movements may be observed. The primary dystonias characteristically have an insidious onset and are progressive in nature. Initially, the movements may be action induced, later occurring at rest and producing fixed and sustained postures. The disorder ultimately plateaus in severity. Five criteria for the diagnosis of primary dystonia were established by Herz in 1944 and are still applicable. These include (a) the development of dystonic movements or postures; (b) a normal perinatal and developmental history; (c) no precipitating illnesses or exposure to drugs known to cause dystonia; (d) no evidence of intellectual, pyramidal, cerebellar, or sensory deficits; and (e) negative results of investigation for secondary causes of dystonia (particularly WD). Two factors are indicators of a poor prognosis: onset in childhood and onset in a crural distribution. Poor prognosis in dystonia refers to increased disability because life span is not shortened. A majority of patients with crural dystonia have onset of disease in childhood or early adulthood (referred to collectively as early-onset disease). The clinical presentation is heterogeneous.

The classical early-onset primary dystonia is DYT1 dystonia. It is the most severe and the most common form of hereditary early-onset dystonia. Oppenheim, who first described the syndrome in 1911, called this disorder dystonia musculorum deformans. It has been suggested that this disorder be renamed Oppenheim's dystonia. It also has been referred to as idiopathic torsion dystonia. DYT1 dystonia is inherited in an autosomal dominant pattern, with a 30% to 40% penetrance. The gene is located at chromosome 9q34. The gene abnormality is a unique three-base pair GAG deletion in the coding portion of the transcript in exon 5. The resulting protein, torsin A, is characterized by the loss of one of a pair of glutamic acid residues in a conserved region of a novel adenosine triphosphate (ATP)-binding protein. The function of this protein and its role in altering basal ganglia function to cause dystonia remain unknown. However, the protein is expressed in the substantia nigra pars compacta, origin of dopaminergic neurons projecting to the basal ganglia. It has homology to the ATPases and heat shock proteins. The wild-type protein is found in the cell body and colocalizes with endoplasmic reticulum and vesicular markers. The mutant protein leads to the formation of cyto-plasmic inclusions. These findings suggest that the torsin A protein plays a role in maintaining endoplasmic reticulum integrity and membrane trafficking. There is a high prevalence of early-onset dystonia in Ashkenazi Jewish families, with more than 90% resulting from a single founder mutation in the DYT1 gene. This mutation has been traced back more than 350 years to Lithuania, and the current gene frequency is approximately 1 in 2,000. In 50% to 60% of non-Jewish ethnically diverse families with early-onset dystonia, the disease results from the same DYT1 mutation that has arisen independently in varied populations. Thus, apparently, only one variation in the encoded protein can give rise to the DYT1 phenotype.

The clinical spectrum of early-onset DYT1 dystonia is similar in all ethnic populations. Onset of symptoms occurs at an average age of 12 years, but most patients have onset before age 27. The initial presentation is with limb onset, usually leg (crural dystonia). The presence of leg or foot dystonia is the best predictor of a DYT1 mutation. The foot often is twisted and plantar flexed while ambulating, and the patient usually toe-walks. All patients ultimately have leg involvement. The disorder may start in the arm (possibly as writer's cramp), although less frequently. In these cases, the age of onset is a little older than crural onset and the patients are less likely to end up with generalized dystonia. Generally, early-onset dystonia progresses by spreading across or down/up, and this occurs over approximately 5 years, with 50% of patients becoming either bedridden or wheelchair bound. Intellectually they are normal, and no other neurologic abnormalities are seen. Spasmodic dysphonia occurs in about 5%, cervical involvement is rare, and cranial involvement is generally not seen. Onset in the neck or vocal cords in early-onset patients, even if they are of Ashkenazi Jewish descent, rarely is caused by the DYT1 gene. These patients rarely generalize. Late-onset (older than 26 years old) craniocervical dystonia generally indicates that the patient does not have DYT1 dystonia. In adult life, the patient often stabilizes and may even improve to some degree, but the disorder does not spontaneously remit. There may be remissions early in the disorder, and these may last hours to years. Most, if not all, recur, usually in the same distribution.

Genetic testing is available for DYT1 dystonia. It should be considered for all primary dystonias with age of onset younger than 26 years and patients with later onset who have a family history of early-onset generalized dystonia. The specificity of using age 26 as a cut-off age is 63% for Ashkenazi Jews and 43% for non-Jews.

Linkage studies involving several large families with adult- or mixed-onset dystonia of a variety of distributions have excluded the DYT1 locus. However, dystonia families have been linked to other possible genes. DYT6 has been linked to chromosome 8p in two Mennonite families from the midwestern United States with an autosomal dominant form of dystonia with incomplete penetrance. The phenotype of these families includes a broader age of onset (5 to 38 years; mean, 19) and an onset distribution that includes limbs and cervical or cranial areas. There is frequent spread to cranial muscles, and there are apparently few patients whose dystonia becomes generalized. In some, the dystonia remains focal. Thus, while some of the patients appear identical to those with DYT1 dystonia, there are obvious differences when examining the complete family. In addition, there are differences from typical adult-onset craniocervical dystonia because DYT6 dystonia that starts in these regions commonly spreads to the limbs, but the former syndrome does not.

The DYT7 gene has been linked to chromosome 18p in a family from northwest Germany. This family has an autosomal dominant form of adult-onset craniocervical dystonia with incomplete penetrance. The average age of onset was 41 years (range 28–70 years), and most patients had focal cervical dystonia. Some had cranial or laryngeal involvement as well, and postural hand tremor also was seen. In the same town, apparently sporadic cases of spasmodic torticollis also were studied, and they shared allelic characteristics with the family, suggesting that they also had an autosomal dominant form with reduced penetrance. One other family was designated DYT13 and linked to chromosome 1p36. This was an Italian family with focal and segmental dystonia usually affecting the craniocervical region. Some had early-onset disease and generalized, indicating a mixed presentation. Other inherited forms of dystonia are listed in Table 11.1.

ADULT-ONSET SPORADIC DYSTONIA

Adult-onset primary dystonia is the most common of all types of dystonia. It presents more commonly with brachial, truncal, and craniocervical dystonia and only rarely with crural dystonia. Only 18% of these patients progress to generalized dystonia, with even a smaller percentage becoming wheelchair bound or bedridden. The dystonia usually remains in the body part where it presented as a focal dystonia, but it may spread to a contiguous body part on rare occasions, becoming segmental in distribution. The course is typically benign, and remissions occur in approximately 10% of patients.

CRANIOFACIAL DYSTONIA

Blepharospasm–oromandibular dystonia syndrome was first described by Henry Meige in 1910 and often is referred to as Meige's syndrome. Blepharospasm and oromandibular dystonia may occur independently in this syndrome, but the combination is more frequent. It also may be accompanied by pharyngeal, laryngeal, or cervical dystonia. Blepharospasm in isolation (referred to as essential blepharospasm) is more common than oromandibular dystonia. Blepharospasm often is preceded by eye irritation, photophobia, and increased blinking frequency. It may start in one eye and spread to the other, or it may start in both. Approximately 12% of these patients are functionally blind because of their inability to voluntarily open their eyes. Features that aggravate blepharospasm include looking upward, feeling stress, being fatigued, watching television, walking, driving, talking, and even yawning. Sensory tricks used by patients to open their eyes include forced raising of the eyelids, applying pressure on the superior orbital ridges with a finger, and rubbing the eyelids. In addition, some find that forced jaw opening, neck movements, whistling, and wearing dark glasses are helpful. Some patients use eyeglasses with eyelid crutches to hold the lids open.

Oromandibular dystonia frequently is accompanied by lingual involvement. It may be aggravated by talking, chewing, or swallowing. Sensory tricks used include pressing on the lips or teeth with fingers, pressing on the hard palate with the tongue, or putting a finger in the mouth. Meige's syndrome affects women more commonly than men and presents in the sixth decade of life. It often begins with blepharospasm, which is followed by oromandibular, lingual, and pharyngeal dystonia. Other dystonic movements in other body parts may occur in some patients, and hand tremor similar to ET also may be an associated problem. The severity of the dystonia fluctuates from day to day and disappears with sleep. Spontaneous remissions have been observed but are rare.

CERVICAL DYSTONIA (SPASMODIC TORTICOLLIS)

Cervical dystonia is the most common of adult-onset focal dystonias, making up about 40% (Fig. 11.1). The age of onset is in the fourth or fifth decade (mean age, 41 years) and women are affected more frequently than men by about 3 to 1. The disorder is characterized by abnormal involuntary neck movements, abnormal postures of the neck and shoulders that are often painful, and hypertrophy of involved neck muscles. Pain is present in about 80% of patients, and hypertrophy is seen in all. Initially, some patients do not perceive their dystonia, and it is brought to their attention by others. This suggests that a problem with perception of head position exists. The movements may be intermittent at first and associated with specific actions. Most patients deteriorate during the initial 5 years and then stabilize. The condition may be characterized ultimately by dystonic postures that

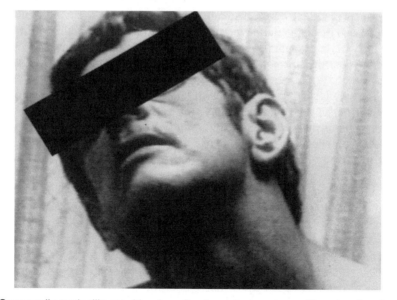

FIG. 11.1. Spasmodic torticollis resulting in a fixed cervical posture with extension, lateral flexion, and rotation to the right.

are present at rest, worsen with action, and improve in sleep. Spontaneous remissions occur in 10% to 30%, most commonly in the first year. All patients relapse but few have a second remission. Rotation of the neck (torticollis) is the most common posture seen (with neither side being particularly more common), with lateral flexion (laterocollis), anteflexion (anterocollis), and extension (retrocollis) also occurring in various combinations. Spasmodic (dynamic) movements are not present in all patients despite the commonly used term spasmodic torticollis. In fact, they occur in only 10% to 15%. Factors that may exacerbate cervical dystonia include emotional stress, fatigue, walking, working with the hands, and attempting to look in the opposite direction of the dystonic contractions. When the patient tries to overcome the movements and look in the opposite direction, he or she may experience a high-amplitude, jerky tremor referred to as dystonic tremor. Some patients present with bidirectional torticollis because at varying times the head may turn in different directions and muscles of both sides of the neck may be involved. Many of these patients present with head tremor (40%). The tremor varies in amplitude, and if there is little directional change in the neck along with tremor, the patients frequently are misdiagnosed as having ET. The distinction is important because dystonia does not respond to tremor medications but does respond to botulinum toxin and other dystonia therapies. This tremor can be distinguished from essential head tremor by the presence of subtle changes in posture, a jerky non-rhythmic quality, and muscle hypertrophy along with improvement with sensory tricks. Sensory tricks usually involve the use of a light touch or pressure to the chin or cheek with fingers (geste antagonistique) or other objects such as a pen or eye glasses and holding the back of the head with the hand or leaning the head against a wall or a headrest. This lessens the head tilt and tremor and relaxes the muscles for variable durations of time. After a while, the tricks lose their effectiveness. Cervical dystonia may be associated with Meige's syndrome, writer's

cramp, and ET, and it also has been observed in patients with generalized dystonia. Complications of prolonged torticollis occur in one-third to one-half of patients and include degenerative osteoarthritis of the cervical spine along with the expected sequelae of radiculopathy and myelopathy. These may represent emergent situations that potentially could lead to permanent neurologic deficits.

WRITER'S CRAMP

Writer's cramp (Fig. 11.2) is a dystonic spasm that is induced by a specific task (action-induced or task-specific dystonia). When these cramps occur with a single type of action (such as writing), they are referred to as simple writer's cramp, but when the spasms occur with a variety of activities, they are referred to as dystonic cramps. Writer's cramp occurs in both men and women, and the age of onset ranges from 20 to 70 years. These patients present with a change in handwriting that becomes sloppy and illegible. Some patients squeeze the pen tightly and press down hard on the writing surface, which results in a jerky writing motion and tearing of the paper. In others, the fingers splay and pull away from the pen involuntarily. The act of writing is painful in most patients. Initially, the dystonic contraction occurs with persistence of task, but as the disorder progresses, it occurs with initiation of the task. Initially, other tasks performed with the same hand are normal, but later these too may become involved. The disorder is usually asymmetric at first, but in those patients who learn to write with the opposite hand, the disorder may become bilateral (about 25% of patients) years after the change in hands. When some patients write with the unaffected hand, the affected hand exhibits involuntary spasms—so-called mirror dystonia. Writer's cramp may be associated with ET and may be related to the syndrome of primary writing tremor, which is thought by some to be a variant of ET. Some other occupational cramps that have been reported include pianist and violinist palsy, golfer's palsy, and dart-thrower's palsy. The

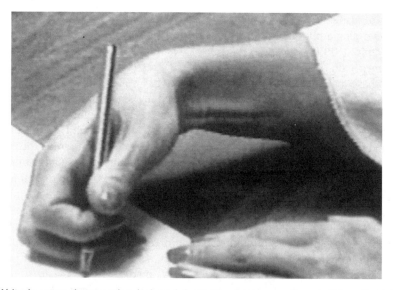

FIG. 11.2. Writer's cramp is an action-induced dystonic spasm, resulting, in this patient, in wrist flexion, metacarpophalangeal joint extension, extension of the thumb, and flexion of the distal interphalangeal joints, leaving the patient with an inability to continue writing.

common factor in all of these disorders is the occurrence during the performance of a well-learned motor (manual) task and perhaps the overuse of the hand with that particular task. In writer's cramp, there appears to be co-contraction of agonist and antagonist muscles, perhaps related to loss of reciprocal inhibition. Patients generally have an otherwise normal neurologic examination, and this disorder is usually resistant to therapy.

DOPA-RESPONSIVE DYSTONIA

One form of dystonia plus syndrome that warrants discussion is DRD (DYT5). DRD is characterized by childhood (mean = 6) or adolescent onset, female predominance (four times that of males), foot dystonia in childhood, and parkinsonism in adults and a diurnal fluctuation. Patients function well in the morning and deteriorate as the day wears on. They improve with sleep. Purely dystonic presentations involving the limb are most common, although cranial distribution can be seen. Some patients have mixed dystonia and parkinsonism, and the parkinsonism becomes more prominent with age. The clinical spectrum has expanded to include developmental delay and spasticity mimicking cerebral palsy. The most characteristic feature is profound and sustained response to levodopa (<300 mg/day). So profound is the response, and sustained, that it is recommended that all individuals with symptoms within the spectrum of DRD initially be treated with levodopa.

DRD has been linked genetically to two chromosomes. The most common is chromosome 14q11-24.3—the gene codes for an enzyme in the rate-limiting step in the biosynthesis of tetrahydrobiopterin (GTP cyclohydrolase I), a cofactor in dopamine synthesis, and is dominantly inherited. It is most commonly related to a point mutation in this gene, but a large number of mutations have been reported in all exons. The other link is to a rare defect seen on chromosome 11p15.5—the gene codes for tyrosine hydroxylase, the rate-limiting step in catecholamine metabolism—and is recessively inherited. This defect seems to be more commonly associated with an akinetic-rigid syndrome or spastic paraplegia. The resulting deficiency of biopterin, a cofactor in catecholamine synthesis, leads to decreased levels of dopamine, which explains the long-term responsiveness of patients to levodopa. Dopamine transporter single-photon emission computed tomography (SPECT) scanning is normal in patients with DRD, and this helps differentiate these patients from those with early-onset Parkinson's disease. Currently, genetic testing is not available commercially for diagnosis. Diagnosis of DRD is based on clinical profile and response to levodopa.

SECONDARY DYSTONIA

To make a diagnosis of primary dystonia, one must rule out known causes of dystonia (i.e., secondary or symptomatic dystonias [Table 11.2] and hereditary degenerative diseases [Table 11.1]). Clues to the diagnosis of a secondary dystonia can be uncovered with a thorough history and physical examination and radiologic and laboratory testing. Usually, there are examination findings in addition to the dystonia suggestive of dysfunction of other parts of the central nervous system (CNS), including the cranial nerves, pyramidal system, cerebellar system, and higher cortical function. There is often an abrupt onset to the dystonia, and dystonia is present at rest from the start in secondary cases. The presence of hemidystonia suggests a focal lesion such as a tumor, infarction, abscess, or arteriovenous malformation in the basal ganglia. In those patients with a single non-progressive event such as an infarction or trauma, the dystonia will stabilize and not be progressive. The examiner should be cautious because secondary dystonia may mimic idiopathic dystonia. For instance, stroke in the basal ganglia may cause typical-looking torticollis and neuroleptic-induced (tardive) dystonia in adult patients and may be symptomatically identical to adult-onset primary dystonia. Clues that tardive dystonia is more likely include more retrocollis, a more phasic or dynamic form of torticollis, and the co-occurrence of choreiform movements. These patients also report less effectiveness of tricks and do not often have head tremor. A lack of muscle hypertrophy also suggests drug-induced dystonia.

An important feature of secondary dystonia, which physicians must consider, is that dystonia may have a delayed onset after a cerebral insult. In adults, the most frequent cause of delayed-onset dystonia is cerebral infarction. The duration of the delay can vary from weeks to years and often is associated with an improvement of the original neurologic deficit. In children, the most frequent cause of delayed-onset dystonia is perinatal trauma or hypoxia. The reason for the delay is unclear, but it has been postulated that the dystonia in these circumstances is a result of neuronal sprouting stimulated by the original injury. A history of perinatal difficulties must be ruled out if a diagnosis of primary dystonia is made.

The most important disorder to rule out in a new-onset dystonia patient, particularly young onset, is WD. A screen for WD and an imaging study of the brain should be performed on all patients with dystonia, and then the rest of the workup should be tailored to the individual patient's needs. It has been suggested that secondary dystonia occurs mainly in genetically susceptible individuals. This was thought to be particularly true in tardive dystonia because it appears to be very similar clinically to primary dystonia. However, it has been demonstrated that these patients are not carriers of the DYT1 gene, suggesting that genetic susceptibility is not a necessary component of tardive dystonia. Similar work needs to be done for other, particularly adult-onset, dystonia genes.

PATHOLOGY AND NEUROCHEMISTRY

Dystonia is considered to be the result of basal ganglia dysfunction. Because there have been few neuropathologic examinations of patients with dystonia reported (most were without abnormality), the pathologic–anatomic basis of this movement disorder has been related almost exclusively to cases of symptomatic dystonia. Location of abnormalities reported include the putamen and, to a lesser extent, the caudate nucleus and the thalamus. These findings have been supported by radiologic studies. In those rare cases of dystonia with pathologic abnormalities, the microscopic changes were observed in the brainstem. In one case of generalized dystonia, neurofibrillary tangles were found in the locus ceruleus and other brainstem nuclei. In one case of Meige's syndrome, neuronal loss was observed in multiple brainstem nuclei. Whether these abnormalities relate directly to the clinical syndrome is unclear. In Lubag, the X-linked dystonia–parkinsonism syndrome (DYT3) seen most commonly in the Philippines, the characteristic pathology is gliosis in a mosaic pattern seen primarily in the putamen and caudate nucleus. These patients have severe craniocervical dystonia, and many of them generalize. This finding supports the concept that dystonia is a basal ganglia disorder.

The neurochemical basis of dystonia is also unclear. It has been suggested that the abnormality in this disorder is in the dopamine or acetylcholine systems. Clinical evidence to suggest these hypotheses include the onset of dystonia after treatment with dopamine receptor antagonists and the response of dystonia to anticholinergic medications. In addition, the discovery that DRD is acutely responsive to small doses of levodopa and that it is caused by two genes involved in the biosynthesis of dopamine support a dopaminergic hypothesis. Finally, the expression of torsin A (DYTI) in the substantia nigra pars compacta also implicates the dopamine system. A noradrenergic imbalance in the lower portion of the brainstem involving the lateral tegmentum of the medulla oblongata and locus ceruleus also has been hypothesized (based on a single case of dystonia). In some areas, norepinephrine is elevated, whereas in others the levels are diminished. Norepinephrine is a neurotransmitter that, among other actions, inhibits cholinergic neurons. A deficiency in norepinephrine might explain the response of dystonia to anticholinergic medications. This finding is particularly interesting because the location of the DYT6 gene is in a region of chromosome 8 that contains the genes for alpha-1 and beta-3 adrenergic receptors. Other theories include alterations in gamma-amino-butyric acid (GABA) or cerebral somatostatin. GABA alterations in the motor cortex have been implicated in the abnormalities of activation and inhibition in this region demonstrated by physiologic testing and positron emission tomography (PET).

Another hypothesis suggests that dystonia may be the result of a deficiency in activity of mitochondrial complex I, the first protein of the respiratory chain. This was considered a possibility because a mitochondrial complex I deficiency was seen in the hereditary disorder Leber's optic neuropathy with dystonia. Several different studies have been reported on platelet mitochondrial function in the primary dystonias with varied results. One study indicated that the deficiency was in all types of dystonia and severity of dystonia correlated with severity of the deficiency. Another reported that the complex I deficiency was present only in the focal dystonia. A third indicated that no deficiency was present in this or any dystonia group. Further studies are required to clarify the role of mitochondrial dysfunction in dystonia.

TREATMENT

In the absence of a clear understanding of the etiology and neurochemistry of dystonia, medical treatment has been less than satisfactory. As a result, a number of therapeutic modalities have been tested and varied responses have been observed. Generally the approach is to treat patients empirically with one agent at a time (Table 11.3). Ultimately various combinations may be tried. It is interesting that none of these agents has been tested in large, multicenter, controlled trials. Less than half of dystonic patients respond to medical therapy. Because of the dramatic effect levodopa has on DRD, it is recommended that each patient with dystonia be treated with this agent first. Usually, patients with DRD will respond rapidly to low doses (<300 mg/day). It is recommended that the dose be pushed to 600 mg/day over 2 to 3 weeks. If there is no benefit, withdraw it and move on. Anticholinergics are the most

TABLE 11.3. *Medical Treatment of Dystonia*

Drug Name	Initial Daily Dose	Usual Daily Dose Range
Levodopa	100	300–600 mg
Trihexiphenidyl	2	12–24 mg
Baclofen	10	60–120 mg
Clonazepam	0.5	3–6 mg
Reserpine	0.1	1–3 mg
Tetrabenazine	25	100–200 mg
α-methyl tyrosine (Metyrosine)	250	250–1,000 mg
Mexilitine	150	300–600 mg

frequently used agents to treat primary dystonia. In an open-label trial using gradually increasing doses in children and adults with primary dystonia, significant improvement was seen in 61% of children and 38% of adults. The average daily dose of trihexyphenidyl in children and adults was 41 mg and 24 mg, respectively. Adults were less tolerant of the anticholinergic side effects than the children. Side effects include blurred vision, dry mouth, urinary difficulties, constipation, sleep pattern alteration, forgetfulness, weight loss, personality changes, and psychosis. Severity of disease is not a good predictor of response to the anticholinergics, but patients with hemidystonia (as a result of a focal lesion) did not respond well. The earlier in the course of disease patients were treated, the better they did. Pyridostigmine, a peripheral cholinesterase inhibitor, can be used to treat cholinergic side effects. Tetrabenazine, a dopamine-depleting agent, is effective in patients with Meige's syndrome and a variety of other movement disorders including other types of dystonia. This drug is not yet available in the United States but can be obtained in the UK. However, reserpine, another dopamine-deleting drug, is available and effective in approximately 30% of patients. The side effects of most concern with dopamine-depleting agents include depression (which can be severe, come on suddenly, and have a protracted course), Parkinsonism, orthostatic hypotension, and gastrointestinal problems. The effectiveness of dopamine antagonists such as haloperidol has been inconsistent, and studies using these drugs have been inconclusive. Because of the threat of TD, these drugs should be avoided. Mixed results with

baclofen, carbamazepine, benzodiazepines (particularly clonazepam and diazepam), mexiletine, and clozapine have been observed, but these are used frequently nevertheless, especially in patients unresponsive to anticholinergics. In patients failing medical and botulinum toxin therapy (see below), surgical techniques, including both central and peripheral procedures, have been used with less than adequate results. Central procedures are used mainly for generalized dystonia. Of the central procedures, stereotaxic thalamotomy with the ventral tier of the thalamus as the target was once the most commonly used technique. The ventralis oralis posterior and ventralis intermedius (VIM) are the main targets. Between 30% and 70% of patients demonstrated improvement, and some had long-term effects. Those with posttraumatic hemidystonia had the best result. Modern techniques include the use of stimulation (deep brain stimulation [DBS]) and electrophysiologic microelectrode cellular recording and mapping to improve localization. These techniques have improved morbidity and mortality and are one of the reasons these surgical techniques enjoy resurgence. Bilateral ablative procedures of this type result in serious complications in more than 20%, including pseudobulbar palsy, dysphagia, and gait disorder. Although thalamotomy fell out of favor, it was shown that stereotactic posteroventral pallidotomy could eliminate dyskinesia and dystonia in patients with advanced Parkinson's disease. This prompted the evaluation of this technique in patients with generalized dystonia. This surgery is safer than thalamotomy, and results in a small number of patients have been significant (up to 70% of patients with improvement). In one particular case the improvement was delayed and reached a maximum in 3 months. As with Parkinson's disease, ablative surgical procedures have given way to DBS. In this case, stimulation electrodes are left in the region of interest. Stimulation is adjustable and reversible as opposed to the ablative counterparts. Recent studies on a small number of patients have demonstrated that pallidal DBS is associated with better outcomes. This procedure rapidly is becoming the surgery of choice in this disease, but still only a small number of cases have been reported in the literature and more information is needed. Of the results published, about 80% had an improved global outcome. Even focal dystonia cases are being treated with this technique with some success. Response to DBS often is delayed. Better outcomes are seen when bilateral procedures are performed.

A peripheral procedure used in blepharospasm and Meige's syndrome includes myectomy of the orbicularis oculi, but results are mixed. The surgery consists of the extirpation of the lid protractors and strengthening of the lid retractors. Recurrence of blepharospasm weeks to months after this procedure is not unusual. In cervical dystonia, selective peripheral denervation is a technique under investigation at numerous institutions. In this procedure denervation of specific muscles is the goal. Results have indicated that the primary posture of the neck improves, but there is a decrease in range of motion and muscle atrophy occurs. Some patients experience a recurrence of the dystonia with involvement of different cervical muscles. One other technique used to treat generalized dystonia is intrathecal baclofen. With this technique baclofen is delivered to the intrathecal space through an inserted catheter with a continuous pump. This has been highly effective in treating spasticity of spinal and cortical origin. In the small number of patients with dystonia treated to this point, results have been modest at best. There has been the occasional case of severe dystonic crisis that improved dramatically with this treatment. Secondary dystonia seems to respond better than the primary type. Possible side effects include respiratory depression from baclofen overdose, catheter malfunction, and pump infection.

Intramuscular injection of botulinum toxin (BoNT) remains the treatment of choice for focal dystonias, particularly in the craniocervical distribution. BoNT is one of the most lethal toxins known to man. Of eight subtypes produced by the anaerobic organism clostridia botulinum, three have been linked to human botulism: types A, B, E. BoNT A (Botox) has been used therapeutically since the mid 1980s. At that time, its usefulness in strabismus was demonstrated. In 1990, BoNT A was approved by the U.S. Food and Drug Administration (FDA) for treatment in blepharospasm, strabismus, and hemifacial spasm secondary to CN VII compression; in 2000 it was approved for cervical dystonia. BoNT B (Myobloc) also was approved for use in cervical dystonia in 2000. There is also a second form of BoNT A under investigation in the United States (Dysport). The use of these toxins is now more widespread than these indications because they are used routinely to treat all types of focal dystonia, including blepharospasm, oromandibular dystonia, spasmodic dysphonia, and limb dystonias (among other things). BoNTs act presynaptically at the cholinergic neuromuscular junction. The toxin attaches to an acceptor protein that is specific for each type of BoNT and is endocytosed into the nerve terminal. It then blocks the release of acetylcholine from vesicles by cleaving one of the three docking proteins. BoNT type A and B cleave different proteins. The toxins are made up of a heavy chain that binds to the acceptor and the light chain that is a zinc-dependent protease that cleaves the docking protein once in the cell. The blockade of the neuromuscular junction results in weakness and atrophy of the muscle and a decrease in muscle spasms, but the effect is transient, lasting 3 to 6 months. Repeated injections are necessary. BoNT is administered by direct intramuscular injection. All side effects are local, secondary to its primary effect of weakening muscles. The dosing for each formulation of BoNT is individualized, but guidelines for initial dosing and ranges have been published. There are no established dosing equivalencies between BoNT A and B. In blepharospasm, the toxin is injected into the orbicularis oculi with two injections in the upper lid, one injection in the canthus, and one or two injections in the lower lid. In addition, one or two injections are given in the frontalis muscle in the forehead, if necessary. The standard total dose of type A is 15 to 40 units; for type B it is 500 to 2,000 per eye. After 3 to 14 days improvement is seen, with moderate to marked functional improvement in 70% to 90% of patients. The response lasts 2 to 4 months so that treatment is needed three or four times per year. Side effects include ptosis, diplopia, and increased tearing, all of which are transient. Cervical dystonia is probably the most common disorder treated with BoNT. Multiple studies with both toxins have shown significant improvement in a majority of patients. Treatment requires an average of about 260 units per treatment for type A and 15,000 units for type B. All patients should be started at lower doses and titrated according to need. As with blepharospasm, response occurs in 3 to 14 days and lasts 3 to 6 months. Patients require two to four treatments per year. Neck muscles injected are chosen based on the presence of pain and hypertrophy and spasm and in relation to the posture itself.

Some investigators have suggested using electromyography techniques (EMG) as an additional guide to injection; however, not all treating neurologists find it necessary. Some physicians use EMG in complicated cases and in patients who do not experience an adequate initial response. In the treatment of cervical dystonia, up to 90% respond and response is dose dependent. Side effects are transient and include neck weakness, dysphagia, dry mouth, and a "flulike" syndrome. Spasmodic dysphonia of the adductor type, previously poorly responsive to any therapy, responds dramatically to BoNT. Both unilateral and bilateral techniques have been used. The bilateral method is preferred because lower doses (0.65 to 5 units per side of type A) can be used. The thyroarytenoid muscles are approached through the neck with EMG guidance. The only adverse effects are a breathy, whispery voice and dysphagia, which improve over days to weeks. Injection is required two to four times per year. Treatment of oromandibular dystonia is also frequently successful. Injections can be made into the pterygoid muscles (medial or lateral) with EMG guidance, the masseters, temporalis and digastric muscles in varied combinations depending on whether the patient has jaw opening, closing or lateral deviation as the main manifestation. Dosing for oromandibular dystonia range from 50 to 400 units of type A. Of patients, 70% to 90% of patients improve, and side effects are dysphagia and weakness of the soft palate that allows fluid to be regurgitated through the nose. Limb dystonias (writer's cramp) respond with less consistency because the resulting weakness of the hand muscles may be more troublesome than the cramps themselves. Nevertheless, some patients find them useful, especially if specific isolated actions and muscles are causing the problem. Controlled clinical trials have supported the use of both types of BoNT for dystonia. In addition, some studies examined the effect on quality-of-life measures and found that there was a significantly positive impact. Most neurologists feel that BoNT is the treatment of choice for most focal dystonias because of greater efficacy than standard medical therapies and fewer side effects. Secondary immunoresistance to the toxins has been a concern for years, especially in patients with cervical dystonia who receive higher doses. It is believed that patients may develop antibodies that neutralize the toxin and make it ineffective. Not all resistant patients have measurable levels of antibodies. The frequency of secondary resistance remains unclear and, based on retrospective studies, appears to be approximately 10% for type A. Risk factors for the development of resistance include frequent injections, booster injections, higher cumulative doses, and younger age. Although there is a commercially available test for antibodies to type A, the best way to assess resistance for type A is to clinically evaluate the patients after treatment. For example, the sternocleidomastoid can be injected with 75 to 100 units and examined 2 weeks later for atrophy. If no atrophy occurs, then the patient is resistant. A similar test involves the injection of a frontalis muscle (one side). After an injection of 15 units, if the folds on the forehead remain the same (and symmetric) and the patient can raise his or her eyebrow and wrinkle the forehead, they are resistant. It seems that the various types of toxins are antigenically distinct so that resistance to one does not mean resistance to all. Patients resistant to BoNT A can use BoNT B, and the reverse is also true.

A small percentage of patients have primary non-responsiveness—that is, they never respond. The mechanism for this is unknown. Physicians administering BoNT should be very familiar with the disorders treated, mechanisms of action and effective doses in each disorder, and the anatomy of the area injected. The disorders treated with BoNT have expanded beyond dystonia and include spasticity, achalasia, anal and urethral sphincter disorders, hyperhydrosis, sialorrhea, and others. BoNT A also has been approved for cosmetic use for facial wrinkles.

There are no alternative medical therapies with proven effect on dystonia. Physical therapy can be a useful adjunct; however, if it is too rigorous, it actually can aggravate the dystonia. Still, it may be useful for maintaining mobility and preventing contractures. Some devices have been used that take advantage of the usefulness of "trick."

When to Refer to a Neurologist

Dystonia is a complicated disorder. Neurologists, especially movement disorder specialists, would be best suited for addressing the issues of diagnosis, genetic testing, and therapy. In particular, referral should be made to a neurologist well versed in the use of BoNT.

Special Challenges for Hospitalized Patients

Most hospital staff will be unfamiliar with dystonia, and because of the bizarre movements, cessation with sleep, and exacerbation with anxiety, they are likely to assume or suspect that the movements are psychogenic in origin. This can lead to frustration and anger on the part of the patient. Staff education is required. Patients may be unable to stay still for testing and procedures, and mild sedation may be necessary.

ESSENTIAL TREMOR

Tremor may be characterized by its prominence only in certain activities or postures, and it may be the sole manifestation of a disorder or a symptom of a disease. It generally is classified by its anatomic location; frequency; etiology; or, most frequently, in relation to rest, posture, and action. Resting tremor refers to tremor while the body part is at rest. The classical rest tremor is that seen in Parkinson's disease. Postural tremor refers to tremor occurring while the body part is maintaining posture against gravity, the most common being that seen in ET. Finally, kinetic tremor refers to tremor during goal-directed movements, as typically seen in cerebellar disease. Recognizing these differences can be helpful in making a diagnosis. A listing of tremors classified by position is provided in Table 11.4. Because ET

TABLE 11.4. *Differential Diagnosis of Tremor*

Rest tremors
Parkinson's disease
Secondary parkinsonism
Hereditary chin quivering
Severe essential tremor
Drug-induced (neuroleptics)
Postural tremors
Physiologic tremor
Essential tremor
Neuropathic tremor (Roussy-Lévy syndrome)
Cerebellar head tremor (titubation)
Dystonic tremor
Drug-induced tremor (lithium, valproate, neuroleptics, caffeine, theophylline, tricyclic antidepressants, amphetamines)
Action tremors
Classical cerebellar tremor (multiple sclerosis, infarction)
Primary writing tremor
Mixed tremors
Wilson's disease
Rubral tremor
Psychogenic tremors

is the most common cause of tremor and is a disorder primarily of tremor, it will be the subject of this discussion.

CLINICAL FEATURES

ET is a disorder of the nervous system that occurs in a sporadic or familial form with autosomal-dominant inheritance. The term senile tremor, referring to patients with tremor onset after age 65 years, refers to late-onset ET and is a term no longer used. ET is considered to be the most common movement disorder, occurring in up to 6% of the population. It occurs equally in men and women and is characterized by a postural tremor, with or without a kinetic component, that is most evident in the upper extremities. The kinetic component is seen in finger-to-nose testing, although it is often not as dramatic as in cerebellar disorders, and tremor at rest occurs rarely (in 5% to 10% of patients) in the most severe cases where the patient has a long duration of disease. The frequency of tremor ranges from 4 to 12 Hz.

A maneuver to potentiate tremor during physical examination is to have patients hold the fingertips of their two open hands close together under the chin without touching while holding their elbows out like wings. This maneuver can also bring out a more proximal distribution. One also could perform a cup test: the patient holds a full cup of water and pours it into another cup or takes a drink. The tremor is often worse as the hand approaches the face. The onset of ET can be at any age from early childhood to age 90, with a mean of 45 years. Those patients with a family history appear to have an earlier age of onset (age 40) when compared to sporadic cases (age 51). ET usually affects the fingers and hands first and then moves proximally. Tremor onset may occur bilaterally in the hands or in one hand at a time. When bilateral, it may be symmetric or asymmetric. Although hemitremor has been observed, it occurs only rarely. When tremor is asymmetric, it usually is worse in the dominant hand. Handedness in ET is distributed according to population norms.

Tremor may spread to the head and neck. Approximately 50% to 60% of patients with ET have head involvement, and in some instances head tremor is the sole manifestation. Head tremor may present as a vertical nod (yes-yes) or as a horizontal nod (no-no). Voice tremor occurs in approximately 25% to 30% of patients with ET. The voice is characterized by rhythmic alteration in intensity at the same frequency as the hand tremor. Head and voice tremor tend to be more frequent and severe in women than in men. Tremor in the head or voice should strongly suggest a diagnosis of ET and not Parkinson's disease because both are very uncommon in the latter. Less frequently, tremor occurs in the jaw, face (lips, tongue), trunk (if present while standing only, this is referred to as orthostatic tremor), and legs (15%). There are also a variety of task-specific tremors (i.e., primary writing tremor), which many believe to be variants of ET. One other non-tremor feature in patients with ET has been deterioration of tandem walking. This feature worsens with advancing age.

ET is a slowly progressive disorder that remains stable in some patients for decades, or it progresses continuously. It is not unusual for patients to seek medical advice after having the tremor for one or two decades. Initiation of a specific posture may aggravate the tremor early in the course. Later, it is aggravated by many different movements or postures. The tremor disappears during sleep and worsens with anxiety, fatigue, temperature changes, local pain, caffeine ingestion, aminophylline ingestion, and possibly hunger. Alcohol characteristically improves the tremor (in 74% of those who drink any alcohol). A substantial proportion of patients are functionally disabled, with 20% having impaired job performance and requiring early retirement. This is why the term benign has been eliminated from the name. Other patients are very embarrassed by the tremor and impose social isolation on themselves.

ET is a clinically heterogeneous disorder that may go unnoticed by the patient; may simply represent an embarrassment; or actually may be disabling, leading to difficulties with writing, drinking, or using kitchen utensils. Approximately 5 million people in the United States have this disorder. As many as 13% of individuals older than age 65 probably have ET. There are many people with this problem who have not bothered to seek medical care and therefore are not diagnosed.

GENETICS

ET is an autosomal dominant disorder with 100% penetrance. At least 60% of cases have a clear genetic component. This may be an underestimate because some sporadic cases may represent non-recognition. Genetic mapping has resulted in the linking of ET to genes on two different chromosomes. In one study, 16 small families with 75 affected individuals from Iceland were examined using a genome-wide scan with 350 markers. The result was linkage to chromosome 3q13. The mutation in this gene (referred to as FET1) apparently accounts for the disease in 80% of Icelandic families with ET.

The second study evaluated one large American family that originally hailed from the Czech Republic. This family had 18 affected members with pure ET. Using similar methods, the study authors discovered linkage to a locus on chromosome 2p22-p25. This has been confirmed in three other families. Genetic anticipation was suggested in the family because onset in each successive generation was progressively younger. Anticipation usually is associated with a CAG trinucleotide repeat, and, in fact, repeat expansion detection analysis in this family revealed the presence of just such a mutation, but it remains unclear if there is a direct linkage between this CAG repeat and the ET gene. These findings indicate that a single highly penetrant gene is sufficient to cause ET. It also demonstrates that ET may be a genetically heterogeneous disorder.

PATHOLOGY AND PATHOPHYSIOLOGY

Because ET is neither life threatening nor life shortening, the opportunity for a post-mortem examination of the CNS is not frequent. In those patients who have been examined pathologically, there is no distinctive CNS pathology. PET studies have demonstrated an increase in regional cerebral blood flow in the cerebellum (bilateral) and red nucleus, indicating that the neuronal circuitry involving these regions may be the location of the abnormality. One study also demonstrated increased glucose metabolism in the inferior olivary nucleus of the medulla. This structure may be the source of the rhythmic discharge causing the tremors. This notion is supported by the fact that lesions in the cerebellum and thalamus may stop tremor.

Another interesting pathophysiologic postulate is that ET represents an exaggeration of physiologic tremor. Physiologic tremor is a normal phenomenon that can be recorded in all people by the use of an accelerometer and can be observed clinically in some normal individuals (8 to 12 Hz). Physiologic tremor can be seen in almost everyone when the hands are held out and a sheet of paper is placed over the fingers. The tremor starts at a frequency of 6 Hz and increases to a frequency of 8 to 12 Hz in childhood. It then decreases again with age. Possible physiologic mechanisms include inherent properties of motor neuron firing, oscillations in the stretch reflex causing synchronization of motor neuron discharges, or a supraspinal rhythmic input to the motor neurons. This tremor is exacerbated by anxiety, emotional stress, thyrotoxicosis, caffeine intake, and intake of other stimulants. Some believe that physiologic tremor may be a forme frust of ET and that both originate from the same neuronal oscillators. Thus, ET begins as enhanced physiologic tremor and then progresses in severity over time. However, evidence has been presented that physiologic tremor and ET are different. This controversy remains unresolved.

DIFFERENTIAL DIAGNOSIS

The diagnosis of ET is a clinical one (Table 11.4). The most common misdiagnosis in ET patients is Parkinson's disease. The two disorders usually can be differentiated by careful history and physical examination. The tremor of Parkinson's disease occurs at rest, whereas the tremor of ET is a postural and kinetic tremor. Patients with parkinsonism have rigidity, bradykinesia, micrographia, and postural and gait difficulties, and ET is associated with none of these. Other than the tremor, neurologic examination in ET is normal. The handwriting of a patient with ET is usually large and tremulous (Fig. 10.1 from Chapter 10). Sometimes a handwriting sample alone can lead to the correct diagnosis because in Parkinson's disease the handwriting is small. Some studies demonstrated increased prevalence of Parkinson's disease in families of patients with ET, increased prevalence of ET in parkinsonian patients, and increased prevalence of Parkinson's disease in patients with ET, suggesting that an association of some kind exists. The nature of this association remains a mystery.

Postural tremor frequently is present in patients with ITD. This tremor can be indistinguishable from ET. A family history of ET is not uncommon in both of these disorders. Some investigators have indicated that this frequent association between postural tremor and dystonia is indicative of a link between ET and idiopathic dystonia, but linkage of ET to the DYT1 gene has been ruled out. Tremor is particularly frequent in patients with spasmodic torticollis and Meige's syndrome. In spasmodic torticollis, head tremor is present in approximately 40% of patients, and misdiagnosis is frequent. In addition, approximately 20% of torticollis patients have a hand tremor similar to that seen with ET. It is important to differentiate between these disorders because treatments differ.

Postural and kinetic tremor secondary to cerebellar lesions can be differentiated from ET because of the presence of other signs of cerebellar dysfunction and the difference in severity (cerebellar tremor is generally much more disabling). There are three types of cerebellar tremor: (a) the classical cerebellar kinetic tremor, (b) cerebellar outflow rubral tremor, and (c) head titubation. The classical tremor appears with goal-related movements most evident at the beginning and end of the movement. It is much slower than ET, 2 to 5 Hz, and of wider amplitude. The lesion usually includes the dentate nucleus (most common in stroke patients). Outflow tremor is present at rest, when maintaining posture, and with action. Amplitude and frequency are similar to the classical tremor, and the lesion includes the outflow pathway from dentate nucleus to the thalamus, with the most common location of the lesion in the midbrain including the red nucleus. This type of tremor is seen most commonly in young patients as a manifestation of multiple sclerosis and in the elderly as the result of a stroke. Finally, titubation is a head tremor similar to the head tremor of ET. It is generally the result of bilateral cerebellar lesions.

EVALUATION

The diagnosis of ET is based on findings in the history and examination. If the patient presents with the typical history and findings, then no laboratory or imaging studies are necessary except for thyroid function studies. Hyperthyroidism can worsen an already-existing tremor or cause an enhanced physiologic tremor that may appear similar to ET. Any patient with a sudden-onset tremor, unilateral tremor, or other complex features that do not appear to fit with ET or Parkinson's disease should be studied further with imaging studies and screening for WD. The diagnosis of Wilson's is extremely important because it is fatal if undiagnosed (see page 184). All patients under the age of 50 years with an atypical ET presentation should have an evaluation for Wilson's. Finally, any person presenting with tremors must have his medications examined carefully, as many can induce tremors of varying types.

TREATMENT

Medical treatment of ET can be helpful in improving function and relieving embarrassment in a substantial portion of patients. How-

TABLE 11.5. *Medical Therapy for Essential Tremor*

Drug Name	Initial Daily Dose	Usual Daily Dose Range
First-line agents		
Propranolol	20	60–320
Primidone	25	50–750
Benzodiazepines		
Alprazolam	0.25	0.75–3 mg
Clonazepam	0.5	1.5–6 mg
Carbonic Anhydrase Inhibitors		
Acetazolamide	125	250–750 mg
Methazolamide	50	100–200 mg
Anticonvulsants		
Gabapentin	300	900–3600 mg
Topiramate	50	100–400 mg
Phenobarbital	30	60–120 mg

ever, effectiveness often is limited (for review of medical therapy of ET see Table 11.5). The two agents considered firstline treatment for ET are propranolol and primidone. Propranolol (standard and long-acting formulations) is a beta blocker that has been known to be effective for more than 20 years. It is particularly useful in controlling postural and kinetic tremor in the upper extremities and may make a significant difference to the patient in terms of being able to feed himself or write legibly. This may be true although propranolol usually does not abolish the tremor but may only decrease its amplitude, having little or no effect on frequency. There are often markedly inconsistent therapeutic results, with 40% to 70% of patients showing a decrease in amplitude of 50% to 60%. There does not appear to be a correlation between plasma concentration of propranolol or its metabolites and a reduction in tremor. There are no apparent features that separate responders and non-responders. The dosage of propranolol may range from 60 to 320 mg/day but usually is less than 120 mg/day. It exerts its effect in 2 to 6 hours after a single dose, and the effects may last as long as 8 hours. Withdrawal from propranolol may result in a rebound increase in amplitude of the tremor, which may last longer than a week. The site of action of propranolol, whether central or peripheral, has not been fully established. There are certain groups of patients with ET in whom the use of propranolol is relatively contraindicated. They include patients with diabetes mellitus, chronic obstructive

lung disease, and asthma; propranolol can cause dyspnea and wheezing in these patients. In these instances the substitution of a different beta antagonist, metoprolol, may result in amelioration of the tremor and no bronchospastic symptoms. Metoprolol is a beta receptor antagonist that is relatively selective in its action; however, patients who do not respond to propranolol also do not respond to metoprolol, and propranolol is superior to it. It has been suggested that the selectivity of this agent is lost when higher doses are used, and at higher doses bronchospastic symptoms may reemerge. Acute side effects of beta blockers include bradycardia and syncope; chronic problems include dizziness, fatigue, impotence, and depression. Propranolol also rarely causes hallucinations.

Primidone, an anticonvulsant, may be as effective as propranolol in the treatment of ET. The major problem has been acute adverse effects that are frequent (30%) and include vertigo, a general ill feeling, unsteadiness, nausea, ataxia, and confusion. These side effects clear spontaneously after 1 to 4 days so patients can be encouraged to stick with the drug during this time. It has been observed that lower doses (50 to 250 mg/day) are as effective as higher doses and are better tolerated. As with propranolol, response has varied from patient to patient; the reason for this is unknown. However, many patients prefer primidone to propranolol. Plasma levels of primidone and its metabolites do not correlate with responsiveness. It is likely that a combination of primidone and propranolol will be more effective than each drug used alone.

A majority of patients respond to either propranolol or primidone. However, patients who do not respond or who are unable to tolerate these agents are difficult to manage.

Several other drugs have been used in the treatment of ET. One feature in the clinical history that an adult with ET will volunteer is the salutary effect of alcohol on the tremor. In fact, alcohol may be the most effective agent—75% of patients respond quickly and dramatically. The occasional use of alcohol in patients with ET is a reasonable recommendation. Benzodiazepines, particularly alprazolam and clonazepam, also have been demonstrated to be successful in treating ET. Alprazolam is the only one found to be effective in controlled trials and induced significant reduction in tremor. This drug can be useful when others are not. Some literature suggests clonazepam is particularly useful in kinetic predominant tremor. A major side effect of this class of medications is sedation. Alprazolam has a less sedating effect than clonazepam.

Other agents useful in some patients with ET include methazolamide and acetazolamide, gabapentin, phenobarbital, clozapine, and topiramate. Clozapine seems to have a general tremorolytic action improving tremors in ET, Parkinson's disease, and multiple sclerosis. At low doses (<50 mg/day) there was reduction in tremor amplitude and frequency. The major disadvantage of using this drug is the need to monitor white blood counts because 1% of patients develop agranulocytosis. It is also very sedating. Topiramate and gabapentin are both antiepileptic agents reported to be helpful in ET. The dose of gabapentin was up to 3600 mg/day, but typical dosing schedules range from 300 to 600 mg tid. It can cause sedation, dizziness, slurred speech, and gait imbalance. Topiramate is more recently reported to have tremorolytic activity. Although it is also an anticonvulsant that enhances GABA activity, it is also a carbonic anhydrase inhibitor. It has been reported to be effective in tremor suppression in two small trials in dosages not exceeding 400 mg/day. Topiramate is currently the subject of a multicenter, double-blind, randomized, placebo-controlled trial. This is the first such trial of its kind for ET. Adverse effects include ataxia, fatigue, dizziness, poor concentration, slowing down, weight loss, paresthesias, nausea, and renal stones. The data on carbonic anhydrase inhibitors methazolamide and acetazolamide have been conflicting. In our experience these drugs provide no useful effect. Mirtazapine has been suggested as an alternative treatment for ET; however, this is based on a small open trial and requires confirmation.

Several studies have indicated that BoNT A (Botox) injection directly into contracting muscles may be useful in dampening tremor. Pilot studies have been completed in patients with head, hand, and voice tremors with moderate to marked functional improvement and tremor reduction in approximately 70% of patients. It is not used often for hand or arm tremor because of the tradeoff related to weakness. However, it is very useful for the treatment of head and voice tremor. Type B botulinum toxin (Myobloc) probably has the same effect but has not yet been tested.

Of patients 30% to 60% do not respond to medications, and the rest have only a partial response. Many have severe tremor and it is these patients in whom surgery needs to be considered. Stereotaxic thalamotomy of the VIM nucleus has been used for 30 years with varying levels of success. Some patients experience a dramatic resolution of tremor, but in about 20% of patients recurrence is observed. Persistent side effects from unilateral thalamotomy are uncommon but include dysarthria, dysphagia, and limb paresis. Complications from bilateral thalamotomy occur in more than 25% of cases and include speech impairment, mental status change, involuntary movements and gait disorder. This bilateral procedure is not recommended.

During thalamotomy, stimulation was used to optimize placement of the lesion. It was found that stimulation reduced tremor. This finding led to the evaluation of chronic VIM stimulation as a treatment for tremor. This procedure is known as deep brain stimulation

(DBS) and has replaced the ablative counterpart. Chronic stimulating electrodes are implanted through a burr hole in the skull and placed in the thalamus using stereotactic techniques and magnetic resonance imaging (MRI) or computed tomography (CT) imaging. It is tested in the operating room for effectiveness while the patient is awake. Once the correct location is found the wire is tunneled under the skin and connected to a pulse generator placed under the clavicle in the pectoralis muscles. In some patients, placing the electrode alone will reduce tremor as the result of a microthalamotomy. The stimulator can be adjusted and reprogrammed with a special computer, and the patient can turn the stimulator on and off with an external magnet. It is recommended that patients keep it off at night to avoid the development of tolerance and to preserve the battery. Significant improvement has been observed in blinded evaluations and maintained for 1 year. In one study efficacy was seen up to 8 years. More than 30% of patients with ET experience complete resolution, and 90% demonstrate moderate to marked improvement. This magnitude of response is not seen with any medications. It improves writing, pouring, drinking, and other activities. DBS improves all types of tremor—resting, postural, and kinetic—and improvement of disability correlated most closely with improvement of kinetic type. Surgical complications have included intracerebral hemorrhage, subdural hematoma, and postoperative seizure. Stimulation-related complications include transient paresthesias, which occur in nearly all patients at the time the stimulator is turned on; headache; gait disequilibrium; limb paresis; dystonia; and dysarthria. These problems may disappear with time. Bilateral implants are not associated with the high morbidity of thalamotomy. The stimulation parameters (voltage, frequency, and pulse width) do not require significant adjustments over time. The advantages of DBS over thalamotomy include reversibility (minimal destructive lesions), adaptability (can change stimulus parameters to improve efficacy and decrease side effects), and safe implantation of bilateral stimulators with much less risk.

Drawbacks include the cost of the stimulators; implantation of a foreign object; need to replace battery (every 3–5 years depending on the parameters); and possibility of breakage, malfunction, and infection. One study compared thalamic DBS and thalamotomy in 68 patients with Parkinson's disease, ET, and multiple sclerosis in a prospective randomized fashion. DBS resulted in greater functional status improvement and a greater number of patients who experienced complete or almost complete tremor suppression. The overall improvement of tremor was not dramatically different in the two groups. However, thalamic DBS was associated with fewer adverse effects.

There are no alternative therapies that are useful for ET. Occupational therapy suggestions include using either wrist weights to decrease the amplitude of tremor or weighted cups and utensils.

When to Refer to a Neurologist

Most patients are well controlled by taking propranolol or primidone. However, if tremor is severe and unresponsive to these agents, referral to a neurologist is necessary. This is particularly true if surgery is being considered. The referral should be to a specialty center performing DBS. If BoNT injection is being considered, then referral should be made to a neurologist with experience with this modality of therapy. Finally, if the tremor is complex and diagnosis is unsure, referral to a movement disorders center is suggested.

Special Challenges for Hospitalized Patients

Education of hospital staff is useful to let them know that patients with severe ET may require either assistance in feeding themselves or special utensils.

HUNTINGTON'S DISEASE

HD is a chronic degenerative disorder of the CNS characterized by involuntary movements (most notably chorea), psychiatric symptoms, and progressive cognitive deterioration. Prevalence in the United States is approximately 12 per 100,000 population. There are two places in the world where it is much more frequent: Maracaibo, Venezuela (where most of the genetic research was conducted) and Moray, Scotland. It is inherited in an autosomal dominant pattern and commonly presents in adult life. It is named for George Huntington, who eloquently described several generations of the disorder in his only medical publication. The word chorea is derived from the Greek word for dance *(choreia)* and originally was used to describe the dancelike gait and continual limb movements of infectious forms of chorea (Sydenham's chorea). The term chorea now is applied to a class of abnormal involuntary movements defined earlier. Choreiform movements disappear during sleep and often are exacerbated by nervousness and emotional distress.

CLINICAL FEATURES

A patient with HD may manifest his or her disease initially with chorea, psychiatric features, or dementia, although eventually all of these abnormalities are seen. HD may begin any time from the first to seventh decade but most commonly presents between the ages of 35 and 42 years. The onset of chorea is almost always insidious with a few irregular movements of the face and limbs. Patients find themselves to be fidgety and clumsy. The typical history includes slight clumsiness or restlessness that progresses to "piano playing" movements of the fingers and facial grimacing. Family members will notice a peculiar gait associated with irregular involuntary hand movements. The patient may try to mask the involuntary facial movements by chewing gum and the limb movements by sitting on their hands. The muscles remain strong and the ability to initiate movements remains preserved, but the carrying out of a continuous movement frequently is impeded by the superimposition of the chorea. The reflexes are frequently brisk, but patients rarely have the

Babinski sign until the final stages of the disease. The voice often is affected by this condition, and abnormalities of respiratory and articulatory muscles may lead to severe dysarthria and erratic, sometimes explosive, speech. As the disorder progresses, the chorea may diminish and rigidity and dystonia may ensue. On some occasions, other movement disorders, including dystonia, parkinsonism, and myoclonus, may predominate instead of chorea.

Approximately 5% of patients have onset in childhood. Of these patients, 60% have parkinsonian features, not chorea. This has been referred to as the Westphal variant. There is an increased incidence of seizures in children with HD (30% to 60%). These patients progress more rapidly than adult cases and die in an average of 9 years. Childhood-onset cases more frequently inherit the disease from their fathers, and this relates to the type of genetic abnormality found in the HD gene.

Progressive intellectual and psychiatric deterioration can be manifested as a personality change, depression, or dementia. Some patients show more emotional than intellectual decline, becoming irritable, agitated, excitable, or even apathetic. Inattention, poor concentration and judgment, and eventual memory loss progress until the patient is overtly demented. Other psychiatric features include psychosis and obsessive-compulsive disorder (OCD).

Voluntary movement difficulties include abnormal ocular motor function, gait difficulties, and loss of finger and hand dexterity. The ocular motor difficulties include impairment of fixation, increased ocular reaction time with an obvious latency before the movement is initiated, loss of smooth pursuit movements, and an inability to look toward an object without accompanying head movements and blinking. Optokinetic nystagmus is generally abnormal. These findings frequently are observed early in the course of the disease. The gait abnormality is not solely the result of choreiform movements. The gait, which has characteristics of both basal ganglia and cerebellar dysfunction, has a stuttering and dancing character to it. The patient also exhibits a wide-based stance, swaying motions, decreased arm swing, spontaneous knee flexion, and a variable cadence. One other interesting feature of HD is the inability to maintain tongue protrusion. Finally, weight loss can be a serious issue for these patients. Studies demonstrate that the change in weight starts early in the course and may relate to metabolic changes.

In general, patients with HD live from 10 to 30 years (average, 17) with the disease and usually die from pulmonary causes (aspiration pneumonia), cardiac disease (ischemic heart disease), trauma-related injuries (subdural hematoma) from multiple falls, or nutritional deficiencies. Slower progression of disease is associated with an older age of onset of HD and heavier weight at onset. Patients inheriting the disease from their mothers also tend to have a slower progression. Since the discovery of the gene, it has been shown that HD is more clinically heterogeneous than originally thought. For instance, patients with late-onset chorea and no dementia have been shown to have the HD gene. The final stages of the disease include a loss of ambulatory function, severe dysarthria, dysphagia with the threat of aspiration, and dementia. The loss of functional capacity and rate of progression can be correlated in some patients with the degree of caudate nucleus atrophy seen on CT or MRI scan and caudate nucleus hypometabolism as measured on PET.

The clinical picture of HD is variable, and some patients have more chorea than mental changes, but the reverse is also possible. This can lead to difficulties with diagnosis. Because HD is an inherited, progressive, debilitating disorder with no cure, accurate diagnosis is of the utmost importance. In the patient with adult-onset chorea, dementia, and a positive family history, the diagnosis can be made easily. However, in patients with chorea and even dementia who have no family history, the diagnosis of HD requires a diagnostic gene test. If a patient has chorea but a definite lack of family history, the chorea may result

from some other etiology. However, studies of patients with a sporadic form of chorea resembling HD have shown that a majority of these patients do indeed have the HD gene. A follow-up study of 49 patients suspected to have HD on clinical grounds but without family history revealed that 75% do have the disease. This finding is less common in patients with atypical features. Dementia and emotional symptoms are not essential for the diagnosis and are not considered sufficient evidence of HD in a family, but a history of family members hospitalized for these reasons in middle age or because of neurologic problems helps to raise the index of suspicion in patients with typical choreiform movements. There are a number of disorders that present with chorea and make up the differential diagnosis for HD (Table 11.6).

Since the discovery of the gene, presymptomatic patients have been studied in an attempt to find out when the earliest features begin. It is interesting to note that these patients can be perfectly normal even with psychometric testing. Subtle changes in motor skills, including movement time, movement time with decision, and auditory reaction time, have been described in patients considered to be at-risk, asymptomatic gene carri-

TABLE 11.6. *Differential Diagnosis of Huntington's Disease*

1. Benign hereditary chorea
2. Senile chorea
3. Familial Alzheimer's disease with myoclonus
4. Creutzfeldt-Jakob disease
5. Wilson's disease
6. Neuroacanthocytosis
7. Tardive dyskinesia in a psychiatric patient
8. Basal ganglia or subthalamic infarction
9. Patients with Parkinson disease treated with levodopa
10. Dentato-rubro-pallidal-luysian atrophy (DRPLA) (chromosome 11)
11. Choreoathetotic cerebral palsy
12. Chorea gravidarum
13. Recurrence of Sydenham's chorea in adulthood
14. Other drug-induced choreas (oral contraceptives, anticonvulsants, stimulants, antidepressants, anticholinergics, calcium channel blockers, buspirone)
15. Hyperthyroid chorea

ers. Cognitive changes (measured via psychometric testing) also have been described in some reports as very early features in patients otherwise considered to be asymptomatic. The CAG trinucleotide repeat length significantly correlated with these test performances.

GENETICS

HD is inherited as an autosomal dominant disorder with 100% penetrance. Children of an affected parent have a 50% risk of developing the disease. The emotional impact of the disease on children is profound. They must watch as a parent deteriorates slowly, inexorably, while facing the prospect of inheriting the same disorder. Enormous advances have been made in the last decade regarding the genetics of HD. In 1993, the HD gene was discovered, and this lead to the development of genetic testing. The availability of such a test has raised a number of ethical questions, most fundamental of which is the following: Why should predictive testing be performed for an illness that has no effective therapy? The impact of revealing to a young healthy person the rather bleak future of HD may be devastating. The results could be marital difficulties leading to disruption of the family and divorce, loss of employment, and psychiatric problems including suicide. However, positive reasons for genetic testing are numerous. In symptomatic patients, genetic testing is the gold standard for diagnosis. Its use will avoid a very costly workup for other causes of chorea. In asymptomatic individuals, genetic testing allows for personal and family planning and relieves uncertainty, and in both groups it will prepare patient and physician for treatment possibilities (e.g., clinical trials or new treatment). There are now realistic hopes that research in genetics and pathogenesis will lead to disease-modifying therapies. There are also legal and social issues related to predictive testing that need to be addressed. Early studies showed that approximately 75% of at-risk patients would be interested in participating in predictive testing, but with the advent of such testing this was found to be a gross overestimation. Experience has demonstrated that less than 5% of at-risk individuals actually request the predictive test.

HD genetic testing is extremely serious. One can imagine the devastating effect of a positive result on a young asymptomatic person and his or her family, but, surprisingly, a negative result also can cause havoc. Some people live their lives and make decisions based on the probability that they will develop HD. When it is discovered they do not carry the gene, they experience regrets, and this can have a significant impact on family relationships. In addition, there is guilt for being gene negative while other family members suffer with the disease. This may cause the subjects to either spend inordinate amounts of time helping the affected siblings or to distance themselves.

The testing process needs to be performed at a testing center staffed with the appropriate team of personnel in genetics, neurology, psychiatry, psychology, social work, speech therapy, and nutrition, for both testing and treatment. The goals of such a program are to ensure that an informed decision is made, to prepare the subject for the result, and to ensure that an adequate support system is in place. The program must have maximal control over whether the patient and his or her family receive this irrevocable information (because of its profound impact), it must provide the opportunity for the subject to withdraw, and it must be able to ensure confidentiality. In most centers, the process of genetic testing for asymptomatic patients begins with an initial visit with a genetics counselor followed by evaluations from neurology, psychiatry, speech therapy, and sometimes psychology. This takes place over a 4- to 8-week period. Occasionally, a second genetic visit is required. Once all evaluations are complete, the team meets and addresses whether the patient is already symptomatic and decides if testing can be performed safely or if it needs to be delayed. The subject then comes in for blood to be drawn and returns for results. Results are never given by phone or mail. In early symptomatic patients, the process is the same, but in advanced cases, and where a diagnosis is not clear, many of the steps are skipped depending on decisions made by the testing team. In some centers prenatal testing is performed, but this leads to a whole new set of issues. For instance, a positive test may reveal simultaneously the carrier status in the parent and child (if the parents' status is not known). Counseling regarding the option of terminating the pregnancy becomes important. Testing should be avoided under the following circumstances: when not requested by the patient but requested by an employer, insurance company, prison, court, or the military; if the subject is younger than 18 years of age (debatable); if there is no informed consent; and if the subject has a poor support system.

The HD gene is on chromosome 4p16.3 and is referred to as IT15 (IT = interesting transcription). The gene product is a protein designated as huntingtin. The abnormality within the gene is a polymorphic trinucleotide repeat sequence [(CAG)n] that is expanded and unstable and located on exon 1 of 67. The instability leads to variations (expansion) in length between generations, especially if the father carries the gene. In normal individuals, this sequence repeats up to 29 times. Repeat lengths of 30 to 34 could lead to paternal transmission if expansion occurs, and lengths of 35 to 39 represent an intermediate or a reduced penetrance as well as expansion in offspring. In HD, there are 40 or more copies and every person with this sequence ultimately is affected. Longer segments (55 or greater) appear in juvenile cases, suggesting that there is an inverse correlation between repeat length and age of onset of symptoms. This is a statistical correlation, but any given expansion may be associated with a broad range of onset ages and thus is not predictive. The repeat length also appears to expand with each additional generation if the affected parent is the father. This could lead to the phenomenon of anticipation, when the disease occurs at younger ages with each generation. There is also a correlation of repeat length and severity of disease and severity of pathology. There

are no differences in repeat length in those patients presenting with neurologic or psychiatric symptoms. A small number of families have been reported with the HD phenotype but no expansion on chromosome 4. These disorders have been referred to as HD-like diseases.

PATHOLOGY, NEUROCHEMISTRY, PATHOGENESIS

Postmortem examination of brain tissue from patients with HD reveals characteristic pathologic abnormalities. Grossly, the caudate nucleus, putamen, and cerebral cortex are atrophied. In advanced cases brain weight may decrease as much as 30%. On microscopic examination, there is severe neuronal loss (especially GABAergic medium spiny neurons) and gliosis in the striatum, with the caudate nucleus being more affected than the putamen. Neuronal loss and gliosis also are seen in layers III, V, and VI of the cerebral cortex and in the thalamus, substantia nigra pars reticulata, hypothalamus, and deep cerebellar nuclei. Neuronal intranuclear inclusions are seen in these regions. Although it has been suggested that early features of disease are related to striatal degeneration, it has been demonstrated that widespread neuronal degeneration occurs early. Occasionally, patients come to postmortem examination with well-documented chorea and no pathologic changes.

Postmortem studies also have revealed that levels of many neurotransmitters, biosynthetic enzymes, and receptor binding sites are abnormal. Those that appear to have the most significance, as far as pathophysiology is concerned, will be discussed. GABA levels are diminished in the striatum and globus pallidus. The levels of glutamic acid decarboxylase (GAD), the synthetic enzyme of GABA, also have been found to be reduced in the same areas. Both localize to the medium spiny neurons of the striatum. Levels of both are normal in other parts of the brain. GABA is an inhibitory transmitter that is released by the striatonigral pathways to modulate the outflow of dopamine from the nigrostriatal pathway. The result of the diminished GABA levels is a relative increase in dopamine activity. GABA is also the transmitter in neurons projecting from striatum to the globus pallidus. There are two projections: one to the external segment (the so-called indirect pathway) and the other to the internal segment (the direct pathway). The projection to the external segment (also containing enkephalins) appears to be first to degenerate in typical HD. The result is decreased activity of the major output nucleus of the basal ganglia, the internal segment of the globus pallidus. This leads to the presence of a hyperkinetic movement disorder. In juvenile cases, where parkinsonism is the main clinical feature, both direct and indirect pathways degenerate at the same time.

Somatostatin is widely distributed throughout the brain including the basal ganglia and cerebral cortex. A threefold to fivefold relative increase in this neurotransmitter has been discovered in the caudate, putamen, and globus pallidus in patients with HD compared to controls, indicating that the neurons containing it are spared. This indicates that cell death is selective both in terms of regions and cell type. Striatal cholinergic interneurons also appear to be spared. Other neurochemical abnormalities include diminished levels of substance P, cholecystokinin, met-enkephalin, and angiotensin-converting enzyme, plus an increase in neuropeptide Y. All these abnormalities are seen in the basal ganglia.

The pathogenesis of the selective neuronal degeneration in the striatum remains unknown. However, there is an increasing body of evidence pointing to a defect in mitochondrial energy metabolism and excitotoxicity. The evidence for mitochondrial abnormalities include: (a) glucose hypometabolism in the brain; (b) increased lactate concentrations in the basal ganglia and cortex; (c) decreased activity of mitochondrial complex II–III (55%) and IV (25%) in caudate and putamen, with sparing of this activity in other brain and nonbrain regions; (d) increased lactate-to-pyruvate ratios in cerebrospinal fluid (CSF) of pa-

tients with HD; and (e) abnormal energy metabolism in muscle of some patients with HD via ^{31}P MRI spectroscopy.

Evidence for the excitotoxicity model includes quinolinic acid lesions in animal models which reproduce selective cell loss in the striatum and a movement disorder.

The two mechanisms of excitotoxicity and mitochondrial dysfunction are closely linked. The energy defect may mediate cell death through excitotoxicity and possibly free radical formation. Progressive mitochondrial impairment results in increased vulnerability of neurons to normal endogenous levels of glutamate. Presumably, the decreased ATP formation in the mitochondria leads to failure of the sodium–potassium pump (ATPase), membrane depolarization, and persistent activation of the n-methyl-d-aspartate (NMDA) type of glutamate receptors by ambient levels of glutamate. This results in an influx of calcium ions and nitric oxide production, triggering the formation of free radicals, including the highly damaging peroxynitrite from the nitric oxide and superoxide, which the mitochondria can no longer take up, and oxidative cellular damage is initiated. This, in turn, leads to further mitochondrial inhibition and damage and decreased formation of ATP, increasing susceptibility to excitotoxic damage. In animal models, the cell damage caused by mitochondrial toxins is blocked by NMDA antagonists, which supports this concept. An increase in markers for oxidative damage in HD supports the notion that free radicals play some role. However, some investigators suggest that mitochondrial dysfunction and free radical formation are precipitated by excitotoxicity and enhanced by a self-amplifying cycle. The pattern of enzymatic change, which occurs in parallel with the pathologic change, supports the presence of free radical generation and excitotoxicity. Excitotoxicity also leads to triggering a series of kinases that ultimately results in apoptotic cell death.

The study of the pathophysiology of HD has made great progress. The development of transgenic animals where the human gene is placed in the animal genome has allowed investigators to study the disease process in animal models and to carefully examine the function of huntingtin. The normal function of huntingtin and the effect of the mutation on that function remain unknown, but progress has been made. There are now several forms of transgenic animals including mice, fruit flies, and worms. The mice are studied most extensively to this point, and several renditions of the model have been developed each with different properties. The key finding in these mice is that they parallel the human disease closely, with some variations. Clinically they develop a progressive disease with weight loss and a movement disorder, and the pathology is characterized by neuronal loss, gliosis, and neuronal intranuclear inclusions in the striatum. In fact, it was the animal model that brought attention to the inclusions in the human disease. In addition, there is increasing evidence that excitotoxicity, mitochondrial dysfunction, and free radical formation play a role in the pathophysiology of cell death in the animal model. Specifically, mitochondrial complex IV activity is decreased in the animals and nitric oxide is increased.

The CAG trinucleotide repeat expansion in the gene results in a polyglutamine (polyQ) stretch within the huntingtin protein near the N-terminus. The protein is necessary for normal growth and development as demonstrated by the fact that knockout animals (not expressing the gene) do not survive. Its role in cell survival may be the result, in part, of enhancement of the transcription of brain-derived neurotrophic factor stimulation. It has been suggested that the mutant gene is less efficient at this task, leading to decreased levels of the nerve growth factor and the development of apoptosis. Huntingtin, in the wild-type form, normally is ubiquitous, being expressed in the cytoplasm of most cells in the body. In the brain, it primarily is seen in neurons and is associated with several organelles including endoplasmic reticulum, microtubules, vesicles, and mitochondria. The widespread location of the protein begs the question of how selective neuronal degeneration occurs in disease. Protein interactions

may be the explanation. The protein contains several caspase cleavage sites. It also interacts with several proteins, including huntingtin-associated protein (HAP-1) and PSD95 (postsynaptic density protein 95). The later protein acts by anchoring receptor proteins to membranes, including the NMDA receptor. Mutant huntingtin does not bind as well as wild type, and this leads to hypersensitivity of NMDA and other glutamatergic receptors, which would lead to excitotoxicity. HAP-1 and caspases are associated with the process of apoptosis, and interaction with mutant huntingtin appears to be proapoptotic, leading to enhanced cell death. It appears that wild-type huntingtin can protect cells against the mutant protein.

The mutant protein is found in the cytoplasm and the nucleus where it forms aggregates. When the mutant enters the nucleus it is cleaved by caspases, making the protein more susceptible to aggregate formation. The interaction between huntingtin and caspases is an important step in neuronal toxicity. It appears that the nuclear aggregates themselves are toxic to cells; in fact, it is suggested that penetration of huntingtin into the nucleus is a necessary step for toxicity. The presence of aggregates disturbs proteolysis within cells. An increased number of polyQ repeats correlates with the number of aggregates. Huntingtin also binds (via the polyglutamine stretch) to an important glycolysis enzyme (glyceraldehyde-phosphate dehydrogenase), which may lead to decreased mitochondrial function; decreased ATP formation; and, in turn, increased glycolysis and increased lactate. Some additional roles of huntingtin include iron homeostasis, maintenance of perinuclear organelle structure, trafficking of secretory membranes, and gene expression.

To summarize, mutant huntingtin potentially affects several pathways to cell death. These include alteration of brain-derived neurotrophic factor activity, excitotoxicity, free radical formation, reduction of energy production, activation of apoptosis, and disruption of gene transcription through varied protein interactions. Huntingtin entrance into the nucleus and caspase-induced cleavage and aggregation seem to be important steps in cellular toxicity. The potential of these mechanisms in the progression of disease has lead to the testing of possible disease-altering agents in transgenic animals. Free radical scavengers, glutamate antagonists, creatine, and caspase inhibitors (including minocycline) have prolonged life by 20% in mice. These findings have lead to the examination of possible disease-modifying agents in patients with HD.

TREATMENT

Disease-Modifying Agents

The goal of therapy is to find an agent (or agents) that will stop or slow the disease process. The study of transgenic mice has led to several trials in patients. Glutamate antagonists have been examined most frequently as potential disease-modifying therapy. Baclofen, remacemide, riluzole, and lamotrigine all failed. However, remacemide, riluzole, and amantadine have antichoreic effects. Amantadine is easily available, and at doses of 200 to 400 mg/day improvement of the chorea can be seen. This drug is better tolerated than neuroleptics in most patients. Free radical scavengers and energy boosters also have to be examined in HD. Vitamin E, OPC 14117, and idebenone all failed to alter HD. However, one study demonstrated possible effects from the dietary supplement coenzyme Q10. This compound occurs naturally in mitochondria and shuttles electrons between complexes I, II, III, and it functions as an antioxidant and a respiratory chain activator. Coenzyme Q10 was examined in a 30-month, double-blind trial in 360 patients to examine its potential disease-modifying effects. The primary endpoint was change in the total functional capacity (TFC) scale portion of the Unified Huntington's Disease Rating Scale. Patients on coenzyme Q10 demonstrated a 13% slowing in TFC decline, which was not significantly different from other groups but represented an interesting trend. Coenzyme Q 10 (600 mg/day) was safe

and well tolerated. There are current plans to examine higher doses in a larger cohort of patients. Safety and tolerability studies examining minocycline and creatine have been completed and the results are pending. Over the next few years, it is expected that other caspase inhibitors, NMDA receptor blockers, and other novel agents will be examined.

The potential for reversal of the disease has been demonstrated using a "conditional" transgenic mouse. This model allows the huntingtin gene to be turned on and off pharmacologically. The investigators demonstrated that, if the gene is turned off even after disease progression, the disease does not just stop progressing but actually improves and pathology reverses. Thus, interrupting the action of the huntingtin gene potentially could lead to reversal of the disease process, the ultimate goal. Once such an agent is available, presymptomatic patients also will be targeted for treatment.

Symptomatic Therapy

The symptomatic management of HD involves a multidisciplinary approach. HD clinics usually include neurologists, psychologists, psychiatrists, speech therapists, physiotherapists, nutritionists, and social workers. From the neurologic standpoint the only feature that is amenable to symptomatic therapy is the movement disorder. Historically, the mainstay of therapy for chorea has been dopamine receptor antagonists. Phenothiazines (e.g., chlorpromazine) and the butyrophenones (e.g., haloperidol) share the property of dopaminergic receptor blockade and may be required for relief of chorea. It should be kept in mind that improvement in chorea may not be helpful in improving functional ability or quality of life. Frequently a patient with gait disorder and chorea will be treated with neuroleptics, but often the gait worsens because of the development of parkinsonism. The treatment of chorea should be limited to those in whom it is severe and troublesome. Atypical antipsychotics may have a role because of their potential for fewer extrapyramidal effects. Clozapine has been examined in several trials. In doses ranging from 25 mg/day to 500 mg/day, some improvement in chorea was reported, often associated with sedation and sometimes with no improvement in quality of life. Experience with risperidone in HD for symptomatic treatment of chorea is even more limited. It appears to have an effect similar to haloperidol when used at doses between 1 mg/day and 6 mg/day. There is no significant literature regarding the use of other atypical agents in HD. However, experience in practice has demonstrated that risperidone and olanzapine can be used in a manner similar to standard neuroleptics for the treatment of chorea. Quetiapine has less effect. Atypical agents should be used prior to standard neuroleptics in the treatment of chorea. Other agents that decrease striatal dopaminergic activity include reserpine, alpha-methylparatyrosine, and tetrabenazine. Historically, reserpine was the first agent reported to be of use in the treatment of chorea. A rauwolfia alkaloid, reserpine acts to block intravesicular neurotransmitter reuptake and depletes the brain of dopamine. Because it also acts to deplete central norepinephrine and serotonin, reserpine's activity is not specific, but it still is used in the treatment of HD at doses of 0.5 to 3 mg/day because it has a less severe side-effect profile than dopamine antagonists. Tetrabenazine is another dopamine depletor that is a reversible vesicle uptake inhibitor that may be useful in HD. It also has minor dopamine receptor–blocking effects but has not been reported to cause TD. Tetrabenazine adverse events (hypotension and shorter duration of depression) are less severe than those of reserpine. The typical dose is 50 to 200 mg/day. Tetrabenazine is not yet available in the United States. Alpha-methylparatyrosine inhibits tyrosine hydroxylase and prevents the synthesis of dopamine and norepinephrine. After intravenous administration of this agent, amelioration of choreic movements in patients with HD has been noted. Amantadine (NMDA receptor antagonist) is another agent that can be used to treat chorea. The effective

dose is 200 to 400 mg/day. It appears to be well tolerated by patients with HD with no cognitive changes. One other antichoreic agent is valproic acid, which in a small number of patients improved chorea.

Patients with onset at a younger age may develop parkinsonism instead of chorea as a manifestation of their HD. Some will respond to doses of carbidopa–levodopa.

Psychiatric symptoms need to be treated aggressively in patients with HD, and pharmacologic therapy may be very helpful. For psychosis atypical antipsychotics should be the first agents used. Quetiapine, olanzapine, risperidone, and clozapine all have been shown to be effective in treating HD-related psychosis. These agents also may be of benefit for agitation and irritability. For depression, anxiety, and obsessive-compulsive symptoms serotonin reuptake inhibitors are effective and well tolerated. For depression, particular care should be taken in assessing whether the patient is at risk for suicide. In addition to pharmacotherapy, many of these issues can be addressed with psychologic approaches.

There are several other issues that are addressed routinely at clinic visits. These include physical disability, speech disorders and dysphagia, nutritional status and weight loss, and home safety. These problems require the assessments of physical and speech therapists, nutritionists, and social workers. The goals are improved quality of life and a safe environment in the home. The most difficult decisions surround the need for feeding tubes and nursing home placement. There are some nursing homes that specialize in HD care and should be contacted at the appropriate time.

When to Refer to a Neurologist or Other Specialist

All patients with HD should be referred to a neurologist or psychiatrist who is involved in a multidisciplinary clinic to provide comprehensive care. This is particularly true for those with more advanced disease. At-risk patients (affected parent or sibling) who request presymptomatic testing should be referred to a testing center.

Special Challenges for Hospitalized Patients

Hospital staff should be educated regarding variability of chorea and the relationship of severity of chorea to stress. Behavioral abnormalities are frequent in these patients, and staff should be aware of this problem.

WILSON'S DISEASE

WD, or hepatolenticular degeneration, is a rare neurologic disorder of copper metabolism with a prevalence of approximately 5 to 20 per million; its prevalence is higher in countries with increased consanguinity, but it is present throughout the world. Accumulation of copper ultimately causes signs and symptoms that are neurologic (most notably movement disorders), psychiatric, hepatic, or ocular in nature, but they may occur in variable combinations, making WD a difficult disorder to recognize. The importance of recognizing WD cannot be overstated because it is a treatable and often reversible disorder that, if not diagnosed, inevitably results in death. There is no question that the only way to make the diagnosis is to always keep it in mind. Approximately 75% of deaths from WD result from a lack of diagnosis.

CLINICAL MANIFESTATIONS

Approximately 40% of patients with WD present with neurologic signs and symptoms. The most common are speech or extrapyramidal disorders beginning at 18 to 20 years of age. WD has a slowly progressive course, often with a single symptom predominating for months or even years before other manifestations appear. However, there may be a sudden dramatic worsening of what appears to be a stable neurologic deficit. Incoordination involving fine finger movements such as handwriting and typing is frequently an early manifestation. It may be subtle at first but worsens

as the disorder progresses. Resting tremor is a common early manifestation, and when associated with rigidity, bradykinesia, and/or gait difficulty, WD may mimic Parkinson's disease. The tremor also may be postural or kinetic. When severe, it takes on a flapping quality at the wrist with high-amplitude oscillations and a "wing beating" appearance at the shoulder, often resulting in significant disability. Some patients present with just bradykinesia and rigidity without tremor. Focal or generalized dystonia is also a common and predominant symptom of WD. Chorea is rare but may result in movements and a gait disorder that resemble HD. Spasticity and ataxia are seen rarely. Dysarthria is a consistent feature of WD. It sometimes is associated with dysphagia, and frequently patients show frustration because of their difficulty communicating. Often patients develop a characteristic facial expression with retraction of the upper lip, the mouth constantly agape, and upper teeth protruding. This gives the patient the appearance of grinning, or a "vacuous smile." Approximately 6% of patients have generalized seizures. A majority of the symptoms are exacerbated by emotional stress and ameliorated by calm and sleep. There is also an acute dystonic form of WD. These patients appear ill, and they have a high fever, significant muscle rigidity, rapid emaciation, and confusion, a picture that can be confused with a neuroleptic malignant syndrome. This acute presentation could be a preterminal event so diagnosis is of utmost importance. Because of the protean nature of WD, it is very important to consider this diagnosis in all patients under the age of 40 years presenting with movement disorders.

Approximately 25% of patients with WD are seen first by psychiatrists for a wide range of emotional difficulties. At least 50% of patients have early psychiatric manifestations. There are no psychiatric manifestations that are specific for WD, and diagnoses may range from adolescent adjustment reactions to depression and schizophrenia. The most common features include abnormal behavior, such as irritability, incongruous behavior, aggression, and personality change. Depression and cognitive impairment are also common, but schizophreniform psychosis is rare. Isolated psychiatric problems may be seen without neurologic deficits, making differentiation from the primary psychiatric disorders quite difficult. However, there frequently are neurologic findings in association with the psychiatric symptoms, and this clinical situation should raise the index of suspicion that WD may be the cause of the patients' problem. Some patients with psychiatric manifestations treated with neuroleptics, who later develop movement disorders, are misdiagnosed as having a primary psychiatric disorder and TD. Again, a raised index of suspicion is required. In one study, personality change and irritability appeared to be more frequent in patients with bulbar and dystonic features. To diagnose this treatable illness, some have advocated that all patients admitted to psychiatric wards under the age of 30 should be screened for WD.

Hepatic disease may be superimposed on neurologic manifestations or may be the presenting problem in 30% to 50% of patients. Hepatic disease usually presents at an earlier age than the neurologic symptomatology of WD (approximately age 10). There are four different presentations for hepatic WD. First, there may be a transient acute hepatitis that resolves spontaneously. This often is misdiagnosed as infectious mononucleosis or viral hepatitis because patients present with the typical hepatic symptoms and signs such as jaundice, malaise, and anorexia. The second presentation is fulminant hepatitis, which is seen in adolescents and which presents with sudden onset of jaundice and ascites progressing relentlessly to hepatic failure and death. A history of fulminant hepatitis in a sibling of a patient suspected as having WD is significant. Third, and most common, is chronic active hepatitis that presents with weakness, anorexia, jaundice, malaise, and abnormal liver function tests. Finally, patients may present with cirrhosis. A family history of cirrhosis may be an important diagnostic point. Nearly all patients have some residual cirrhosis. Hepatic patients with WD may be psychologically and neurologically normal.

All patients with WD and neurologic symptoms exhibit a Kayser–Fleischer (KF) ring in the cornea. This is a golden or greenish-brown ring that represents copper deposition in Descemet's membrane (Fig. 11.3). The ring is seen easily around the limbus in patients with light-colored or blue eyes but may be quite difficult to see in those with brown eyes. A slit lamp examination should be performed by an experienced ophthalmologist to accurately diagnose a KF ring in all those suspected of WD. Although a KF ring is not pathognomonic for WD, its presence is im-

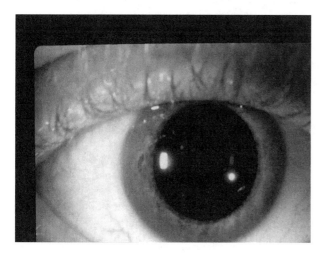

FIG. 11.3. Kaiser-Fleischer ring in a patient with Wilson's disease.

portant in the diagnosis. It fades with adequate chelation therapy.

Another unusual ocular manifestation of WD is the sunflower cataract. This is a disc-shaped opacity with frondlike radiations that often are described as a "cataract like the rays of the sun."

Other possible manifestations of WD include Coomb's-negative hemolytic anemia; skeletal changes, including pathologic fractures from metabolic bone disease and hypertrophic osteoarthropathy; renal disease, including gross hematuria, stones, tubular and glomerular disease, and the Fanconi syndrome; and cardiac symptoms including arrhythmia and cardiomyopathy.

NEUROPATHOLOGY

The lenticular nuclei are involved bilaterally and symmetrically. The lesions vary from softening and discoloration to frank cavitation. Other areas less significantly involved include the subcortical white matter, cerebellum (most commonly the dentate nucleus), and other nuclei that make up the basal ganglia. Excess copper is distributed throughout the CNS. Neuronal loss is observed in the basal ganglia and, to a lesser extent, in the cerebral cortex.

PATHOGENESIS AND GENETICS

Excessive accumulation of copper as a result of poor copper excretion leads to organ system dysfunction and clinical stigmata of WD. Ceruloplasmin, a copper-containing polypeptide, is deficient in 95% of patients with WD. The relationship between deficient ceruloplasmin, the pathogenesis of WD, and the WD gene mutation is beginning to unfold. Biliary excretion of copper in WD is impaired and copper accumulates in the liver, binding to thiol and carboxyl groups on copper-storage proteins. The copper binding alters both structure and function of storage proteins, disrupting normal cellular activity in a variety of ways. When storage reaches capacity, excess copper begins to move into extrahepatic stor-

age sites, particularly the eye and brain. This explains why KF rings are not seen in 50% of patients with hepatic WD.

WD is an autosomal recessive disorder with the gene locus located on chromosome 13q14-q21. In 1993 the WD gene was cloned, and the mutant gene frequency is 0.6% with a carrier frequency of 1 in 90. The gene codes for a copper-transporting p-type ATPase called ATP7B. ATP7B functions in copper transport coupled with the synthesis of ceruloplasmin in the Golgi apparatus. The abnormal protein from the mutated gene leads to decreased function, which causes failure of the liver to excrete copper into the bile. Nearly 200 gene mutations already have been identified, most being point mutations or small deletions. Some mutations leave some residual transporter function, whereas others leave none at all. It is believed that those with residual function have a later onset of disease (neurologic or psychiatric), whereas patients with no transporter function have earlier (hepatic) onset. The most common mutation is the H1059Q, which leads to a mean age of onset of 20 years.

Genetic diagnosis is not commercially available. However, if the mutation of a family member is known, the subject's gene status can be determined.

DIAGNOSIS

It can never be said enough that a high index of suspicion is very important in making the diagnosis of WD. This is especially true when evaluating patients 40 years or younger who present with extrapyramidal disorders, psychiatric disorders (especially when associated with neurologic signs and symptoms), and hepatic disease. In addition, a family history of WD (particularly a sibling) or hepatic disease at a young age should alert the physician to a possible diagnosis of WD. Once suspected, the diagnosis of WD can be confirmed using four tests: (a) a slit lamp examination for KF rings (the specificity of KF rings for patients with neuropsychiatric WD is nearly 100%); (b) a serum ceruloplasmin level (usually low in 80% of patients with WD); (c) 24-hour urinary copper excretion (elevated in WD to more than 100 ug); and (d) a liver biopsy with quantitation of copper concentration—the most definitive of all tests (copper levels higher than 250 µg/g of dry tissue are considered diagnostic). Clinical evaluation and the first three tests are usually sufficient to make the diagnosis of WD in symptomatic patients, and liver biopsy is generally not required. A normal serum ceruloplasmin (often used to screen for WD) by itself should not convince the treating physician that WD is ruled out because 5% to 20% of patients with WD have normal levels. In a patient with a neuropsychologic presentation, absence of a KF ring indicates that he probably does not have WD. If ceruloplasmin level is low, examination for KF ring and 24-hour urine copper excretion must be performed. If ceruloplasmin is normal and KF ring is present, a liver biopsy should be performed to make the diagnosis. Hepatic WD is the most difficult presentation to diagnose because ceruloplasmin

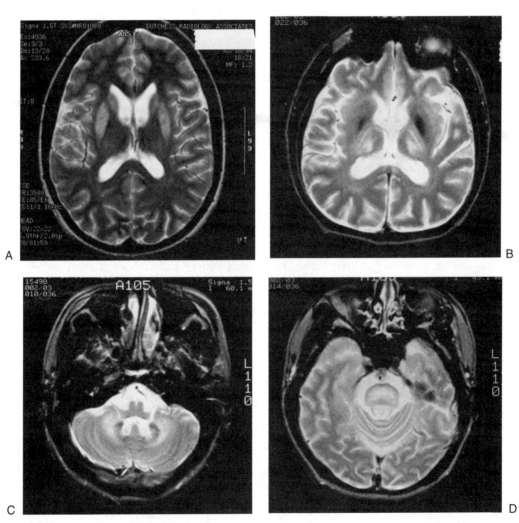

FIG. 11.4. A: T2-weighted magnetic resonance imaging (MRI) scan of a patient with early symptomatic Wilson's disease, demonstrating hyperintensity in the caudate nucleus and putamen. **B:** T2-weighted MRI scan of a more advanced patient with hypointensity in the striatum. The same scan as seen in *B,* showing hyperintensity in the dentate nucleus of the cerebellum *C* and the pons *D.*

may be falsely elevated or normal in WD hepatitis and a KF ring may be absent. If confusion remains after serum ceruloplasmin levels, slit lamp examination, and 24-hour urinary copper concentration, liver biopsy is required.

WD is inherited as an autosomal recessive disorder, so each sibling of a patient with WD has a 25% chance of having the disease. All siblings of patients with WD should be screened. If they have WD, treatment will prevent onset of clinical stigmata. The at-risk siblings should have slit lamp examination and 24-hour urinary copper and ceruloplasmin determination, along with physical and neurologic examinations at regular intervals. If a KF ring is present, ceruloplasmin level is low, and urinary excretion of copper is elevated, the diagnosis of WD is clear and liver biopsy is not required. However, if the serum ceruloplasmin level is low but KF ring is absent, the patient may be a heterozygote for WD and liver biopsy will be necessary to make a definitive diagnosis. Of heterozygotes, 10% to 20% have low serum ceruloplasmin levels, but these patients do not require treatment. With the recent discovery of multiple polymorphic DNA markers close to the gene on chromosome 13, multilocus linkage analysis makes possible accurate and informative testing of potential carriers in families with WD in whom the mutation has been found. With these techniques, one could discriminate between carriers and presymptomatic patients. Advantages of this technique include its noninvasive nature and early (possibly prenatal) diagnosis. Neuroimaging techniques are not diagnostic in WD, but typical lesions can be observed. On CT scanning, cortical and brainstem atrophy are seen in nearly all patients. Hypodensity of the head of the caudate and putamen is seen early, and cavitation of the putamen is seen late. Sometimes, hypodensities are seen in other areas including cerebellum, brainstem, thalamus, and cerebral cortex. These lesions do not enhance with contrast. On MRI scanning, hypointense lesions are observed in the lenticular nucleus, thalamus, caudate nucleus, cerebellum, brainstem, and subcortical white matter on T1-weighted images; hyperintensity ae observed on T2 (Fig. 11.4). The accumulation of copper leads to areas of hypointensity adjacent to the hyperintense regions (Fig. 11.4B). These changes are seen in all patients with neurologic symptoms and represent edema, gliosis, or cystic lesions.

TREATMENT

Once the diagnosis of WD is confirmed, treatment should be instituted without delay. There is now a choice of agents including chelating agents such as D-penicillamine, trientine, or zinc acetate, all of which are now FDA approved (Table 11.7). There is also an experimental agent that shows great promise, tetrathiomolybdate (TTM). D-penicillamine, a potent chelating agent with thiol groups to bind copper and remove it from organ systems via urinary excretion, had been the treatment of choice for decades. However, zinc acetate is becoming the treatment of choice because of penicillamine's toxicity and the risk of worsening of neurologic symptoms associated with its use. Penicillamine has a rapid action in mobilizing and clearing copper through the urine. Four divided doses of 1 to 2 g should be given 30 minutes before or 2 hours after meals to ensure maximal absorp-

TABLE 11.7. *Medical Treatment of Wilson's Disease*

Drug Name	Initial Daily Dose	Usual Daily Dose Range
Penicillamine	125 mg qid	250 mg qid
Trientine	250 mg qid	250 mg qid
Zinc acetate	50 mg tid	50 mg tid
Tetrathiomolybdate	20 mg 6 times	20 mg 6 times[a]

[a]Currently experimental.

tion. Pyridoxine, 25 mg/day, should be added because of an antipyridoxine effect of penicillamine. Improvement begins from 2 weeks to 1 year after the institution of therapy. The variation in response results from the size of the abnormal body pool of copper, variation in initial penicillamine dose, patient compliance, and variation in strength of copper binding from patient to patient. There is no set pattern as to which symptoms clear first, but dystonia tends to be more resistant than tremor, whereas dysarthria and the characteristic smile typically remain. Improvement of psychiatric manifestations is unpredictable. Sequelae resulting from irreversible structural damage to the liver or brain will remain unchanged and generally are known by 2 years after the initiation of therapy. Of patients with WD, 75% to 80% respond successfully to penicillamine. In the first 2 months of therapy, complete blood count, urinalysis, and liver enzyme levels should be examined frequently. Some patients may initially worsen with penicillamine therapy. The actual frequency of this occurrence is unknown but is suggested to be as high as 50%. For some the worsening is permanent. In addition, a small percentage of patients with WD continue to progress and die despite treatment.

Adverse effects of penicillamine are many and occur early and late. Early adverse effects include hypersensitivity reactions, fever, rash, adenopathy, leukopenia, thrombocytopenia, collagen vascular disorders, and bone marrow suppression. If any of these reactions are severe, therapy should be interrupted until symptoms subside. Then prednisone should be given, followed by the reinstitution of penicillamine or a change to another agent. Late adverse effects occurring after a year of therapy include nephrotic syndrome, agranulocytosis, thrombocytopenia, Goodpasture's syndrome, pemphigus, myasthenia gravis, elastosis perforans serpiginosa, and dermopathy. Serious intolerance to penicillamine occurs in only 3% to 5% of patients, and these patients require alternative therapy.

Trientine, like penicillamine, is a copper-chelating agent and is the alternative chelation therapy of choice. The dosage is 1 to 1.5 g/day 30 minutes before or 2 hours after meals. Adverse effects include collagen vascular disorders and iron-deficiency anemia. Two newer therapies have changed the approach to these patients. Zinc acetate, approved by the FDA in 1997, induces excretion of copper via the gastrointestinal tract by increasing the concentration of metallothionein in the bowel mucosa by 25-fold. As the tissue content of this protein increases, the proportion of copper in the cells increases. Then, as the mucosal cells are sloughed and lost in the stool, copper is excreted. Metallothionein levels also increase in the liver; this increases liver copper levels, but the copper is stored in a nontoxic form. Initially, zinc has a slower effect on copper excretion than the chelating agents. The dose is started at 50 to 100 mg three times a day 1 hour after or before food or beverage in adults and 50 mg twice a day in children, and the ultimate daily dose ranges from 300 to 1200 mg/day. Patients are monitored by following urinary copper levels. Monitoring should be performed within the first 2 weeks, and if no change is seen the dose is increased. The final dose is individualized. Zinc is less toxic than penicillamine and does not cause paradoxical worsening of symptoms as penicillamine can. The side effects include gastrointestinal irritation, elevation of serum amylase, and decreased high-density lipoprotein. Rarely, copper deficiency can occur, leading to leukopenia and anemia. It has been used successfully as both initial treatment and maintenance.

The newest treatment is tetrathiomolybdate. When given with meals it prevents absorption of copper, and when given between meals it is absorbed into the blood and forms complexes with copper and albumin, rendering the copper non-toxic. It has a rapid action in relation to copper metabolism and does not cause worsening of symptoms. It has been studied for initial therapy but not for maintenance. The daily maintenance dose is 20 mg six times a day, three doses with and three without meals. One side effect is a reversible anemia. The drug is experimental and has limited availability.

Initial treatment of WD has recently become controversial. Some argue that the old reliable treatment of penicillamine chelation therapy, based on decades of experience (since the 1950s), should not be abandoned. Others argue that zinc is the appropriate choice because it is equally effective, is much better tolerated, and does not cause paradoxical worsening. For hepatic presentations, it is suggested that zinc and a chelating agent be used concurrently. Some suggest trientine because it is less toxic than penicillamine. For neuropsychiatric presentations, zinc and a chelating agent should be initiated unless TTM is available. For maintenance, zinc is the treatment of choice. There have been no formal controlled trials to examine this issue. Zinc has become the treatment of choice in presymptomatic and pregnant patients. Copper-rich foods should be avoided, particularly shellfish and liver.

Frequently, patients whose neurologic symptoms have resolved will be tempted to stop their chronic medication. It may become difficult for asymptomatic patients to connect their good health to their chronic medication. Discontinuing chelation therapy invariably results in disaster for these patients, many of whom die of fulminant hepatitis within 3 years. It is the physician's job to reinforce the need for medication and to inform these patients of the disastrous results that lie ahead should the medication be stopped. Response to medication should be monitored using 24-hour urinary copper levels. Chelating agents will cause an increase in urinary copper output before a decrease.

For patients with liver failure the standard measures should be taken including lactulose, neomycin, and protein restriction. Liver transplant is sometimes the only treatment alternative in patients with fulminant hepatitis and cirrhosis with liver failure. The 1-year survival rate is about 80% and the 5-year survival rate is 40% to 70%. These numbers are quite respectable, especially in this situation in which all patients will otherwise die without treatment.

There is no role for alternative therapies in WD. However physical, occupational, and speech therapy may play a role. Speech therapy and assistive devices can be helpful for the dysarthria that characterizes WD. Physical therapy may be useful for treating dystonia and gait disorders, perhaps with the addition of assistive devices such as walkers. Occupational therapy can help patients who have dystonia and tremor to continue to function.

When to Refer to a Neurologist or Other Specialist

WD is a complex disorder with regard to diagnosis and assessment of siblings. Any patient with neuropsychiatric symptoms should be referred to a neurologist. Treatment is also a complicated matter best handled by a neurologist with experience. When the diagnosis is suspected and an evaluation for a KF ring is sought, it should be performed by an experienced ophthalmologist. Finally, all patients should have an evaluation by a gastroenterologist.

There are no special challenges for hospitalized patients in the case of WD.

GILLES DE LA TOURETTE'S SYNDROME

GTS is a hereditary movement disorder dominated by tics—the cardinal feature—and various behavioral abnormalities. It is seen in approximately 1% to 3% of school children and is three times more common in males than females. Tics are defined as sudden, brief, intermittent involuntary movements or sounds. They are classified according to whether they are motor or vocal, simple or complex. Simple motor tics are abrupt, brief, purposeless, isolated (single muscle or muscle group) movements that are jerky or clonic and emerging out of a background of normal activity. Examples of simple motor tics are eye blinks, head or limb jerks, and shoulder shrugs. Complex motor tics are more coordinated, sequential, and complicated movements or gestures that almost appear purposeful but are inappropriately intense and timed. Examples of complex motor tics include eye deviation, facial grimacing, hand shaking, waving arm movements, muscle flexing and posing with isometric or tonic movements, touching, jumping, hitting, kicking, squatting, truncal bending or gyrating, copropraxia (making obscene gestures), and echopraxia (mimicking the movements of others). Sometimes, a cluster of simple tics will appear to be complex. In extreme cases tics may be so forceful as to cause self-injurious behavior such as cervical injury with neck tics or lip biting. Simple vocal (phonic) tics are a variety of inarticulate noises and sounds. Examples include sniffing, snorting, barking, throat clearing, and grunting. Complex vocal tics are actually linguistically meaningful utterances. They can include the utilization of words ("no-no"), phrases ("oh boy"), or even sentences. Classical forms of complex vocal tics include palilalia (involuntary repetition of words or sentences), echolalia (involuntary repetition of words or sentences just spoken by another person), and coprolalia (involuntary utterances of curse words). This latter phenomenon is perhaps the best known feature in GTS, but it occurs in less than 10% of patients. Coprolalia is distinguished from emotionally-driven swearing by its cadence, volume, and context. Vocal tics in general tend to occur at phrase junctions in speech and can cause blockage or hesitation of speech patterns.

Although motor tics are commonly clonic or rapid in nature, when they are slow, twisting, and result in brief sustained postures (resembling dystonia), they are referred to as dystonic tics. A common type involves slow shoulder shrugging with rotational scapular movements. Others include blepharospasm, ocular deviations, and torticollis. Sensory tics (premonitory sensations) are patterns of somatic sensations that have been variously described as a pressure, a tickle, a temperature change, paresthesias or an uncomfortable feeling, localized to specific body regions, and resulting in dysphoric feelings. These uncomfortable sensations may provoke a motor or a vocal tic such as limb stretching, blepharospasm, and throat clearing. This indicates that the tic itself actually may be a voluntary movement (sometimes referred to as "unvoluntary"). The uncomfortable sensation usually is relieved by this movement, but relief is only temporary, leading to repeated movements.

Tics have a number of characteristic features that help to differentiate them from other movement disorders. They are suppressible to some extent. Often, when patients with GTS come into the physician's office, their history of tics is a better indication than just observation because patients can suppress their tics in the office. In addition, tics tend to wax and wane, so they can vary in intensity over time and occur in bouts. They also tend to change location over time. More frequently, tics begin in the eyes with eye blinking and then move so that there are neck movements or shoulder shrugs or other types of movements. Patients often will describe an inner tension or urge that is transiently relieved by the tic itself. When patients suppress the tics, the inner tension grows and there often will be a flurry of tics once the suppression is released. Patients often will give a history of having few tics during work but having a flurry of them once they return home at the end of the day. Tics, in general, increase with stress, anger, and excitement and decrease with relaxation, concentration, distraction, and sleep. The urges or sensations may be disabling by themselves.

Tics usually begin between the ages of 3 and 8 years, although GTS is defined by onset prior to age 21. They start as facial movements, especially blinking, and then move to other regions including neck and shoulders. Vocal tics typically occur after the motor tics. Tics reach peak severity in the early to mid second decade and then diminish by the beginning of the third. By 18 years, up to 50% of patients may be tic free. In the rest the movement disorder persists into adulthood but with diminished severity. There are occasional cases with adult-onset tics. The severity of tics in childhood has no bearing on severity in adulthood because even the most severe cases can improve or even disappear. Moderate to severe tics in late adolescence, however, can be an indication that patients will have more severe tics in adulthood. Despite difficulties in school at younger ages, most people with tics are employed or go on for further education as young adults and become very well adjusted. The need for treatment diminishes in adulthood.

CLINICAL SPECTRUM OF TIC DISORDERS

Tic disorders represent a continuum from a mild transient form to a potentially devastating neurobehavioral disorder. Studies of large families have indicated that various types of tic disorders occur in individual families and that they all appear to represent varied severity of a single disease. Transient tic disorder is probably the most common and mildest form of the disorder. It is defined by a duration of less than 12 months. As such, the diagnosis is often retrospective. In these patients, tics are usually the simple motor type. Chronic multiple tic disorder is a more severe form than transient tic disorder. In this case, patients have multiple motor or vocal tics but not both. Multiple motor tics are much more common. The duration of this disease is longer than 1 year. GTS represents the full expression of the disorder. Estimates of the prevalence of this disorder are probably significantly lower than actual prevalence because, in the milder cases, a large percentage are unaware that they have a tic disorder and in many the tics are not bothersome so they do not seek medical assistance.

ASSOCIATED BEHAVIORAL DISTURBANCES

OCD is present in 20% to 60% of cases. This behavioral disorder appears to be linked genetically to GTS and, in fact, may represent an alternate expression of this disorder. Symptoms can result in significant stress and disability. Examples of compulsive symptoms include ordered arranging habits; rituals of decontamination, including repeated hand washing; checking rituals (locks on doors or cars and stove switches); and ritualistic counting. Obsessive thoughts often can intrude on conscious thoughts and interrupt daily routines. Examples include fears and images of injuries to loved ones; fear of contamination with germs, dirt, or disease; feelings of responsibility for misfortune of others; feelings of doubt that one has performed tasks that are already completed; and need for exactness and symmetry. Obsessive thoughts can lead to slowed cognitive function. Compulsive behavior and tics, particularly complex ones, can overlap and they may be difficult to differentiate. OCD symptoms, like tics, wax and wane and increase with stress.

Another common behavioral disturbance is attention deficit hyperactivity disorder (ADHD). In these patients, the disorder can result in a short attention span, restlessness, poor concentration, diminished impulse control, and hyperactivity. It may be present in 40% to 70% of children with GTS, and it is not uncommon for ADHD to precede the onset of tics. ADHD seems to be more common in those patients with severe tic disorder. Increased irritability, rage attacks, vulnerability to drug abuse, depression, and antisocial behavior are common in those with notable ADHD. ADHD occurs in the earliest stages of the disease, whereas OCD emerges in the late teen years; both continue over time. Stimulant medications that are used for primary ADHD for years have been believed to provoke or exacerbate tics. A study by the Tourette Study Group using methylphenidate dispelled that myth and demonstrated that methylphenidate can be used in this population with no concern of inducing tics.

Other behavioral abnormalities include learning disabilities, oppositional defiant disorder, anxiety (separation anxiety), depression, mania, conduct disorders, self-injurious behavior, phobias (simple, social, agoraphobia), dyslexia, and stuttering. These disorders have been found to be 5 to 20 times more common in GTS than in the general population. It is difficult to know whether these disorders are secondary to the primary aspects of the disease (tics, OCD, ADHD) or whether they are neurobiologically linked. Finally, sleep disorders are present in about half the patients. Problems include somnambulism, night terrors, nightmares, sleep initiation, and maintenance.

DIAGNOSIS AND DIFFERENTIAL DIAGNOSIS

The diagnosis of GTS is based on clinical symptoms; there are no diagnostic laboratory tests. Because the features can be so varied, there is often a delay in diagnosis, perhaps for years. Many patients diagnose themselves based on what they see on television or read on the Internet. It is when patients recognize their own symptoms that they seek a medical opinion. The Tourette Syndrome Classification Study Group formulated diagnostic criteria for GTS. They are as follows: (a) both multiple motor and one or more phonic tics must be present at some time during the illness, not necessarily concurrently; (b) tics must occur many times per day, nearly every day, for a period of more than a year; (c) the anatomic location, number, frequency, type, complexity, or severity of tics must change over time; (d) the onset is prior to age 21 years; (e) the symptoms must not be explainable by other medical conditions; and (f) the tics should be witnessed by a reliable examiner at some point.

There are other diseases that cause tics. Tics have been seen in patients with stroke, tumor, head trauma, peripheral trauma (neck or face), encephalitis (and postencephalitic syndrome of encephalitis lethargica), and carbon monoxide poisoning. Locations of lesions in these disorders include frontal lobe, temporal lobe, and basal ganglia. The most common cause of secondary tics is chronic use of neuroleptic medications (tardive tics). These patients usually have onset in adulthood and a clear history of neuroleptic exposure prior to the onset of the disorder. Other drugs that cause tics include anticonvulsants (phenytoin, carbamazepine), stimulants (including cocaine), and antihistamines. Finally, tics can be a manifestation of chronic neurodegenerative disorders; examples include HD and neuroacanthocytosis. They also can be a manifestation of developmental diseases or chromosomal disorders; examples include Klinefelter's syndrome, Down's syndrome, and Fragile X disease.

GENETICS AND PATHOPHYSIOLOGY

Evidence from the study of multiple large families and twins has suggested that GTS is an autosomal dominant disorder. It has variable expressivity, including transient tic disorder, chronic multiple tic disorder, GTS, and OCD, and is sex influenced because males are affected more than females. Several methods have been used to isolate genes linked to GTS. They include segregation analysis in large affected families, sib pair approach, identity-by-descent, twin studies, and the examination of candidate genes; although linkage has been found in some studies to several chromosomes such as 11q, 4q and 8q, the nature of GTS genes that lead to the development of the disorder remains elusive. Other disease aspects suggest a genetic pattern different from a major dominant gene and that it is more likely to be a complex polygenetic pattern. Bilineal transmission is apparently common in this disorder (~25%). It probably occurs because of a phenomenon referred to as assortative mating, in which people with the same clinical features are attracted to one another, perhaps because they do not find their clinical symptoms unappealing. Second, it has been suggested that genomic imprinting, in which gene expression is altered by whether the gene is inherited from the father or mother, may play a role in GTS. This phenomenon remains to be proven. GTS appears to be genetically heterogeneous, relating to the interaction of several genes and influenced, to some extent, by non-genetic factors.

Despite clear genetic influences, there appear to be non-genetic developmental factors that influence the form and severity of the disorder. Such factors include maternal life stresses during pregnancy, gender of the child, severe nausea and/or vomiting in the first trimester, and birth weight.

One other possible environmental cause of GTS that is currently a matter of debate involves a relationship with streptococcal infection. It is proposed that an antibody response results in the development of cross-reactive antibodies against neuronal substrates, so-called antineuronal antibodies. Some have argued that the development of tics or OCD falls into the spectrum of childhood-onset disorders called PANDAS (Pediatric Autoimmune Neuropsychiatric Disorders Associated with Streptococcal infection). Although some patients with GTS have been found to have antistreptococcal antibodies and antineuronal antibodies in the sera, the connection between the two remains to proved. There is no association between antibody titre and severity of tics and no occurrence of inflammatory related symptoms such as polyarthritis or mitral valve disease. Although it is possible that tics may result from a postinfectious process much the way chorea does (Sydenham's chorea), it seems unlikely that this is the cause of GTS in most patients.

The neuroanatomic location of the abnormality resulting in GTS is unknown. It is suspected from cases of secondary tic disorders and imaging such as PET, SPECT, and MRI studies that the basal ganglia (particularly striatum), midbrain, frontal and medial temporal lobes, and limbic structures may be involved. One particular PET study suggested that basal ganglia–limbic circuitry is most important. The types of MRI studies have used volumetrics and functional MRI to decipher the lesion. Volumetric studies have suggested that there is loss of the normal asymmetry in the basal ganglia, increased volume of cingulated gyrus, and altered cortical systems. Functional MRI studies showed aberrant activity in several circuits correlating with tic severity including sensorimotor, prefrontal, and paralimbic circuits.

The biochemical basis of GTS is also not clearly understood. However, there is evidence to suggest that increase in activity of the dopamine systems is directly involved. This evidence includes: (a) response to dopamine antagonist medications, (b) response to dopamine-depleting medications (reserpine, tetrabenazine), (c) the occurrence of tardive tics, (d) the presence of alterations in dopamine metabolites in the CSF of patients with GTS, and (e) possible increased density of presynaptic dopamine transporters and postsynaptic D2 receptors. Two hypotheses related to this increase in dopamine stimulation have been suggested. The more prominent one is that there is dopamine receptor supersensitivity in the basal ganglia, similar to that described in TD. There is also the possibility that there is an increase in dopamine input into the striatum. However, the recent discovery that dopamine agonist medications actually may alleviate tics has placed the hyperdopaminergic hypothesis in question. Further studies are required. Pathologic studies, which are few, have demonstrated various neurochemical alterations in the brain. Dynorphin levels (from the opiate system) have been found to be reduced in the lateral globus pallidus, serotonin levels are low in the brainstem, and glutamate was found to be diminished in the globus pallidus.

TREATMENT

Effective pharmacologic treatment is available for GTS and its many behavioral manifestations. Multidisciplinary treatment including a neurologist, psychiatrist, and social worker is the best approach. Many patients with this disorder do not need treatment because their symptoms are mild. If symptoms are not disruptive or disabling, patients should be treated supportively. Some patients may do well with behavioral therapy such as relaxation training and self-monitoring. However, benefits of such therapies are usually only temporary. Nevertheless, they may be useful when used in conjunction with pharmacotherapy. Pharmacologic treatment should be used only in those patients who are severely troubled by their symptomatology. The team approach to evaluating patients can dictate which group of symptoms requires treatment (i.e., tics or behavioral disorder). Treatment should be individualized and directed toward those specific symptoms that are most troublesome (Table 11.8).

With regard to tics, dopamine antagonists (neuroleptics) historically have been the most frequently used and effective drugs available. Doses of haloperidol ranging from 0.25 to 2.5 mg/day at bedtime can be effective in up to 80% of patients. Side effects, however, can be limiting and include sedation, dysphoria, weight gain, TD, acute movement disorders (akathisia, acute dystonia, parkinsonism), depression, poor school performance, and school phobias. Other neuroleptic medications with fewer side effects are now available. Pimozide can be used at a dose of 1.5 to 10 mg/day. This drug can cause prolongation of the QT interval, which ultimately can lead to cardiac dysrhythmias. An electrocardiogram is required at baseline and should be repeated periodically. In recent years atypical neuroleptics have been available. Clozapine, the first of this group, has been used in a limited number of patients with GTS with mixed results. Risperidone has demonstrated efficacy in several case reports, short-term open trials, and placebo-controlled trials in treating motor tics and perhaps OCD. Approximately 30% to 60% of patients had tic improvement. A 12-week, double-blind, randomized comparison with pimozide was reported in 50 patients with GTS. The final mean doses were 3.8 mg/day for risperidone and 2.9 mg/day for pimozide. Both treatments resulted in a significant improvement in tic measures with no

difference between groups. In a global severity rating scale, 54% of patients taking risperidone showed a substantial improvement (only mild or no tics seen), and the same was true for 38% of patients treated with pimozide. Results were similar for children and adults. Extrapyramidal symptomatology (EPS) was reported in 15% of patients treated with risperidone and 33% of patients in the pimozide group. Somnolence, fatigue, weight gain, and depression were seen with both therapies. These results indicate that risperidone improves tics as well as OCD to an equal or better level than pimozide and causes fewer EPS. This may suggest that when a neuroleptic is needed, risperidone may be the treatment of first choice.

Olanzapine, ziprasidone, and quetiapine all have been reported to suppress tics but to a lesser extent and only in case reports and open trials. Further studies are needed with all three of these drugs.

Neuroleptics are the most potent therapeutic agents for tics; however, adverse events suggest they should be used with caution. Neuroleptics should be used in children with severe tics and avoided if possible in adults, particularly women who are at greatest risk for TD and other extrapyramidal effects. Clonidine is a useful alternative for GTS. This drug is an alpha-2 adrenergic agonist that inhibits presynaptic norepinephrine release. It

TABLE 11.8. *Medical Therapy for Tics*

Drug Name	Initial Daily Dose	Usual Daily Dose Range
Neuroleptics		
Haloperidol	0.25	0.25–5
Pimozide	1	1.5–10
Atypical Antipsychotics		
Risperidone	0.5	0.5–4
Olanzapine	2.5	2.5–10
Ziprasidone		20–40
Clonidine	0.1	0.1–0.3
Guanfacine	1	1–4
Clonazepam	0.25	0.5–3
Topiramate	25	25–100
Donepezil	5	10–15
Pergolide	0.05	0.05–0.4
Baclofen	10	30–120

can be useful for tics but also for behavioral aspects of the disorder. Daily doses range from 0.15 to 0.5 mg. It is available as oral medication or transdermal patches. Guanfacine is a similar class agent. Adverse events include sedation, dry mouth and eyes, headaches, and postural hypotension. Clonidine is a good firstline drug because of its better side-effect profile.

It is surprising that the use of the dopamine agonist pergolide may be helpful in the treatment of GTS. In a double-blind, placebo-controlled trial in 57 patients, this drug led to a 30% improvement in tic severity. It also improved behavioral problems related to ADHD. This effect was noted with a dose of less than 0.5mg/day. The drug was well tolerated.

Other agents used with some success, which have not been studied in controlled trials, include clonazepam, reserpine, selegiline, baclofen, donepezil, topiramate, nicotine patches, and opiate antagonists. For facial and neck tics, especially dystonic tics, carefully placed intramuscular BoNT injections may be useful. In some patients the injections decrease the tic number and severity, eliminate the associated urge to perform the tic, and decrease the pain that results from the tics. This has been confirmed in a small double-blind study in which a 37% reduction in tics was reported.

When treating OCD, behavioral-modification techniques can be useful; however, pharmacologic intervention is often necessary. Selective serotonin reuptake inhibitors are the treatment of choice for this behavioral disorder. Fluoxetine, a bicyclic antidepressant, can be extremely useful at doses of 20 to 60 mg/day. Clomipramine, sertraline, paroxetine, venlafaxine, citalopram, and fluvoxamine are other selective serotonin reuptake inhibitors that have been used in primary OCD with favorable results and may be useful in GTS. These drugs also may be effective in treating associated anxiety, depression, and social phobias. ADHD can be disabling in GTS. The standard therapies for primary ADHD, stimulant medications, such as methylphenidate (MPH), dextroamphetamine, and pemoline have been associated with worsening of tics

and were relatively contraindicated in these patients. However, a multicenter, double-blind trial has modified this notion and actually shed new light on the use of both MPH and clonidine. The design of this study randomized 37 children to MPH, 34 to clonidine, 33 to clonidine and MPH, and 32 to placebo. ADHD significantly improved in all three active groups, with the most significant change in the combination group. Clonidine was most useful for impulsivity and hyperactivity; MPH was most useful for inattention. A similar degree of tic worsening was seen with MPH and placebo, and tic severity actually lessened in all active groups. Therefore, there is no reason to avoid MPH in patients with GTS. In patients with GTS with ADHD and tics the treatment of choice is MPH plus clonidine. Selegiline, a monoamine oxidase B inhibitor that is metabolized to methamphetamine, has been found to be useful in treating ADHD and tics. The same is true for tricyclic antidepressants.

There are no data to support the use of alternative medications or physical therapy for GTS.

When to Refer to a Neurologist

Tic disorders are often complex clinically, especially with the associated behavioral disorders, and may represent diagnostic and therapeutic dilemmas. Simple tics are quite common, often do not require treatment, and need not be referred. If the movements are more severe and associated with behavioral problems, patients should be referred to a neurologist or psychiatrist for diagnostic clarification and treatment.

Special Challenges for Hospitalized Patients

The hospital is a stressful place for patients. Stress can make tics worse so physicians should anticipate an escalation. This is particularly pertinent to those who have had surgery. Wound infection and tearing of sutures is not unusual. Proper arrangements should be made to avoid these problems.

TARDIVE DYSKINESIA

TD is an iatrogenic movement disorder related to treatment with dopamine receptor antagonist drugs (neuroleptics and antiemetics). The term tardive was coined to describe two features of the illness: (a) that it occurs after chronic therapy with these drugs (the cutoff has been arbitrarily set at 3 months for patients younger than age 60 years and 1 month for those older than 60) and (b) that the disorder is persistent. In recent years, the chronic exposure requirement has come into question because some cases have occurred shortly after initiation of therapy. Relative persistence of the dyskinesia remains a characteristic feature. It has become clear that a number of variants of TD exist. The most common is the classical TD syndrome, characterized by stereotypic or choreiform movements, which constitutes at least half of all tardive syndromes. Others are classified by the movement disorder that dominates the clinical picture—tardive dystonia, tardive akathisia, tardive tics, and tardive myoclonus. Although all these variants occur and can be present at the same time, there are clear differences beyond clinical phenomenology (including natural history and pharmacology). Separation of these syndromes is important from a practical standpoint as well as for research protocols. It is the classical TD syndrome that is discussed here.

CLINICAL FEATURES

With standard neuroleptic therapy, TD occurs in approximately 20% (0.5%–56%) of patients. The incidence of new cases increases 5% per year. Approximately 10% of patients can be severely disabled. The incidence and prevalence with the newer atypical antipsychotics is unknown, especially because some of them (i.e., risperidone) behave similarly to standard agents and most patients treated with atypical antipsychotics have been treated previously with typical neuroleptics. Classical TD is characterized by patterned, stereotypic orobuccolingual (OBL) chewing-type movements or dyskinesias. The tongue often has a writhing-type movement that will result in pushing out the cheeks (bon-bon sign), but there also may be stereotypic repetitive protrusions (referred to as fly catcher's tongue). The movements range in severity from extremely mild (in which the patient may be totally unaware of the movements and the movements simply look like an exaggeration of normal movements such as lip wetting) to severe enough to cause dysarthria and dysphagia to the point of requiring a feeding tube. On examination, the tongue movements tend to decrease with protrusion. In addition, patients can have jaw movements (opening, closing, deviations), facial grimacing, blepharospasm, cheek retraction and puffing, pouting, puckering, and lip smacking. Choreiform movements also may be present in limbs (piano playing movements of the fingers) and in the axial regions (with dancelike movements). Involvement of intercostal and diaphragm musculature results in respiratory dyskinesia. These patients have grunting, sighing, air gasping, and belching sounds as part of their picture, and they may become short of breath because of irregular breathing patterns. Respiratory dyskinesia usually occurs in conjunction with OBL and affects about 15% of patients with TD. Another interesting type of choreic movement involves pelvic thrusting and twisting movements (so-called copulatory dyskinesia). TD movements may be exacerbated by activating tasks such as testing dexterity maneuvers (finger or toe tapping, rapid alternating movements), having the patients walk and perform cognitive tasks. Anxiety and fatigue also increase the movements.

The natural history of TD is that it reaches its maximal levels fairly quickly. In 50%, the movement disorder is persistent. In those patients in whom the inciting agent is removed, TD may disappear gradually, but this may take years (as long as 5 years). The course may be one of persistence or fluctuations in severity. In some patients with choreiform movements, the continued administration of neuroleptics will result in progression. In these patients, isolated OBL dyskinesias may spread to involve the axial, limb, or diaphragmatic musculature. Another example of progression might be an increase in the severity and amplitude of the individual choreiform movements. For these reasons, as well as some theoretical reasons to be discussed under prevention and treatment of TD, the use of a neuroleptic to treat TD is unwarranted. The fact that many patients who develop this syndrome have an irreversible problem is an indication of the serious nature of this disorder.

One form of TD occurs only when the neuroleptics are withdrawn—so-called withdrawal emergent dyskinesia. Although the phenomenology of these movements is the same as TD, some suggest it is a different disorder that is always reversible and not necessarily related to TD. This remains to be elucidated.

TD can occur in any patient who is chronically exposed to dopamine-blocking agents, including those who are neurologically and psychiatrically normal. Nevertheless, there are factors that seem to increase a patient's risk for the development of this disorder. Age is the most consistent risk factor for TD. After age 40, there is a dramatic rise in relative risk. There appears to be a direct relationship between age and severity and an inverse correlation between age and remission rate. Other possible patient-related risk factors include female gender, diagnosis of affective disorders, history of drug-induced parkinsonism, concomitant use of anticholinergics, and presence of diabetes mellitus. There are also a number of treatment-related risk factors, including the use of depot formulations of neuroleptics and duration of exposure to these drugs. Genetic risk factors also have been the subject of study; TD is associated with mutations in the cytochrome P450 2D6 (CYP 2D6) gene, a major drug-metabolizing enzyme.

PATHOPHYSIOLOGY

Based on models of basal ganglia function, it has been shown that hyperkinetic movement disorders (e.g., chorea) are the result of a decrease in the activity of the internal segment of the globus pallidus with a resulting loss of inhibition of the thalamus and increased stimulation of the motor cortex. This may relate to changes in the nigrostriatal dopamine system where dopamine can have stimulatory or inhibitory effect on D1 and D2 receptors, respectively. Investigations have focused on alterations in dopaminergic function as a possible mechanism for TD. It has been proposed that the chronic administration of neuroleptics results in a chronic blockade of striatal dopamine receptor sites and that this chronic blockade ultimately induces alterations in the sensitivity and number of dopamine receptors. Clinical data that support this notion include the exacerbation of TD with dopaminergic medications, suppression of TD with dopamine antagonists, and enhancement of the movements with anticholinergics. In addition, the study of atypical antipsychotics has demonstrated that those with the lowest risk (apparent) for extrapyramidal side effects are those atypical antipsychotics that do not chronically bind to dopamine receptors. Clozapine and quetiapine bind loosely to these receptors and are easily dissociated by the presence of endogenous dopamine. This phenomenon is referred to as loose binding or fast dissociation and equates to lower binding affinity. In the simplest conceptual terms, it has been proposed to be a form of chemical denervation supersensitivity. Although choreiform movements may begin when the neuroleptic is chronically administered without a change in dosage, the most common clinical setting in which the movement disorder emerges is after the dosage is lowered or discontinued entirely. This latter setting is in keeping with the postulate of lowering the pharmacologic blockade of the dopamine receptor and allowing normal dopaminergic mechanisms to resume their interaction with the already hypersensitized receptor. Although there is much evidence in animal models to support this notion, there have been inconsistencies. For this reason, examination of other neurotransmitter abnormalities and mechanisms related to TD have been evaluated, such as a decrease in

GABA activity in the basal ganglia. Both animal and human studies have indicated that this is a possibility. An increased release of GABA from the external globus pallidus neurons innervating the subthalamic nucleus ultimately could result in decreased output from the globus pallidus. Some studies have indicated that an overactivity of norepinephrine is present and that decreased activity of serotonin (both of which modulate dopamine transmission) and increased glutamatergic transmission also may occur. Finally, there has been some suggestion that a decrease in acetylcholine activity in the striatum might play a role.

Another possible pathophysiologic mechanism for TD is direct neurotoxicity of neuroleptic medications. It has been theorized that the blockade of dopamine receptors results in an increase in dopamine turnover. This, in turn, results in the formation of increased free oxyradicals that ultimately damage striatal neurons. Neuroleptics also may be toxic to mitochondrial complex I. Finally, a comparison of the pharmacology of typical neuroleptic medications with atypical neuroleptics that do not cause TD (e.g., clozapine) has led to other theories, including the uncoupling of D1 and D2 receptors.

PREVENTION

As in all iatrogenic disorders, prevention is better than treatment. This is especially true for TD, in which the symptoms and signs may be irreversible. There are a series of simple steps that may help to limit the development of TD in the general population. First of all, the number of subjects at risk should be limited. This implies that standard neuroleptics should be used only to treat appropriate illness including schizophrenia, psychosis and GTS syndrome. These agents should not be used for minor episodes of anxiety, restlessness, insomnia, or other minor psychiatric disturbances. The development of TD does not depend on any preexistent brain damage or psychiatric history, and patients who are normal psychiatrically can develop TD if exposed to neuroleptic agents. A second and a third means of decreasing the incidence of TD would be to limit the dose of neuroleptic used and to limit the duration of treatment with neuroleptics. Finally, if an antipsychotic agent is needed, then the choice should be one with less risk of extrapyramidal side effects—atypical agents. These include olanzapine, quetiapine, aripiprazole, and clozapine. Although data suggest a lower frequency of extrapyramidal side effects with these drugs, it should be remembered that the frequency is not zero. All of these recommendations are commonsense approaches and seem realistic, although there is little clinical information in the literature to confirm these concepts. It is usually wise to limit the dose of a pharmacologic agent to the symptoms being treated or controlled. Neuroleptic administration is no exception, and the dose of neuroleptic administered should be tailored to each patient. This is also true for the atypical agents. When neuroleptics are totally withdrawn from patients with relapsing psychosis, the relapse rate is significant. However, an initial episode of psychotic behavior does not necessitate chronic lifelong administration of neuroleptics. Another point in attempting to decrease the incidence of TD in the population is to avoid the concomitant use of anticholinergic and neuroleptic administration on a chronic long-term basis. The problem of chronic administration of neuroleptics and anticholinergics concomitantly is that there is some retrospective clinical evidence that patients who are taking both have a slightly greater risk for the development of TD than those taking neuroleptics alone. The only reason for the concomitant use of anticholinergics and neuroleptics is to treat drug-induced parkinsonism. Drug-induced parkinsonism is a transient phenomenon that usually resolves within 3 months. If the patient develops parkinsonism and is treated with anticholinergics, at the end of 3 months the anticholinergic should be withdrawn slowly to assess whether continued therapy is required. In addition, if the drug-induced parkinsonism has abated, there is no point in administering a pharmacologic agent that is no longer indicated. Because the use of anticholinergics is directed toward the treatment of drug-induced parkinsonism, and because drug-induced parkinsonism is usually transient and reversible, it seems unwise to chronically administer an anticholinergic with a neuroleptic, even if the concomitant use of these drugs represents only a small increase in the risk for the development of TD.

An additional approach that may limit the development of TD is the early recognition of the syndrome and discontinuation of all neuroleptics, if psychiatrically possible, when the first abnormal movements are detected. The continued administration of neuroleptics in the face of developing TD may result in progression and permanence of the syndrome. The best chance of both stopping progression and reversing TD resides in early detection of abnormal movements. Patients should be monitored routinely for the emergence of abnormal movements. A final approach to the prevention of TD relates to the use of antipsychotic agents that are associated with a lower risk of TD—atypical antipsychotics. Clozapine, the first of this class of drugs approved in 1990, appears to have lower affinity for dopamine receptors, has similar preference for D1 than D2 receptors, and has a strong affinity for D4 receptors. Clozapine does not appear to cause D2 dopamine receptor supersensitivity and causes significantly fewer chewing-type movements than standard neuroleptics in animal models. Clinical trials have demonstrated that this drug is much less likely to cause TD. There has not been a case of de novo TD in a patient treated with clozapine who never received treatment with a standard neuroleptic. Clozapine has been approved for use in patients who have psychosis that does not respond to typical neuroleptics and in cases where typical neuroleptics are contraindicated. The presence of TD is a contraindication. If these movements are found early and the neuroleptics are stopped, TD could reverse and disappear. If clozapine is used, TD can be prevented. There are drawbacks to this medication. The most important

is agranulocytosis. For this reason, a weekly white blood count is required for patients taking this drug for the first 6 months, and then blood counts are required every other week. Other atypical antipsychotics approved in the United States for treatment of psychosis since 1990 include olanzapine, quetiapine, ziprasidone, and aripiprazole. It is too early to know if these medications carry the same low risk for TD that clozapine does. As these agents are used more as firstline drugs and fewer patients are treated with standard agents, we will be able to investigate whether the use of atypical antipsychotics is truly preventative. Currently, the prevalence and incidence of TD have not actually changed.

TREATMENT

The management of a patient who has developed TD is a difficult clinical task. Medical therapies are frequently inadequate. In particular, the longer TD is present the less likely it is to respond. The first approach to these patients should be careful review of whether the neuroleptics that have been and are being administered are psychiatrically indicated. In many instances, there is no major psychiatric indication for the use of these agents. If this is true, these neuroleptic agents should be tapered off gradually. In many patients, the movement disorder initially becomes worse when the neuroleptics are discontinued. This should not be surprising because, if TD is related to increased dopamine receptor site sensitivity secondary to chronic neuroleptic blockade, and if the patient is having involuntary movements (indicating dopamine receptor site sensitivity alteration is already present) while on the neuroleptics, and the drug is discontinued with abolition of the blockade, the abnormally hypersensitive dopamine receptor would be exposed to normal dopaminergic physiology. This results in increased involuntary movements. This time period is often difficult to manage because the patient becomes worse. This should not be confused with worsening of the disease process itself, and generally this rebound of TD on withdrawal of the neuroleptic may persist for only 2 to 6 weeks. At the end of this time, assessment of the extent of the baseline disorder is possible.

TD has been reported to be irreversible in 30% to 50% of cases, depending on the age of the patient. Pharmacologic intervention in this choreiform movement disorder is based on pathophysiologic mechanisms that indicate that agents that decrease dopaminergic activity within the brain will decrease chorea. Consequently, agents such as reserpine or tetrabenazine, which deplete the brain of dopamine, will ameliorate chorea seen in TD. Doses of reserpine from 1 to 5 mg/day are reached with a gradually increasing dosage schedule. Side effects of these agents are of concern and include orthostatic hypotension, parkinsonism, depression, and gastrointestinal problems. This is frequently the first line of treatment in TD. Tetrabenazine differs from reserpine because it is shorter acting and causes fewer side effects, particularly orthostatic hypotension and depression. The dose is 50 to 200 mg/day. Reserpine-induced depression can last months, whereas tetrabenazine use leads to short-term symptoms. Other major drugs that interfere with dopaminergic activity include neuroleptics. However, despite the fact that if the neuroleptic dosage is raised the chorea in TD can be ameliorated, this is an incorrect approach because it will place the treating physician in a position of using the etiologic agent to treat the disorder. This situation should be avoided. The only time that neuroleptics should be used to treat TD is if the TD is life threatening, and this is rare. Atypical antipsychotics may have a therapeutic effect. There are some data on clozapine. Clinical trials evaluating the effectiveness of clozapine in psychosis not only suggested that the drug is less likely to cause TD, but they also indicated that there may be therapeutic potential in treating TD. In a trial of clozapine and chlorpromazine in 126 patients with schizophrenia with treatment-resistant psychosis, abnormal involuntary movements also were studied and found to improve over the 6 weeks of the study. Mean abnormal involuntary movement scores (AIMS) improved more in the clozapine group. However, because patients had been treated with haloperidol until 2 weeks before the trial, distinguishing the effects of haloperidol's wearing off from new drug effects is difficult.

Since then, a series of papers including single case reports and larger studies have addressed the therapeutic usefulness of clozapine in TD. Results of publications have been varied with some documenting dramatic improvement and others reporting clozapine as "less effective than 'typical' neuroleptics in suppression of TD." In one open-label trial all 24 patients had improved AIMS scores of at least 50%, with three patients apparently "cured" when evaluated 1 year later and no longer taking clozapine. In another open-label study 37 patients treated for psychosis (30 of whom had TD) with clozapine were followed. Sixteen (43%) had a decrease in AIMS of 50% or more, and 34% of the patients had complete resolution within 2 years of clozapine therapy. It was noted that the mean TD scores decreased significantly within the first 12 weeks and then remained stable without recurrence or worsening of TD over the next 33 months. An additional paper reported 32 patients with moderate to severe TD treated in a blinded protocol with randomization to clozapine and placebo or haloperidol and benztropine. This was followed by 12 months of clozapine therapy and a 1-month withdrawal period. At the end of the treatment period patients taking clozapine demonstrated an improvement in TD, whereas the haloperidol group did not. The improvement began after 4 months of therapy. It is interesting that during a 4-week drug withdrawal after 12 months of treatment, the haloperidol-treated group suffered worsening (withdrawal emergent) dyskinesias and the clozapine treated group did not.

Review of these and other studies indicates that some patients appear to show improvement of TD with clozapine, indicating an active therapeutic effect. Variability of response may relate to the heterogeneity of TD. However, considerable caution must be taken when interpreting results of this literature because of methodologic limitations. The studies were open-label treatment protocols with inadequate controls. Properly controlled double-blind studies will be necessary before definitive conclusions can be made. Still, the use of clozapine is strongly recommended as treatment of choice in psychotic patients with TD, with discontinuation of all standard neuroleptics. The recommended dosage ranges from 100 to 900 mg/day, and the side effects more commonly seen include sialorrhea, orthostatic hypotension, weight gain, and seizures.

Dopamine-agonist medications, such as levodopa or bromocriptine, also have been used based on "down regulating" dopaminergic hypersensitivity. Studies have shown variable results with these agents, and they should be used with caution. Other pharmacologic approaches to the treatment of TD are based on manipulation of other neurotransmitter systems that may be abnormal in TD. Increasing cholinergic activity often will decrease chorea, and interfering with cholinergic activity (anticholinergics) may increase chorea. On one hand, anticholinergic medications have no role in the treatment of TD. On the other hand, there has been interest in the use of cholinergic agents in the treatment of chorea. Several attempts at precursor-loading strategies have been made using drugs such as choline and lecithin. These agents have not provided effective therapies. There are no data on cholinesterase inhibitors used for the treatment of Alzheimer's disease. The use of a variety of GABA-agonist medications, including valproate, diazepam, clonazepam, and baclofen, also has been disappointing: some patients do respond, but who will do so cannot be predicted. Noradrenergic antagonists, such as propranolol and clonidine, have been somewhat successful in some patients, but this needs to be confirmed in larger controlled studies. Propranolol decreases neuroleptic blood levels, and clonidine decreases the release of norepinephrine. These drugs are safe and reasonable choices in the treatment of TD. Glutamatergic agents such as amantadine may

be very helpful in controlling the movements. Finally, facial and neck distribution (especially if the tardive movements are dystonic) movements are amenable to intramuscular BoNT injections.

One alternative medication, vitamin E, an antioxidant, has been shown to improve TD symptoms. This may occur through blockade of free radical damage to cells that may result from long-term neuroleptic use. The effects have been demonstrated in several small double-blind studies using a dose of 400 mg tid. However, results have varied. Because of its safety, vitamin E is a choice for firstline treatment, although it is often not helpful. The roles of physical, occupational, and speech therapy are varied depending on patient needs, but they can be helpful.

When to Refer to a Neurologist

TD is often complex clinically and may present diagnostic and therapeutic dilemmas. Patients with TD should be referred to a movement disorder specialist for diagnostic clarification and treatment. In mild cases medication can be withdrawn and the patient can be observed, but in those in whom the symptoms are troublesome, referral for appropriate therapy is recommended.

Special Challenges for Hospitalized Patients

Because the movements can be bizarre in appearance and influenced by stress and anxiety, staff education is required so that all understand that this is a neurologic disorder.

QUESTIONS AND DISCUSSION

1. Match the neurologic term with the appropriate description:

A. Tremor1. Excessive, spontaneous movements irregularly timed, nonrepetitive, randomly distributed and "dancelike"

B. Chorea2. An abnormal sustained posture

C. Dystonia3. Involuntary, rhythmic, oscillating movement resulting from alternating or synchronous contraction of reciprocally innervated antagonist muscles

D. Tic4. Patterned sequence of coordinated movements that may be simple or complex

The correct matches are (A) and (3), (B) and (1), (C) and (2), (D) and (4).

2. A patient presents with sustained involuntary eye closure and forced involuntary mouth opening. Which diagnosis (or diagnoses) is to be considered?

A. Meige's syndrome

B. Primary adult-onset dystonia

C. Adverse effect of neuroleptic medication

D. Wilson's disease

E. All of the above.

All answers are correct. The description is that of Meige's syndrome. Meige's syndrome may be a manifestation of adult-onset primary dystonia or an adverse effect of neuroleptics. The latter may mimic the former quite closely. Dystonia may be a manifestation of Wilson's disease, a diagnosis that should be considered if the patient is younger than 30 years old when the syndrome occurs.

3. A 19-year-old patient complains of the recent onset of shaking, which occurs when he lifts a cup to drink or tries to retrieve food with a fork. When his index fingers are approximated, the tremor worsens. A sister has a history of liver disease. This description suggests:

A. Essential tremor

B. Huntington's disease

C. Wilson's disease

D. Parkinson's disease

The answers are (A) and (C). The description is that of a postural and kinetic tremor. This may be seen in ET, which may be familial or sporadic and frequently occurs in adolescence or early adult life. Wilson's disease also must be considered in all patients under the age of 50 with any movement disorder, especially if there is a family history of liver disease.

4. Agents that might be effective in abating essential tremor would include:

A. Alcohol

B. Gabapentin

C. Amphetamine

D. Propranolol

E. Primidone

The answers are (A), (B), (D), and (E). The last two agents are frequently used treatments for essential tremor. Amphetamines may induce a tremor similar to essential tremor or worsen an already-present tremor.

5. A patient presents with a generalized choreiform disorder that began at the age of 45 years. He denies any neurologic or psychiatric problems prior to the onset of his current problem and never received neuroleptic medications. He denies a family history of any similar movement disorder, but his mother was institutionalized at the age of 55 for psychiatric reasons. What is this patient's possible diagnosis?

A. Huntington's disease

B. Parkinson's disease

C. Essential tremor

D. Primary dystonia

The answer is (A). Huntington's disease is an autosomal dominant disorder with onset typically in middle age. Although psychiatric symptoms are insufficient for making a diagnosis of Huntington's, a family history of a parent with psychiatric disease in a patient with a choreiform disorder may be very suggestive. The diagnosis can be made through genetic testing.

6. Which of the following is not inherited in an autosomal dominant fashion?

A. Primary childhood-onset (Oppenheim's) dystonia

B. Huntington's disease

C. Essential tremor

D. Wilson's disease

E. Gilles de la Tourette's syndrome

The answer is (D). Wilson's disease is inherited as an autosomal recessive disorder.

7. Botulinum toxin is used in therapy for which of the following?

A. Spasmodic torticollis

B. Strabismus

C. Tics

D. Blepharospasm

E. Tremor

The answer is all of the above. Botulinum toxin therapy is accepted as safe and effective in strabismus, focal dystonias, and dystonic tics. Recent studies suggest that it is also useful in tremor.

SUGGESTED READING

Blanchet PJ. Antipsychotic drug-induced movement disorders. *Can J Neurol Sci* 2003;30(Suppl 1):S101–S107.

Brewer GJ. Wilson's disease: current treatment options in neurology 2000;2:193–203.

Gasser T, Bressman S, Durr A, et al. Molecular diagnosis of inherited movement disorders: Movement Disorders Society Task Force on Molecular Diagnosis. *Mov Disord* 2003;18:3–18.

Goetz CG. Therapies in movement disorders. *Arch Neurol* 2002;59:699–702

Goldman JG, Comella CL. Treatment of dystonia. *Clin Neuropharmacol* 2003;26:102–108.

The Huntington Study Group. A randomized, placebo-controlled trial of coenzyme Q10 and remacemide in Huntington's disease. *Neurology* 2001;57:397–404.

Jankovic J. Tourette's syndrome. *N Engl J Med* 2001;345:1184–1192.

Lang AE, Weiner WJ. *Drug-induced movement disorders.* Mount Kisco, NY: Futura, 1992.

Leckman JF. Tourette's syndrome. *Lancet* 2002;360:1577–1586.

Louis ED. Essential tremor. *N Engl J Med* 2001;345:887–891.

Nemeth AH. The genetics of primary dystonias and related disorders. *Brain* 2002;125:695–721.

Schuurman PR, Bosch DA, Bossuyt PMM, et al. A comparison of continuous thalamic stimulation and thalamotomy for suppression of severe tremor. *N Engl J Med* 2000;342:461–468.

SuttonBrown M, Suchowersky O. Clinical and research advances in Huntington's disease. *Can J Neurol Sci* 2003;30 (suppl 1):S45–S52.

The Tourette's Syndrome Study Group. Treatment of ADHD in children with tics: a randomized controlled trial. *Neurology* 2002;58:527–536.

Young AB. Huntingtin in health and disease. *J Clin Invest* 2003;111:299–302.

12

Neurologic Complications of Alcoholism

Winona Tse and William C. Koller

Alcoholism is associated with a diverse range of neurologic disorders. The neurologic complications of alcoholism have been classified by Victor under the five headings contained in Table 12.1. This review examines the typical clinical features, the principles guiding proper diagnosis and evaluation, and the treatments currently available (Table 12.2).

ALCOHOL INTOXICATION

The manifestations of acute alcoholic intoxication are well known. Although alcohol is a central nervous system depressant, initially intoxication is associated with varying degrees of excitation and uninhibited behavior. Speech is increased and often slurred. The gait becomes ataxic. With further drunkenness, drowsiness, stupor, and coma may oc-

TABLE 12.1. *Neurologic Complications of Alcoholism*

Alcohol intoxication
  Drunkenness
  Coma
  Pathologic intoxication
Withdrawal syndrome
  Tremulousness
  Hallucinosis
  Seizures
  Delirium tremens
Nutritional disease secondary to alcoholism
  Wernicke–Korsakoff syndrome
  Polyneuropathy
  Optic neuropathy
  Pellagra
Disease of uncertain pathogenesis associated with
   alcoholism
  Cerebellar degeneration
  Marchiafava–Bignami disease
  Central pontine myelinolysis
  Cerebral atrophy
  Myopathy
Neurologic disorders associated with cirrhosis
  Hepatic stupor and coma
  Chronic hepatocerebral degeneration

cur. It should be stressed that alcohol intoxication can cause coma and even death.

In a certain population of patients, alcohol has an even more excitatory effect. This reaction has been variously labeled a pathologic intoxication or an acute alcoholic paranoid state. Although this state is not well studied, it is said to consist of irrational and destructive behavior that follows the ingestion of only small amounts of alcohol. The patient usually has no recollection of the episode. The mechanism underlying this paradoxical reaction is not known.

Most symptoms of alcohol intoxication are related to its depressive action on neural function. The early stimulatory effect of alcohol is thought to be caused by depression of subcortical structures that inhibit cerebral activity, thus resulting in stimulation. The usual manifestations of intoxication require no specific therapy. Mild stimulants (coffee, analeptics) may be of some help. Coma caused by alcohol intoxication requires the maintenance of respiration and blood pressure, if necessary. This supportive care is no different from that required in the treatment of coma from other causes. Pathologic intoxication requires the use of restraints and the parenteral administration of sedatives (e.g., phenobarbital or amobarbital).

ALCOHOL WITHDRAWAL SYNDROME

A variety of neurologic symptoms may occur in the chronic drinker after a period of relative or absolute abstinence from alcohol, termed the abstinence or withdrawal syndrome.

The most common manifestation of the withdrawal syndrome is tremulousness or

TABLE 12.2. *Treatments for Alcohol-Related Neurologic Syndromes*

Syndrome	Treatment (See Text for Full Discussion)
Alcohol withdrawal syndrome	1. Maintain fluid intake and electrolyte balance. 2. Prescribe thiamine in the dose of 50–100 mg IV and IM acutely and then 100 mg po or IM for 3 days thereafter. Patients should be maintained on oral thiamine as well as multivitamin supplements. 3. Treat metabolic abnormalities. 4. Control agitation—chlordiazepoxide may be given at 25–100 mg IM q 3–4 hours as needed to achieve sedation (also may be given po or IV).
Wernicke's encephalopathy	Thiamine supplementation (please see above for dosage). Also, multivitamin supplementation should be given, including vitamin B complex.
Alcohol amblyopia	Balanced diet, B vitamins, and multivitamin supplement.
Pellagra	Niacin 40–250 mg q day and balanced diet.
Alcoholic myopathy and neuropathy	Multivitamin, B vitamins, balanced diet. In myopathy: prevention of renal failure from myoglobinuria with administration of intravenous fluids.
Hepatic encephalopathy	Protein-free or protein-restricted diet and lactulose 30 ml q 6–12 hours with titration to yield 2–4 loose stools q day, orally or by retention enema. Alternatively, neomycin may be given at 1 g QID po or by retention enema. (Please note that chronic administration of neomycin can produce hearing loss and renal impairment, as well as other side effects.)

IV, intravenously; IM, intramuscularly.

"the shakes." This occurs after several days of drinking and frequently appears in the morning after the short abstinence that occurs during sleep. Associated symptoms consist of general irritability, mild autonomic hyperactivity, anorexia, nausea, and vomiting. The patients are clear mentally, although they tend to be inattentive with poor recollection of past events. Tremor is generalized and of a fast frequency. The severity of the tremor tends to increase with activity and emotional stress and to decrease in a quiet environment. The tremor, hyperalertness, and autonomic instability may last for several days.

The second major symptom of the withdrawal syndrome is disordered perception and hallucinosis. This may occur in 10% to 25% of tremulous patients. Initially, there may be nightmares and disturbances of sleep. Illusions occur as sensory and visual information are distorted and misinterpreted. True hallucinations may be purely visual or auditory in type, mixed visual and auditory, and occasionally tactile or olfactory. Visual hallucinations often take the form of human, animal, or insect life. The feeling that bugs are crawling on oneself (formications) is an example of such hallucinations. Auditory hallucinations may be either acute or chronic. They are usually vocal in nature, with God or friends often speaking directly to the person. The voices most often are maligning and reproachful and may disturb and threaten the individual. Suicide may even be attempted in an effort to escape the verbal abuse. Hallucinations usually begin during the first day after the cessation of drinking and may last as long as a week. Initially, most patients do not recognize that they are hallucinating and it is only when the hallucinations cease that they acknowledge their previous hallucinations.

Chronic auditory hallucinosis presents a unique feature of this condition. In a small number of patients, the auditory hallucinations continue, and a schizophreniform personality evolves, with paranoid ideations and disordered thoughts. It has been suggested that repeated attacks of acute auditory hallucinosis may lead to the chronic form.

The third main symptom of the abstinence syndrome is withdrawal seizures. The majority of seizures, or "rum fits," occur within 8 to 48 hours of the cessation of drinking, with a peak incidence between 12 and 24 hours. Most often, withdrawal seizures are single, but several in a row also may occur. The seizures are usually generalized motor seizures with loss of consciousness. Rarely, status epilepticus may occur. A focal seizure in a patient with alcoholism should lead to a search for focal disease (e.g., subdural hematoma). It also should be mentioned that people with a seizure tendency may have their seizures potentiated by a short abstinence period (e.g., overnight) after drinking. During the period of high-risk seizure activity, the electroencephalogram (EEG) may be transiently abnormal. The patient may be unusually sensitive to stroboscopic stimulation and may respond with either generalized myoclonus (photomyoclonus) or a generalized seizure (photoconvulsion). Other patients show diffuse abnormalities compatible with a mild encephalopathy.

Treatment of withdrawal seizures does not in most cases require anticonvulsants. The seizures are usually brief and do not recur. The long-term administration of anticonvulsants in patients with generalized withdrawal seizures is not reasonable because of poor patient compliance and because starting a drinking spree usually also means the abandonment of all medications. Because sudden withdrawal from drugs can be associated with withdrawal seizures, cessation of drugs as well as alcohol actually may increase the risk of seizures.

The fourth manifestation of the withdrawal syndrome is delirium tremens. This term should be reserved for the rare, serious state of profound confusion, with vivid hallucinations, tremors, sleeplessness, and signs of increased autonomic nervous system activity, including fever, tachycardia, dilated pupils, and profuse sweating. Of 266 consecutive admissions of patients with alcoholism to the Boston City Hospital, only 5% had delirium tremens. Although this can be a serious condition with a mortality rate of 5% to 10%, delirium tremens in most cases is benign and short-lived, lasting several days. The patient usually has no recollection of the events of the delirious period. Hyperthermia and peripheral vascular collapse are the usual causes of death. Intercurrent infection or injury tend to worsen the prognosis.

The mechanism of the withdrawal syndrome is unknown. Nutritional deficiency does not appear to play a primary pathogenic role. A depression of serum magnesium often is found during the withdrawal period and may increase the susceptibility to seizures, although it is probably not responsible for the entire syndrome.

The management of alcohol withdrawal begins with a careful search for infection or associated injury, such as subdural hematoma or meningitis. Lumbar puncture, a brain scan, and often an EEG are indicated. The major medical complications include water and electrolyte imbalance, vascular collapse, pneumonia, cirrhosis, gastritis, and hyperthermia. Specific treatment includes the following:

Maintenance of fluid intake and electrolyte balance. High volumes of fluids can be lost because of hyperthermia and sweating. Careful and continuous monitoring of intravenous fluid needs must be continued for several days.

Thiamine and multivitamin administration. Thiamine in a dose of 50 to 100 mg intramuscularly may be given, and thiamine may be added to the intravenous bottles. When the patient is on a diet, 100 mg thiamine once a day orally is recommended.

Hypoglycemia. Blood glucose must be checked frequently because hypoglycemia is a complication of alcoholic binges, especially in the patient with inadequate hepatic function.

Control of agitation. The hallucinating, agitating patient can be dangerous to himself as well as to hospital personnel. A well-lighted room and the presence of a responsible family member helps to maintain the patient's contact with reality. Sedatives may be needed to control agitation: chlordiazepoxide often is recommended in doses of 25 to 100 mg intramuscularly every 3 to 4 hours as needed. It is important to check to see if the patient is awake before administering sedatives, and sedative orders should not be written on a continual basis.

Accumulative dose effect can be seen with delayed metabolism of such drugs. These drugs are administered to calm the patient without putting him to sleep, so no sedative should be given to the sleeping patient.

NUTRITIONAL DISEASES

Several of the neurologic complications of alcohol on the nervous system are thought to be caused by the nutritional deficiency that occurs secondary to chronic alcoholism. These diseases include Wernicke's encephalopathy, Korsakoff's psychosis, polyneuropathy, alcohol amblyopia, and pellagra. In the patient with alcoholism, caloric intake is supplied by alcohol, and there is an increased demand for B vitamins, which are necessary to metabolize the carbohydrate load imposed by alcohol. These nutritional diseases also can be seen in the nonalcoholic person in a variety of settings and hence are not seen exclusively in this patient population.

WERNICKE–KORSAKOFF DISEASE

Wernicke's disease is a neurologic syndrome characterized clinically by the triad of eye movement disorders, ataxic gait, and mental status changes. The ocular disturbances usually consist of nystagmus, paralysis of the lateral recti, or paralysis of conjugate gaze. Nystagmus, which may be either vertical or horizontal, is the most frequent abnormality. When cranial nerve VI paralysis occurs, it is usually bilateral, although not symmetric. The ataxia involves both stance and gait, and it may be so severe in the acute stages that the patient cannot stand up. The walk is broad-based and ataxic; heel-to-shin testing is severely compromised. Three main types of mental symptoms may be observed. First, the most common change is that of a quiet, confusional state. The patient is apathetic, inattentive, and indifferent to his surroundings. Spontaneous speech is minimal, and communication is difficult. Second, the symptoms of delirium tremens or its variants may be present (i.e., disorders of perception).

Third, there may be a selective abnormality of memory, termed Korsakoff's psychosis (see later in this chapter).

The principal pathologic changes consist of paraventricular lesions in the thalamus and hypothalamus, in the mammillary bodies, in the floor of the fourth ventricle, and in the periaqueductal region of the midbrain. These lesions tend to be symmetric. Microscopic examination reveals capillary proliferation, often with necrosis of parenchymal structures and at times discrete hemorrhages, particularly in the mammillary bodies.

Korsakoff's psychosis is characterized by a selective memory deficit. The disordered memory is manifested by an impaired ability to recall events and other information that had been well established before the onset of the illness and a dramatically impaired ability to acquire new information. Remote memory tends to be better preserved than recent memory. Cognitive impairment (e.g., of mathematic skills and abstract thinking) also may be present. The patient may show little spontaneity and initiative. Confabulation, although frequently referred to as a main symptom of Korsakoff's psychosis, is not essential for the diagnosis.

The biochemical basis of Wernicke–Korsakoff disease appears to be a thiamine deficiency. The ophthalmoplegia, nystagmus, and ataxia can be reversed by the administration of thiamine alone. The ocular signs are the most sensitive to thiamine. Although the confusional state appears to clear with thiamine treatment, the memory deficit and confabulation are much less responsive. These symptoms recover slowly, if at all. Korsakoff's psychosis has a poor prognosis, with only 20% of patients having significant recovery. An index of thiamine deficiency can be estimated by the blood transketolase activity. Transketolase is one of the enzymes in the hexose monophosphate shunt and requires thiamine-dependent cocarboxylase as a cofactor. Treatment with thiamine should be started immediately with 50 mg intravenously and 50 mg intramuscularly.

It also should be mentioned that Wernicke's syndrome can be precipitated by giving patients with alcoholism intravenous solutions containing sugar without any vitamin supplements. The carbohydrate load may diminish marginal thiamine stores and induce the syndrome. As a rule, patients with alcoholism seen in an emergency room or office should be given thiamine in an attempt to prevent the Wernicke–Korsakoff syndrome.

POLYNEUROPATHY

A common effect of chronic alcoholism is peripheral neuropathy. The extent and severity of the polyneuropathy in alcoholism is extremely variable. Some patients are asymptomatic, although sensory and motor loss and hyporeflexia may be found on examination. Many patients complain of weakness, paresthesia, and pain. Other patients may be so severely affected that they cannot walk. Symptoms usually evolve insidiously, with initial distal symptoms that progress proximally. The legs are affected exclusively, or they are affected more severely and earlier than the arms. Both motor and sensory symptoms often occur concomitantly. Paresthesias may be described as burning or as dull and constant. Examination discloses various degrees of motor, sensory, and reflex loss. Typically, signs are symmetric, more severe in the distal portions of the limbs, and often confined to the legs. The main pathologic change in alcoholic neuropathy is degeneration of the peripheral nerves. Both myelin and axons are destroyed. There are no specific histologic changes that distinguish this type of neuropathy from that of other causes.

The pathogenesis of polyneuropathy in alcoholics may be the result of a nutritional deficiency because neuropathy does not occur in chronic alcoholism if the diet is supplemented by B vitamins. The precise nutritional factor responsible has not been fully identified. Patients with alcoholism with neuropathy should be treated with daily B vitamins. Physical therapy may be helpful. Even with these therapies, recovery from alcoholic neuropathy is often slow and incomplete.

ALCOHOL AMBLYOPIA

Alcohol amblyopia is characterized by the complaint of blurred vision and the finding on examination of a reduction of visual acuity and the presence of central scotomas indicative of an optic neuropathy. These changes develop gradually over several weeks and are always bilateral and generally symmetric. If untreated, irreversible optic neuropathy may occur. This type of amblyopia also may be seen during nutritional deficiency from other causes (e.g., in prisoners of war). Deficiency of several B vitamins (riboflavin, thiamine, vitamin B_{12}) has been implicated. Although pathologic changes have not been well documented, reported changes include degeneration of the optic nerves and at times degeneration of the chiasm and optic tract. Treatment should consist of a good diet and the administration of B vitamins. Improvement usually occurs with this regimen, although in long-standing cases the response may be minimal and the patient remains with severe visual compromise.

PELLAGRA

The neurologic complication of pellagra is an encephalopathy. Fatigue, insomnia, and irritability commonly occur, and occasionally a confusional psychosis is present. Alcoholic pellagra, like pellagra of other causes, is known to be caused by a deficiency of nicotinic acid. Since the enrichment of bread with niacin began, this condition has become rare.

Pathologic changes consist of degeneration of the large cells of the motor cortex. Other central nervous system areas, such as the spinal cord, also may show changes. Treatment consists of a nutritious diet and the administration of niacin.

ALCOHOLIC DISEASES OF UNKNOWN PATHOGENESIS

There is a diverse group of neurologic and muscle disorders of unknown etiology associated with chronic alcoholism. These disorders do not specifically appear to be caused by nutritional deficiency.

ALCOHOLIC CEREBELLAR DEGENERATION

Alcoholic cerebellar degeneration is a common and highly characteristic syndrome. This disorder occurs most frequently in men. Clinically, patients demonstrate a wide-based gait, varying degrees of trunkal instability, and ataxia of the legs with relatively preserved upper-extremity coordination. Infrequently, other neurologic symptoms such as nystagmus and dysarthria occur. Most often the syndrome evolves subacutely over a period of several weeks and then stabilizes. In general, these cerebellar symptoms cannot be distinguished from the ataxia associated with Wernicke's disease, although they are usually more chronic and severe and are not associated with the behavioral signs of the latter condition.

The pathologic changes are as distinctive as the stereotyped clinical syndrome. Marked and restricted degeneration of all neurocellular elements, particularly the Purkinje cells, occurs in the anterior cerebellar lobe and superior aspects of the vermis. In more advanced cases, there are additional paravermal changes in the anterior lobe. Although cerebellar degeneration is thought by some to be caused by a nutritional deficiency, vitamin therapy is usually of no benefit.

MARCHIAFAVA–BIGNAMI DISEASE

Marchiafava–Bignami disease is a rare complication of chronic alcoholism. Although it first was described in Italian men addicted to red wine, it may occur in a variety of settings, including in the nonalcoholic person. The clinical features are varied. For the most part, symptoms resemble those of frontal lobe disease with dementia, confusion, seizures, and apathy. Bilateral frontal lobe signs, such as a grasp-and-suck reflex, may occur, and rigidity and tremor also may be present. The clinical picture is therefore one of a gradual

and progressive dementia. The diagnosis usually is made at autopsy because of the particular degeneration of the central portions of the corpus callosum. Other fiber tracts also may be affected. This is a rare condition, and many more common causes of altered mental states in patients with alcoholism exist (hepatic encephalopathy, cerebral cortical atrophy, Wernicke–Korsakoff disease, subdural hematoma, and so forth).

CENTRAL PONTINE MYELINOLYSIS

Central pontine myelinolysis is a distinctive syndrome that occurs as a rare complication of chronic alcoholism, as well as in other conditions such as carcinoma. Clinically, spastic bulbar paralysis and quadriplegia occur. This syndrome tends to occur in undernourished patients with alcoholism who usually have weight loss, nausea and vomiting, and electrolyte disturbances (particularly hyponatremia).

The pathologic picture consists of a large symmetric lesion of necrosis at the center of the basis pontis. Nearly all myelin sheaths are destroyed, with the axis cylinders being preserved. Thus, like Marchiafava–Bignami disease, the lesion consists mainly of demyelination. In the past, the diagnosis of central pontine myelinolysis was made at postmortem examination.

CEREBRAL CORTICAL ATROPHY

Postmortem neuropathologic examination in patients with alcoholism frequently discloses diffuse cortical atrophy and ventricular enlargement. These changes often can be visualized with computed tomography. The clinical correlate of these structural changes is imprecise. Although many of such patients are demented, some show very little cognitive or neurologic impairment.

ALCOHOLIC MYOPATHY

Alcohol is able to cause dysfunction of both cardiac and skeletal muscle. Several different types of myopathic syndromes affecting skeletal muscle exist and can be divided into acute and chronic myopathies. In the acute group, the first involves painless proximal weakness that develops during or shortly after heavy drinking and is associated with hypokalemia. Treatment with potassium supplements will reverse the disorder. The more dramatic myopathy involves sudden, severe pain; tenderness; and diffuse edema of the muscles. Renal damage and hyperkalemia usually exist. Myonecrosis is reflected in high serum muscle enzymes (creatine phosphokinase, aldolase) and myoglobin in the urine. Recovery usually occurs, but renal damage may be permanent. Another myopathic syndrome is characterized by muscle cramps without marked weakness and may be rather asymmetric. Muscle enzyme levels are elevated. The chronic form of myopathy associated with alcohol is uniform. It presents as a slowly progressive and painless weakness with atrophy of the proximal muscles as the hallmark. If the patient stops drinking alcohol and eats a normal diet, this condition often improves.

DISORDERS SECONDARY TO CIRRHOSIS OF PORTAL SYSTEMIC SHUNTS

Two neurologic disorders (hepatic coma and acquired hepatocerebral degeneration) often occur in the presence of severe alcohol-induced liver disease.

Hepatic Encephalopathy and Coma

Hepatic coma, or acute hepatic encephalopathy, is an episodic disorder of consciousness associated with severe liver disease (i.e., cirrhosis). Initial mental confusion precedes progressive drowsiness and coma. The confusional state frequently is associated with characteristic liver flap or asterixis. The sign may be observed in a variety of metabolic encephalopathies, and although common in hepatic encephalopathy, it is not diagnostic.

The EEG, which is frequently abnormal in the early stages of the disease, may show characteristic paroxysms of bilaterally synchronous slow waves. Triphasic waves, an indication of a metabolic disturbance, may be present.

The pathogenesis of hepatic encephalopathy is poorly understood. A disturbance of nitrogen metabolism with an increase in ammonium often is present because protein metabolism is altered by liver disease. However, the severity of the hyperammonemia often correlates poorly with the extent of the mental status changes. Neuropathologic changes in hepatic coma reveal a diffuse increase in the number and size of the protoplasmic astrocytes in the cerebral cortex, lenticular nuclei, thalamus, substantia nigra, and dentate and pontine nuclei. Nerve cells basically are unaffected.

The treatment of hepatic encephalopathy aims to reduce the intestinal production of ammonia. If gastrointestinal bleeding is present, it must be arrested as quickly as possible. Gastric aspiration is indicated if the bleeding is from the upper gastrointestinal tract, and cleansing enemas may be of additional value. Administration of any narcotics, sedatives, or tranquilizers containing ammonia or amino compounds should be stopped. The diet must be altered to a low protein content with an adequate calorie supply. Multivitamins should be given as well. Oral administration of poorly absorbed antibiotics decreases the intestinal bacteria and hence diminishes ammonia production and absorption. Neomycin, 4 to 6 g/day in divided doses, may be given orally for this purpose. The poorly absorbed ketohexose lactulose has been reported to be effective in decreasing encephalopathic symptoms. The drug is thought to act by producing a more acidic colonic pH, thus enhancing the movement of ammonia from blood into stool. Importantly, infections, especially those of the central nervous system, should be searched for vigorously because patients with hepatic encephalopathy may have additional secondary causes of central nervous system compromise. Electrolyte imbalance, especially hypokalemia and alkalosis, must be avoided, so careful monitoring of fluid and electrolyte balance is essential. Levodopa has been reported to result in transient clearing of consciousness in patients with hepatic encephalopathy. It has been proposed that levodopa crosses the blood–brain barrier and alters central neurotransmitter concentrations, producing a more normal transmitter profile.

ACQUIRED HEPATOCEREBRAL DEGENERATION

This condition refers to the symptoms that may develop after a patient has experienced several episodes of hepatic coma. Clinical features include tremor, asterixis, choreic movement, myoclonus, dysarthria, ataxia of gait, and impairment of intellectual function. The condition may evolve over months or years with increasing neurologic deficit. The EEG usually reveals a diffuse slow-wave abnormality. Hepatic function in these patients is grossly abnormal, with jaundice, ascites, esophageal varices, and elevated serum ammonium levels being present. Portacaval shunts always are present. Although the symptoms may resemble those of Wilson's disease, the lack of family history, Kayser-Fleischer rings, or disordered copper metabolism facilitates differentiation. Although the pathogenesis of this condition is unknown, there appears to be a close relationship between the acute form of hepatic coma and the chronic irreversible hepatocerebral lesions. Many attacks of hepatic coma usually precede the development of the hepatic cerebral syndrome. Astrocytic hyperplasia occurs in both conditions. Hyperammonemia is common to both disorders.

Pathologic findings are localized mainly to the cortex and consist of necrosis and gliosis. Microscopically, there is hyperplasia of protoplasmic astrocytes seen in many areas of the brain. Nerve cells may appear swollen with chromatolysis (Opalski cells). Similar cells are seen in Wilson's disease.

WHEN TO REFER PATIENTS TO A NEUROLOGIST

Urgent neurologic consultation should be obtained in patients with alcoholism with al-

tered mental status and/or coma to evaluate for possible emergent causes of an encephalopathic state (i.e., subdural hematoma). Any focal neurologic signs warrant further investigation by a neurologist to determine whether the central or peripheral nervous system is impaired. Patients with multiple or prolonged seizures or focal seizures deserve a neurologic consultation emergently to evaluate the possibility of an underlying and treatable central nervous system lesion and also to guide evaluation and treatment for status epilepticus. Patients with alcoholism who present with acute-onset ataxia also should be evaluated immediately by a neurologist to rule out emergency causes of acute ataxia such as cerebellar hemorrhage.

Patients with alcoholism with neuropathy or myopathy should be evaluated by a neurologist to exclude other possible causes of nerve or muscle dysfunction. In these cases, further blood testing to rule out metabolic conditions, such as hypothyroidism and electrophysiologic testing, may be helpful to further elucidate the etiology of the condition. These cases generally are evaluated as an outpatient.

SPECIAL ISSUES IN HOSPITALIZED PATIENTS

The primary concern for hospital staff caring for a patient with alcoholism is alcohol withdrawal. Whereas some hospitals permit alcohol, this policy is infrequent in the United States. Because many alcoholics may deny or not even consciously recognize their physical dependence on alcohol, hospital staff should know the signs of alcohol withdrawal and be ready to consider the diagnosis in all patients. If withdrawal signs, especially agitation and dysautonomia, develop in this context, hydration and metabolic and electrolyte balance should be assured and chlordiazepoxide treatment should be considered. Because alcoholism crosses all gender, age, racial, and economic categories, all hospitalized patients should be considered potentially at risk for alcohol withdrawal.

REHABILITATION THERAPIES AND ALTERNATIVE TREATMENTS IN ALCOHOL-RELATED NEUROLOGIC SYNDROMES

Physical therapy for alcohol-related neuropathy and myopathy may be helpful in improving mobility and preventing the development of contractures. Passive range-of-motion techniques may be useful initially if the patient is incapacitated or bedbound. Patients with severe paralysis should have molded splints applied to the arms, hands, legs, and feet while resting in bed. Padded splints should be used on heels and elbows to avoid excessive pressure on those areas while the patient is lying supine. A stay in an inpatient rehabilitation unit for a period of time may be indicated when gait is severely impaired. At this time, no alternative treatments are known for the alcohol-related neurologic syndromes.

QUESTIONS AND DISCUSSION

1. A 30-year-old man, a known alcoholic, comes to the emergency room complaining of abdominal pain, and a diagnosis of pancreatitis is made. An intravenous solution of dextrose 5% in water is started, and the patient is admitted to the hospital. Hours later, the patient is noted to be confused, and nystagmus and ataxia now are noted on physical examination.

i. The clinical picture of confusion, nystagmus, and ataxia fits with the diagnosis of Wernicke's encephalopathy.

ii. Intravenous glucose can lower marginal body thiamine stores.

True statement(s) is/are:

A. i. only
B. ii. only
C. i. and ii. are correct
D. None are correct.

The answer is (C). It is probable that the patient developed Wernicke's syndrome from intravenous glucose administration, which further decreased his marginal stores of thiamine. Thiamine deficiency is responsible for Wernicke's syndrome. It is important that patients with alcoholism be given thiamine, and multi-

vitamins should be added to all intravenous solutions for patients with alcoholism.

2. A routine neurologic examination of a patient with alcoholism admitted 10 days previously for detoxification now reveals the following findings: no ankle jerk, loss of vibratory sensation in the lower extremities, mild distal weakness in the legs, inability to perform tandem gait, and dysmetria on heel-to-shin examination. What neurologic syndrome fits with these findings?

A. Spinal cord damage (myelopathy), especially anteriorially
B. Brainstem degeneration, involving midbrain and pons
C. Sensorimotor neuropathy with midline cerebellar impairment
D. Muscle disease (myopathy), most likely with rhabdomyolysis

The answer is (C). Examination revealed evidence of a sensorimotor neuropathy (hyporeflexia, motor and sensory abnormalities) and a midline cerebellar syndrome (poor tandem gait). These abnormalities are common in chronic patients with alcoholism and are so characteristic that other causes are much less likely. The patient should be given multivitamins, although full functional recovery would not be expected.

3. A chronic alcoholic patient has focal involuntary shaking of the left side of the face and the left arm, lasting several minutes. These spells began 1 week after admission to the hospital. The patient was admitted originally for tremulousness and hallucinosis. Those symptoms were gone by the sixth day of hospitalization. These focal left-sided behaviors best fit with the diagnosis of:

A. Withdrawal seizures
B. Focal seizures
C. Pellagra
D. Wernicke's encephalopathy

The answer is (B). Withdrawal seizures or "rum fits" characteristically occur between 8 and 48 hours after the cessation of drinking. The majority occur 12 to 24 hours after the reduction of drinking, and seizures are of the generalized motor type without a focal character. Focal seizures always should raise the possibility of focal pathology (e.g., subdural hematoma, tumor, and so forth), and the patient should undergo radiographic evaluation (i.e., computed tomography of the head). The case is not typical of either pellagra or Wernicke's encephalopathy.

4. Which is true of alcoholic myopathy?

A. Acute painful myopathy usually is associated with hyperkalemia.

B. Necrosis of muscle is associated with low levels of creative phosphokinase and myoglobin.

C. Chronic alcoholic myopathy affects distal muscle with prominent atrophy of the fingers and feet.

D. Myopathy is one of the diagnostic criteria for Marchiafava–Bignami disease.

The answer is (A). Painful myopathy is usually rapid in onset and associated with high potassium levels. If muscle damage occurs, myoglobinemia and high CK levels are typical. Myopathies usually affect proximal muscles, whereas neuropathies affect distal strength. Marchiafava–Bignami disease affects the corpus callosum of the brain and has nothing to do with muscle damage.

SUGGESTED READING

Adams RD, Foley JM. The neurological disorder associated with liver disease. *Res Publ Assoc Res Nerv Ment Dis* 1953;32:198.

Adams RD, Victor M, Mancall EL. Central pontine myelinolysis. *Arch Neurol Psychiatry* 1959;81:154.

Dreyfus PM, Victor M. Effects of thiamine deficiency on the central nervous system. *Am J Clin Nutr* 1961;9:414.

Goetz C, Pappert E. *Textbook of clinical neurology.* Philadelphia: WB Saunders, 1999.

Kinsella LJ, Riley DE. Nutritional deficiencies and syndromes associated with alcoholism. In: Goetz CG, ed. *Textbook of clinical neurology,* 2nd ed. Philadelphia: WB Saunders, 2003.

Morris J, Victor M. Alcohol withdrawal seizures. *Emory Med Clin North Am* 1987;5:827.

Ragan JJ. Alcohol and the cardiovascular system. *JAMA* 1990;264:377.

Spillane JD. *Nutritional disorders of the nervous system.* Baltimore: Williams & Wilkins, 1947.

Victor M. The alcohol withdrawal syndrome. In: Seixas F, Eggleston S, eds. Alcoholism and the central nervous system. *Ann NY Acad Med* 1973;215:210.

Victor M. The pathophysiology of alcoholic epilepsy. *Res Publ Assoc Res Nerv Ment Dis* 1968;46:431.

Victor M, Adams RD. The effect of alcohol upon the nervous system. *Res Publ Assoc Res Nerv Ment Dis* 1953;32:526.

Victor M, Adams RD, Collins GH. *The Wernicke–Korsakoff syndrome.* Philadelphia: FA Davis, 1971.

Victor M, Adams RD, Mancall E. A restricted form of cerebellar degeneration occurring in alcoholic patients. *Arch Neurol* 1959;1:577.

13

Peripheral Neuropathy

Morris A. Fisher

CLINICAL FEATURES AND SCIENTIFIC BACKGROUND

The peripheral nervous system (PNS) starts as the pia arachnoid ends, at the level of the intervertebral foramina and therefore encompasses those parts of the nervous system that lie outside the confines of the brain, brainstem, and spinal cord. As such, it consists of those portions of the primary sensory neurons, lower motor neurons, and autonomic neurons that are outside the central nervous system (CNS). By definition, therefore, the PNS includes the cranial nerves, the spinal nerves with their roots and rami, the peripheral nerves, and those aspects of the autonomic nervous system that are outside the CNS. There are disease processes that preferentially involve primarily the PNS, and it is therefore useful to consider this system as a nosologic entity.

All parts of the PNS are associated with Schwann cells or the comparable ganglionic cells, the satellite cells. This anatomic commonality may account for some of the pathologic aspects of the PNS. More significantly, the normal functions of all parts of the PNS are dependent on the normal functioning of the nerve cell bodies from which the motor and sensory axons originate. For example, the foot is supplied by nerve fibers whose cell bodies lie at the level of the lower thoracic/upper-lumbar vertebrae. A motoneuron and its associated motor axon innervating a foot muscle are one cell, and the complexities involved in maintaining normal nerve function of this cell extending from the lower back to the foot are considerable. There is retrograde constant transport system from the nerve cell bodies to their most distal axonal projections, and this system is necessary for maintaining normal nerve (and muscle) function. There is

also transport so that the cell bodies are influenced by distal events. This system provides the conduit by which agents such as herpes virus may reach the nerve cell body. Given the complexity and length of the structures involved, it is not surprising that the normal functioning of the PNS frequently is disturbed.

ANATOMY

Except for the cranial nerves, peripheral nerves separate at the level of the roots. The dorsal roots contain afferent ("sensory") fibers that are located either preganglionic or postganglionic to the dorsal root ganglion on their way to the spinal cord. The ventral roots consist of efferent ("motor") fibers that originate from the lower motor neurons. The resultant mixed ("motor" and "sensory") nerves are the structures for providing information to and from the CNS throughout the body. In the thoracic and upper-lumbar region, these nerves are joined by sympathetic fibers after these fibers have synapsed in the ganglionic chain adjacent to the vertebral column. The parasympathetic outflow originates either in the cranial region (cranial nerves III, VII, IX, and X) or in the sacral region passing distally as the pelvic splanchnic nerves (Fig. 13.1).

Individual muscles and areas of skin are supplied not only by particular nerves but also by fibers that originate in particular roots. The PNS distribution in the limbs is superficially complex because of the routing that occurs in the brachial and lumbosacral plexuses involving the upper and lower limbs, respectively.

Individual nerves are composed of bundles of individual nerve fibers called fascicles, which, in turn, are surrounded by connective tissue. All of the motor fibers and many of the

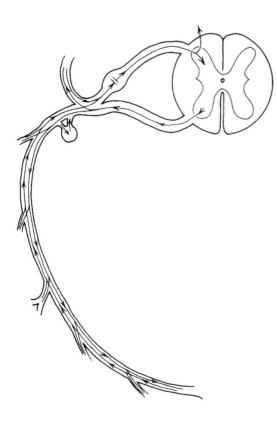

FIG. 13.1. Drawing of peripheral nerve originating from *(1)* ventral root with cells of origin in the anterior horn of the spinal cord and *(2)* dorsal root with a dorsal root ganglion. The postganglionic dorsal root fibers pass to the dorsal horn or more superiorly in the spinal cord. The posterior primary ramus extends dorsally, whereas the anterior primary ramus is the main extension of the peripheral nerve. Sympathetic fibers join the peripheral nerve by way of the sympathetic ganglion.

sensory fibers are surrounded by myelin. Myelin is formed by foldings of Schwann cell membranes. These supporting cells are ubiquitous throughout the PNS. In myelinated fibers, the junction of sheaths from two adjacent Schwann cells occurs at what are referred to as nodes of Ranvier. Most sensory fibers and all autonomic fibers are either poorly myelinated or unmyelinated. Even unmyelinated nerve fibers, however, are ensheathed by Schwann cells.

Nutrient arteries that arise from adjacent blood vessels supply nerves. The arterial supply is richly collateralized both to and within the nerves themselves. The result is a system resistant to large-vessel ischemia.

INDICATIONS OF NEUROPATHIC INJURY

The symptoms and signs of neuropathic injury can be predicted from the preceding discussion. If nerves to muscles are disrupted,

weakness may be present, and atrophy of muscle fibers can occur. Cramping with fatigue is a common symptom. Reflexes may be decreased or absent if the afferent or efferent nerves that subserve the reflex are disturbed.

A wide range of sensory disturbances are found. With complete loss of innervation, there may be total loss of feeling–anesthesia. This rarely happens because of the considerable overlap of sensory nerve supply. More commonly, alterations in sensation are found. Unusual feelings such as "pins and needles" are called paresthesias, and unpleasant sensations such as burning are called dysesthesias. A decrease in sensation on examination is referred to as hypoesthesia; an increase is called hyperesthesia. A decrease in perception of position and vibration indicates dysfunction in larger fibers, whereas diminished pinprick and temperature sensation indicates abnormalities in smaller fibers. The effects of autonomic dysfunction include cardiac, vasomotor, and gastrointestinal disturbances as well as alterations in sweating. The skin may become smooth and glossy, hair may decrease (or occasionally increase), and the nails may become thickened. Because of loss of feeling, repeated injury and inadequate repair can result in permanent losses in limbs as well as of function of joints (Charcot joints).

ANATOMIC DISTRIBUTION

Motor and sensory changes caused by PNS disease occur in the distribution of nerve roots or the peripheral nerves themselves. Charts are readily available that show these distributions. The information has been obtained indirectly based on root or nerve injury. Although superficially complex, with practice the information becomes readily usable. There is some variability between different charts, and one should not attempt to fit each patient into a rigidly circumscribed view of normal. Patterns of root and nerve distribution in a broad sense are reliable, and it is important to try to identify these patterns clinically (Fig. 13.2).

The muscles of the shoulder girdle are innervated mainly by the C5 root, those of the arm by C5 and C6 (triceps brachii, C7), those of the forearm by C7 and C8, and those of the hand by C8 and T1. In the lower extremity, the thigh muscles are supplied by the L2, L3, and L4 roots. Those muscles of the anterior leg are innervated by L4 and L5 roots, those of the posterior leg by S1, and the small muscles of the foot by S1 and S2.

The root sensory distribution can be visualized with the individual in the anatomic position. In general, C1–C4 innervate the back of the head, the neck, and the shoulder region; C5 innervates the lateral aspect of the arm; C6 innervates the lateral portion of the forearm extending into the hand involving the thumb and

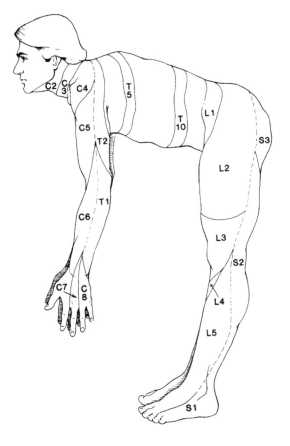

FIG. 13.2. Sequential nature of the cutaneous root distribution as shown with the individual in the quadruped position.

index finger; C7 innervates the midportion of the hand and ring finger; and C8 innervates the more medial portion of the hand including the little finger. The posterior aspect of the upper extremity then is supplied by T1 and T2, and the torso is innervated sequentially by T2–L1, with T5 at about the level of the nipples and T10 at the umbilicus. The anterior thigh is supplied by L1, L2, and L3; the anterior leg and foot are supplied predominantly by L4 and L5; the posterior aspect of the lower extremity is supplied by S1 and S2; and the region of the anus is supplied by S3, S4, and S5.

The three main terminal nerves of the brachial plexus in the upper extremity are the radial, median, and ulnar nerves. The radial nerve innervates the extensor muscles and provides much of the cutaneous supply to the extensor surface of the arm, forearm, and hand. The median nerve is the predominant nerve innervating the forearm flexors as well as the muscles of the thenar eminence controlling thumb movement. The ulnar nerve innervates the remaining intrinsic hand muscles. The median and ulnar nerves supply the cutaneous sensibility to the hand. The ulnar territory characteristically encompasses the little finger, half

of the ring finger, and the adjacent palmar surface, whereas the median nerve provides the remaining cutaneous innervation (Fig. 13.3).

In the lower extremity, the femoral nerve supplies the knee extensors in the thigh in addition to the cutaneous branches for the anterior thigh and medial aspect of the leg and foot (by way of the saphenous nerve). The posterior thigh muscles controlling knee flexion, as well as all the muscles of the leg and foot, are innervated by the sciatic nerve. The peroneal (anterior tibial) branch of the sciatic nerve supplies the anterior compartment of the leg—namely, those muscles that affect dorsiflexion of the ankle and toes as well as foot eversion. The tibial portion of the sciatic nerve innervates those muscles producing plantar flexion. The cutaneous distribution is comparable. Branches of the peroneal nerve supply the anterior leg and dorsum of the foot, whereas the posterior aspect of the leg and plantar aspect of the foot are innervated by branches of the tibial nerve. The medial plantar aspect of the foot and toes is supplied by the medial plantar nerve, whereas their more lateral aspect is supplied by the lateral plantar nerve. The medial and lateral plantar nerves

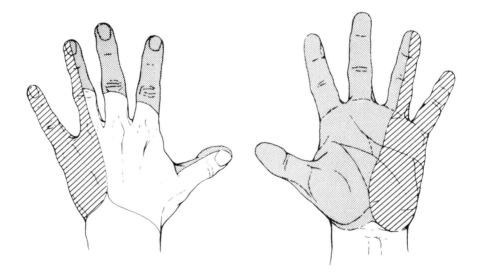

FIG. 13.3. Cutaneous innervation of the hand by the radial *(clear section),* median *(stippled section),* and ulnar *(diagonal lines)* nerves.

are the terminal equivalents of the upper-extremity median and ulnar nerves, respectively.

Table 13.1 indicates selected muscle movements with their main innervation, and Table 13.2 shows a schema of the cutaneous innervation of the limbs. These tables and the preceding discussion are designed to provide a framework for the clinical evaluation of peripheral nerve disorders. To do the examination well requires considerable experience. Obtaining the necessary information from the patients can be demanding, and the examination itself must be an active process looking for patterns of abnormality. As such, neurologic consultation for the evaluation of peripheral nerve disorders is frequently helpful.

TABLE 13.1. *Selected Muscle Movements and Their Innervation*

Joint Movement Muscles[a]	Peripheral Nerves[a]	Spinal Segments[a]
Upper Extremity		
Shoulder	Abduction Deltoid	Axillary C5
Lateral (external) rotation	Infraspinatus	Suprascapular C5
Elbow Flexion	Brachialis	Musculocutaneous C5, C6
Biceps brachii Extension	Triceps brachii	Radial C7
Radial-ulnar	Supination Biceps brachii	Musculocutaneous C6
Supinator	Radial	
Pronation	Pronator teres	Median C7
Wrist Dorsal flexion (extension)	Extensor carpi radialis longus and brevis	Radial C7
Palmar flexion	Flexor carpi radialis	Median C7
Flexor carpi ulnaris	Ulnar	
(Thumb) Palmar adduction	Interossei	Ulnar T1
Palmar abduction	Abductor pollicis brevis	Median C8
Extension	Extensor pollicis longus et brevis	Radial C7, C8
Opposition	Opponens pollicis	Median T1
(Finger) excluding thumb	Adduction Palmar interossei	Ulnar T1
Abduction	Dorsal interossei	Ulnar T1
Extension	Extensor digitorum	Radial C7, C8
(metacarpophalangeal joints)		
Extensor indicis		
Extensor digiti minimi		
Lower Extremity		
Hip Flexion	Iliopsoas	Femoral L2
Extension	Gluteus maximus	Inferior gluteal S1, S2
Adduction	Adductor magnus	Obturator L2, L3
Adductor brevis		
Adductor longus		
Abduction	Gluteus medius	Superior gluteal L4, L5
Knee	Extension Quadriceps	Femoral L3, L4
Femoris		
Flexion	Biceps femoris	Sciatic S1
Semitendinosus		
Semitendinosus		
Ankle Dorsiflexion	Tibialis anterior	Peroneal L4
Plantar flexion	Gastrocnemius	Posterior tibial S1, S2
Soleus		
Inversion	Tibialis posterior	Posterior tibial L5
Tibialis anterior	Peroneal L4	
Eversion	Peroneus longus et brevis	Peroneal L5
(Large toe) Extension	Extensor hallucis longus	Peroneal L5

[a]Only main controlling muscle, nerve, and roots listed.

Joint action listed because (a) it can be easily tested and (b) muscle, nerve, and root control are relatively simple. Parentheses indicate action at more than one joint.

Note: Terminal divisions of the brachial plexus can be tested at the thumb. Hip action controlled by muscles innervated by L2-S2 roots.

TABLE 13.2. *Schematic Cutaneous Innervation of the Limbs*

Extremity[a]	Lateral	Anterior	Medial	Posterior
Upper				
Arm	C5 Axillary radial		Medial cutaneous nerve of arm T2	
Forearm	C6 Musculocutaneous		Medial cutaneous nerve of forearm T1	
Hand and fingers[b]	Thumb Index C6 C6		Middle Ring Little C7 C8 C8	
Lower				
Thigh	Lateral femoral cutaneous	Femoral L2, L3	Obturator	Posterior cutaneous nerve of the thigh S2
Leg	Peroneal L5		Saphenous L4	Sural S1, S2
Foot		Peroneal L5		Plantar nerves S1

[a]Portions of the posterior midline areas of the arm and forearm are supplied by branches of the radial nerve.
[b]For cutaneous distribution, see Figs. 13.2 and 13.3.

PATTERNS OF ABNORMALITY

Derangements of motor, sensory, and autonomic function may be present with lesions at the level of the roots, plexuses, or peripheral nerves. Sensory loss, for example, involving the lateral aspect of the leg combined with weakness of dorsiflexion of the toes would be consistent with a lesion of the L5 root; motor and sensory changes in the distribution of both the axillary and radial nerves would be compatible with injury to the posterior cord of the brachial plexus; and weakness and atrophy of intrinsic hand muscles combined with sensory loss involving the medial aspect of the palmar surface of the hand, the little finger, and adjacent half of the middle finger would indicate an ulnar nerve lesion.

The most common pattern of PNS disease is a symmetric polyneuropathy. Sensory, usually more than motor, signs and symptoms are present in a more or less symmetric, predominantly distal distribution. The signs and symptoms start distally in the legs and progress proximally. Clinical findings in the legs and arms are related to the distance from the spinal cord (i.e., from C7 in the arms and T12–L1 in the legs). Sensory loss should extend to the mid-legs, for example, before such findings are present in the arms. Diabetic polyneuropathy, uremia, and drug or toxic ex-

posure are common examples. One possible cause for this distribution may be the greater vulnerability of longer nerve fibers to disturbances in nutrient transport.

Damage to a single nerve is called a mononeuropathy. An example would be the carpal tunnel syndrome as a result of median nerve injury at the level of the wrist. Compressive injury is a frequent cause.

A mononeuropathy multiplex indicates dysfunction of multiple single peripheral nerves. This patten is common in diabetes as well as vasculitides such as polyarteritis nodosa.

Plexopathies refer to injury at the level of the brachial, lumbar, or sacral plexuses. Idiopathic brachial neuritis, traumatic injury to the brachial plexus, and retroperitoneal or apical lung tumors are common causes. Radiculopathies are caused by injury to the roots. Sensory loss is then in a dermatomal rather than peripheral nerve distribution. Disc and vertebral bone disease are among the associated conditions.

An important clinical distinction is whether a process is diffuse or multifocal. In multifocal neuropathies, the length-dependent basis of nerve dysfunction in neuropathies is not necessarily present. Cranial nerves may be involved, the arms may be more affected than the legs, and there may be prominent differences in the degree of injury between similar nerves on the right or left or between nerves (e.g., tibial and peroneal) in comparable areas of a limb.

PATHOLOGY

Pathologic processes affecting nerves usually involve both myelin and axons, although at times the physiologic effects predominantly may reflect to one or the other of these structures. In demyelinating processes, myelin may be lost diffusely (e.g., inherited demyelinating neuropathies) as well as segmentally (e.g., acquired demyelinating neuropathies). There may be marked slowing and blocking of conduction. The axons may be relatively well preserved. As such, clinical recovery in the acquired demyelinating neuropathies such as the Guillain-Barré syndrome can be both rapid and complete if remyelination occurs.

Prominent axonal degeneration is more common than primary demyelination. This is characteristic of neuropathies as a result of a large number of exogenous toxins and metabolic derangements. These processes may affect the nerve cell bodies as well as the axons and may be manifest as a dying back of the distal portion of the axon. Secondary demyelination occurs in those fibers with axonal damage. Recovery occurs by regeneration of axons, which often must then reinnervate denervated structures. As a result, recovery may be relatively slow and incomplete.

With physical injury to nerves, the injury may be limited to focal (paranodal) demyelination with associated conduction block and rapid recovery (neuropraxia). If axons are interrupted (axonotmesis), degeneration (Wallerian) of the axons and myelin may occur distal to the site of injury. If the Schwann cell basal lamina and endoneurial tissue remain intact, axonal regeneration commences promptly after injury. If both the axon and surrounding connective tissue are disrupted (neurotmesis), Wallerian degeneration is inevitable and axon regeneration may be disrupted by intervening connective tissue. Neuromas and aberrant regeneration may occur.

The potential pathologic processes that affect the PNS are similar to those that affect other systems. Metabolic or toxic derangements (e.g., vitamin deficiencies, uremia, alcoholism, heavy metals, industrial solvents, and certain medications) frequently result in nerve dysfunction. Vascular abnormalities affecting nerves usually involve the medium and small arteries, and these abnormalities may be found in rheumatoid arthritis, polyarteritis nodosa, and temporal arteritis. Diabetic mononeuropathies are probably vascular in origin, and the primary pathologic process in diabetic polyneuropathies maybe a vascular-based ischemia. Idiopathic polyneuritis (Landry-Guillain-Barré syndrome) is representative of an inflammatory process. This probably has an immunologic basis, as do the neuropathies seen in paraproteinemias and paraneoplastic syndromes. Leprosy is a common infectious process affecting nerves, as are some of the neuropathies associated with human immunodeficiency virus (HIV) infection. A genetic basis for PNS dysfunction such as peroneal muscular atrophy (Charcot-Marie-Tooth disease) is also not uncommon. Schwannomas and neurofibromas are representative tumors. Trauma is a frequent cause of nerve injury. This includes entrapment neuropathies—namely, mononeuropathies resulting from vulnerability because of anatomic features of the nerves. Carpal tunnel syndrome is the most common entrapment neuropathy, but other common injuries include the ulnar nerve at the elbow and the peroneal nerve at the fibula head.

Neuropathies are common. An approach to evaluating these problems is essential in all areas of medicine. Even under the best of circumstances, the cause for a neuropathy may not be established in about one-third of these patients. As in other areas of medicine, often the important thing for management to determine is what is not the cause as much as what is the cause.

DIAGNOSIS

As in other areas of neurology, the physical examination remains a powerful tool for the evaluation of disorders of the PNS. The examination need not be subtle, but it must be accurate. Motor and sensory distributions of a polyneuropathy, mononeuropathy, or radiculopathy often can be appreciated.

The action of individual muscles should be tested and rated as to strength. Strength may be normal (5), mildly decreased (4), moderately decreased (3) (i.e., no movement against gravity), markedly (1–2) decreased, or absent (0). Muscle strength testing should be concentrated in those areas that aid in the analysis of the particular problem.

The sensory examination need not be tedious, but it must be accurate. Again, concentration on areas relevant to the diagnostic question is important. The patient often can best outline a circumscribed area of sensory deficit. This area then can be analyzed in more detail for light touch and pain sensations using a finger and a sharp instrument such as a safety pin, respectively. (Separate pins should be used for each patient so as not to spread hepatitis.) A distal to proximal area of sensory change can be outlined in a similar fashion. Moving relevant joints can test position sense. Slight movements of distal joints should be appreciated accurately. A 128-cycles-per-second (cps) tuning fork with the base placed on bony prominences is used for testing vibration. In neuropathies, vibration is characteristically more affected than position. The examination should start from the most distal area of abnormality. Then one should test vibration in more proximal locations only if the patient does not perceive the full duration of the vibration at the more distal site. A finger of the examiner touching the same bony region as the tuning fork helps evaluates the patient's sensitivity.

As mentioned previously, the sensory examination may be difficult and confusing. A primary care physician should have a low threshold for seeking consultation if it could be helpful.

The most valuable ancillary study for analysis of PNS disorders is electromyography (EMG). This is best viewed as an extension of the neurologic examination. Although an EMG is harmless, it does entail some discomfort. Reliable information obtained in an efficient fashion is crucial, and this, in turn, will depend on the experience and skill of the electromyographer.

EMG consists of two basic parts. The first is an evaluation of the conduction in nerves. The second part involves analysis of the electrical activity in muscles—the EMG per se. The data can define the location of a lesion and aid in understanding the pathophysiology.

Conduction in motor fibers is determined by stimulating electrically and recording the resultant evoked motor response. Muscle fiber contraction is associated with electrical activity caused by the movement of charged ions across membranes, and this electrical activity can be recorded. Latency refers to the time from the stimulus to the onset of the electrical activity. The latency will be shorter if the stimulus is closer to the muscle than if it is more distant. The time difference between a distal and a more proximal latency divided by the distance between the two stimulating points enables a conduction velocity to be determined—that is, distance/time = conduction velocity (CV). When recording from muscle, a CV can be determined only if stimulation is performed at least two points. The unknown time for transmission in slow-conducting terminal nerve fibers as well as across the junction between the nerve and the muscle then is "subtracted out" (Fig. 13.4).

Electrical responses from afferent (sensory) fibers also may be recorded. Because the amplitudes of these evoked afferent responses are several orders of magnitude less than the evoked motor responses, the sensory potentials are more difficult to record. At the same time, a meaningful CV can be obtained from a single latency because a CV may be calculated from the time taken to traverse a particular distance because there is no unknown time in the region of the neuromuscular junction.

The amplitude of evoked motor or sensory responses is a less accurate indicator of normality than is the latency. Amplitude may be affected by the site of the recording as well as by the amount of tissue between the electrical-activity generator in the muscle or nerve

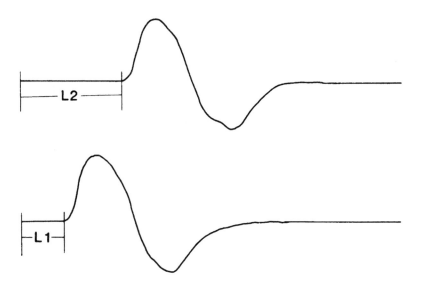

$$cv = d/L2-L1$$

FIG. 13.4. Evoked motor responses with the shorter-latency L1 resulting from stimulation closer to the recording site, in comparison with the latency L2 resulting from stimulation of the nerve at a more proximal site. The conduction velocity (CV) in the nerve is determined by dividing the distance (d) between the stimulating sites by the latency differences.

and the recording electrodes. Nevertheless, the amplitudes of the evoked efferent or afferent responses reflect the amount of electrical-activity-generating tissue. Decreased amplitude responses can be defined, and side-to-side comparisons of response amplitudes can be particularly helpful.

The different fibers in a particular nerve conduct impulses at different rates. There is a linear relation between fiber size and conduction velocity, with the largest fibers conducting at the fastest velocities. If activity in the largest fibers is lost, then conduction will be slowed. The maximum degree of slowing that may be present with axon loss alone, however, is considerably less than that which may be found with demyelination.

In addition to slowed conduction and decreased amplitude, nerve injury can produce altered configuration and dispersion of evoked responses. These changes in evoked responses can define the location of focal nerve dysfunction. Temporal dispersion is characteristic of demyelinating injury, as is

conduction block. In the latter, the size of the response is meaningfully decreased or even absent during stimulation proximal to the block. The result may be a striking picture in which nerve function is lost but conduction studies distal to the region of conduction block are entirely normal because those portions of the nerve distal to the block may be entirely normal.

Studies are available (i.e., H reflexes and F responses) that monitor conduction in nerve fibers to and from the spinal cord. These studies are important because proximal nerve injury may be present even in the absence of injury to the more distal nerves.

The electrical activity generated by muscle contraction can be recorded from the muscle surface but is best evaluated by recording from a needle electrode inserted in the muscle itself. The resultant electrical activity then can be monitored, amplified, and displayed.

At rest, there is no electrical activity. Some activity usually is seen as a needle is moved through muscle ("insertional activity"), but these responses stop when needle movement stops. As a muscle contracts, there is increasing activity. This consists of the firing of motor units. A motor unit is composed of a lower motor neuron in the anterior horn of the spinal cord, its motor axon, and the muscle fibers innervated by that axon. Increasing force of contraction results primarily from the recruitment of more units, although an increased rate of firing also contributes to the increase in muscle tension. This increased muscle activity with increasing force of muscle contraction is readily appreciated during routine EMG. More electrical activity is seen; the amount of visible baseline without motor unit activity decreases; and the audio amplification of the muscle activity becomes increasingly prominent (Fig. 13.5).

Each motor unit is composed of muscle fibers scattered widely throughout a particular muscle. The number of muscle fibers in a motor unit varies with the fineness of control required. For example, there may be only six muscle fibers per motor unit in the eye muscles but up to several thousand in some of the large postural muscles. The simultaneous contraction of all the muscle fibers in a motor unit results in the usual integrated smooth, triphasic electrical response (Fig. 13.6). Motor unit size varies not only between muscles but also within muscles. The larger motor units have more muscle fibers, and, therefore, with discharge they will generate more electrical activity than smaller units. Thus the larger units generally will be of larger amplitude. During normal reflex or voluntary recruitment, motor units are activated sequentially according to size, with the smaller units discharging first. As a muscle contracts, more, larger units are activated. The amplitude of a particular motor unit is, however, a relatively poor indicator of motor unit size because of (a) the potential variation of muscle fiber organization within a particular motor unit and (b) the relation of the recording needle to those muscle fibers. Motor unit duration provides a better estimate of relative motor unit size because motor unit duration reflects the dispersion of the muscle fibers in an individual motor unit within a muscle; larger motor units have larger motor unit durations.

When there is a disruption of the normal connection between nerve and muscle (i.e., denervation), abnormalities appear at rest 1 to 3 weeks after injury, and EMG can detect

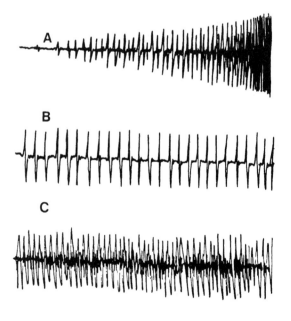

FIG. 13.5. Drawings of motor unit recruitment patterns. **A:** Normal pattern with increasing number and size of motor units with increasing force of muscle contraction. **B:** Repetitive firing of a single large motor unit characteristic of neuropathies. **C:** A "rich" pattern of many small motor units even at low levels of muscle tension seen in myopathies. Amplitude calibrations in the ratio of 1:5:0.5 for A:B:C.

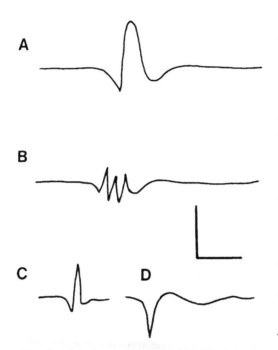

A

B

C   D

FIG. 13.6. Tracings of **A,** normal triphasic motor unit potential; **B,** polyphasic potential; **C,** fibrillation; and **D,** positive sharp wave. Calibrations: vertical (microvolts)—*A* and *B*, 500; *C* and *D*, 50; horizontal (milliseconds)— *A* and *B*, 5; *C* and *D*, 2.

them. Individual muscle fibers may discharge at rest, and this type of electrical activity is referred to as fibrillations or positive sharp waves. This activity is not visible clinically. Other types of abnormal spontaneous activity may be present, such as runs of complex potentials (complex repetitive discharges). Irregular contractions of entire motor units may appear; these are called fasciculations. They are visible clinically and can be present in normal individuals, especially with fatigue. They also occur with axonal injury and are characteristic in disorders of the motor neuron such as amyotrophic lateral sclerosis (ALS).

EMG using special electrodes can record electrical activity from single muscle fibers. This technique is particularly useful for defining abnormalities of the neuromuscular junction such as myasthenia gravis. Similar abnormalities also may be seen in rapidly progressive neuropathic injury or with reinnervation.

In neuropathies, there is a loss of functioning axons. Fewer motor units than normal may be found on voluntary activation of a muscle. At its most extreme, only a single motor unit may be seen to discharge within the recording field of the electrode, even with maximum muscle contraction. In association with these changes, the motor units may be larger than normal. The muscle fibers that have been denervated may be reinnervated by the remaining viable axons of remaining motor units. As a result, these motor units may be larger than normal and also more complex in configuration. Small, complex (polyphasic)-appearing motor unit potentials, however, also may be found. Although these potentials are considered more characteristic of myopathies as a result of loss of functioning muscle fibers, they also are seen in neuropathic injury during reinnervation. As motor axons grow into muscle that has lost its innervation, new motor units are formed, and these new units initially will be small and polyphasic because they include a relatively limited number of muscle fibers. A reduced number of motor units, especially if they are large and associated with electrophysiologic evidence of denervation, would be characteristic of a neuropathic process.

These may be the only electrophysiologic findings in those neurogenic processes caused by loss of motoneurons such as ALS. More commonly in neuropathies, slowing of conduction is present and provides evidence of nerve dysfunction. Prominent slowing with no or relatively little denervation and preserved response amplitudes would be consistent with a demyelinating process. Borderline to mildly slowed conductions associated with clear and relatively diffuse axonal injury would indicate predominant axonal injury. Low-amplitude evoked responses are most characteristic of axonal dysfunction because of loss of functioning nerve or muscle tissue.

The patient's symptoms may not correlate with the degree of nerve injury found on EMG. The usual electrodiagnostic studies monitor function only in large fibers. Disabling dysesthesias as a result of small fiber dysfunction may occur with unremarkable or relatively minor EMG abnormalities. At the same time, severe, diffuse nerve abnormalities may be accompanied by few complaints because of preservation of sufficient, even if decreased, nerve fibers. In general, electrodiagnostic findings will correlate better with motor symptoms and signs (weakness) than sensory dysfunction. Electromyographic studies can provide information not only about the severity and duration of a neuropathic process but also about the prognosis of nerve injury.

Normal conduction and lack of denervation several weeks after the onset of nerve dysfunction could indicate a good prognosis because this pattern would be consistent with functional, but not necessarily structural, abnormalities of the nerve. This is a common clinical consideration, for example, in Bell's palsy caused by disruption of facial nerve function.

At their best, electrodiagnostic studies should be considered not only for establishing the presence of a neuropathy—this is often apparent on examination—but primarily for establishing the pattern of abnormality. This includes not only whether a process is demyelinating or axonal; this distinction in fact is usually less easily established than one might think from reading the literature. Equally important is the degree of symmetry or asymmetry. If one can establish diffuse versus multifocal axonal or demyelinating patterns, the differential diagnosis can be focused. For example, diffuse demyelinating patterns are characteristic of some inherited neuropathies, multifocal demyelinating patterns are characteristic of acquired neuropathies such as the Guillain-Barré syndrome, diffuse axonal patterns suggest toxic neuropathies, and multifocal axonal patterns suggest vasculitic neuropathies such as occur in collagen diseases.

Nerve biopsies can be performed. The sural nerve is biopsied most commonly. At times, the information may be pathognomonic, such as in infiltrative neuropathies (e.g., amyloidosis and metachromatic leukodystrophy). In other circumstances, the information may be important for patient management (e.g., defining the presence of chronic demyelinating inflammatory injury). "Teased" fiber preparations allow an examination of individual fibers and thereby more accurate analysis of the pathology of nerve injury. Immunologic staining can define the type of antibody and abnormal cells present in nerves. Nerve biopsy itself is performed under local anesthesia and is essentially a benign procedure, although there can be transient uncomfortable residua. Sophistication also is required for determining when a nerve biopsy is indicated. As such, a nerve biopsy should probably only be performed in consultation with someone with expertise in neuromuscular disorders.

Antibody testing is increasingly being performed for evaluation of peripheral neuropathies. This stems from the increasing recognition that antibodies can be present in patients with neuropathies that may be pathogenetic for the neuropathies. This is particularly true for those antibodies against neural gangliosides. The anti-GQ1b antibody is present in about 95% of patients with a particular variant of the Guillain-Barré syndrome (the Fisher syndrome). An immunoglobulin M (IgM) GM1 antibody is present in about 50% of patients with a variant of a chronic inflammatory demyelinating neuropathy (multifocal motor neuropathy), and a relatively specific neuropathic syndrome is present in those with an IgM monoclonal gammopathy and antibodies to myelin-associated glycoprotein. Nevertheless, the circumstances where these antibodies will be present and clinically useful are small. There is no reason to order these studies routinely. Given their expense and low yield, these studies are probably best ordered by one knowledgeable about their limitations and possible clinical usefulness.

Given the large number of causes for neuropathies, how one approaches the evaluation of neuropathies will depend on the patients being seen. If one works in an area with a large industrial base, the main concerns may be entrapment and toxic neuropathies. If one deals with an elderly population, the concerns would include diabetes, hypothyroidism, monoclonal gammopathies, and paraneoplastic neuropathies. B$_1$2 deficiency may present in a subtle fashion and is worth evaluating in those with unexplained neuropathic sensory disturbances.

Management

If the underlying cause of a neuropathy can be established, treatment of this cause can improve the neuropathy. The neuropathies associated with hypothyroidism, carcinoma, and vitamin deficiencies, for example, improve with treatment. Uremic neuropathies can resolve after transplantation, and nerve dysfunction related to drugs (vincristine, heavy metals [lead], and industrial solvents [n-hexane, acrylamide]) can improve by removing the offending agent. A representative list of systemic disorders and toxic causes associated with peripheral neuropathy is presented in Table 13.3. Disulfiram, dapsone, and vincristine all can cause peripheral neuropathies, but they are used to treat conditions in which peripheral neuropathy is a common presentation—alcoholism, leprosy, and carcinoma. Inherited neuropathies such as Charcot-Marie-Tooth disease are common. Two specific neuropathies and their management are discussed in the following sections—acquired inflammatory polyradicular neuropathies and diabetic neuropathies.

TABLE 13.3. *Disorders of the Peripheral Nervous System*

Systemic Diseases	Vitamin Deficiency	Exogenous Toxins
Diabetes mellitus	Thiamine	Alcohol
Hypothyroidism	Pyridoxine	Chloramphenicol
Renal failure	Niacin	*Cis*-platinum
AIDS	Riboflavin	Dapsone
Intestinal malabsorption	Folic acid	Diphenylhydantoin
Acute intermittent porphyria	Vitamin B$_{12}$	Disulfiram
Amyloidosis		Ethionamide
Acromegaly		Glutethimide
Leprosy		Gold
Diphtheria		Hydralazine
Lyme disease		Isoniazid
Mycoplasma		Metronidazole
Rheumatoid arthritis		Nitrofurantoin
Systemic lupus erythematosus		Nitrous oxide
Paclitaxel (taxol)		
Polyarteritis nodosa		Perhexiline maleate
Wegener's granulomatosis		Pyridoxine (lack or excess)
Carcinoma		Thalidomide
Waldenströms macroglobulinemia		Vinca alkaloids
Multiple myeloma		*Heavy Metals*
POEMS (polyneuropathy, organomegaly, M protein, skin changes)		Lead
Cryoglobulinemia		Thallium
Paraproteinemia		*Industrial Agents*
(Monoclonal gammopathy of uncertain significance—MGUS)		Solvents:
Sarcoidosis		*n*-Hexane
Whipple's disease		Methyl-*n*-butyl-ketone
		2,5 Hexanedione
		Carbon disulfide
		Trichlorethylene
		Acrylamide
		Dimethylaminopropionitrile
		Dichlorophenoxyacetic acid
		Triorthocresyl phosphate
		Organophosphorus compounds
HIV		
Syphilis		

Treatment of neuropathies also may be symptomatic. Consultations with physiatrists and occupational therapists can be rewarding. Bracing, for example, may help a foot drop. Canes, walkers, and motorized wheelchairs can be helpful for those with gait problems. Useful implements can be made for those with limited finger and hand movement. Painful neuropathies are common, and pain is often the reason a patient with a neuropathy seeks medical attention. Neuropathic pain can be treated with medications. Representative medications and their dosages are shown in Table 13.4. The tricyclic antidepressants commonly are used for aching discomfort. The exact mechanism by which these drugs alleviate pain is unknown. However, they must be given in high enough doses and for a long enough period (i.e., several months) to ascertain whether they will be effective.

The anticonvulsants are more commonly used for "positive" symptoms such as paresthesias and dysesthesias. The latter reflect abnormal discharges in diseased nerves, and anticonvulsants presumably help by decreasing these discharges. Opiates can be helpful. Given their potential for abuse, a program of opiates is probably best instituted in conjunction with neurologic consultation. The exception may be tramadol because it has a relatively low potential for abuse. Nevertheless, it is important to be sensitive that tramadol is an opioid and has produced problems with addiction. The natural history for painful neuropathies is for improvement—either because of progression of the neuropathy and loss of pain fibers or because the neuropathies improve. Patients often are puzzled by the presence of pain and loss of feeling in the same area, such as the feet. This is common and reflects the differing effect of nerve injury on different nerve fibers.

ACQUIRED INFLAMMATORY POLYRADICULONEUROPATHY

Of remitting polyneuropathies, acute inflammatory polyradiculoneuropathy (AIPN), also known as the Guillain-Barré syndrome, is the most common, estimated to occur at a rate of 1.5 per 100,000 people. AIPN occurs most commonly in young adulthood and early middle age, preceded in almost half of patients by an antecedent infectious illness that usually clears before neurologic dysfunction begins. The etiology is thought to be immunologic. Of the patients, 20% to 30% have antiganglioside antibodies (GM1, GD1a) to neural antigens. The hallmarks of the syndrome are progressive, often profound, weakness; complete tendon areflexia; high spinal fluid protein; possible cranial nerve and respiratory compromise; and substantial or complete spontaneous recovery. Weakness develops over hours to days but should not progress longer than 4 weeks. The severe motor compromise, short duration of progression, and elevated cerebrospinal fluid (CSF) protein with few (<10 mononuclear cells/mm^3) are features that distinguish this syndrome. Sen-

TABLE 13.4. *Drug Treatment of Painful Neuropathies*

Drug	Suggested Starting Dose	Usual Maximum Dose
Tricyclic Antidepresssants		
Amitryptyline	10–25 mg HS; inc 10–25 mg Q7 days	150–200 mg HS
Nortriptyline	10–25 mg HS; inc 10–25 mg Q7 days	100–150 mg HS
Anticonvulsants		
Carbamazepine	100–200 mg bid; inc 100–220 mg Q3–7d	1200 mg/d as tid
Gabapentin	300–400 mg QD; inc 300–400 mg Q3–7d as tid	3600 mg/d as tid
Toprimate	50 mg QPM; inc 50 mg Q7d as bid	400 mg as bid
Opioids		
Tramadol	50 mg QD; inc 50 mg Q3–4d as qid	400 mg as qid

sory loss may be mild but should be looked for carefully because abnormalities of sensation help differentiate this syndrome from other conditions that may appear similar, including hypokalemia, botulism, and poliomyelitis. Pathologically, there is widespread inflammatory segmental demyelination, most prominent proximally and presumably immunologically mediated. Prominent axonal injury and marked decrease in evoked motor response amplitudes argue for a slow recovery.

Although there are characteristic clinical features, the variability of clinical presentation in actual practice should be emphasized. These include the Miller Fisher syndrome (ataxia, ophthalmoplegia, and hyporeflexia) as well as limited findings such as facial diplegia with cardiac arrhythmias indicative of focal injury to the facial and vagal nerves. The CSF protein may not be elevated initially, and repeated lumbar punctures may be necessary to demonstrate an increased protein with the associated characteristic dissociation between protein and cells. Autonomic instability may be a prominent feature and may result in morbidity and occasional mortality. EMG studies may reveal prominent slowing of nerve conduction, but evidence of conduction block associated with segmental demyelination and proximal conduction abnormalities may be the only findings. The EMG examination can have prognostic implications.

AIPN is considered idiopathic in origin. Syndromes similar to AIPN, however, may be found in conditions such as acute intermittent porphyria and Hodgkin's disease and less commonly with other neoplasms, hepatitis, infectious mononucleosis, Lyme disease, and recently acquired HIV infection. Certain toxic neuropathies such as with thallium may be similar.

Although recovery may be slow, the characteristic history of AIPN is one of almost complete improvement. As such, the most important treatment is symptomatic, particularly respiratory support and monitoring autonomic dysfunction. Steroids have been advocated, but they have not been beneficial and are possibly detrimental. Plasmapheresis or intravenous immunoglobulins (IVIG) can hasten recovery and appear particularly indicated for those with severe respiratory compromise and if used within 7 days of onset. A total of three to five courses of plasmapheresis usually is given every other day; the standard dose for IVIG is 0.4 g/kg/day for a total of 5 days.

A syndrome similar to AIPN sometimes may occur in a chronic (CIP) or a chronic relapsing (CIRP) form. In these patients, the symptoms progress for more than 4 weeks. In comparison to AIPN, the onset is often more gradual; antecedent infections are less common; and sensory symptoms and signs are more frequent. As in AIPN, the basic pathologic process is an inflammatory segmental demyelination, but there is also a loss of myelinated fibers. Onion bulbs are found as a result of repeated episodes of demyelination with remyelination. The CSF again shows high protein and relatively few cells at some stage in the illness, but it may be normal at the time of a particular examination. EMG studies characteristically show slowed conduction. Nerve biopsy may be helpful for the diagnosis. In contrast to AIPN, steroids are thought helpful in CIP and CIRP. Immunosuppressive agents also have been used, and plasmapheresis and IVIG have produced a temporary improvement. The clinical presentation of patients with chronic acquired neuropathies can be quite variable; there are no firm diagnostic EMG criteria. The treatments are costly and can have serious side effects, such as with high-dose steroid therapy. As such, the diagnosis and management of this condition should be in conjunction with those experienced with these problems.

NEUROPATHIES ASSOCIATED WITH DIABETES MELLITUS

Diabetes mellitus is common and often is associated with nerve dysfunction. Diabetic neuropathies are probably now the most common neuropathies in the Western world. The reported incidence of neuropathic abnormalities in diabetes has varied widely, most likely as a result of differing criteria and techniques used to diagnose PNS injury in these patients. A balanced view probably would indicate a prevalence of 50% to 60% of some form of neuropathy in patients with diabetes. The prevalence increases with the duration of the disease, but diabetic nerve dysfunction may be the initial sign of diabetes. Given the various presentations and probable pathogenesis, it is best to think in terms of diabetic neuropathies rather than in terms of a single entity.

Polyneuropathies, mononeuropathies, plexopathies, radiculopathies, and autonomic neuropathies all are found individually or in combination in diabetes, and diabetes therefore can be associated with abnormalities at any level of the PNS. Patients with asymptomatic diabetes may show decreased nerve conductions that can normalize with improved control of blood sugar. A distal sensory or sensorimotor polyneuropathy is the most common type of diabetic neuropathy. Although commonly described as "symmetric," careful examination of these patients frequently reveals some, even if limited, asymmetry. Describing the findings as "stocking glove" in distribution is actually somewhat misleading. The findings are related to the distance in the limbs from the spinal cord; sensory loss limited to the hands and feet would be consistent with spinal cord injury, not peripheral nerve. A loss of position, vibration, and light touch as well as decreased reflexes are prominent features of the "large fiber" pattern. Relatively pronounced loss of pain and temperature sensation, in association with pain, indicate predominant "small fiber" injury. The pain may have a dull, aching quality in the limbs and also a distal, burning discomfort most prominent at night. Rarely, there is a pattern of sensory ataxia, pain, and arthropathy (diabetic "pseudotabes"). The "small fiber" and "pseudotabetic" patterns may be associated with autonomic dysfunction, including an involvement of the gastrointestinal, cardiovascular, and genitourinary systems. Autonomic dysfunction also can occur without other evidence for a neuropathy. Postural hypotension, diarrhea, impotence, urinary retention, and increased sweating are examples of symptoms that may be caused by a diabetic autonomic neuropathy. The painful, asymmetric, proximal weakness of the legs found in diabetes (diabetic amyotrophy) is probably a result of the involvement of the lumbar plexus and frequently is found in the context of a history of weight loss. Clinical patterns of a polyradiculopathy may occur. Mononeuropathies can affect almost every major peripheral nerve as well as the cranial nerves, particularly the extraocular muscles. The onset of symptoms in mononeuropathies is characteristically abrupt and frequently painful. Diabetes may present as peroneal palsies.

The pathogenesis of diabetic neuropathies is varied. Metabolic derangements have been cited as the basis for the polyneuropathies. There is experimental evidence, however, that edema secondary to structural changes in endoneural blood vessels with associated ischemia may be the primary cause. This may account for the asymmetric clinical findings in patients with "symmetric" diabetic neuropathies. The abrupt onset of painful, focal lesions in the diabetic mononeuropathies is similar to that of other vascular neuropathies and has led to the concept that these neuropathies are the result of occlusion of the small, nutrient blood vessels supplying nerves. This finding, however, has not been confirmed pathologically.

The natural history of diabetic mononeuropathies, amyotrophies, and polyradiculopathies is one of improvement, even if slow. The course of diabetic polyneuropathies varies: some diabetic neuropathies improve, many plateau, and some steadily progress. A severe disability is the exception. The pseudotabetic variety is generally progressive and more disabling. Pain, particularly distal burning dysesthesias, can be a major problem. Although the manifestations of the autonomic neuropathy may be subclinical, they are not infrequently incapacitating. The prognosis for the autonomic neuropathy is among the worst of the diabetic neuropathies.

Good metabolic control is probably helpful for both preventing and ameliorating diabetic neuropathies, and good control of blood sugar therefore should be a goal in these patients. Exercise should be encouraged. Other therapies are symptomatic. An eye patch is helpful in patients with the self-limited diabetic ophthalmoplegia, and bracing may be helpful in those with peroneal palsy. Medications have been helpful in the painful sensory neuropathies (Table 13.4), and analgesics are reasonable for the acute pain associated with mononeuropathies. Trophic ulcers of the feet may require changes in shoe size, debridement, and antibiotics. Standard medical regimens should be tried for autonomic dysfunction. These regimens include codeine phosphate and diphenoxylate for diarrhea, support stockings and fluorocortisone or midodrine for postural hypotension, and regular voidings assisted by suprapubic pressure in those with bladder atony. Nighttime lights can assist walking in those patients with sensory loss by preserving visual cues.

FUTURE PERSPECTIVES

Our understanding of peripheral nerve disorders and their management remains unsatisfactory. There is the potential for an increased understanding of peripheral neuropathies. Newer techniques of histopathologic evaluation, including electron microscopy, teased fiber preparations, and morphometric analysis of nerves, already have added meaningfully to our understanding of both normal and abnormal nerves. Similarly, more sophisticated forms of electrophysiologic analysis should allow for a better evaluation of nerve dysfunction. These techniques include recording from single muscle fibers (single fiber EMG); computer analysis of motor unit firing, clinically applicable techniques for evaluating changes in ion conductances in nerves, and increasing routine study of a wider range of electrophysiologic responses and more sophisticated analysis in EMG studies. The recording of cortical responses evoked by peripheral nerve stimulation (somatosensory evoked responses) not only allows for a more detailed evaluation of certain peripheral nerve injuries but also provides a possible technique for evaluation at the interface between peripheral and CNS dysfunction. Immunologic studies are becoming increasingly important for understanding the pathogenesis of nerve disorders and for providing guides to therapy. Patients with a clinical picture similar to ALS but with conduction block on electrophysiologic examination and frequently elevated titers of anti-GM_1 antibodies have been treated successfully with immunosuppressive agents. Finally, basic research in the physiology, biochemistry, immunobiology, and axonal transport of nerves provides a dynamism and makes an interest in peripheral nerves rewarding.

QUESTIONS AND DISCUSSION

1. A 64-year-old patient with a 10-year history of insulin-dependent diabetes mellitus complains of burning dysesthesias in the feet. Examination reveals a mild decrease in strength at the toes and ankles; absent Achilles reflexes; decreased pinprick, touch, and vibration sensitivity to the knees; and decreased position sense in the toes. Electrodiagnostic studies indicate slowed motor conduction velocities and absent sensory potentials in the legs with evidence of denervation distally in the lower extremities on needle EMG examination. Sensory conductions in the upper extremities are slowed.

Four weeks later, the same patient develops weakness in the left leg associated with some pain in the region of the left knee. An examination 3 weeks after onset reveals relatively more prominent decreased pinprick and touch sensation in the lateral aspect of the left leg and dorsum of the left foot, as well as lack of dorsiflexion and eversion of the left ankle. EMG examination shows no evoked motor response stimulating at the fibula head and denervation in the left tibialis anterior, peronei, and extensor digitorum brevis muscles.

Is the history in the first or second part of the first question indicative of a polyneuropathy, mononeuropathy, or radiculopathy? Are both of these histories compatible with a diabetic etiology?

Answer: The description in the first part of the first question would be characteristic of a polyneuropathy. The clinical and electrodiagnostic examinations reveal a diffuse sensorimotor neuropathic process most prominent distally.

The history and findings in the second part, by contrast, would indicate a mononeuropathy of the left peroneal (anterior tibial) nerve. Clinically, there is sensory loss, motor weakness, and EMG abnormalities in the distribution of that nerve.

Diabetes mellitus can produce both a polyneuropathy and a mononeuropathy, not infrequently in the same patient. The pathogenesis of the polyneuropathy is probably multifactorial, including metabolic derangements and ischemia, whereas the mononeuropathy may be secondary to vascular infarction of the peroneal nerve.

A diabetic polyneuropathy argues for good diabetic control. Diabetic mononeuropathies usually resolve with time because of the partial nature of the nerve injury secondary to the ischemic insult. A short leg brace to aid in dorsiflexion of the left ankle could be helpful for this patient during the recovery period.

2. A 50-year-old woman has a 6-month history of progressive pain in her right wrist. A diagnosis of hypothyroidism recently has been made. This pain awakens her at night, usually within several hours of falling asleep. She has noticed clumsiness in the use of that hand and complains of paresthesias radiating into the thumb and index fingers. Recently, she has noted some discomfort in the left wrist. An examination reveals paresthesias and pain radiating to the fingers on tapping the wrists bilaterally (positive Tinel's signs); weakness of the right abductor pollicis brevis muscle; and numbness involving the right thumb, index finger, and middle finger as well as the adjacent one-half of the ring fin-

ger. There is also numbness involving the lateral half of the palmar surface of the right hand.

This history most likely represents mononeuropathy of which nerve? Where is the lesion located? Is the process probably unilateral or bilateral? EMG examination reveals a prolongation of the median distal motor latencies and a lack or slowing of median sensory potentials, more prominent on the right. Are these findings consistent with your diagnosis?

Answers: The case presentation would be compatible with a diagnosis of a carpal tunnel syndrome (CTS). This syndrome is a mononeuropathy caused by "entrapment" of the median nerve as it passes through the carpal tunnel at the wrist. A positive Tinel's sign is a common clinical finding in an area of partial nerve injury, and progression of this sign distally can be used to follow regeneration after a nerve has been severed. Characteristic electrodiagnostic findings in the CTS are those that indicate median nerve dysfunction at the level of the wrist—that is, prolonged motor conduction stimulating the nerve at the wrist and recording from median-innervated thenar hand muscles as well as prolonged median sensory conductions with the level of injury at the wrist. The history would suggest a bilateral process—an assumption confirmed by the electrodiagnostic studies. Bilateral involvement in the CTS is present in approximately 25% of the cases. This syndrome is frequently part of several systemic illnesses including hypothyroidism. A CTS may be the presenting complaint in a patient with abnormal thyroid function.

Initial treatment would consist of therapy for the hypothyroidism as well as splinting the wrists to limit movement. If these measures failed, the transverse carpal ligaments probably should be surgically sectioned. Steroid injections can produce symptomatic relief, but the long-term effectiveness and the possible harm of this therapy have been debated.

3. A 55-year-old patient undergoing vincristine therapy has developed progressive weakness over several weeks, resulting in an

inability to walk. An examination reveals decreased vibration in the legs, decreased pin sensation to the upper legs and in the fingers, preserved position sense, absent reflexes in the legs, and moderate to marked weakness in the legs and mild to moderate weakness in the arms, most marked distally. Electrodiagnostic studies reveal borderline, slow motor conduction velocities with considerable evidence of denervation, again most prominent distally.

Does this polyneuropathy involve primarily axons or myelin, and what is the appropriate treatment?

Answers: The history and clinical findings would be typical for a polyneuropathy secondary to vincristine therapy. The prominent denervation indicates disruption of the normal connections between nerve and muscle. Combined with the borderline slowing of conduction velocities, the primary disease is of axons rather than of myelin—that is, an axonal type of neuropathy. The treatment is to stop the vincristine.

4. A 35-year-old man has a 6-month history of weakness in the hands that now involves the legs. An examination reveals atrophy and fasciculations in the intrinsic muscles of the hands, weakness that is distally more prominent in the upper than in the lower extremities, hyperactive reflexes, and extensor plantar responses bilaterally. Sensory testing is unremarkable. Electrodiagnostic examination reveals normal motor and sensory conduction studies in the presence of denervation and decreased activation of motor units in all four extremities. Many of the motor units are both large and polyphasic. A cervical myelogram has been unremarkable.

Questions

This would be characteristic of a neuropathic process at what level of the motor unit? What is the most likely diagnosis? Would a sural nerve biopsy be helpful for the evaluation of this neuropathy?

Answers: The history and findings are consistent with a diagnosis of ALS. The extensor

plantar responses and hyperactive reflexes would indicate some involvement of the long motor system tracts in the CNS, but the atrophy and fasciculations would be consistent with involvement of the lower motor neurons. This is confirmed by the electrodiagnostic studies, which indicate a chronic motor neuropathic process not readily explained by a process primarily affecting peripheral nerves, plexuses, or roots. The normal conduction velocities indicate preservation of at least some of the fast-conducting (i.e., largest) motor axons. Because the pathologic process involves strictly efferent (i.e., motor) fibers, a sural nerve biopsy would not be helpful. The sural is a sensory nerve and therefore contains only afferent fibers.

Nerve dysfunction may involve either motor or sensory fibers only. In ALS, the primary pathology is at the lower motor neuron level in the anterior horns of the spinal cord. It may be argued this is not an illness of the PNS. Conversely, because ALS involves the cell bodies of efferent fibers with resultant abnormalities in nerve and muscle, the illness might be considered a prototypical axonal neuropathy.

SUGGESTED READING

Blume G, Pestronk A, Goodnough LT. Anti-MAG antibody–associated polyneuropathies: improvement following immunotherapy with monthly plasma exchange and IV cyclophosphamide. *Neurology* 1995;45:1577.

Brown WF, Bolton CF, Aminoff MJ, eds. *Neuromuscular function and disease: basic, clinical, and electrodiagnostic aspects.* Vols. 1 and 2. Philadelphia: WB Saunders, 2002.

Cros D, ed. *Peripheral neuropathy: a practical approach to diagnosis and management.* Philadelphia: Lippincott Williams & Wilkins, 2001.

Donofrio PD, Alber JW. Polyneuropathy: classification by nerve conduction studies and electromyography. *Muscle Nerve* 1990;13:889.

Dyck PJ, Thomas PK, Griffin JW, et al, eds. *Peripheral neuropathy,* Vols. 1 and 2. Philadelphia: WB Saunders, 1993.

Kimura J. *Electrodiagnosis in diseases of nerve and muscle.* Philadelphia: FA Davis, 2001.

Latov N. Pathogenesis and therapy of neuropathies associated with monoclonal gammopathies. *Ann Neurol* 1995; 37(Sl):S32.

Mendell JR, Kissel JT, Cornblath DR, eds. *Diagnosis and management of peripheral nerve disorders.* Oxford: Oxford University Press, 2001.

Notermans NC, Lokhurst JIM, Franssen H. Intermittent cyclophosphamide and prednisone treatment of polyneuropathy associated with monoclonal gammopathy of undetermined significance. *Neurology* 1996;47:1227.

Parry JG. *Guillain-Barré syndrome.* New York: Thieme, 1993.

Pestronk A. Motor neuropathies, motor neuron disorders, and antiglycolipid antibodies. *Muscle Nerve* 1991;14:927.

Ropper AH, Gorson KC. Neuropathies associated with paraproteinemia. *N Engl J Med* 1998;338:1607.

Saperstein DS, Katz JS, Amato AA, et al. Clinical spectrum of chronic acquired demyelinating polyneuropathies. *Muscle & Nerve* 2001;24:311–324.

Schaumberg HH, Berger AR, Thomas PK. *Disorders of peripheral nerves.* Philadelphia: FA Davis, 1992.

Stalberg E, Trontelj JE. *Single fiber electromyography.* Old Woking, England: Miravalle Press, 1994.

Tuck RR, Schmelzer JD, Low PA. Endoneurial blood flow and oxygen tension in the sciatic nerves of rats with experimental diabetic neuropathy. *Brain* 1984;107:935.

14

Vertigo and Dizziness

Judd M. Jensen

Of all the reasons patients seek medical attention, few engender more frustration on the part of physicians and more anxiety on the part of patients than the complaint of dizziness. The physician's frustration seems to be rooted in the perceived difficulties of establishing an accurate diagnosis and providing effective therapy. The patient's fears are grounded in the significant discomfort associated with many of these syndromes and the subsequent assumption that whatever is wrong must be equally horrible. However, the majority of the syndromes discussed below are benign and not life-threatening. The physician's first step—and often an important one—in treating patients who are dizzy is the explanation of this fact and the conveyance of an understanding of the disease process. This chapter will attempt to provide a logical approach to the evaluation of patients with vertigo and dizziness so that an accurate diagnosis and subsequent prognosis can be made. Effective therapies for some of these syndromes have been developed, and these will be discussed in detail.

LET THE PATIENTS TELL THEIR STORY

In assessing patients with dizziness syndromes, it is important that physicians keep their questions open ended during history taking. Beginning the interview with direct questions alters the spontaneity and character of the patient's replies and, thus, reduces their diagnostic value. The best approach is to coax the patient to first describe his or her symptom complex in his or her own words. An accurate diagnosis often can be made in the first few minutes of the encounter by using this

method. Later, specific and important questions that were not addressed by the patient, such as symptom frequency and duration, precipitating body positions, and associated symptoms, can be asked. By using this approach, the history is diagnostic in the majority of cases. At the very least, the patient's symptom complex can be placed into one of the three following categories.

DEFINITIONS AND CATEGORIES

Vertigo

Patients who have vertigo experience a false sensation of movement. Most commonly, they report that their environment is spinning around them. However, the sensations of tilting, swaying, and being impelled forward, backward, or to either side are also vertiginous. Nausea, vomiting, and some degree of imbalance typically are associated as are autonomic signs such as diaphoresis, pallor, and tachycardia. These patients have a disorder of either the peripheral or central vestibular system. Peripheral vestibular disorders comprise approximately 90% of cases. Patients with peripheral or central vestibular disorders seek medical attention with either an acute episode of vertigo or with a history of recurrent attacks of vertigo (Table 14.1).

Presyncope

Patients who have presyncope describe their dizziness as "lightheadedness" or "feeling like I'm going to faint." This sensation usually is associated with generalized weakness, visual blurring or blackout, diaphoresis, shortness of breath, or palpitations. The patient usually looks pale to an observer. It

TABLE 14.1. *Distinguishing Peripheral and Central Vestibular Disorders by Bedside Examination*

	Peripheral	Central
Presence of headache and/or alteration in level of consciousness	Never	Frequent
Type of spontaneous nystagmus	Mixed, unidirectional, suppressed by fixation	Pure, multidirectional, unsuppressed by fixation
Gait ataxia	None or mild	Moderate or severe
Appendicular ataxia	Absent	Often present
Presence of hearing loss or tinnitus	Occasional	Never
Presence of other focal neurologic symptoms or signs[a]	Never	Frequently
Positive head thrust test (see text)	Usually	Never

[a]Diplopia, dysarthria, dysphagia, Horner's sign, hoarseness, hiccoughs, unilateral or bilateral facial or extremity weakness or numbness.

should be noted that occasionally patients with presyncope report vertigo during their episodes, presumably because of inadequate perfusion in the brainstem vestibular nuclei. This can lead to diagnostic confusion with the primary vestibular syndromes, although the remainder of the clinical picture usually distinguishes the two types of dizziness. Presyncope is typically episodic and is caused by a transient reduction in global cerebral perfusion. Therefore, it is a primary cardiovascular problem rather than a neurologic one.

Disequilibrium

Disequilibrium is a more complex category than the previous two. Whereas patients with vertigo and presyncope tend to have episodic symptoms or attacks, patients with disequilibrium typically have more continuous symptoms. The key historical feature is that these patients are dizzy primarily when standing or walking and tend to improve when seated or supine. They often have difficulty describing what they feel. Responses such as "bad balance," "poor equilibrium," or "I'm just dizzy" are common. Disequilibrium is the result of dysfunction at one or more points in the complex system required for bipedal balance and ambulation. The causes of this dysfunction are many and varied, as will be discussed.

VERTIGO SYNDROMES

Anatomy, Physiology, and Pathophysiology

Vertigo is a symptom of disease in the vestibular system. This system usually is divided into peripheral and central components. The peripheral vestibular apparatus includes the labyrinth, which is located in the petrous portion of the temporal bone, and the vestibular portion of the eighth cranial nerve, which connects the labyrinth to the brainstem and is located in the internal auditory canal and cerebellopontine angle. The labyrinth is divided into three semicircular canals that sense head rotation and the otoliths (utricle and saccule) that sense head position relative to gravity. The central vestibular apparatus consists of vestibular nuclei at the pontomedullary junction in the brainstem. These nuclei receive impulses from the eighth cranial nerve and have rich connections with the nuclei controlling eye movements and the cerebellum. Normally, the paired labyrinths supply balanced tonic impulses to the central nervous system (CNS) regarding the position of the head and its movements. Vertigo occurs when a pathologic process acutely disrupts the input from one labyrinth. The remaining unbalanced contralateral input produces the false sensation of movement. With time, the CNS will adjust to unilateral input. Vertigo is thus typically acute and episodic. A pathologic process that slowly disrupts the input from one labyrinth either will be asymptomatic or will produce a disequilibrium syndrome such as those that follow.

Neighborhood Signs

The physician must determine whether a patient's vertigo is of central or peripheral origin. The presence of one or more neighborhood signs and symptoms may be helpful in making this distinction. The most important neighborhood symptoms in peripheral vestibular lesions are hearing loss and tinnitus. These occur in diseases affecting the cochlea, the middle ear, and the acoustic portion of the eighth cranial nerve. Processes that disrupt the vestibular portion of the eighth nerve in the cerebellopontine angle or in the internal auditory canal usually also affect the acoustic portion. Likewise, labyrinthine processes also may affect the cochlea or middle ear. Central processes affecting the brainstem and cerebellum rarely cause hearing loss or tinnitus. However, it should be noted that there is one peripheral vestibular disorder related to cerebrovascular disease. Occlusion of the internal auditory artery typically causes sudden, profound, unilateral hearing loss and vertigo.

Eighth cranial nerve and cerebellopontine angle mass lesions (i.e., acoustic neuroma) often present with progressive hearing loss and/or tinnitus and can have associated facial weakness, facial sensory loss, and/or a depressed corneal reflex. However, it is distinctly unusual for such lesions to produce either an acute vertigo syndrome or recurrent attacks of vertigo. When acoustic neuroma and other mass lesions of the eighth nerve and cerebellopontine angle produce dizziness, it is more commonly a disequilibrium syndrome related to slow destruction of the vestibular portion of the eighth cranial nerve or pressure on the brainstem vestibular nuclei.

The vertigo seen in central vestibular syndromes frequently is accompanied by one or more neighborhood symptoms and signs. It is important to note that it is often the presence of such additional findings that clearly defines the vertigo as central in origin. The list of possible neighborhood signs and symptoms includes diplopia, cortical blindness, homonymous hemianopsia, dysarthria, dysphagia, Horner's sign, hiccoughs, hoarseness, bilateral extremity weakness or sensory symptoms, and unilateral or bilateral facial weakness or numbness.

The degree of gait ataxia is an important distinguishing feature in vertigo syndromes. Patients with peripheral vestibular syndromes usually can stand, although they typically complain of feeling unsteady and often will lean to one side when standing. Patients with central vestibular disorders often are unable to stand at all. In addition, prominent appendicular ataxia in the form of finger-to-nose or heel-to-shin dysmetria is suggestive of a central process, usually a cerebellar infarction or hemorrhage (Table 14.1).

Nystagmus

Nystagmus is present in virtually all patients during the acute experience of vertigo. It typically subsides as soon as the vertigo resolves in peripheral vestibular syndromes. However, the nystagmus may persist longer than the vertigo in central syndromes. Nystagmus is often difficult to appreciate in a vertigo syndrome of peripheral vestibular origin. Part of the reason for this has to do with the way physicians typically examine eye movements. By having the patient focus on the index finger while it moves side to side as well as up and down, the physician is requiring visual fixation. Such fixation tends to suppress nystagmus of peripheral vestibular origin. The optimal way to examine such patients is by watching their eye movements while fixation is prevented. This is ideally done with the use of Frenzel lenses. These are +30 diopter binocular lenses, which the patient wears during the examination. These lenses prevent visual fixation on the part of the patient but allow the examiner to see the eye movements. If such lenses are unavailable, there is a simple bedside technique that may be used to demonstrate nystagmus in peripheral vestibular lesions. While the examiner is performing a funduscopic examination on one eye with an ophthalmoscope, the contralateral eye is alternately covered and uncovered. When the eye is uncovered, the patient is asked to fixate on an object in the room. If the patient has a peripheral vestibular syndrome, the examiner should be able to detect an increase in the amplitude of the nystagmoid jerks (by watching the movement of the optic disk) when the contralateral eye is covered (fixation prevented) as opposed to when it is uncovered and the patient is able to fixate.

There are other ways of distinguishing central and peripheral nystagmus. Nystagmus of peripheral origin is unidirectional—that is, the fast component of the nystagmus always beats in the same direction, no matter which direction the patient is looking. For example, with a left peripheral vestibular lesion, the fast component of the nystagmus will be to the right on left lateral gaze, right lateral gaze, or vertical gaze. Nystagmus of peripheral origin also is mixed—that is, it typically has both a horizontal and a rotatory or torsional component. Nystagmus of central origin is typically multidirectional (i.e., the fast component of the nystagmus changes with the direction of gaze). Pure horizontal, pure vertical, or pure rotatory nystagmus is almost always central. Unfortunately for diagnostic purposes, nystagmus of central origin can mimic peripheral nystagmus by being unidirectional or of a mixed form. Peripheral lesions, however, almost never produce multidirectional or pure forms of nystagmus. Perhaps the best means to distinguish central from peripheral nystagmus is by the response to fixation. Central nystagmus is not suppressed and frequently is enhanced by fixation. In general, the nystagmus of central vestibular disorders is more prominent and more persistent than the nystagmus of peripheral vestibular origin.

Head Thrust Test

The head thrust test can be very helpful in distinguishing peripheral and central vestibular disorders. It can be performed quickly and easily at the bedside. The examiner holds each side of the patient's head with his or her hands. The head is turned 10 degrees to the right or left of primary position. The patient is asked to keep his or her eyes fixed on the examiner's nose. The examiner then quickly turns the patient's head 10 degrees back to the primary position. In a normal response, the patient's eyes remain fixed on the examiner's nose. If there is a unilateral peripheral vestibular lesion, the patient's eyes will move with the head and then make a corrective return to the examiner's nose after the movement is over. The test should be repeated with the head 10 degrees to the opposite side. A unilateral abnormal response indicates an ipsilateral peripheral vestibular injury.

Electronystagmography

Electronystagmography (ENG) can be a useful test in evaluating patients with disorders of the vestibular system. The technique takes advantage of the rich connections between the vestibular and ocular motor nuclei. This examination requires skill and experience to perform and interpret. Unfortunately, the results do not always provide the clinician with definitive answers. At best, ENG can determine the presence of vestibular dysfunction, establish the unilateral or bilateral nature of the dysfunction, and distinguish central from peripheral vestibular dysfunction.

CAUSES OF RECURRENT EPISODES OF VERTIGO

Benign Paroxysmal Positional Vertigo

Clinical Syndrome

Benign paroxysmal positional vertigo (BPPV) is the most common diagnosis in patients who seek medical evaluation for vertigo. It is also the most common cause of recurrent vertigo by a wide margin. The history is characteristic: the patients report that a few seconds after assumption of a certain head position (usually supine in bed), they experience the sudden onset of vertigo, which lasts 15 to

60 seconds and then resolves. The patients also may note that if they put their heads in the same position a second or a third time (within a relatively brief interval), the vertigo will be less intense each time. The key historical features are the characteristic head position (there can be more than one), the brief latency to onset of vertigo, and the fatigability of the vertigo with repeated trials.

The patient's symptom complex frequently can be reproduced in the office with the Dix-Hallpike maneuver (Fig. 14.1). This maneuver begins with the patient sitting on the examination table. His head is turned 45 degrees to the right, and then he is quickly put in the supine position with his head hanging over the edge of the table and extended approximately 30 degrees. If the vertigo does not begin within 30 seconds, he is returned to the sitting position, his head is turned 45 degrees to the left, and the patient is again made supine with his head extended. If this maneuver is performed during one of the patient's symptomatic periods, it almost always produces vertigo associated with nystagmus that has a prominent rotatory or torsional character.

This syndrome is most commonly idiopathic but can be seen after head trauma; an acute peripheral vestibulopathy; or, rarely, with a variety of other structural posterior fossa lesions. The pathophysiology of this syndrome is thought to be an accumulation of calcium carbonate crystals that form a plug, usually in the posterior semicircular canal. When the patient places his head in the recumbent position with the affected canal down, the calcium carbonate plug acts as a plunger and stimulates the labyrinth, thus producing the vertigo. The latency reflects the time required for the plunger to move in the canal and stimulate the system. The fatigability reflects dispersion of the calcium carbonate crystals in the canal with repeated movement.

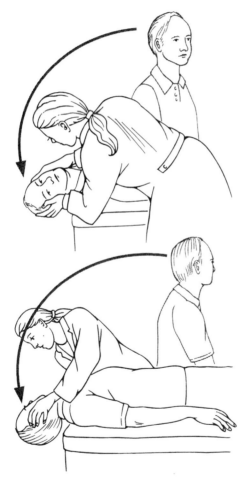

FIG. 14.1. Dix-Hallpike positional test for benign positional nystagmus. Patient is moved rapidly from the sitting to the head-hanging position. (Redrawn from Baloh RW, Halmagyi GM, eds. *Disorders of the vestibular system.* Copyright 1996 by Oxford University Press, Inc. Used by permission.)

Treatment of Benign Paroxysmal Positional Vertigo

The treatment of this syndrome is directed at moving the calcium carbonate crystals from the posterior semicircular canal into the utricle by either a canal-particle-repositioning maneuver called the modified Epley maneuver (Fig. 14.2) or by a series of bedside exercises (see Brandt and Daroff's *Physical therapy for benign paroxysmal positional vertigo*). The Epley maneuver should be performed until it no longer produces vertigo. This may require two to five repetitions of the maneuver at the time of initial treatment. The patient then should be instructed to sleep up-

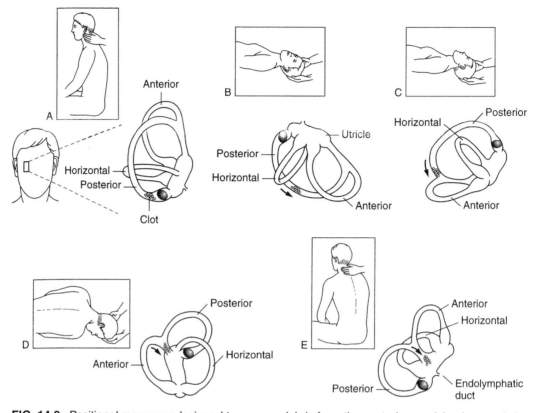

FIG. 14.2. Positional maneuver designed to remove debris from the posterior semicircular canal. **A:** In the sitting position the clot of calcium carbonate crystals lies at the bottommost position within the posterior canal. **B:** Movement to the head-hanging position causes the clot to move away from the cupula, producing an excitatory burst of activity in the ampullary nerve from the posterior canal (ampullofugal displacement of the cupula). **C:** Movement across to the other head-hanging position causes the clot to move further around the canal. **D:** The patient then rolls onto the side facing the floor, causing the clot to enter the common crus of the posterior and anterior semicircular canals. **E:** Finally, the patient sits up, and the clot disperses in the utricle. The maneuver is repeated until no nystagmus is induced, and the patient then is instructed not to lie flat for 48 hours (to prevent the debris from reentering the canal). (Redrawn from Epley JM. The canalith repositioning procedure: for treatment of benign paroxysmal positional vertigo. *Otolaryngol Head Surg* 1992;107:399, with permission.)

right for the next two nights and to wear a soft cervical collar continuously for 72 hours. Both the Epley maneuver and the bedside exercises are effective treatments in the majority of patients. The natural history of this disorder is typically a waxing and waning course over months to years. The treatments will put most patients into a "remission," but the symptoms may recur at some point. Most cases eventually resolve. Rare cases are unremitting, debilitating, and unresponsive to treatment. In such cases, surgical division of the posterior ampullary nerve or occlusion of the posterior semicircular canal can be considered. No data are available on the treatment of BPPV with alternative medications.

In a clinically typical case of BPPV (with characteristic head position, latency, and fatigability) with a normal neurologic examination and a positive Dix-Hallpike maneuver, no brain imaging is necessary. The only workup required is a screening audiogram. Significantly asymmetric sensorineural hearing loss, especially high tone loss, would require that the patient have a magnetic resonance imaging (MRI) scan of the posterior fossa. This entity is not associated with hearing loss, tinnitus, or other vestibular system neighborhood signs. The presence of any of these should prompt a search for an alternate diagnosis, and such patients should have MRI of the brain and posterior fossa.

A Word of Caution

Movement-related vertigo (MRV) can be a source of confusion and occasionally is misinterpreted as BPPV. MRV typically occurs after a patient has had a prolonged episode of vertigo (i.e., acute peripheral vestibulopathy, vertebrobasilar ischemia) but can occur *de novo*. In MRV, almost any head or body movement produces vertigo. In addition, there is no latency or fatigability as in BPPV. It is this lack of specificity of head movement and the absence of latency and fatigability that distinguish MRV from BPPV. MRV can be seen in any peripheral or central vestibular process.

Ménière's Disease

Clinical Syndrome

Ménière's disease is a syndrome characterized by recurrent attacks of vertigo, hearing loss, tinnitus, and aural fullness. Classically, the patient experiences the entire symptom complex with each episode. However, there is considerable variability and there are atypical cases of Ménière's that have only vestibular symptoms (i.e., vertigo) without cochlear symptoms (hearing loss and tinnitus) and others with cochlear symptoms and no vertigo. Attacks of vertigo can be as short as a few minutes and rarely last longer than 4 or 5 hours. The hearing loss fluctuates and usually improves after the vertigo resolves. However, over time there is progressive loss of hearing. The pathologic findings associated with this syndrome are referred to as endolymphatic hydrops. However, the pathophysiology that leads to this pathologic endpoint is not understood. It is possible that there are multiple causes that lead to this common endpoint. Serial audiograms are very helpful in the diagnosis and management of these patients. As noted, fluctuating hearing loss is typical. Low-frequency hearing is lost first, but eventually there is a global loss of auditory function. All patients should have an MRI of the posterior fossa. Symptoms typically begin in one ear but ultimately become bilateral in nearly 50% of patients. Approximately 80% of patients go into remission within 5 years, although most of these will be left with significant hearing loss and some with a chronic disequilibrium syndrome.

Treatment of Ménière's Disease

Salt restriction has been shown in some studies to reduce the frequency of the attacks of vertigo and hearing loss. This treatment should be initiated with a restriction of 1 to 2 g of sodium per day. If this level of restriction is ineffective, then sodium should be reduced to less than 1 g/day. Thiazide diuretics and acetazolamide also have been reported to be helpful in some patients. Smoking and consumption of caffeinated beverages exacerbate Ménière's disease and should be avoided. Some patients have frequent, disabling attacks of vertigo. Historically, surgical ablative procedures, such as labyrinthectomy and vestibular neurectomy, have been offered in such patients. More recently, endolymphatic-mastoid shunts have been used with some success. There also has been increasing interest in the use of intratympanal gentamicin. This modality seems to prevent the recurring attacks of vertigo and often maintains some auditory function. Most authors feel that this is now the treatment of choice. No data are available on the treatment of Ménière's disease with alternative medications.

Migraine

The vestibular nuclei in the brainstem receives its blood supply from branches of the basilar artery, so it is not surprising that migrainous vasospasm of the basilar artery can produce vertigo. Other neurologic symptoms such as scintillating scotoma, homonymous hemianopsia, cortical blindness, diplopia, dysarthria, ataxia, paresthesias, and quadriparesis also may be seen with vertigo in this syndrome. Hearing loss and tinnitus also may be associated with basilar artery migraine.

These patients are usually young, and the history typically is dominated by the severe headache that follows the vertigo. In some patients, however, the headache may not be prominent, whereas in others the headache may not always follow the vasospastic component of the syndrome. This latter phenomenon is called a migraine equivalent and should be considered in a patient with isolated attacks of vertigo who also has a history of vertigo followed by headache. The treatment of basilar artery migraine is similar to the treatment of other migraine syndromes and is not discussed here.

Perilymph Fistula

The perilymph fistula syndrome results from an abnormal communication between the perilymphatic space of the inner ear and the pneumatized middle ear. It usually is caused by head trauma or barotrauma. The latter can be obvious, as in the case of a deep-sea diver, or quite subtle, as after straining at stool or a hard cough. The patients experience a variable symptom complex that can include episodic vertigo, fluctuating hearing loss, tinnitus, and a disequilibrium syndrome. The symptoms usually are triggered by Valsalva, exertion, or further barotrauma. There is no completely satisfactory diagnostic test for this disorder. Findings on pneumatic otoscopy can be helpful, but they are not specific or sensitive enough to be definitely diagnostic. The most reliable diagnostic method is the elicitation of a history of an appropriate inciting event and the reproduction of symptoms with Valsalva or repeated barotrauma. Initial treatment should include at least 4 to 8 hours of strict bed rest with the head elevated and avoidance of any activity that would increase intraabdominal pressure (i.e., bending, lifting, straining). If this fails to result in improvement, then surgical grafting of the oval and round windows can be considered.

Temporal Lobe Epilepsy

Rarely, vertigo can be experienced as part of a temporal lobe seizure, typically representing the aura of the seizure. However, the clinical picture usually is dominated by other manifestations of the seizure, including alteration of consciousness, automatisms, and postictal disorientation. On very rare occasions, the patient may experience frequent auras without the remainder of the seizure. In this circumstance, this syndrome could conceivably be confused with a vestibular disorder. However, an electroencephalogram (EEG) is not considered part of the routine workup of patients with vertigo syndromes. A positive head thrust test usually can be elicited.

CAUSES OF A SINGLE ACUTE EPISODE OF VERTIGO

Acute Peripheral Vestibulopathy

Clinical Syndrome

Acute peripheral vestibulopathy is the second most common cause of vertigo for which patients seek medical attention. Vestibular neuritis, vestibular neuronitis, and labyrinthitis are terms frequently used to refer to this syndrome, although the last should be used only when there is associated hearing loss. The pathophysiology of this disorder is incompletely understood. Although it is thought to have a viral or postviral etiology, the proof of this pathogenesis is lacking. This syndrome is an acute disorder of the peripheral vestibular system and is benign in its prognosis. However, it must be distinguished from ischemic or hemorrhagic vertebrobasilar vascular disease, which will be discussed.

Despite the confusing nomenclature and uncertain pathophysiology, the clinical syndrome is well known to most clinicians. In the typical acute peripheral vestibulopathy, the vertigo is gradual in onset, peaks in several hours, and resolves by 24 to 48 hours. Patients remain fairly incapacitated during the experience of vertigo and usually have associated nausea, vomiting, and gait ataxia. They typically prefer to remain motionless during this time because any head or body movement tends to exacerbate the vertigo. A disequilibrium syndrome often follows the resolution of the vertigo and may persist for days, weeks, or even months. This disequilibrium is caused by a mismatch between the aberrant input to the brain from the affected vestibular apparatus and the normal tonic input from the unaffected contralateral side. The disequilibrium eventually will resolve in the vast majority of patients regardless of whether there is complete recovery of the affected vestibular apparatus. This recovery is the result of CNS compensation for the imbalance in vestibular tone.

The neurologic examination during the vertigo phase is remarkable only for nystagmus of the type seen in peripheral vestibular lesions (as described earlier). A positive head thrust test usually can be elicited. There may be mild gait ataxia, with the patient tending to veer to the side of the affected vestibular apparatus. However, prominent gait ataxia, extremity ataxia, or other vestibular neighborhood signs should raise the question of a brainstem or cerebellar infarction or hemorrhage. During the period of disequilibrium, after the vertigo resolves, the neurologic examination may be quite normal despite the patient's complaints of persistent dizziness and imbalance.

A typical case in a young healthy adult requires no brain imaging. However, in older patients and in those with risk factors for vascular disease, an urgent noncontrast computed tomography (CT) scan of the brain is necessary to exclude a cerebellar hemorrhage. Ischemic disease of the cerebellum and brainstem is poorly imaged by CT. Therefore, MRI may be necessary in these patients (see later).

Treatment of Acute Peripheral Vestibulopathy

Therapy for acute vertigo consists of bed rest, intravenous fluids, phenothiazines, antihistamines, and benzodiazepines (Table 14.2). The use of corticosteroids and antiviral agents has been studied in patients with acute vestibular syndromes of presumed viral etiology. No clear benefit has been discerned. Patients who develop a prolonged disequilibrium syndrome can be treated with vestibular exercises (discussed later in "Therapy for Disequilibrium"). There are no data on treatment of acute vertigo with alternative medications.

TABLE 14.2. *Pharmacologic Treatments for Acute Vertigo Syndromes*[a]

Drug	Starting Dose	Maintenance Dose	Potential Drug Interaction
Promethazine (Phenergan)	25 mg IM, IV PR, or PO	12.5–50 mg Q4–8 h	Tranquilizers, antiparkinsonian medications
Prochlorperazine (Compazine)	10 mg IM, IV, PR, or PO	5–20 mg Q4–12 h	Tranquilizers, antiparkinsonian medications
Droperidol[b] (Inapsine)	2.5 mg IM or IV	2.5–10 mg Q3–4 h	Tranquilizers, antiparkinsonian medications
Dimenhydrinate (Dramamine)	50 mg IM, IV, or PO	25–100 mg Q4–8 h	Sedatives, tranquilizers, antidepressants
Meclizine (Antivert)	25 mg PO	12.5–50 mg Q4–8 h	Sedatives, tranquilizers, antidepressants
Diazepam (Valium)	5 mg IM, IV, or PO	2–10 mg Q4–8 h	Sedatives, antidepressants
Lorazepam (Ativan)	1 mg IM, IV, or PO	0.5–2 mg Q4–8 h	Sedatives, antidepressants

IM, intramuscularly; IV, intravenously; PR, by rectum; PO, by mouth.
[a]All of these medications are useful for acute vertigo. However, they may exacerbate the chronic disequilibrium syndrome that often follows vertigo syndromes.
[b]Should not be administered to patients with known or suspected prolonged QT syndrome.

Vertebrobasilar Vascular Disease: Posterior Circulation Vascular Events

Clinical Syndrome

Vertigo is a cardinal symptom in several of the posterior circulation stroke syndromes. These diagnoses should be considered in any patient with persistent vertigo who has risk factors for vascular disease (hypertension, diabetes mellitus, heart disease, hyperlipidemia, tobacco abuse) or in any elderly patient regardless of the presence of risk factors. One study suggested that up to 25% of patients who present to the emergency room with isolated vertigo and who have risk factors for vascular disease may have inferior cerebellar infarctions.

The vertigo in these vascular syndromes usually is abrupt in onset and maximal at the beginning, unlike peripheral vestibular syndromes, in which the vertigo typically worsens over several hours. Gait ataxia is usually a prominent feature in posterior circulation stroke, and many patients are unable to stand. Similarly, appendicular ataxia in the form of finger-to-nose or heel-to-shin dysmetria is often prominent. The most ominous posterior circulation disorder is cerebellar hemorrhage. This potentially fatal condition is important to recognize because surgical decompression often is required and is life saving. These patients usually are identified by the presence of prominent headache and some degree of altered level of consciousness. However, headache and lethargy can be absent initially and then develop hours later when edema from the hemorrhage begins to produce brainstem compression. To complicate matters further, headache occurs in several of the posterior circulation ischemic strokes. Cerebellar hemorrhage can be diagnosed accurately by a noncontrast CT scan of the brain. Patients with this disorder require an urgent neurosurgical evaluation and intensive care unit (ICU) monitoring.

The ischemic vertigo syndromes, in general, have a more benign prognosis. However, because of the increasing effectiveness of secondary or recurrent stroke prevention, these are important diagnoses to make. The most common ischemic syndromes are those of the vertebral artery (VA) and the posterior inferior cerebellar artery (PICA). After the VA enters the skull, it gives rise to the PICA and then supplies perforating branches to the lateral medulla before joining with the other VA to form the basilar artery. The PICA gives variable branches to the lateral medulla before supplying the inferior surface of the cerebellum. Occlusion of the VA typically produces a lateral medullary infarction. However, depending on the site of the occlusion, there also may be ischemia in the PICA distribution and, thus, an inferior cerebellar infarction. Similarly, primary occlusion of the PICA produces ischemia to the inferior cerebellum but also may cause infarction of the lateral medulla. Thus, there are many similarities in the vascular syndromes produced by disease of these two vessels.

Lateral medullary infarction is the most common brainstem ischemic stroke and usually is referred to as the Wallenberg syndrome. The vertigo in this syndrome can be associated with a wide variety of symptoms including dysarthria, dysphagia, hoarseness, hiccoughs, Horner's sign, diplopia, facial pain or numbness, and gait and limb ataxia. Most patients will have loss of pain and temperature sensation on the face ipsilateral to the infarction regardless of whether they complain of facial numbness. Most patients also will have loss of pain and temperature sensation on the contralateral side of the body. These patients are usually not aware of this deficit, so it must be sought by the examiner in all suspected cases of vertigo of ischemic origin. The typical Wallenberg syndrome has two or three of these symptoms and signs. The entire clinical picture is seen only rarely. In inferior cerebellar infarction, vertigo, ataxia, nausea, and vomiting are the only symptoms. A small percentage of these patients develop significant edema in the area of cerebellar infarction with resultant brainstem compression. This group of patients, like those with cerebellar hemorrhage, may require surgical decompression.

The anterior inferior cerebellar artery (AICA) supplies the lateral pons, the vestibular and cochlear structures via a branch called the internal auditory artery, and the anterior inferior portion of the cerebellum. Occlusion of the distal portion of this vessel can produce a cerebellar infarction that is clinically identical to that seen in the PICA syndrome. Occlusion of the internal auditory artery produces sudden, profound hearing loss and severe vertigo. Finally, occlusion of the more proximal portion of the AICA produces a brainstem syndrome with ipsilateral facial weakness, resembling a Bell's palsy. There may be associated hearing loss, and vertigo if the ischemia extends into the internal auditory artery.

The vertigo in these vascular syndromes tends to last longer than the vertigo seen with peripheral vestibular lesions. Moreover, the ataxia and nystagmus seen in central lesions tend to persist well beyond the resolution of the vertigo. This does not occur with peripheral vestibular disorders. Finally, the nystagmus seen with these posterior circulation vascular syndromes has the character of central nystagmus discussed previously.

Any of the ischemic stroke syndromes that can cause vertigo also can present as transient ischemic attacks. These episodes can be difficult to distinguish from a peripheral vestibular syndrome because the patient usually is not examined until after the symptoms have resolved. As a general rule, any episode of vertigo lasting less than 30 minutes in a patient with risk factors for stroke should be considered a possible transient ischemic attack. Vertigo lasting seconds is unlikely to be ischemic in etiology and probably is related to a peripheral vestibular process.

MRI is the optimal diagnostic tool for evaluating patients with posterior circulation stroke syndromes. Specifically, MR diffusion-weighted imaging often will demonstrate an ischemic lesion less than 1 hour after onset of symptoms. However, this examination is not required in all patients. As mentioned, any patient with persistent vertigo who is older than age 60 or has risk factors for vascular disease should have a noncontrast CT scan of the brain to rule out a cerebellar hemorrhage. CT will not demonstrate most ischemic posterior circulation strokes. In patients with a vertigo syndrome where a clear distinction between a peripheral and a central etiology cannot be made, MRI should be performed. Evaluation for vertebrobasilar vascular stenosis can be done by either MR angiography (MRA, an imaging technique that does not require the injection of contrast material) or by transcranial Doppler ultrasonography (TCD). TCD is not available at many institutions. MRA generally is available wherever MRIs are performed. Both techniques have advantages and disadvantages. MRA produces a multidimensional image of the vessels being examined but often has a tendency to overestimate the degree of stenosis. TCD is very sensitive for the detection of significant stenosis in the vertebrobasilar system, but this technique can be limited by neck thickness and vessel tortuosity. These two noninvasive studies correlate best with standard angiography when they are in agreement.

Treatment of Posterior Circulation Vascular Events

Neurosurgical decompression is required for many patients with cerebellar hemorrhage and some patients with large ischemic cerebellar infarctions. Otherwise, the acute management of posterior circulation stroke is similar to that of hemispheral stroke syndromes: avoidance of overaggressive blood pressure management, prevention of dehydration, swallowing evaluation when appropriate, deep-vein thrombosis prophylaxis, and antiplatelet agents. There is no proven role for anticoagulation in posterior circulation ischemia caused by atherosclerotic disease of the vertebrobasilar system. Patients with posterior circulation stroke as a result of cardiogenic embolism should be considered for anticoagulant therapy. If a cardiac or aortic cardiac source of embolism is suspected, transesophageal echocardiography is the diagnostic test of choice. Otherwise, risk-factor modification is the mainstay of secondary stroke prevention. Carotid endarterectomy is not indicated for secondary stroke prevention in posterior circulation ischemia.

Multiple Sclerosis

Vertigo is one of the cardinal symptoms of multiple sclerosis. It can occur as the presenting symptom or in a patient with an established diagnosis. The clinical syndrome can mimic acute peripheral vestibulopathy. The character of the nystagmus may be the only distinguishing feature. Hearing loss is rare but does occur in this disease. Any young person who presents with an acute vertigo syndrome should be questioned about past neurologic symptoms. The long-forgotten optic neuritis or the transient extremity paresthesias that were thought to reflect a pinched nerve may be a clue to the etiology of their vertigo syndrome. MRI is the diagnostic test of choice for multiple sclerosis. Although it may not always demonstrate brainstem or cerebellar lesions, the periventricular white matter lesions usually are present. Therapy consists of pulse oral or intravenous corticosteroids.

SPECIAL CONSIDERATIONS FOR HOSPITALIZED PATIENTS

Many patients with prolonged episodes of vertigo will require hospitalization because of severe discomfort and/or protracted vomiting. For patients with peripheral vestibular disorders, the symptomatic medications listed in Table 14.2 combined with fluid and electrolyte replacement are the mainstays of therapy. It is important to reassure the patient and family regarding the benign and self-limited nature of the disease because many patients are fearful their symptoms will be prolonged or reflect some life-threatening process. Education of the patient regarding the disequilibrium syndrome that often follows the resolution of the vertigo and instruction on vestibular exercises are also important. Patients should be cautioned about resuming their full level of activity prematurely.

Patients with posterior fossa and vascular events often do not require as much symptomatic treatment as those with peripheral vestibular syndromes. However, the workup and treatment options are more complex, as discussed earlier. All patients with cerebellar hemorrhages who have had surgical evacuation and all patients with ischemic cerebellar infarctions require close observation for changes in the neurologic status. In particular, change in level of alertness is an early sign of brainstem compression and should be dealt with on an emergent basis. Most of these patients should be monitored in an ICU setting with frequent neurologic checks for at least 72 hours. Intravenous fluids should be kept to a minimum, vomiting should be controlled, sedatives should be avoided, and the head of the bed should be raised to 30 degrees.

WHEN TO REFER PATIENTS WITH VERTIGO TO A NEUROLOGIST OR OTHER SPECIALIST

For recurrent episodes of vertigo, if the primary care physician is inexperienced or uncomfortable performing the Epley maneuver and the patient with BPPV has not responded to the bedside exercises, then referral to a neurologist or otolaryngologist who has experience performing the Epley maneuver should be made.

All patients with suspected Ménière's disease should be evaluated and followed by either a neurologist or otolaryngologist with an interest in vestibular disorders. All patients whose history suggests the presence of a perilymph fistula should be seen by an otolaryngologist.

Any acutely vertiginous patient who has risk factors for vascular disease or is older than age 50 years should be evaluated by a neurologist. Similarly, any patient with vertigo accompanied by headache, a change in level of alertness, or findings on neurologic examination that suggest a central vestibular process requires a neurologic evaluation.

PRESYNCOPE

After vertigo, the second category of dizziness is presyncope. Presyncope is a primary cardiovascular problem with neurologic symptoms. Lightheadedness, visual blurring or blackout, facial or extremity paresthesias, and generalized weakness result from a global reduction in cerebral perfusion from either a decrease in systemic arterial pressure, failure of cardiac output, or diffuse cerebral vasoconstriction. Diaphoresis, palpitations, and nausea often are present as the autonomic nervous system becomes activated in an attempt to restore cerebral perfusion. Most patients with presyncope will have their symptom complex reproduced by hyperventilation even if hyperventilation syndrome is not the cause of their symptoms. This can be useful in the bedside evaluation of patients with dizziness. Hyperventilation results in a drop in arterial P_{CO_2} with subsequent cerebral arterial vasoconstriction and global reduction in cerebral blood flow. The procedure can be performed by holding a handkerchief or tissue 12 inches in front of the mouth and having the patient breath rapidly and deeply for up to 3 minutes. The handkerchief or tissue must be displaced significantly with each exhalation to ensure hyperventilation. If this procedure exactly reproduces the patient's dizziness, the physician can be confident of a presyncopal syndrome.

Presyncope is caused by a global reduction in cerebral perfusion and, therefore, it is not a transient ischemic attack, which is always the result of a focal area of brain ischemia. Although presyncope occasionally can be difficult to distinguish from a vertebrobasilar transient ischemic attack, this syndrome cannot be the result of carotid ischemia. Finally, presyncope is not a type of seizure, and an EEG is not a useful part of the diagnostic evaluation of patients with this syndrome.

Causes of Presyncope

Hyperventilation Syndrome

Hyperventilation syndrome is a common cause of presyncope and occurs in two forms. The patient with high-grade hyperventilation tends to have acute episodes of dizziness that are precipitated by stressful situations or panic attacks. These patients usually have the complete syndrome, including visual blurring, perioral and digital paresthesias, and generalized weakness. They often are aware of breathing rapidly or feeling short of breath. The patient with low-grade hyperventilation has a more protracted and insidious form of dizziness. The symptoms tend to wax and wane over longer periods. Visual blurring, paresthesias, and generalized weakness usually are absent. Patients are almost never aware that they are overbreathing, and they do not feel short of breath. This syndrome occurs in anxious, pressured, driven individuals. They may exhibit frequent sighing during the office interview.

The symptom complex of both high-grade and low-grade hyperventilators can be reproduced easily by the technique of artificial hyperventilation, as described earlier. In fact, these patients tend to be very sensitive to even short periods of induced hyperventilation. Reassurance regarding the etiology and benign nature of their symptom complex is the most important aspect of treatment for these patients. The high-grade hyperventilator may be helped by placement of a paper or plastic bag over the mouth during the attacks. Supportive psychotherapy or counseling may be helpful in some patients. Anxiolytic agents may be appropriate in selected patients.

Orthostatic Hypotension

Orthostatic hypotension is also a common cause of presyncope, particularly in the elderly. The symptoms almost always occur when the patient is standing and are frequently maximal just after the patient rises from the sitting or supine position. Gravity decreases venous return to the heart, resulting in a decline in left heart filling. The autonomic nervous system normally is able to adjust peripheral resistance, cardiac rate, and contractility so that cardiac output and blood pressure are maintained. However, if the patient is hypovolemic from fluid loss or diuretic therapy, if he has been pharmacologically vasodilated, or if his compensatory autonomic responses are blunted by medication or disease, cardiac output and blood pressure may fall sufficiently to produce presyncopal symptoms. In these patients, a significant drop in blood pressure usually can be demonstrated at the bedside and this procedure often will reproduce the patient's symptom complex. The blood pressure always should be checked as the patient goes directly from the supine to the standing position. It is important to note that asymptomatic but demonstrable orthostatic blood pressure changes are common in the elderly. If the patient's history does not suggest orthostatic hypotension and the orthostatic maneuver does not reproduce the symptoms, then the observed drop in blood pressure may not be the cause of the dizziness.

The most common causes of orthostatic hypotension are diuretic and other antihypertensive medications. Other causes of this syndrome include autonomic neuropathy, primary orthostatic hypotension, and Shy–Drager syndrome.

Symptomatic orthostatic hypotension from antihypertensive medications should be treated by adjusting the patient's medication regimen. The "neurologic" causes of chronic orthostatic hypotension have several possible treatments. Raising the head of the patient's bed by 30 degrees can be very helpful. Elastic stockings are another simple initial treatment. If these maneuvers do not provide adequate symptomatic relief, then sodium chloride tablets can be added judiciously if they are not contraindicated by hypertension, congestive heart failure, hepatic disease, or renal failure. The mineralocorticoid fludrocortisone acetate can be used in difficult cases. The initial dose is 0.05 mg (half a tablet) three times a week. This may be increased gradually as tolerated. Blood pressure and serum electrolytes must be monitored closely. The new alpha agonist midodrine also can be used in selected patients.

Vasodepressor or Vasovagal Presyncope

Vasovagal presyncope is probably more correctly called neurocardiogenic presyncope. The patient's history is usually diagnostic. The episode of dizziness occurs either in a hot crowded room or in the setting of sudden pain or strong emotion. The patient always is standing and may have premonitory symptoms of yawning, diaphoresis, and pallor. The reduction in blood pressure and cerebral blood flow are caused by sudden, reflux dilation of the resistance arterioles. This syndrome usually occurs in young, otherwise healthy adults but can occur in the elderly. Hot, crowded rooms favor a vasodilation and could produce symptomatic hypotension in an elderly patient with otherwise compensated mild orthostatic hypotension. The only treatments for this syndrome are reassurance and avoidance of the precipitating circumstances.

Cardiac Presyncope

Cardiac presyncope usually is caused by an arrhythmia that produces a sudden decrease in cardiac output and a subsequent decrease in cerebral perfusion. Common offending arrhythmias include sick sinus syndrome, paroxysmal supraventricular tachycardia, atrial fibrillation-flutter, complete heart block, and ventricular tachycardia. This diagnosis should be strongly considered in any patient whose presyncope occurs in the sitting or supine position. Workup includes an electrocardiogram and Holter monitoring, although it sometimes requires repeated or prolonged monitoring to document the arrhythmia. Exercise-related presyncope may be caused by aortic stenosis or idiopathic hypertrophic subaortic stenosis. An echocardiogram is used for the diagnosis of these conditions. Finally, paroxysmal episodes of lightheadedness and dizziness can be a manifestation of coronary ischemia. These episodes sometimes are called angina equivalents because the patients may not experience chest pain. This diagnosis should be considered in any patient with unexplained episodes of presyncope and the appropriate risk factors.

Carotid Sinus Hypersensitivity

Carotid sinus hypersensitivity is primarily a disorder of the elderly in which the carotid sinus in the neck becomes abnormally sensitive to pressure and produces episodes of bradycardia and reduced cardiac output. Classically, this syndrome was described in men who wore tight collars. However, such a history will not be present in most patients with this disease. It should be suspected in middle-aged or elderly patients with ongoing bouts of presyncope or syncope. The diagnosis is made by carotid massage under strictly controlled conditions (i.e., the presence of a crash cart and personnel skilled in cardiopulmonary resuscitation). The treatment is placement of a permanent pacemaker.

Hypoglycemia

Although this metabolic derangement does not cause a reduction in cerebral blood flow, its symptom complex is similar to that seen in presyncope. Thus, it should be considered in evaluating patients with episodic dizziness.

Most patients with symptomatic hypoglycemia are insulin-dependent diabetics who either did not consume an adequate caloric load for their insulin dose or took an excessive dose of insulin. Oral hypoglycemic agents are occasionally unpredictable in their action and can produce symptoms of hypoglycemia. Early diabetics who are not yet on therapy can have reactive hypoglycemia from surges of insulin. This typically occurs 2 to 5 hours after eating and is more often manifested by diaphoresis and palpitations than lightheadedness and other "neurologic" symptoms. The diagnosis is made by documenting serum hypoglycemia while the patient is symptomatic. In general, a serum glucose less than 50 mg/dl is necessary to produce CNS symptoms. Insulin-secreting tumors can present with repeated episodes of hypoglycemia.

When to Refer the Patient with Presyncope to a Neurologist

Because syncope is cardiologic in origin, the neurologist is not a final referral expert. If questions of vertebrobasilar cerebral ischemia occur, the neurologist will help in defining brainstem signs or symptoms.

SPECIAL CONSIDERATIONS FOR HOSPITALIZED PATIENTS WITH PRESYNCOPE

The stress and anxiety of hyperventilation can augment hyperventilation, and prolonged bedrest can enhance orthostatic hypotension, so hospital staff must be aware of these causes of presyncope. Dehydration and constipation can enhance vasovagal presyncope, and nursing staff should be educated on alert surveillance for these frequently encountered hospitalization problems.

DISEQUILIBRIUM

After vertigo and presyncope, disequilibrium is the third category of dizziness to consider. Disequilibrium is a common problem in the elderly but can be seen in younger patients after an acute vertigo syndrome or mild head trauma. Unlike the vertigo in presyncope syndromes, the dizziness tends to be more constant and is typically maximal with standing and ambulation. These patients often complain of feeling off balance and are insecure when walking. They tend to reach for walls or furniture when ambulating at home or in the office. They may feel even more uncomfortable when outside.

There are a number of etiologies of disequilibrium, and some patients have more than one contributing cause. Before these causes are discussed, a review of the physiology of human balance mechanisms will be presented.

NORMAL MECHANISMS OF EQUILIBRIUM

Gravity and environmental stimuli are constant challenges to bipedal locomotion. Several coordinated events must occur to ensure proper maintenance of an upright posture and smooth ambulation. First, the CNS must get adequate sensory input regarding the position of the head and body in space relative to the earth and the pull of gravity. Second, the CNS must be able to correctly process the sensory input. Third, an appropriate motor response must be mounted to meet the gravitational and environmental challenge. Deficits in one or more of these physiologic functions result in imbalance or disequilibrium.

Four sensory inputs provide information regarding the position of the head and body in space. The most important of these inputs is vision. Visual loss alone (even complete blindness) does not usually produce disequilibrium. However, the visual system is an important compensatory mechanism when there are other sensory or motor deficits. Therefore, visual loss in the setting of such additional deficits can be disabling for the patient and can produce significant balance difficulties. Whereas visual loss alone does not usually produce disequilibrium, visual distortion often does. Such distortion typically occurs when the visual input from one eye is significantly different from the other.

The vestibular system is the second most important sensory input for balance. It provides information regarding movement and the relationship of the head to the pull of gravity. Acute, unilateral vestibular disturbances produce vertigo, but slowly progressive, bilateral, or healing vestibular lesions produce a disequilibrium syndrome. Position sense or proprioception in the joints and muscles of the lower extremities is the third input necessary for normal balance. Hearing is the fourth sensory modality necessary for normal equilibrium.

PROCESSES THAT DISTURB EQUILIBRIUM

A broad range of diseases can interfere with sensory input, central integration, or motor response and therefore produce disequilibrium. Some patients with this syndrome have disease at only one level. However, many patients have disease at multiple levels or with multiple facets of the same level (i.e., multiple sensory deficits).

Abnormalities of Sensory Input

As mentioned, diseases that distort vision tend to cause disequilibrium more commonly than those that produce visual loss alone. Many patients with sudden ophthalmoplegia and resultant diplopia feel off balance during ambulation. Some corneal and retinal diseases that produce significant asymmetry of visual input also can produce disequilibrium.

A wide variety of diseases of the vestibular system can produce disequilibrium. As mentioned, many patients recovering from an acute peripheral vestibulopathy will have residual dizziness for as long as several weeks. Likewise, patients with recurrent peripheral vestibular dysfunction, as in Ménière's syndrome, may have persistent disequilibrium between their acute attacks of vertigo and hearing loss. A number of drugs are known vestibulotoxins. Anticonvulsants and benzodiazepines produce reversible vestibular dysfunction. Aminoglycoside antibiotics and cisplatin produce vestibular injury that is often not reversible. These drugs tend to produce a disequilibrium syndrome rather than acute vertigo. Slow-growing neoplasms of the posterior fossa (e.g., acoustic neuroma) may produce a feeling of imbalance as well as hearing loss, facial numbness, and facial weakness. There are a variety of congenital and hereditary vestibular disorders that can produce progressive disequilibrium. Finally, idiopathic degenerative vestibular dysfunction is a recognized cause of disequilibrium in elderly patients.

Peripheral neuropathy can produce proprioceptive loss in the lower extremities and subsequent disequilibrium. This is probably most commonly seen with diabetic polyneuropathy but can result from any cause of peripheral neuropathy. Spinal cord disease, particularly when involving the posterior columns, can produce significant proprioceptive loss in the lower extremities and subsequent disequilibrium.

Hearing loss alone does not usually produce disequilibrium. However, in the presence of other deficits of sensory input, it can contribute to a patient's feeling of imbalance.

Abnormalities of Central Integration

Any process that produces a global impairment in CNS function can produce disequilibrium. Many patients complain of dizziness after minor head trauma. This syndrome may be the result of mild, diffuse, cerebral dysfunction from the head injury. Medications, particularly those with sedative side effects, may impair central integration. Likewise, patients with metabolic encephalopathy of any etiology may have a disruption of central integrative processes and disequilibrium.

Abnormalities of Motor Response

There are three major elements in the human motor system: the pyramidal system, the extrapyramidal system, and the cerebellum. Disturbance in any one of these elements can produce a disequilibrium syndrome. Parkinson's disease, a degenerative disorder of the extrapyramidal system, produces bradykinesia, rigidity, flexed posture, and a loss of postural reflexes. Patients with Parkinson's disease occasionally complain of dizziness and feeling off balance because they are unable to mount a smooth motor response to their environmental challenges.

The pyramidal system can be involved with disease at multiple levels. Degenerative frontal lobe dysfunction can produce significant gait apraxia. Likewise, hydrocephalus and frontal lobe neoplasms can interfere with normal motor function. At the spinal level, cervical spondylitic myelopathy is a common cause of lower-extremity stiffness and spasticity. All of these syndromes can interfere significantly with gait and cause a feeling of imbalance.

The cerebellum is involved significantly in the coordination of gait and can be affected by a wide variety of disease processes. These would include primary and alcoholic degenerative syndromes, cerebellar neoplasms, paraneoplastic syndromes, cerebellar infarction, and demyelinating disease. Any of these processes can produce a disequilibrium syndrome.

DIAGNOSTIC EVALUATION IN PATIENTS WITH DISEQUILIBRIUM

A review of the patient's medication regimen and a careful neurologic examination are the first steps in the evaluation of these patients. Medications that are vestibulotoxins should be discontinued if possible. Likewise, medications with significant sedative side effects should be reduced in dosage or discontinued.

If the patient offers complaints that suggest visual distortion, then an ophthalmologic evaluation should be obtained. A history of hearing loss or tinnitus should be sought. The unilateral presence of these symptoms should lead to a posterior fossa evaluation by MRI. Most patients who have had an acute peripheral vestibulopathy with vertigo will provide that history, but all patients with disequilibrium should be quizzed about past episodes of vertigo.

A careful and complete neurologic examination should be performed in all patients with disequilibrium. Proprioceptive function in the feet can be tested by having the patient close his eyes while the examiner moves the first toe of each foot up or down. The patient should be able to appreciate movements of 1 cm or less. The Romberg maneuver is a test of proprioceptive function in the lower extremities. However, this test also can be abnormal in patients with cerebellar or vestibular disease. Tone should be tested carefully in all extremities. The presence of cogwheel rigidity suggests the presence of an extrapyramidal syndrome. Spasticity in the lower extremities suggests either a spinal cord or frontal lobe dysfunction. These syndromes usually are associated with hyperactive deep tendon reflexes and bilateral Babinski signs. Observing the patient's gait is probably the most important part of the examination. Parkinson's disease produces a shuffling gait with a flexed posture and reduced movements in the upper extremities. Frontal lobe dysfunction produces a stiff gait with short steps. The patient may have difficulty initiating steps or getting through doorways. Feet may appear stuck to the floor. Spinal cord disorders tend to produce a spastic gait. Cerebellar disorders typically produce a wide-based, often staggering gait.

Patients with frontal lobe dysfunction will need either a CT or an MRI scan of the brain.

Patients with cerebellar syndrome should be evaluated by MRI because CT is not reliable for imaging of the posterior fossa. Patients with spinal cord syndromes require MRI scan of the cervical spine. All patients with frontal lobe or cerebellar dysfunction require a thyroid battery to rule out hypothyroidism.

WHEN TO REFER PATIENTS WITH DISEQUILIBRIUM TO A NEUROLOGIST

A high percentage of these patients will have one or more neurologic diagnoses. Therefore, the great majority of these patients should have at least an initial evaluation by a neurologist.

THERAPY FOR DISEQUILIBRIUM

Patients with Parkinson's disease can be treated effectively with dopaminergic agents that can improve their gait and reduce the feeling of disequilibrium. There is no definitive therapy for the degenerative frontal lobe disorders. Patients with hydrocephalus potentially can be treated with ventricular shunting. Frontal lobe and cerebellar neoplasms often can be effectively treated with surgical excision. Alcohol cerebellar degeneration may improve somewhat with abstinence. Paraneoplastic cerebellar degeneration has been reported to improve after treatment of the underlying neoplasm. Cervical spondylitic myelopathy potentially can improve with surgical decompression.

Patients with peripheral neuropathy may improve with the use of a light cane, which can provide some adjunctive proprioceptive input through the hand. Patients with degenerative vestibular disorders sometimes benefit from the use of a soft cervical collar (best worn with the Velcro clasp in front). By reducing head movement, this modality dampens aberrant vestibular input.

Patients who are experiencing disequilibrium after an acute vestibular syndrome, with a chronic vestibular syndrome such as Ménière's disease, with drug-induced vestibular toxicity, or after an episode of minor head trauma may experience benefit from vestibular exercises. The goal of these exercises is to accelerate the process of central vestibular compensation. The program should include exercises to improve ocular stability and balance. Eye and head coordination exercises begin with slow oscillations of the head from side-to-side while maintaining visual fixation on a stationary target. As the patient begins to improve, exercises that provide stronger stimulation to the central vestibular centers should be used. The eyes are kept stationary in the primary position and the head is moved back and forth or up and down over an excursion of at least 90 degrees. This exercise is done slowly at first and then more rapidly as the patient's tolerance increases. As further improvement is noted, these head movements should be performed while the patient is standing and walking. Patients should be advised that these exercises will likely transiently increase their sense of disequilibrium. However, they ultimately will result in more rapid resolution of their syndrome.

Balance exercises can be performed in the home or anywhere that a straight walkway 20 to 30 feet in length can be found. The patient begins the exercise by walking. The feet should be spread wide apart, and the arms should be outstretched laterally and parallel to the floor. The patient should walk up and down the walkway, narrowing the distance between the feet with each pass until the balls of the feet touch with each step. The procedure then is repeated with the arms held tightly at the side. It then is performed a third time with the arms outstretched in front of the patient, parallel to the floor. When this procedure is completed, the whole exercise is repeated with the eyes closed. The entire procedure should take 20 to 30 minutes and should be performed twice a day.

Finally, meclizine often is used to treat patients with the various disequilibrium syndromes. With the exception of an occasional patient with a chronic vestibular disorder, this drug is ineffective and actually may exacerbate the disequilibrium for some patients by its sedative side effects.

QUESTIONS AND DISCUSSION

1. J.D. is a 42-year-old man who experienced the sudden onset of vertigo, nausea, vomiting, and ataxia 3 weeks ago. The vertigo, nausea, and vomiting resolved in 48 hours, but the patient still complains bitterly of "dizziness" and states that he cannot go back to work because "I walk like a drunk." When questioned, he admits that his dizziness is present only when he is standing or walking and seems to resolve when he is sitting or supine. He denies hearing loss and tinnitus. There is no associated visual blurring, diaphoresis, or pallor. His neurologic examination is normal except that he tends to veer to the right when walking. How would this patient's current symptom of dizziness be categorized?

A. Vertigo
B. Presyncope
C. Disequilibrium
D. Malingering
E. Not classifiable

The answer is (C). The patient's syndrome began with vertigo. However, it has converted to a disequilibrium syndrome. This is a common sequela to acute vestibulopathy, caused by a residual mismatch between the inputs from the paired vestibular systems. The symptoms usually resolve over several weeks, and recovery often is hastened with the use of vestibular exercises.

2. S.T. is a 28-year-old woman who complains of a 2-week history of "everything is spinning around." The episodes are precipitated by any type of head movement in the horizontal or vertical plane. The vertigo begins immediately with each head movement. The patient denies hearing loss and tinnitus but does recall a 2-week episode of "numbness" below her waist about 3 months ago. When she was asked to follow the examiner's finger with her eyes, coarse horizontal nystagmus was noted on lateral gaze bilaterally and vertical nystagmus was present on upgaze. Her neurologic examination was otherwise remarkable only for questionable bilateral Babinski signs. The most likely diagnosis is:

A. Depression
B. Benign paroxysmal positional vertigo
C. Ménière's disease
D. Multiple sclerosis
E. Perilymph fistula

The answer is (D). This patient's symptoms are typical of movement-related vertigo, a nonspecific symptom that can be seen in any vestibular disorder. The multidirection, pure horizontal, or pure vertical nystagmus that is not suppressed by fixation is essentially diagnostic of a central vestibular disorder. The history of transient neurologic symptoms in the lower extremities would make multiple sclerosis a strong diagnostic consideration. The position-related vertigo of benign paroxysmal positional vertigo usually is produced by a single head position, there is a latency of several seconds to the onset of vertigo, and the vertigo tends to fatigue with repeated trials. Ménière's disease can be associated with movement-related vertigo, but there is also a history of hearing loss and tinnitus. Finally, in both benign paroxysmal positional vertigo and Ménière's disease, the nystagmus would have characteristics of peripheral vestibular disease (i.e., unidirectional, mixed, and suppressed by fixation).

3. H.L. is a 69-year-old man who complains of "dizzy spells." The patient describes 10 to 12 episodes in the last 6 weeks of sudden visual "blackout" and feeling "like I'm going to pass out." His wife notes that he breaks out in a cold sweat during the attacks and looks "glassy-eyed." The episodes last 30 to 60 seconds, and the patient feels "fine" afterward. There is no history of vertigo, hearing loss, tinnitus, or other focal neurologic symptoms. The spells are not related to body position or exercise and have occurred in many different situations including watching TV and eating in a restaurant. The patient's neurologic examination is normal, and 3 minutes of hyperventilation reproduce his symptom complex. The patient's dizziness should be categorized as:

A. Vertigo
B. Presyncope
C. Disequilibrium

D. Vertebrobasilar insufficiency

E. Hypoglycemia

The answer is (B). The patient's symptoms are typical of those caused by globally diminished cerebral perfusion. Vertebrobasilar insufficiency causes focal areas of ischemia and focal neurologic symptoms. The episodes are too brief and too discreet for hypoglycemic attacks.

What is the most likely etiology of this patient's presyncope?

A. Hyperventilation syndrome

B. Vasovagal attacks

C. Orthostatic hypotension

D. Cardiac arrhythmia

E. Aortic stenosis

The answer is (D). Hyperventilation should reproduce the symptom complex in all patients with presyncope so the diagnosis of hyperventilation syndrome must be made by other criteria (i.e., the situations of stress or anxiety in which it typically occurs). Vasovagal or vasodepressor attacks are also situational (i.e., hot, crowded room or sudden emotion) and always occur when the patient is upright. Likewise, orthostatic hypotension occurs only when the patient is standing. The aortic stenosis produces exercise-related presyncope. Most patients with type II symptoms that occur when sitting or supine have a cardiac arrhythmia.

4. Which of the following conditions can produce disequilibrium?

A. Chronic renal failure

B. Diabetes mellitus

C. Aminoglycoside antibiotic toxicity

D. Spondylitic cervical myelopathy

E. All are correct.

The answer is (E); all four conditions can produce disequilibrium. Chronic renal failure is associated with peripheral neuropathy that diminishes sensory input from the lower extremities. In addition, the metabolic encephalopathy of uremia may inhibit proper central integration of the sensory modalities required for balance and thus exacerbate the feeling of disequilibrium. Diabetes mellitus also is associated with a peripheral neuropathy. In addition, this disease also frequently is complicated by retinopathy, which decreases input from the most important sensory modality for balance. Aminoglycoside antibiotics can damage the vestibular portion of the eighth cranial nerve and produce a disequilibrium syndrome. Cervical spinal cord compression can decrease sensory input from the lower extremities and cause spasticity, which impedes the proper motor response for balance and ambulation. Parkinson's disease also prevents a smooth motor response and, therefore, can cause a disequilibrium syndrome.

SUGGESTED READING

Baloh RW. Vestibular neuritis. *N Engl J Med* 2003;348: 1027–1032.

Baloh RW. Vertigo. *Lancet* 1998;352:1841.

Baloh RW. Eposidic vertigo: central nervous system causes. *Curr Opin Neurol* 2002;15:17.

Brandt T, Daroff RB. The multisensory physiological and pathological vertigo syndromes. *Ann Neurol* 1980;7:195.

Brandt T, Daroff RB. Physical therapy for benign paroxysmal positional vertigo. *Arch Otolaryngol* 1980;106:484.

Brandt T. Otolitic vertigo. *Adv Otorhinolaryngol* 2001;58: 34.

Derebery MJ. The diagnosis and treatment of diseases. *Med Clin N Amer* 1999;83(1):163.

Drachman DA, Hart CW. An approach to the dizzy patient. *Neurology* 1972;22:323.

Epley JM. The canalith repositioning procedure for treatment of benign paroxysmal positional vertigo. *Otolaryngol Head Neck Surg* 1992;107:399.

Epley JM. Particle repositioning for BPPV. *Otolaryngol Clin North Am* 1996;29:323.

Furman JM, Cass SP. Benign paroxysmal positional vertigo. *N Engl J Med* 1999;341:1590.

Goebel JA. Management options for acute versus chronic vertigo. *Otolaryngol Clin North Am* 2000;33(3):483.

Hain TC, Micco AG. Cranial nerve VIII: vestibulocochlear system. In: Goetz CG, ed. *Textbook of clinical neurology,* 2nd ed. Philadelphia: WB Saunders, 2003.

Lipsitz LA. Syncope in the elderly. *Ann Intern Med* 1983; 99:92.

Magnusson M, Karlberg M. Peripheral vestibular disorders with acute onset of vertigo. *Curr Opin Neurol* 2002;15:5.

Nelson RL. Hypoglycemia: fact or fiction? *Mayo Clin Proc* 1985;60:844.

Norrving B, Magnusson M, Holtas S. Isolated vertigo in the elderly: vestibular or vascular disease? *Acta Neurol Scand* 1995;91:43.

Rubin AM, Zafar SS. The assessment and management of the dizzy patient. *Otolaryngol Clin North Am* 2002;35: 255.

Sloan PD, Coeytaux RR, Beck RS, et al. Dizziness: state of science. *Ann Int Med* 2001;134:823.

Troost TB. Dizziness and vertigo in vertebrobasilar disease. *Stroke* 1980;11:301.

15

Behavioral Neurology

Christopher G. Goetz and Robert S. Wilson

Bizarre or altered behavioral patterns traditionally are felt to relate to psychiatric disorders or generalized delirium from drugs, toxins, or metabolic imbalances. However, some specific neurologic conditions present with remarkably consistent behavioral abnormalities. These conditions have equally consistent anatomic substrates, and, when identified by an astute diagnostician, they suggest specific causes and treatments. In this chapter, five conditions are discussed, each with a prominent behavioral and seemingly psychiatric presentation but with a pathologic basis related to a specific neurologic dysfunction. These conditions are temporal lobe epilepsy (TLE), fluent aphasia, Wernicke's encephalopathy, transient global amnesia, and herpes encephalitis.

These strange disorders are not rare, and their complexity often relates not to management problems but to accurate identification. The topic is thus particularly pertinent to the non-neurologist, who is most likely to be the first person to interview and evaluate these patients.

ANATOMIC BASIS—PAPEZ CIRCUIT

It is well recognized that the ability to recall and engender memories is intimately linked to the emotional makeup of such memories. Furthermore, several clinical conditions demonstrate combined and prominent memory–emotional alterations, suggesting that the anatomic basis of these two functions may be linked. In 1937, the neuroanatomist Papez published a treatise describing an anatomic circuit that linked those nuclei and paths that appear important to many aspects of emotional–behavioral integration. This circuit, the Papez circuit, is probably the most important circuit for clinicians dealing with behavioral abnormalities; familiarity with it allows them to think systematically about the anatomic foundations of behavioral neurology.

The circuit is diagrammed schematically in Fig. 15.1A, with anatomic nuclei and paths identified in the sagittal brain section of Fig. 15.1B. As indicated, the pathway is circular, providing continual reintegration of information. The two focal cortical areas most prominently involved are the cingulate cortex and the hippocampus of the temporal lobe. Diffuse cortical impulses travel into the hippocampus, an area felt to be particularly important to memory and emotional expression. This information travels forward in the fornix path to the mammillary bodies of the hypothalamus and continues to the anterior lobe of the thalamus, and further to the midline cingulate cortex, which finally projects diffusely to cortical regions.

Familiarity with this circuit is useful because disease anywhere along the pathway can be expected to result in aberrant emotional behaviors, although not necessarily the same patterns. This knowledge allows the clinician to focus immediately on a finite number of nuclei and connecting paths to explain abnormal behavioral symptoms that may have a focal anatomic basis. The term diffuse cortical input is important because toxic and metabolic encephalopathy often present with agitated behavior or a change in personality. The other areas, however, are focal, and identification of disease at these levels can lead to rapid intervention. Reference will be made to this circuit throughout this chapter.

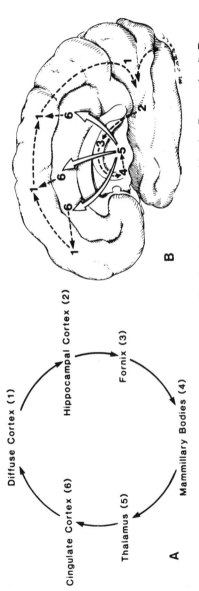

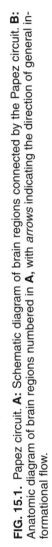

FIG. 15.1. Papez circuit. **A:** Schematic diagram of brain regions connected by the Papez circuit. **B:** Anatomic diagram of brain regions numbered in **A**, with *arrows* indicating the direction of general informational flow.

Diffuse Cortex (1)

Hippocampal Cortex (2)

Fornix (3)

Mammillary Bodies (4)

Thalamus (5)

Cingulate Cortex (6)

A

B

TEMPORAL LOBE EPILEPSY

Also referred to as psychomotor epilepsy and partial complex seizure, psychomotor or psychosensory variety, TLE may manifest itself with intermittent spells of bizarre behavior, including babbling nonsense and frank visual and auditory hallucinations, all related to organic disease of the central nervous system. Differentiation of this disorder from psychotic disorders such as schizophrenia can be difficult, yet it is essential because their treatments are drastically different. Certain specific characteristics are helpful in establishing abnormal behavioral patterns as probable epilepsy, and they are the focus of this discussion.

TLE represents an abnormal electrical discharge that begins in one temporal lobe and usually crosses rapidly to involve both sides of the brain. To recognize TLE in a patient, the clinician should attempt to elicit specific information in four areas. If information in even one of these areas is characteristic of TLE, the diagnosis is suggested.

1. The distinctive temporal pattern of the spells.
2. The presence of an aura, a distinctive feeling or sensation that regularly precedes or begins the spells.
3. The presence of peculiar motor behaviors called automatisms.
4. The specific type of loss of consciousness.

The distinctive temporal pattern of TLE refers to repeated, but intermittent, and paroxysmal changes in behavior, not necessarily linked to any emotional provocation. The behavioral changes are brief, lasting seconds to minutes. Often, before any visible behavioral change can be appreciated by an observer, the patient experiences a stereotypic and fixed sensation, known as an epileptic aura. The aura represents the beginning of the seizure and can help in localizing the focus, or source, of the seizure activity. The aura may be olfactory, in which the patient suddenly smells a strange, often pungent odor, or it may

be a gustatory sensation or a strange abdominal "butterflies" feeling, also called epigastric rising. Emotional changes of sudden unfamiliarity with one's environment ("jamais vu") or sudden intense familiarity with the surroundings ("déjà vu") are seen, and there may be intense and vivid auditory or visual hallucinations. The aura and the area of the temporal lobe cortex that are felt to relate to the seizure focus are listed in Table 15.1. The presence of this stereotypic aura and sudden unprovoked change in behavior help to quickly identify a patient with TLE. The aura is sensed by the patient and is not identified by the clinician except by interview. The patient may not necessarily link the strange aura to his spells, so that information must be solicited specifically.

The presence of automatisms is also useful in the diagnosis of TLE. These activities appear as the seizure spreads in the amygdala region of the temporal lobe. The movements may range from rather primitive movements (lip smacking, eye blinking, or chewing motions) or may be highly complex (dressing and undressing, piling objects on top of one another). These are stereotypic and rather fixed from one spell to another, so a detailed record of two or more episodes helps to establish the pattern of behavior.

The peculiar characteristic of the loss of consciousness seen in TLE is also helpful. After the aura, which the examiner cannot see unless it involves automatisms, there is a sudden loss of contact with the environment. Un-

TABLE 15.1. *Temporal Lobe Foci and Related Auras*

Focus	Aura
Uncus	Smell, taste
Cingulate cortex	Change in emotional perception—déjà vu, jamais vu, euphoria, sense of sudden doom
Insula	Epigastric rising sensation
Amygdala	Pupillary dilatation, photophobia, automatisms
Association temporal cortex	Auditory, visual hallucinations

like patients who have other generalized seizures, these patients only rarely fall to the floor, shake all over, urinate, or bite their tongue. Instead, when they lose consciousness, they maintain body tone and may walk around but "in a daze, out of contact" with the environment. When the spell is over, the patient is usually amnestic for the seizure, except that he may recall its beginning and be able to recount, if specifically asked, the details of the aura. Immediately after the spell, the patient usually is confused and sleepy. If restrained during this period, he may strike out randomly at people who try to assist. However, these patients are generally not violent in a goal-directed manner, either during or after their seizures. As strange as their behaviors may be, focused violence, such as tracking a person with a gun or retrieving a kitchen knife out of a drawer and stabbing a victim, is far outside the repertoire of TLE.

Two specific examples will help to delineate the methods used in diagnosing TLE.

Case 1. A quiet, 34-year-old right-handed woman is admitted for observation after she suffered head trauma on a city bus. She was the cause of an unprovoked fist fight on the bus and reports, "They said I did it but I don't remember a thing."

The question is whether this patient suffers from (a) head trauma with retrograde amnesia; (b) socially deviant behavior, claiming ignorance to avoid responsibility; or (c) amnesia and bizarre behavior related to TLE. To differentiate TLE from the other two disorders, the interview focuses on the characteristics of TLE.

In discussing this event with the patient, it is found that this is only one of many violent episodes in her life. The episodes are similar in that she cannot understand why she gets into fights, being a quiet, shy person, and she says that the events are never precipitated by an argument. She says she has no warning and that "that's all I remember." However, when specifically asked about smells, taste, sounds, and visions, she states that she usually starts thinking of a peculiar tune that always recurs in her head before a fight and makes her nervous for those last few seconds. It is important to note that this major clue is gleaned only with specific questioning.

When the victim of the fight, who is in the next hospital room, is interviewed, he comments that he and the patient were sitting quietly in the bus when suddenly the patient started fidgeting in her purse, picking at items, and smacking her lips loudly. She then started walking around the bus babbling noises and picking at her clothes. The bus was crowded, and the patient bumped into several passengers. A minute later, she seemed to start swinging randomly at people. The man was hit in the head, fell over, and hit his face on the bus seat. As they were both taken to the hospital, this man noticed that the belligerent woman seemed now considerably confused and sleepy.

The characteristic aura, the paroxysmal quality of the repeated episodes by history, and the automatisms of lip smacking and clothes picking with amnesia all suggest TLE. An electroencephalogram (EEG) demonstrated epilepsy, and anticonvulsant medications have virtually abolished the episodes.

Case 2. A 16-year-old boy on the psychiatric unit with a diagnosis of schizophrenia and hallucinatory behavior is evaluated by the neurologist because of a single generalized seizure. On being interviewed, this patient says, "It's just like before, but this time much worse." Several times each week this patient sees "the man," a blurry but discernible bearded man who beckons him forward verbally. As this happens, everything in the patient's environment becomes suddenly more distinct, clearer, and more colorful, with a clear sense of familiarity and warmth. Then a strange feeling of dread and a "fog" come over the patient, who then appears to lose touch for approximately 5 minutes. He has no recollection of this period of losing touch, but his family says that he walks around in the house mumbling strange noises that are sometimes prayers, and at the same time he bows his head back and forth in a seemingly ritualistic manner. After this, he lies down and sleeps for approximately 2 hours. The same

TABLE 15.2. *Clinical Distinctions Between TLE Behavior and Schizophrenia*

	TLE	Schizophrenia
Environmental precipitants	Rare	Frequent
Duration of attack	0.5–5 minutes	May be days
Aura	Usual	Lacking
Injury to others	Rare and undirected	Unpredictable—may be direct or undirected
Disturbance of consciousness	Present	Lacking or only mind-clouding
Symptoms and signs after attack	Sleepy, confused	Lacking

TLE, temporal lobe epilepsy.

stereotypic pattern occurred immediately before the generalized seizure.

This patient again shows the stereotypic aura, which is hallucinatory this time, along with the sense of emotional familiarly with the environment. Stereotypic repetition of episodes and the automatisms with amnesia and sleepiness afterward strongly suggest TLE. In regard to this latter episode in which there was a generalized motor seizure with bilateral shaking, this pattern can be seen with TLE when the seizure activity spreads throughout both sides of the brain. An EEG study with nasopharyngeal recordings demonstrated abnormal epileptiform activity. On medication the patient has shown remarkable improvement. This case demonstrates the important interface between psychiatric symptoms and clear focal neurologic disease.

Table 15.2 serves as a summary and outlines additional guidelines for differentiating TLE episodes from psychotic bizarre behaviors of schizophrenia. These patterns are clinically useful, although no absolute rules hold true.

Anatomy and Clinical Findings

The anatomic lesions of TLE naturally relate to the temporal lobe and, depending on the area damaged, will give rise to different auras (Table 15.1). As can be seen, some of these nuclei are primary portions of the Papez circuit and the others have direct input into the circuit.

In examining a patient with TLE, static findings may include a homonymous hemianopia, or a homonymous quadrantanopsia, especially in the superior fields (Fig. 15.2). Because these fibers pass through the temporal lobe en route to the occipital cortex, the superior quadrantanopsia should be sought specifically.

Much has been written about psychopathology in patients with TLE. Although the seizures and bizarre behavior are intermittent, interictal or between-seizure abnormalities often are attributed to TLE. Problems such as sedation, inattention, and depressed mood may be seen as dose-related side effects of antiepileptic medications. If toxicity can be ruled out, the

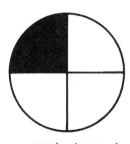

temporal   nasal
LEFT EYE

nasal   temporal
RIGHT EYE

FIG. 15.2. Visual field defect associated with right temporal lobe disease, termed left superior quadrantanopsia.

most common psychiatric problem in epilepsy is depression. Although not specific to TLE, research suggests rates of depression as high as 75% in some clinical samples. Paradoxically, depression may appear after seizure control is accomplished, suggesting that seizures, like electroconvulsive therapy, may serve to elevate mood, possibly through opioid mechanisms.

Aggressive behavior often is attributed to TLE. There is, however, no good evidence of a disproportionate level of aggressive or violent behavior in TLE or epilepsy. Aggressive behavior may be seen following a seizure, but it is typically non-directed and random, occurring when the patient is aroused or restrained. The hypothesis that TLE is characterized by a distinct personality profile has not been supported by recent research. However, psychiatric signs and symptoms in general are seen more commonly in TLE than in other forms of epilepsy, particularly in patients with severe, uncontrolled TLE.

Etiology

TLE often is seen in patients with a history of birth trauma. Brain tumors, both primary and metastatic, also may involve the temporal lobe and present early with characteristic TLE. Subacute onset of TLE with fever should suggest encephalitis, specifically resulting from herpes simplex, which has a predilection for the temporal lobes. EEG findings are discussed in Chapter 8. Treatment drugs useful in the control of TLE are listed in Table 15.3, along with usual doses, plasma levels, and common side effects. There are no specific rehabilitation or alternate medical therapies that are applicable to the treatment of TLE.

When to Refer Patients to a Neurologist

TLE is a complicated neurologic condition, and all patients should be referred to a neurologist at least once to obtain expert opinion on the nature of the condition and its management. The neurologist can provide guidelines to the non-neurologist for drug management and behaviors that fall within and outside the realm of TLE. Because the government guidelines for driving are different in each state, the neurologist also can provide the non-neurologist with the specific rules regarding driving limitations for patients who have seizures.

Special Challenges for Hospitalized Patients

Hospital personnel are unlikely to be familiar with the strange behaviors that typify TLE; therefore, the admitting physician must outline the sequence of behaviors of the seizure

TABLE 15.3. *Drugs Used in the Control of TLE: Dosages, Therapeutic Plasma Levels, and Common or Important Side Effects*

Drug	Adult Dosage (mg)	Plasma Level (microgram/mL)	Toxicity
Carbamazepine	600–1200	4–10	Diplopia, nausea, vomiting, sedation, ataxia
Phenytoin	300	10–20	Ataxia, nausea, vomiting, sedation, folate deficiency
Valproic acid	750–1500	50–150	Tremor, nausea, weight gain
Lamotrigine	300–700	2–15	Dizziness, diplopia, ataxia, insomnia
Phenobarbital	90–180	15–40	Sedation, hyperactivity in children, depression
Gabapentin	900–3000	4–8	Somnolence
Primidone	750–1000	7–15 primidone 20–40 phenobarbital	Nausea, weight gain, vomiting, sedation, depression, impotence
Topiramate	300–700	2–20	Confusion, dysphasia, weight loss
Oxcarbazepine	600–1800	5–50	Diplopia, nausea, dizziness
Zonisamide	200–600	10–40	Confusion, irritability
Levetiracetam	1000–3000	20–60	Irritability, confusion

episodes. Seizure precautions and seizure treatment as outlined in Chapter 8 should be followed throughout the hospitalized period. When patients have surgery and cannot take medications by mouth, alternate routes of medication delivery must be used, as outlined in Chapter 8.

FLUENT APHASIA

Aphasia is a specific language deficit that occurs without weakness of the articulatory muscles, and it is caused by cortical brain disease. The two basic types of aphasia are subfluent and fluent. The former group is not difficult to diagnose and would not be confused with psychiatric disease because in most cases an obvious right hemiparesis accompanies the change in speech pattern. The fluent aphasias, however, are not associated with motor problems, so that these patients present with behavioral alterations in the form of strange speech. The adage taught to young neurologists—when evaluating an acute behavioral change, one always must rule out fluent aphasia—is applicable to all clinicians.

Aphasic problems occur with focal dominant hemisphere disorders. For most people, the left hemisphere is dominant for speech, although in a small percentage of left-handed people the right hemisphere may be dominant. Subfluent aphasias relate to frontal lobe disease, and fluent aphasias relate usually to dominant temporal or temporoparietal damage. Because the temporal lobe is involved in the Papez circuit, behavioral alterations in fluent aphasias are expected and characteristic.

In contrast to the frustration and depressed affect common in subfluent aphasia, patients with fluent aphasia are often seemingly unaware of their deficit and are unconcerned. Patients may not realize that their speech is incomprehensible to others. In extreme cases, these patients may blame their inability to communicate on others to the point of frank paranoia. Impulsivity also is observed. The combination of such behaviors can result in serious management problems.

The evaluation of aphasia is usually rapid and requires no unusual implements. Table 15.4 outlines the manner of examination, which has three focal points. First, by listening to the patient's spontaneous speech, the clinician decides whether the speech is subfluent, slow, and sparse or fluent, rapid, and free flowing. This evaluation makes no judgment on content of speech; instead it judges rhythm and ease of word production. Second, the examiner asks the patient to follow a verbal command— "Show me a spoon," "Raise your left hand," and so forth—which tests ability to comprehend. This integration of auditory information helps to distinguish various aphasias and localizes the disease. The command must be verbal, and the investigator must discipline himself not to use nonverbal communication during this task. Third, the patient is asked to repeat a sentence—first a reasonable phrase, such as "Today is Tuesday; tomorrow I will phone Bill," and then a nonsense phrase, such as "No ifs,

TABLE 15.4. *Major Types of Aphasia with Guides to Their Rapid Identification*

Names	Fluency	Follow Commands	Repeat	Focal Damage	Associative Problems
Broca's	Subfluent	Yes	No	Dominant frontal lobe	Right hemiparesis
Wernicke's	Fluent	No	No	Dominant temporal lobe	Visual field abnormalities, no weakness
Conductive	Fluent	Yes	Yes for short phrases; cannot repeat "no-ifs, ands, or buts"	Dominant connecting fibers between Broca's and Wernicke's area	Visual field abnormalities or mild weakness, decreased sensation on right side of body and face

ands, or buts." These three simple maneuvers can be performed by patients who are confused or intoxicated and by patients with short attention spans. However, they are not performed by patients with aphasia. Furthermore, the pattern of disability in the three tasks isolates the specific areas of dominant cortical dysfunction.

The patient who usually is diagnosed as confused, agitated, and often schizophrenic is the patient with a Wernicke's aphasia (not to be confused with Wernicke's encephalopathy, which is discussed in the next section). The following case history helps to typify this syndrome, and it emphasizes the common confusion between this condition and the word salad of schizophrenia.

Case 3. A 65-year-old hypertensive right-handed woman was well until 3 hours before an evaluation in the emergency room. Her family lived with her and reported that after lunch the patient took a 40-minute nap; on awaking, she "began speaking nonsense—crazy talk." Her past medical and psychiatric histories were negative, and no similar events had ever occurred.

The patient is alert and talkative, but her speech has no discernible sense. Phrases such as "oh, me," "why not," "should we," "what now," and "amen Moses" are spoken rapidly and spontaneously. She can follow no verbal commands nor will she repeat simple phrases. The family feels she may be poisoned or has gone crazy.

The highlights of this case are the patient's age, the acute onset, the characteristic speech pattern, and the easily retrieved results of an accurate aphasia testing screen. It is important to note that in a patient who is 65 years old without prior psychiatric history, the new onset of schizophrenia, regardless of how bizarre the behavior or speech may be, would be exceptional.

Etiology

Wernicke's fluent aphasia usually is seen with dominant temporal lobe disease in the form of cerebrovascular accidents or sometimes tumors. The rapid onset in an elderly in-dividual suggests the former, whereas a more indolent course can be seen with tumors. When this speech pattern is encountered, the clinician immediately should focus attention on the dominant temporal lobe. Associated findings often include the superior quadrantanopsia (Fig. 15.2), and temporal lobe seizures may be an associated phenomenon.

The other fluent aphasia, conduction aphasia, does not appear to be a psychiatric illness; thus it will not be discussed in detail. These patients speak fluently and usually make sense, except that they mix up words or make new words (paraphasic errors). Although they can repeat simple sentences, they have trouble with nonsense phrases such as "no ifs, ands, or buts." This disease localizes to the arcuate fasciculus of the parietal lobe connecting the temporal and frontal speech areas. Strokes and tumors are again the likely causes, although sometimes Wernicke's aphasia, as it resolves, tends to become a conduction aphasia. Anomic aphasia, in which the patient is fluent and behaviorally appropriate but has trouble finding the proper word, is seen as other forms of aphasia resolve.

Treatment

The treatment of aphasia focuses on two elements: rehabilitation of the speech deficit and treatment of the underlying cause. Because patients with fluent aphasia often do not recognize their speech problems, they are difficult rehabilitation patients. Speech therapy is used, but until the patient becomes motivated to communicate more effectively, the speech exercises often are fruitless. No medications or alternate medical treatments are specifically useful. Diagnostic tests, such as MRI scans, will identify the anatomic lesion in the dominant (left) temporal lobe, and the contours of the lesion will help in suggesting a vascular etiology (stroke) from tumor, where there is often extensive edema or multiple discreet lesions. An EEG will help define if there are seizures. The treatments will be directed to the most likely cause; stroke treatment is outlined in Chapter 6, tumor therapy is discussed in Chapter 20, and seizure management is covered in Chapter 8.

When to Refer the Patient to a Neurologist

In contrast to subjects with subfluent aphasia, in which the patient cannot produce speech, patients with Wernicke's aphasia speak excessively and typically are unconcerned about their speech and behavioral abnormalities. The family and medical staff, however, readily recognize the incoherent language, although they may not be able to interpret the problem as an aphasia. Therefore, all subjects with a sudden change in language content should be referred to a neurologist for a consultation. Once the diagnosis and underlying cause are defined, the management often can be directed by the nonneurologist with intermittent consultation back to the neurologist.

Special Challenges for Hospitalized Patients

In the hospital, patients with aphasia are a particular challenge. Usually, they are hospitalized at the onset of the aphasia, and the staff will not understand the language abnormality or its origin. Staff must be educated to be compassionate and solicitous of the patient's needs despite the seemingly nonsensical language. In a patient with a chronic Wernicke's aphasia who must be hospitalized, the family often will be more familiar with the speech deficit than a professional staff, and their aid must be sought to maximize communication efficiency between staff and patient. Because patients with fluent aphasia have specific difficulty understanding language, when the physician or staff need to explain a procedure, treatment, or test, the family member with authority for the patient's care must be included for proper consent.

WERNICKE–KORSAKOFF'S SYNDROME

Wernicke–Korsakoff's syndrome, also known as Wernicke's encephalopathy–Korsakoff's psychosis, represents a neurologic emer-

gency. The important triad of Wernicke's encephalopathy includes behavioral alterations, extraocular movement abnormalities, and ataxia. These symptoms occur to a greater or lesser extent with a selective memory impairment, and when this memory impairment is marked, the syndrome is called Korsakoff's psychosis. The two diseases are the same but are referred to with different terms depending on the degree of memory deficit. The pathogenesis of this syndrome relates to vitamin deficiency in the form of vitamin B_1 (thiamine). The primary patients at high risk for this syndrome are alcoholics who obtain calories through the alcohol but do not receive essential vitamins. Patients with prolonged emesis or with gastric bowel resection also can suffer with thiamine deficiency. Occasionally, voluntary starvation in the form of political protest, psychotic disturbances, or unsupervised treatment of obesity also can induce this syndrome. Finally, and important to surgical patients, hyperalimentation can be associated with Wernicke's encephalopathy when water-soluble B vitamins are not included in the formula.

The behavioral picture of Wernicke's encephalopathy–Korsakoff's psychosis has three different presentations. The patient with acute Wernicke's encephalopathy shows global confusion, and his or her demeanor is usually quiet and apathetic. He or she is alert and responsive but inattentive, and the patient appears fatigued. Occasionally, a patient may be more agitated, especially if he or she is undergoing delirium tremens associated with alcohol withdrawal. The usual presentation, however, is one of an affable but dull affect.

In the partially treated patient or in the early stages of chronic disease, the affect becomes more bright, and the patient becomes more loquacious. The memory deficits become more apparent as the patient is less globally confused. The patient is non-hesitant in his speech, and it is at this point that the famed confabulatory aspects of Korsakoff's psychosis may be seen. Confabulation is not an essential component of Korsakoff's psychosis; the characteristic trait of this condition is the preferential loss of recent memory.

The patient with chronic Wernicke–Korsakoff's syndrome is typically alert and oriented but displays characteristic deficiencies in recent and remote memory. The recent memory deficit is usually profound and consists of an inability to make an enduring record of daily experiences. The remote memory deficit is temporally graded such that more remote events are relatively more accessible to recall. Thus, a patient asked to name presidents since World War II may recall Truman and Eisenhower but not their successors. Confabulation is not typically seen in chronic patients. Behaviorally, such patients are usually apathetic and indifferent, with occasional outbursts of irritability.

In diagnosing this syndrome, the neurologic signs of extraocular muscle palsy or nystagmus and ataxia are important features to recognize. In many ways, the patient with acute Wernicke's encephalopathy looks like a drunkard, in that he or she has trouble walking; he or she may have nystagmus from the alcohol itself; and he or she has an altered affect. Because of the similarity, it is a common adage that a patient seen in the emergency room who is drunk should be given an injection of thiamine (a) to treat possible Wernicke's encephalopathy and (b) to prevent a future episode of the condition. The chronic patient is difficult to manage because, although the extraocular movements improve quickly with thiamine therapy and the ataxia improves to a moderate extent, the memory problems are least abated by thiamine therapy.

Anatomic Basis

The unifying basis for this disorder involves the Papez circuit where there is capillary proliferation at the level of the mammillary bodies. In some cases in which the mammillary bodies are spared, the anterior lobe of the thalamus is involved. Additional pathologic findings may involve cerebellar and diffuse cortical degeneration. Although the clinical picture of Korsakoff's psychosis should immediately suggest vitamin deficiency and disease that at least includes the mammillary bodies, it can be seen in diseases that involve other aspects of the Papez circuit. The same syndrome has been reported in patients who recover from a viral encephalitis with prominent hippocampus involvement. Such clinical overlap again emphasizes the importance of the Papez circuit in localizing diseases that involve both memory and affective disorders.

Treatment

All patients with suspected Wernicke's encephalopathy immediately must receive thiamine. At least 100 mg intravenous thiamine should be given, followed by 100 mg IM daily for 3 to 5 days with then a chronic dose of oral thiamine (50 mg daily) and a multivitamin.

Once thiamine has been given and good nutrition is reestablished, physical and occupational therapy can be recommended to help in gait training and coordination. Full neuropsychologic testing will help in establishing specific mental deficits and provide data that will be useful for discharge planning. No alternative medical therapies are recommended.

There has been new interest in the treatment of memory deficits with presumed cholinergic precursors such as lecithin or choline chloride, but these agents have not been tested extensively.

When to Refer to a Neurologist

The non-neurologist should never hesitate to treat a patient with components of Wernicke's encephalopathy with thiamine. Clear documentation on the chart of the mental status, the presence of nystagmus or ophthalmoplegia, and a description of the gait should be noted. Thereafter, the neurologist can be consulted to corroborate the diagnosis and suggest other treatment or diagnostic evaluations.

Special Challenges for Hospitalized Patients

Because so many patients with Wernicke's encephalopathy are heavy alcohol users, the risk of alcohol withdrawal in the hospital and its consequences including delirium tremens are high. The hospital staff must be aware of these problems and appropriately protect the patient against injury or medical complications of alcohol withdrawal, especially in the first 72 hours of hospitalization, as outlined in Chapter 12. These include a careful attention to the diagnosis of infection or associated injuries, such as meningitis or subdural hematomas. Further, maintenance of fluid and electrolyte balance is essential, as well as a watchful attention to the possibility of hypoglycemia. Control of agitation is essential to avoid patient and staff injury. Specific recommendations are outlined in Chapter 12.

TRANSIENT GLOBAL AMNESIA

The syndrome of transient global amnesia occurs in middle-aged or elderly patients who usually have diabetes or hypertension or who are at high risk for cerebrovascular disease. Physical or emotional stress often precedes the amnestic episode.

When the spell has begun, the patient is unable to learn new information until it is over. His memory for events that day and the preceding day are almost always poor. Memory for prior events will be better, although memory losses sometimes will be detectable even for events that took place years before the amnestic spell. The syndrome is transient and clears completely within 24 hours, except for a permanent amnesia for the episode itself. Significantly, the patient's affect is often bland during the episode, although family members are distressed.

These patients often are brought to medical attention when the family notes that they repeatedly ask the same questions and seem unable to remember the answer and sometimes deny that an answer has been given. At the same time, these patients may perform complex tasks during an episode without difficulty, as long as these tasks were learned prior to the event.

These patients are not globally confused. In testing orientation, however, they may report the wrong answer because they cannot integrate changes in place and time. When asked to do arithmetic calculations or use logical processing, they respond appropriately.

Memory testing during an attack demonstrates a marked inability to establish new memories despite preserved attention, language, and higher cognitive functioning. If the physician leaves the room of a patient with this disorder, he will have to reintroduce himself when he returns. Recent memory function is deficient in such patients regardless of which sensory system is used in the memory tasks, so that visual, tactile, and auditory memories are disturbed. The retrograde amnesia is such that the activities of the previous days may be only dimly recollected during the episode. The retrograde amnesia is occasionally more extensive, affecting memories formed years before the episode. Confabulation is notably lacking in these patients. On recovery, there is no recollection of the episode itself, and there is typically a permanent retrograde amnesia for events occurring in the hour or so prior to the episode.

This syndrome with its peculiar constellation of memory and behavioral features can be highly confusing unless it is recognized. In patients whose amnesic episodes are brief (e.g., less than 1 hour) and/or recurrent, TLE should be considered, and treatment with anticonvulsant medications can be successful. In patients with focal neurologic signs or symptoms during or subsequent to the amnesic episode, tumors and cerebrovascular disease should be considered, and the prognosis may be more guarded. If the amnesia includes additional disorientation and/or inattention, drug ingestion, especially of anticholinergic or sedative drugs, may be the cause.

Transient global amnesia is most often confused with psychogenic amnestic states. Hysterical amnesia may occur abruptly but frequently is associated with a specific precipitating event, with retention of memory for other events within the time interval. One does not see the profound yet selective deficit in recent memory, nor the temporally graded retrograde amnesia.

In the more severe hysterical amnesia, such as in fugue states, there is the characteristic dissociative behavior with an additional loss of personal identity, a feature not seen in transient global amnesia. In contrast to the transient global amnesia patient, the hysterical patient will often acknowledge that the memory is poor but will have an inappropriate affect, "la belle indifférence."

Anatomic Basis

Because the episodes of transient global amnesia tend not to recur, no extensive pathologic studies have been performed on patients. The anatomic basis of this syndrome, however, is felt to relate to temporal lobe disease in the area involved in the Papez circuit. The disorder often is associated with atherosclerotic disease, especially ischemia in the blood vessels that perfuse posterior and undersurfaces of the temporal lobes by the vertebrobasilar arteries. However, seizure activity and migraine attacks also are posited as a mechanism for this syndrome. In many patients, the presence of transient symptoms such as vertigo, nausea, and ataxia occur and suggest alterations in the anatomic structures of the posterior brain and brainstem, but they clear quickly, making them difficult to document by the physician. Special attention to symptoms such as flashing lights or transient homonymous hemianopsia can help to localize the anatomic basis of this syndrome but do not specifically designate a cerebrovascular event from a seizure or migraine episode.

Treatment

For most patients, the dramatic events of transient global amnesia never recur, and therefore treatment is not required. Diagnostic tests to examine for cerebrovascular disease, epilepsy, and migraine are important, and MRI and EEG are both useful tests. A second attack occurs in less than 25% of subjects, and fewer than 5% have more than three episodes. The frequency of seizures or subsequent strokes is not different from that of a comparable age-matched group without a prior episode. Unless a specific etiologic diagnosis is made, no treatment is needed.

When to Consult a Neurologist

The isolated event rarely is seen by the neurologist, and often only the emergency room physician actually witnesses the amnestic episode. In such cases, the neurologist is best utilized as a consultant to interpret the description of events and guide the non-neurologist in the limited diagnostic tests needed and the usual lack of needed intervention. A follow-up appointment after the event with a neurologist is useful to document the absence of static neurologic signs; at this appointment the neurologist can review with the family the relative statistics on recurrence and the signs or symptoms of stroke, migraine, and epilepsy that should alert the family to a second consultation.

Special Challenges for Hospitalized Patients

Most of these patients are seen in emergency room settings; therefore, acute care personnel must be aware of the distinctive features of this syndrome. The combination of sudden memory loss without superimposed confusion and without language abnormalities should alert nurses and physicians to this entity. Very specific and rapid documentation on the memory loss, affect, and preservation of other mental capacities is essential because the syndrome clears quickly. Because of its very good prognosis, transient global amnesia must be considered and specifically diagnosed while the signs are still present, not afterward when the neurologic examination is normal.

HERPES SIMPLEX ENCEPHALITIS

Herpes encephalitis affects primarily the temporal lobes and leads to necrosis and hemorrhagic destruction of brain tissue. The mortality rate in herpes simplex encephalitis has been reduced, but the prevalence of neurologic deficits among survivors remains high. These deficits are almost exclusively in the behavioral realm. Temporal lobe seizures already described are a common presenting feature of this disease. The most common sequela is an amnesia that can be isolated, with sparing of other cognitive functions. The amnesia consists of an inability to form enduring memories. In more severe cases, the deficit in recent memory is accompanied by alterations in language, perception, and intelligence such that global dementia is seen. This linguistic disorder typically resembles a fluent aphasia with poor comprehension and paraphasic or nonsensical speech. Profound perceptual problems also may be seen: patients may be unable to recognize family members or friends (prosopagnosia) or common objects (visual agnosia).

The most striking sequelae of herpes simplex encephalitis, however, are the often bizarre behavioral and emotional changes that, in the extreme, resemble those reported by Kluver and Bucy in primates after bilateral removal of the temporal lobes. In humans, the syndrome sometimes is referred to as a limbic dementia and consists of (in addition to the visual agnosia) emotional placidity, distractibility, and alterations in sexual behavior. Thus, patients are often apathetic with flat affect and may show childlike compliance. In humans, the hypermetamorphosis consists of manual and oral exploration of the environment with placement of objects in the mouth. Episodes of bulimia may be seen along with ingestion of inappropriate material. The sexual changes consist primarily of inappropriate comments and overtures. The Kluver–Bucy syndrome is not diagnostically specific: the symptom complex also may be seen with head trauma, Alzheimer's disease, and Pick's disease. The behavioral alterations in herpes simplex encephalitis are typically less extreme than the full Kluver–Bucy syndrome, and they consist of episodically inappropriate behavior, personality changes, delusions, and hyposexuality. Such behavioral sequelae frequently are viewed as psychogenic by the family and may be resistant to traditional forms of psychiatric treatment.

Anatomic Basis

For unknown reasons, herpes encephalitis has a predilection for the temporal lobes of the brain; therefore the cortical regions of the Papez circuit are involved. The encephalitis is not isolated to the temporal lobe, but the major involvement occurs in this area often in an asymmetric pattern, with one lobe showing more hemorrhagic involvement than the other.

Treatment

Acyclovir is the drug of choice for the treatment of herpes simplex encephalitis, and the standard care is 30 mg/kg/day for a minimum of 14 days. Higher doses and longer courses (3 weeks followed by an oral antiviral agent) are being investigated. Brain biopsy generally is reserved for subjects whose diagnosis remains unclear despite the diagnostic studies that include MRI scans and polymerase chain reaction (PCR) assays of cerebrospinal fluid. Anticonvulsant medications may be needed for seizure treatment or prevention. After recovery, physical, occupational, and speech therapy may be important to maximize rehabilitation. No alternative medical therapies are indicated for this acute infection.

When to Refer the Patient to a Neurologist

The main experts in this condition are infectious disease specialists and neurologists. Rapid consultation is essential to order the appropriate cerebrospinal tests and initiate therapy without delay. With this guidance, the non-neurologist often will manage the case with appropriate reconsultation of these specialists as needed.

Special Challenges for Hospitalized Patients

Most patients with herpes encephalitis are hospitalized during the acute illness, and special attention must be made to the identification of seizures and preherniation syndromes. Nursing staff must be vigilant to the level of consciousness of the patient, vital signs, the strength of arms and legs, and the size of the pupils. Because temporal lobe swelling can occur, the development of a large pupil, contralateral weakness of the arm and leg, and change in level of consciousness are significant neurologic changes and call for emergency intervention. Staff must be educated to observe the patient for involuntary jerking movements, sometimes very subtle, that can indicate seizures.

Future Perspectives

The unifying points of this chapter have been that abnormal behavior can be a manifestation of focal neurologic disease and the lesions responsible for such behaviors mainly are predictably located somewhere in or near the Papez circuit. Using the Papez circuit as the foundation provides two major diagnostic advantages. First, behavior can be analyzed with a systematic, rigorous discipline provided by neuroanatomy. Second, because this is an anatomic circuit, there is the plasticity to integrate diseases that may be of different etiologies or that may affect different nuclei in the brain and yet that present with similar clinical presentations. Future diagnostic tools with greater anatomic precision will help delineate the exact area of involvement in the Papez circuit for the entities discussed. The use of such tools as function magnetic resonance imagery (fMRI) will allow patients to be tested during memory or other tasks to define the functional deficits related to this anatomy. A greater understanding of the neurochemical transmitters that link each nucleus in the circuit will help to design therapies that are more specific to lesions within this neurologic circuit.

QUESTIONS AND DISCUSSION

1. Patients at high risk for developing Wernicke's encephalopathy include:

A. Patients with posthepatitis cirrhosis

B. Hospitalized patients receiving intravenous hyperalimentation

C. Alcoholics

D. Health food advocates who consume large quantities of B vitamins

The answers are (B) and (C). Wernicke's encephalopathy relates to thiamine deficiency. Patients who do not receive vitamins in hyperalimentation eventually will become depleted, as will patients whose dietary caloric intake involves only alcohol. Cirrhosis *per se* is not associated with water-soluble vitamin problems, and patients ingesting megavitamins may develop many other problems but certainly not Wernicke's encephalopathy.

2. A patient says he has a seizure disorder. He is under arrest for having destroyed his friend's apartment and beaten up his girlfriend. He says, "I didn't mean to. I don't remember a thing." This behavior could represent TLE, or it could be antisocial behavior by a patient trying to plead ignorance. Along with an EEG, what facts will help you decide that the patient's behavior is probably related to a seizure?

A. After an argument, the patient raced after his girlfriend, caught her in the parking lot, and beat her up.

B. He was observed to exhibit picking movements of his hands and lip smacking before any belligerent behavior began.

C. The fighting and destructive behavior occurred when the girlfriend tried to restrain the patient from rising out of his chair.

D. The patient says this happened three times before: "I know when I'm going into a spell because I hear a strange buzz in my ears. That's all I remember, everything else is a complete blank."

The answers are (B), (C), and (D). Automatisms like those described in (B) are common in TLE; the aura of primitive auditory sensation is helpful because the primary auditory cortex is in the temporal lobe. The destructive combative behavior should be non-directed—the patient will not chase after someone, but instead will be combative only if restrained or somehow confined. Running after his girlfriend in the midst of an argument and searching for her in a dark parking lot is a highly directed violent activity.

3. Transient global amnesia is felt to relate to vascular insufficiency in the distribution of which cerebral vessel or vessels?

A. Frontal lobe anterior cerebral arteries

B. Parietal lobe middle cerebral arteries

C. Hippocampal posterior cerebral arteries

D. Carotid arteries

The answer is (C). The vertebrobasilar system provides the vascular supply to the hippocampus, specifically by the posterior cerebral artery.

4. Other conditions, besides transient global amnesia, that are part of the differential diagnosis of amnestic syndromes include:

A. Anticholinergic drug effect

B. Psychomotor epilepsy

C. Head trauma

D. Migraine headaches

The answers are (A), (B), (C), and (D). It is important to consider clinically the differential diagnosis of amnestic syndromes.

5. Match the anatomic area of disease most consistently related to each clinical condition.

A. Bilateral hippocampal 1. Psychomotor epilepsy regions

B. Temporal lobe 2. Transient global amnesia

C. Mammillary bodies 3. Wernicke's encephalopathy

D. Dominant 4. Fluent aphasia temporoparietal lobe

The correct matches are (A) and (2); (B) and (1); (C) and (3); and (D) and (4).

6. During or after herpes encephalitis, which of the following occur?

A. Temporal lobe seizures

B. Aphasia

C. Amnesia

D. Childlike affect and hypersexual behavior

The answers are (A), (B), (C), and (D). During the encephalitis, and as a residual, seizures may occur and they may be difficult to control. Because there may not be generalized shaking, tongue biting, or incontinence associated with the spells, they may not be appreciated as epileptic aphasia. Especially fluent forms can occur because the dominant temporal lobe may be diseased, and when both temporal lobes are affected, amnesia and the Kluver–Bucy syndrome may occur.

7. Regarding language recovery from Wernicke's aphasia, which of the following are true?

1. The outcome is better than seen with Broca's aphasia.

2. Patients are usually highly frustrated and depressed during rehabilitation.

3. Paranoid ideations are common.

4. Patients are often unaware of their deficit.

A. 1 and 2

B. 2 and 3

C. 3 and 4

D. 1 and 4

The answer is (C). Patients with Wernicke's aphasia pose major management problems for rehabilitation specialists. In contrast to patients with Broca's aphasia, who are depressed and frustrated over how poorly they communicate, the patient with Wernicke's aphasia is often unaware of the deficit. In addition, there can be thought disorders, including paranoia. For these reasons, the outcome for Wernicke's aphasia is much worse than for Broca's asphasia.

8. Transient global amnesia is characterized by:

A. Severe retrograde amnesia that overshadows anterograde amnesia

B. Quiet affect, patient only speaking when prompted

C. Usually lasting only minutes

D. Causes that include atherosclerotic vascular disease, seizures, and migraine

The answer is (D). Transient global amnesia is primarily anterograde amnesia, and the extent of retrograde amnesia is variable and less pronounced. The patient is usually quite distressed and confused, asking repeatedly "Where am I?" and "What is this?" Typically, the amnesia lasts for hours, not minutes, but it can be short or long, lasting up to several days.

SUGGESTED READING

Benson DF. *Aphasia, alexia, and agraphia.* New York: Churchill Livingstone, 1979.

Benson DF, Ardila A. *Aphasia: a clinical perspective.* New York: Oxford University Press, 1996.

Bogen JE. Wernicke's region—where is it? *Ann NY Acad Sci* 1976;280:834.

Engel J, Caldecott-Hazard S, Bandler R. Neurobiology of behavior: anatomic and physiological implications related to epilepsy. *Epilepsia* 1986;27(Suppl 2):53.

Flor-Henry P. Lateralized temporal-limbic dysfunction and psychopathology. *Ann NY Acad Sci* 1976;280:777.

Gabrieli JDE. Memory systems analyses in aging and age-related diseases. *Proc Nat Head Sci* 1996;93:13534.

Geschwind N. Aphasia. *N Engl J Med* 1971;284:654.

Greenwood R, Bhalla A, Gordon A, et al. Behaviour disturbance during recovery from herpes simplex encephalitis. *J Neurol Neurosurg Psychiatry* 1983;46:809.

Hanibert G. Emotional disturbance and temporal lobe injury. *Compr Psychiatry* 1978;19:441.

Hodges JR, Warlow CP. The aetiology of transient global amnesia: a case-control study of 114 cases with prospective follow-up. *Brain* 1990;113:639.

Kinsella LJ, Riley DE. Nutritional deficiencies and syndromes associated with alcoholism. In: Goetz CG, ed. *Textbook of clinical neurology,* 2nd ed. Philadelphia: WB Saunders, 2003:873–888.

Luria AR, Hutton JT. Modern assessment of the basic forms of aphasia. *Brain Lang* 1977;4:190.

Miller JW, Peterson RC, Metter EJ. Transient global Amer-ica: clinical characteristics and prognosis. *Neurology* 1987;37:733.

Papez JW. A proposed mechanism of emotion. *Arch Neurol Psychiatry* 1937;38:725.

Pierce CJ. The anatomy of language: contributions from function neuroimaging. *J Anat* 2000;197:335–359.

Pincus JH, Tucker GJ. *Behavioral neurology.* New York: Oxford University Press, 1974.

Pritchard PB, Lombroso CT, McIntyre M. Psychological complications of temporal lobe epilepsy. *Neurology* 1980; 30:227.

Roos K. Viral infections. In: Goetz CG, eds. *Textbook of clinical neurology,* 2nd ed. Philadelphia: WB Saunders, 2003:834–859.

Verfaellie M, O'Conner M. A neuropsychological analysis of memory and amnesia. *Seminars Neurol* 2001;20: 455–462.

Victor M, Adams RD, Collins GH. Wernicke– Korsakoff's syndrome—a clinical and pathological study of 245 patients. *Contemp Neurol Sci* 1971;1:1.

Wyllie E, ed. *The treatment of epilepsy: principles and practices,* 3rd ed. Philadelphia: Lippincott Williams & Wilkins, 2001.

16

Alzheimer's Disease and Other Dementias

David A. Bennett and Neelum T. Aggarwal

Loss of cognitive function associated with old age was recognized in antiquity. In the early 20th century, Dr. Alois Alzheimer presented the clinical history of a 54-year-old woman with a progressive dementia that he ascribed to the accumulation of senile plaques and tangles found on postmortem examination. For the next 60 years, the term Alzheimer's disease referred to a relatively uncommon progressive dementia in middle-aged persons. The much more common dementia of older persons was attributed to the effects of cerebral atherosclerosis ("hardening of the arteries") or the inevitable manifestations of aging. Over the past 30 years, however, it has become apparent that most of the older people with dementia have the same condition described by Alzheimer almost 100 years ago.

Only a small proportion of people with dementia are managed in specialized dementia centers. Because physicians often do not look for or recognize the signs of dementia, many people with dementia remain undiagnosed. For example, in community-based studies up to two-thirds of older people with dementia are not detected. Timely diagnosis allows for the patient to be a part of long-term-care decision-making processes. It also permits early pharmacologic and non-pharmacologic intervention. Finally, it can prevent medical emergencies resulting from behavioral disturbances and other superimposed medical problems. Therefore, increased awareness of dementia offers neurologists and non-neurologists an opportunity to improve the lives of patients and their caregivers.

DEMENTIA

Dementia refers to acquired intellectual deterioration in an adult. Evaluating a person for dementia involves determining whether there has been a loss of cognition relative to a previous level of performance. Typically, evidence is obtained through the clinical history from a knowledgeable informant such as a family member or close friend and should be documented by mental status testing. When the clinical history is not adequate or available, test results from a single evaluation can be contrasted with the estimated premorbid level of ability based on the patient's education and occupation. In some cases, formal neuropsychologic performance testing on two or more occasions over a period of 12 or more months may be necessary to document cognitive decline. For clinical purposes, loss of cognition should be sufficiently severe to interfere with an individual's usual occupational or social activities.

MILD COGNITIVE IMPAIRMENT

Because most dementias come on gradually over a period of several years, there must be a phase in which people have mild cognitive dysfunction of insufficient severity to warrant a diagnosis of dementia. The term mild cognitive impairment is being used increasingly to refer to these individuals. Recent data suggest that persons with mild cognitive impairment are at greater risk of death, of developing Alzheimer's disease, and of cognitive decline. Further, they frequently have the pathology of Alzheimer's disease, suggesting that in many cases, mild cognitive impairment represents preclinical Alzheimer's disease.

ALZHEIMER'S DISEASE

Epidemiology

Prevalence estimates suggest that Alzheimer's disease affects about 10% of persons over the age of 65, making it one of the most common chronic diseases of the elderly. The occurrence of Alzheimer's disease is strongly related to age. Therefore, the rapid growth of the oldest population age groups is expected to have a profound effect on the public health problem posed by this disease because Alzheimer's disease is associated with an increased risk of death and institutionalization.

Other than age, there are few well-documented risk factors for Alzheimer's disease. There is some evidence that women may be more likely to develop the disease than men. However, this observation appears to be attributed, in large part, to the fact that women live longer than men. Years of formal education have been associated with a reduced risk of disease in many, although not all, studies. The mechanism linking education to risk of disease is unclear, but recent evidence suggests that participation in cognitively stimulating activities also reduces risk of disease. Diabetes, head trauma, and cerebral infarctions are also possibly associated with an increase in risk. Putative protective factors include postmenopausal estrogen use, use of nonsteroidal antiinflammatory drugs, use of the cholesterol-lowering drugs HMG Co-A reductase inhibitors (statins), and cigarette smoking. Genetic factors are discussed later in this chapter.

Clinical Features

The clinical evaluation for Alzheimer's disease has four objectives: (a) to determine if the person has dementia; (b) if dementia is present, to determine whether its presentation and course are consistent with Alzheimer's disease; (c) to assess evidence for any alternate diagnoses, especially if the presentation and course are atypical for Alzheimer's disease; and (d) to evaluate evidence of other, coexisting, diseases that may contribute to the dementia, especially conditions that might respond to treatment. The clinical history should focus on the temporal relationship between the loss of different cognitive abilities and the development of behavioral disturbances and impairment of motor abilities.

The most common initial sign of Alzheimer's diseases is difficulty with episodic memory, or the ability to learn new information. At the onset, this disease may be almost imperceptible, but it typically will progress to become a more serious problem in a few years' time. The family will report that the patient frequently repeats himself or herself. He or she leaves important tasks undone, such as bills unpaid and appointments not kept. The family members will no longer feel comfortable leaving messages with the patient, and they will have to repeatedly remind him or her about the same things. After the memory disorder becomes apparent, the family will notice other disorders of cognition. Difficulty in balancing a checkbook is a common early complaint. Difficulty in carrying out normal occupational duties also may be seen if the patient is still employed. Confusion in following directions also can be a common earlier symptom, and if the patient is driving a car, he may become lost (an event that frequently precipitates the first evaluation by a physician), have an increase in minor "fender benders," or use poor judgment while driving. Frightening lapses of memory, such as leaving on a gas stove, also may occur.

As the disease progresses, difficulty in communication becomes more apparent. The patient may have difficulty in remembering simple words or names and may be unable to participate in normal conversation. Often family members comment that the patient has become a "listener" instead of actively participating in conversations. Reading and writing also will be impaired, as will simple activities of daily living, such as bathing and dressing. The patient may not recognize family members, which causes the family great distress and dismay. The family will become afraid to leave the patient alone, and the patient will require constant attention.

Agitation, hallucination, delusions, and even violent outbursts may be seen at any time during the course of the illness. Previous personality traits may be exaggerated or may be obscured completely by new behavior patterns. Changes in sleep–wake patterns also may disrupt normal living patterns. These types of symptoms are particularly difficult for the family and place a great burden on the caregiver.

Parkinsonian signs such as unsteady gait and slowed movements are common.

A general physical decline is not seen until the latest stages of the illness. Incontinence may be seen at any time and initially may reflect the patient's inability to find the bathroom. As the illness progresses, there seems to be a true loss of bladder control and ultimately even bowel function. The loss of the ability to walk is also a common occurrence seen at the late stages of the illness. This may result from excessive restraining and tranquilization in an institutional setting, but it is also frequently part of the natural history of the illness. Rarely patients with even the most profound dementia maintain the ability to walk until some type of medical or orthopedic event intervenes. Seizures and an inability or unwillingness to eat also may occur in the later stages of Alzheimer's disease.

The typical history in Alzheimer's disease is a gradually progressive dementia over several years. The average patient with Alzheimer's disease survives about a decade from the time of diagnosis, although the variation may be from a few years to 20 years. There may be plateau periods during which deterioration is not obvious; however, a lengthy plateau would be unusual. There is no clear evidence that the age of onset determines the natural history. Younger patients generally tend to have more speech disorders as the illness progresses, but longevity does not seem to vary significantly with the age of onset. Older patients are more prone to age-related medical problems associated with morbidity and mortality. One question that is asked frequently by the family is whether the physician can predict the course of the illness. No proven methods are yet available to make accurate predictions, but a few guidelines are available. First, clearly, Alzheimer's disease is associated with increased risk of death among patients in institutions. However, in the community, persons with Alzheimer's disease who have mild or moderate cognitive impairment have survival comparable to that of persons without the disease. Finally, patients with any of these three signs—severe cognitive impairment, cachexia, or parkinsonian signs—have a much greater risk of dying than Alzheimer disease subjects without these problems.

Diagnosis

Formal, standardized assessment of cognition is required to make a diagnosis of dementia and Alzheimer's disease. Wide ranges of measures are available for this purpose. Several brief measures (e.g., the Mini-Mental Status Examination and the Blessed Orientation, Memory Concentration Test) are suitable for use at the bedside or in the physician's office. Although they may help distinguish persons with dementia from persons without dementia, they are less effective in distinguishing Alzheimer's disease from other dementias.

In the office or hospital, routine mental status testing should include checking the patient's orientation by asking for his or her full name, the day of the week, the day of the month, the month and the year, where he or she is, and also his or her age and date of birth. Show the patient four or five objects and then ask him or her to name them twice (e.g., a coin, a safety pin, keys, and a comb). Tell the patient that you will ask him or her to recall the objects in a few minutes. Then check the patient's knowledge of common events by asking for the names of well-known public figures (e.g., the president, governor, or mayor). Ask the patient to repeat some numbers (the typical patient can remember six numbers forward and three or four backward). Then ask him or her to do some simple calculations (e.g., multiplication, addition, and "serial sevens"). Ask the patient to repeat a simple phrase, to follow a two-step direction (e.g., "point to the ceiling, then point to the floor"), and to do something with his right hand and then his left hand (e.g., "make a fist with your left hand," followed by "salute with your right hand"). Ask the patient to write his or her name, to write a brief phrase to dictation (e.g., "Today is Monday"), and then to draw something (usually a clock). Also ask the patient to read a simple phrase. Finally, ask the patient to recall the four or five objects that you showed him or her previously.

This mental status test can be administered in a few minutes and should be part of the routine clinical evaluation of all older persons. In a busy office practice, the physician may want to ask an assistant (e. g., a nurse) to administer a formal mental status test. For example, recommended education-adjusted cutoffs have been developed for the Mini-Mental Status Examination. The results can serve as guidelines to direct further evaluation, and they also provide valuable screening information. To make a diagnosis of dementia, a deficit should exist in more than one area of cognition. Patients with early Alzheimer's disease may have profound memory problems with only mild deficits in other aspects of cognition. As the disease progresses, however, language and other aspects of cognitive dysfunction typically become more obvious.

Physical Examination

The most important function of the neurologic examination in evaluating persons with dementia is in diagnosing conditions other than Alzheimer's disease. The general physical examination is usually normal in Alzheimer's disease. The neurologic examination (excluding the mental status testing) is also usually normal. Minor parkinsonian features, myoclonic jerks, frontal lobe signs (grasp reflex, snout and glabellar signs), and similar abnormalities occasionally may be seen on examination, especially later in the course of the illness. Any other significant abnormality of the neurologic examination should alert the physician to the possibility of a diagnosis other than, or in addition to, Alzheimer's disease.

Genetics

As with many other common chronic diseases of older persons, first-degree relatives appear to have a slightly greater risk of inheriting the disease. In rare families, however, Alzheimer's disease is inherited as an autosomal dominant disease in which half of the family members are affected. In these families, the disease has been linked to mutations on one of three different chromosomes: 21, 14, and 1. Chromosome 21 was examined because it was known that nearly all persons with Down's syndrome developed Alzheimer's disease. The mutations on chromosome 21 are in the region that codes for the precursor of the amyloid protein that is deposited in the brains of people with Alzheimer's disease. (This site is adjacent to, but not within, the obligate Down's syndrome region.) The other two genes are called presenilin 1 (chromosome 14) and presenilin 2 (chromosome 1). How these mutations lead to Alzheimer's disease is unknown. Chromosome 19 also is related to Alzheimer's disease because it codes for the apolipoprotein E alleles. Additional mutations and susceptibility genes will be found in the future. It is likely that environmental factors interact with genetics to cause the disease because, although the concordance rate for monozygotic twins greatly exceeds that for dizygotic twins, it is substantially less than 100%. Further, even when both monozygotic twins develop the disease, it is not necessarily at the same age nor do they follow the same course.

There is one well-established genetic polymorphisms associated with disease. The presence of one apolipoprotein E ε4 allele approximately doubles an individual's risk of developing Alzheimer's disease, and the risk is even higher among those homozygous for the allele. By contrast, the apolipoprotein E ε2 allele appears to lower risk of disease. The mechanism whereby this allele causes the disease is unknown, but recent data suggest that it increases the deposition of Alzheimer's disease pathology.

Laboratory Investigation

There is no reliable antemortem diagnostic test for Alzheimer's disease. The purpose of laboratory testing is to identify other conditions that might cause or exacerbate dementia. These tests routinely include a brain scan and blood tests (Table 16.1).

The purpose of morphologic imaging with magnetic resonance imaging (MRI) or computed tomography (CT) is to look for evidence of another disease process that can cause or contribute to cognitive impairment, such as a cerebral infarct or tumor. MRI is superior to CT because it is less subject to artifact, it pro-

TABLE 16.1. *Laboratory Aids in the Differential Diagnosis of Dementia*

Routine Tests	Conditions
Vitamin B$_{12}$	B$_{12}$ deficiency
T$_4$ or TSH	Hypothyroidism
RPR, FTA, MHA-TP	Syphilis
Brain scan (CT or MRI)	Vascular disease (MRI more sensitive but less specific), mass lesions, hydrocephalus, demyelinating diseases, and leukodystrophies (MRI superior)

Other Tests	Conditions
Lumbar puncture	Chronic meningitis, syphilis, inflammatory disease(s)
Electroencephalography	Creutzfeldt–Jacob disease, epilepsy
Single-photon emission computed tomography	Pick's disease and frontal lobe dementias
Drug screen/levels	Delirium due to drug toxicity
Heavy metal screen	Lead, mercury, arsenic, copper poisoning
Sedimentation rate autoimmune profile	Inflammatory disease(s)
Angiography Cerebral biopsy	Chemistry profile Chronic metabolic disturbances, endocrinopathies
Complete blood count	Chronic infections, anemia
HIV	HIV encephalopathy
Ceruloplasmin	Wilson's disease
Long-chain fatty acids	Adrenoleukodystrophy
Arylsulfatase A	Metachromatic leukodystrophy
Chest x-ray	Cardiopulmonary disease, lung tumors
Electrocardiogram	Cardiopulmonary disease

TSH, thyroid-stimulating hormone; RPR, rapid plasma reagin; FTA, fluorescent treponemal antibody; MHA-TP, microhemagglutination assay-*Treponema pallidum*.

vides greater contrast between gray and white matter, and coronal images can provide excellent views of the mesial temporal lobe structures vital to mnemonic function. With agitated patients, however, CT is often the procedure of choice because the image can be obtained more quickly. There is also strong research interest in using morphologic imaging as a direct diagnostic tool for Alzheimer's disease. For example, the volume of the hippocampus (a structure in the medial temporal lobe) on brain MRI is being investigated as a diagnostic aid. Although the technique is widely available, it has not been shown to improve diagnostic accuracy. However, brain MRI still should be used as an adjunct to identify conditions other than Alzheimer's disease that may be causing or contributing to disease.

Several other diagnostic tests for Alzheimer's disease are under investigation, although none of these are at the stage of being suitable for wide clinical use. Although the apolipoprotein E ε4 allele is not a test for Alzheimer's disease, the presence of the allele in a person with dementia of uncertain etiol-

ogy slightly increases the likelihood that the dementia is the result of Alzheimer's disease. Fragments of amyloid or tau proteins in the cerebrospinal fluid (CSF) also are being studied as diagnostic tests, but neither has proven diagnostic value. Finally, examination of cerebral blood flow, oxygen consumption, and the integrity of neural systems using positron emission tomography or single photon emission computed tomography are under evaluation. Currently, it is both more worthwhile and less expensive to refer the patient to the nearest Alzheimer's disease specialist if the diagnosis of dementia is uncertain.

Differential Diagnosis

The differential diagnosis of dementia should emphasize common conditions, such as dementia associated with strokes or Lewy bodies, and potentially treatable disorders that may cause, or exacerbate, dementia. Although reversible disorders are uncommon, their importance justifies a thorough evaluation of each patient.

Vascular Dementia

Vascular dementia includes all dementia syndromes resulting from ischemic, anoxic, or hypoxic brain damage. Thus it is not simply an Alzheimer's-type dementia caused by stroke but a constellation of cognitive syndromes that may or may not mimic Alzheimer's disease. Rather than a course of progressive decline (as seen in Alzheimer's disease), cognitive impairment may fluctuate or even improve in patients with vascular dementia. The concept of multiinfarct dementia (MID) suggests that vascular dementia is caused by the combined effect of multiple, discrete cerebral infarctions. However, other types of brain damage from vascular disease also can cause a dementia syndrome. A history of multiple strokes, an abnormal physical examination with focal neurologic findings, and the presence of vascular risk factors in a person with dementia are all suggestive of vascular disease but do not prove that the dementia is related to cerebrovascular disease. Both Alzheimer's disease and stroke are common among older persons. They often occur in the same individual by chance alone. Therefore, it is important that an attempt be made to temporally relate the onset, or worsening, of cognitive impairment to a stroke. There is no typical neuropsychologic profile of persons with vascular dementia because the behavioral manifestations are dependent on the vascular territory involved, and this may differ widely among patients. However, persons with vascular dementia rarely present with the insidious onset of episodic memory loss that characterizes early Alzheimer's disease.

White matter lesions commonly are found on MRI or CT in elderly persons, but their etiology and significance remain controversial. Many persons with dementia with white matter changes on MRI or CT have Alzheimer's disease at autopsy. Therefore, although the presence of vascular dementia should be supported by evidence of vascular disease on CT or MRI, the presence of these lesions does not necessarily indicate that the dementia is of vascular origin.

Careful control of vascular risk factors such as hypertension and cigarette smoking may alter the natural history of this illness. Other risk factors include coronary disease (including rhythm disturbances such as atrial fibrillation), diabetes, and hyperlipidemia. The value of drugs such as aspirin in preventing the progression of MID is still unknown.

Vasculitides also can cause cognitive dysfunction and psychiatric symptoms, often associated with focal motor signs and seizures. An elevated Westergren erythrocyte sedimentation rate often suggests that further evaluation for a specific immunologic disease is warranted. Further evaluation may require electroencephalography, CSF studies, and/or angiography. In some cases, meningeal and cerebral artery biopsy is necessary for definitive diagnosis.

PARKINSON'S DISEASE AND OTHER CONDITIONS ASSOCIATED WITH LEWY BODIES

The temporal relation between dementia and motor signs of Parkinson's disease is used to distinguish between a variety of related conditions. People with well-established Parkinson's disease who subsequently develop dementia are often simply referred to as having Parkinson's disease with dementia. Although in many cases this is the result of concomitant Alzheimer's disease, persons with Parkinson's disease also can develop a dementia that appears to be the result of the invasion of the limbic system and neocortex with Lewy bodies. In some situations, the dementia and parkinsonian signs appear to develop simultaneously. These cases often are referred to as having dementia with Lewy bodies (DLB), diffuse Lewy body disease, or the Lewy body variant of Alzheimer's disease. These are all rather unfortunate terms because they implicate a specific pathology rather than a dementia syndrome. There have been two workshops on criteria for dementia with Lewy bodies. It remains unclear at this time to what extent this condition simply reflects the coincidental occurrence of two common neurologic diseases of the elderly. Thus histopathologically, DLB is characterized by the presence of cortical and subcortical Lewy bodies in patients, in addition to changes—particularly plaques—that are associated with Alzheimer's disease. In addition to dementia and parkinsonian signs, these patients have fluctuating cognition, depression, REM (rapid eye movement) sleep disturbances, and hallucinations. Finally, many persons with Alzheimer's disease also develop parkinsonian signs. These signs are often the result of concomitant Lewy bodies in the substantia nigra as seen in Parkinson's disease but also can result from Alzheimer's disease changes in the substantia nigra or subcortical ischemic cerebrovascular disease. One feature of DLB is that these patients may be subject to onset of parkinsonian signs and symptoms with modest doses of neuroleptic medications, and use of neuroleptics should be limited.

Mass Lesions

Brain tumors rarely present with a degenerative dementia, and when they do, there are usually other major focal findings and signs of increased intracranial pressure. However, although rare, brain tumors in the "silent" areas of the brain may present exclusively as a change of personality and intellectual decline. Subtle focal findings usually can be demonstrated on the neurologic examination, but they occasionally are lacking. Similar comments may be applied to subdural hematomas, especially in the geriatric age group. Thus, some type of neuroimaging procedure remains warranted for all patients being evaluated for dementia.

Frontotemporal Dementia

The frontotemporal dementias are a rare group of conditions that include Pick's disease, primary progressive aphasia, and motor neuron disease with dementia. They present with neurobehavioral features of frontal and/or temporal lobe dysfunction such as socially inappropriate behavior or a progressive language deficit, as opposed to the amnestic syndrome that characterizes Alzheimer's disease. Patients are typically younger than those with Alzheimer's disease. Patients also frequently have parkinsonian signs. Families with autosomal dominant frontotemporal dementias with parkinsonism and amyotrophy have been linked to mutations in the tau gene on chromosome 17. As a result, these conditions sometimes are referred to as tauopathies.

Prion Diseases

Prion diseases are a heterogeneous group of fatal neurodegenerative conditions of sporadic, infectious, or genetic origin. The transmissible agent appears to be composed solely of the prion protein, encoded by a gene on chromosome 20, without any nucleic acid, making it unlike any other known viral or bacterial agent. Prion protein is a normal glycoprotein. The most common prion disease is Creutzfeldt–Jakob disease (CJD). Sporadic CJD presents as a rapidly progressive dementia with myoclonus, cerebellar dysfunction, parkinsonian signs, and pyramidal tract signs. Iatrogenic CJD can follow corneal or dural transplants or use of implanted stereotactic electrodes or human growth hormone. Several forms of autosomal dominant familial prion diseases can result from mutations in the prion protein gene on chromosome 20. Familial CJD tends to present younger and has a long preclinical period. In its prodromal stage, behavioral symptoms such as mania, paranoia, or psychosis can occur. Gerstmann–Straussler–Scheinker disease is characterized by progressive dementia with prominent cerebellar signs, and fatal familial insomnia is characterized by altered sleep–wake cycles with insomnia and sympathetic overactivity.

Depression

Loss of interest in hobbies and community activities, apathy, weight loss, and sleep disorders may be interpreted by the family as depression, although they actually may be the result of the dementia itself. Among the elderly, depression and dementia coexist and do not always present as two distinct entities. Although it is useful to ask the caregiver about symptoms suggesting dysphoric mood such as crying, complaining, or even suicidal ideation, depression in the elderly may present with agitation or increased irritability. Depression may contribute to impairment of activities of daily living and rarely to the cognitive deficits. If impairment in activities of daily living exceeds what is expected for the severity of cognitive dysfunction, the possibility of a coexisting depression should be considered. Pseudodementia, a syndrome of depression with impaired cognition in which treatment of the depression relieves the cognitive deficit, has been described but is probably rare.

Symptomatic Hydrocephalic Dementia

No other syndrome causing dementia has generated such intense interest (and frustration) among neurologists as normal pressure hydrocephalus. The classic syndrome consists of gait disturbance, dementia, and incontinence, although this triad also is seen commonly in Alzheimer's disease and other degenerative dementias. The onset can progress over months or years. The dementia is mild without the profound episodic memory deficit typical of Alzheimer's disease.

Brain scans typically demonstrate hydrocephalus with enlargement of ventricles out of proportion to sulci. Numerous studies have attempted to determine predictors of improvement following ventricular shunting, without much success. Perhaps the most useful piece of clinical information is a history of a reason for hydrocephalus, such as a history of meningitis or subarachnoid hemorrhage from either a ruptured aneurysm or, more commonly, a previous traumatic head injury. Some patients with gait problems or dementia improve with CSF shunting procedures; however, the insertion of a shunt is not a benign procedure, especially in geriatric patients. Although the diagnosis of normal pressure hydrocephalus rarely, if ever, can be made with complete confidence, an etiology for the hydrocephalus should be sought prior to recommending shunting.

Pathology

Data suggest that the progressive loss of memory and other cognitive abilities from Alzheimer's disease is a complex function of the accumulation of pathology (e.g., amyloid plaques and neurofibrillary tangles) and neurochemical deficits (e.g., cholinergic system), leading to a loss of neurons and synapses within selectively vulnerable neural systems. Grossly, there is atrophy and dilatation of the ventricles and marked atrophy of the hippocampal formation—a feature being exploited, as discussed earlier, to develop a neuroimaging markers of the disease. Microscopically, there are large numbers of neuritic plaques and neurofibrillary tangles. Although both of these lesions can be seen in the brains of older persons without dementia, they are found in greater numbers in the hippocampal formation and neocortex in persons with Alzheimer's disease. The current pathologic criteria for Alzheimer's disease, in fact, are based on the demonstration of a sufficient number of neuritic plaques and neurofibrillary tangles on microscopic examination. Tangles also accumulate in the basal forebrain, the major source of cholinergic neurons that project to the hippocampal formation and neocortex.

Plaques are composed of a central extracellular proteinaceous amyloid core, surrounded by dystrophic axon terminals. Amyloid comes from a larger precursor protein coded on chromosome 21. Processing of this protein by various secretases (alpha, beta, and gamma secretases) can result in either the putative toxic fragment that is deposited in the brain or another smaller, benign fragment.

The major constituents of neurofibrillary tangles are paired helical filaments. Evidence suggests that these tangles are composed of the microtubule associated protein tau, which is in an abnormal hyperphosphorylated state. Cerebrovascular amyloid (amyloid angiopathy) is also a common finding in persons with Alzheimer's disease, as are granulovacuolar degeneration and Hirano bodies.

Treatment

There are many areas in which intervention can improve quality of life for both the patient and the caregiver. Successful intervention requires that the physician work effectively with providers of many other medical and non-medical services. In general, five issues should be discussed with the family: (a) community resources, (b) advocacy, (c) pharmacotherapy, (d) behavior management, and (e) experimental therapies and procedures.

Community Resources

Most patients with Alzheimer's disease in the mild to moderate stage can be cared for at home, assuming a caregiver is available and willing to assume this responsibility. This decision can be made only by the family. It is not appropriate for the physician (or others not involved in daily care) to insist on home care when the family finds this objectionable. Adult day centers provide a structured, comprehensive program in a protective setting. They offer respite for short periods but can provide care up to 7 days a week for 12 hours a day. Most centers serve mixed populations, but some are dementia specific. Many patients do well in the day-care setting, and the use of day centers for patients with dementia results in lower levels of stress and improved psychologic well-being for caregivers. The caregiver's mental and physical health must be maintained. This ultimately benefits the patient because a healthy caregiver can manage a patient with Alzheimer's disease longer and better than one who is overwrought and exhausted. The caregiver must have rest, and other family members should be urged to take turns in caring for the patient. Family support groups, often sponsored by the Alzheimer's Association, are also helpful. The National Adult Day Services Association (866-890-7357 or 703-610-9035) or the Eldercare locator (800-677-1116) have information on local or nationwide day cares.

Special care units (SCUs) have emerged over the last few years in an attempt to maximize the independence of patients by creating a 24-hour supervised environment that is safe for disoriented residents and provide structure. Nursing home placement with dementia care units can exist in rest homes or skilled nursing facilities and often are chosen by most families at the later stages of the illness. The family should be advised to seek out a nursing home where activities and exercise are stressed and where tranquilizers and restraints are minimized.

Alzheimer's disease places a tremendous social, economic, physical, and psychologic burden on the family. The psychologic stress on the family is frequently not dealt with adequately. Stress is placed on the family in general, and particularly on the caregiver. Informal counseling through family self-help groups and formal psychologic counseling may be necessary. The physician should be available and supportive throughout the course of the illness.

Most major cities now have a local chapter of the Alzheimer's Association. The address and telephone number of the local chapter can be obtained from the national headquarters (800-272-3900; Web site: www.alz.org). The association provides information regarding local support services for both the patient and the caregiver from other people facing similar problems. The National Institute on Aging also maintains the Alzheimer's Disease Education and Referral Center (ADEAR) (800-438-4380; Web site: www.alzheimers.org), which has information for both family members and physicians.

Advocacy

Because patients with Alzheimer's disease eventually may lose all decision-making capabilities, it is important that, at the time of the initial diagnosis, the physician alert the patient and family of the need to make decisions regarding advance directives, living wills and trusts, power of attorney, and guardianship. Advance directives should include an open discussion of the patient's wishes regarding nursing home placement and aggressive intervention at the end of life, including feeding tubes, intubations, and resuscitation. The determination of power of attorney or guardianship is fundamental to making economic or ethical decisions regarding the care of the patient. Many patients with mild cognitive impairment are legally competent to execute a valid power of attorney, placing in the hands of another person decisions regarding his or her health and estate. A separate power of attorney for health care and property must be completed. In addition, the power of attorney should be "durable," which means that it remains effective if the patient becomes incompetent. Guardianship must be imposed on a patient who has become incompetent and is no longer able to sign for power of attorney. In the event of family discord, the physician should avoid siding with one family member over another and should refer the family to a competent and sympathetic attorney.

Pharmacotherapy

There are now five agents approved by the U.S. Food and Drug Administration (FDA) for the symptomatic treatment of Alzheimer's disease (Table 16.2). Four drugs work to enhance cholinergic transmission in the brain by reducing the degradation of acetylcholine through inhibition of the enzyme acetylcholinesterase (AchE). Tacrine and rivastigmine inhibit both AchE and butyrylcholinesterase (BuChE), whereas donepezil and galantamine inhibit AchE but have only minimal inhibition of BuChE (Table 16.3). There are several medical contraindications to cholinesterase inhibitors. Patients with serious liver disease or active alcohol abuse are not candidates for treatment with these agents. These inhibitors increase gastric secretions and should not be used in patients with active peptic ulcer disease. They also can increase bronchial secretions and should be avoided in patients with severe chronic obstructive pulmonary disease or asthma. They are vagotonic and can cause bradycardia, and they should not be used in patients with preexisting bradycardia or sick sinus syndrome.

All of them have similar efficacy, although tacrine rarely is used because of hepatotoxicity and the need to monitor liver enzymes. Donepezil administration is once a day, in the evening, starting at 5 mg and increasing to 10 mg after 4 to 6 weeks. Rivastigmine is administered twice daily, starting at 1.5 mg bid, and increased by 3 mg a day every 2 weeks, as tolerated, until a dose of 6 mg bid is reached. Because of significant nausea and vomiting, dose escalation frequently is done more slowly. Galantamine is started at 8 mg bid and increased to 12 mg bid after a couple of weeks. Some drug interactions are known for tacrine. Coadministration of tacrine with theophylline increased plasma theophylline levels by twofold, and use of tacrine with cimetidine can increase the concentration of tacrine in the body. Likewise, donepezil metabolism is inhibited by quinidine and ketoconazole. Medications such as carbamazepine, phenytoin, phenobarbital, rifampin, and dexamethasone may increase donepezil's elimination from the body. Two cases of moderately severe side effects between donepezil and selective serotonin reuptake inhibitor's usage have been reported. None of these drugs are thought to slow the progression of the underlying disease. Thus, patients should be monitored for improvement with both formal mental status testing and discussions with the patient's family and/or caregiver. In addition, none of these medications have proven efficacy among persons with mild memory problems, those who do not have Alzheimer's disease, those with dementia caused by conditions other than Alzheimer's disease, or those with advanced dementia.

The U.S. Food and Drug Administration recently approved memantine for the treatment of moderate to severe Alzheimer's disease. This drug is a low to moderate affinity NMDA (N-methyl-D-aspartate) receptor antagonist. It is

TABLE 16.2. *Pharmacologic Treatments Approved by the Food and Drug Administration*

	Tacrine	Donepezil	Rivastigmine	Galantamine	Memantine
Doses per day	4	1	2	2	2
Initial dose (mg/d)	40	5	3	16	5
Maximum dose (mg/d)	160	10	12	24	20
Given with food	No	No	Yes	No	No
Drug–drug interaction	Yes	Yes	None	None	Yes

TABLE 16.3. *Pharmacokinetic Characteristics*

	Tacrine	Donepezil	Rivastigmine	Galantamine	Memantine
Plasma half life (h)	2–4	73	5	4.4–5.7	60–80
Clearance	Liver	Liver	Kidney	50% kidney, 50% liver	Kidney
Metabolized by CYP450 isoenzymes	Yes	Yes	Minimal	Yes	Minimal
Enzymes inhibited					
AchE	Yes	Yes	Yes	Yes	N/A
BuChE	Yes	Negligible	Yes	Negligible	N/A

thought that overexcitation of NMDA receptors by the neurotransmitter glutamate may play a role in Alzheimer's disease since glutamate plays an integral role in neural pathways associated with learning and memory. Excitotoxicity produced by abnormal levels of glutamate is thought to be responsible for cell dysfunction and eventual cell death observed in Alzheimer's disease. Memantine selectively blocks the excitotoxic effects associated with abnormal transmission of glutamate, while allowing for physiological transmission associated with normal cell function.

The recommended starting dosage is 5 mg/qd with a target dosage of 20 mg/day. Dosages should be titrated in 5 mg increments with a one-week interval between increases. The combined use of memantine with other NMDA antagonists (amantadine, ketamine, and dextromethorphan) have not been systematically evaluated, and caution is advised. Coadministration of memantine with donepezil HCL did not affect the pharmacokinetics of either compound.

Ongoing Clinical Trials for Cognition

Several other agents are in various stages of investigation by the National Institute on Aging-funded Alzheimer's Disease Cooperative Study (ADCS) or by pharmaceutical companies. The ADCS, founded in 1991, is a multicenter consortium of Alzheimer's disease centers with the coordinating center at the University of California, San Diego (see http://adrc.ucsd.edu/ for a list of participating centers). They conducted double-blind clinical trials of estrogen effects among healthy community-dwelling postmenopausal women and a double-blind trial of prednisone. Both of these studies were negative. Many trials are under way and include a trial of donepezil and vitamin E among healthy community-dwelling persons with mild cognitive impairment (to see if time to develop Alzheimer's disease can be delayed) and the use of divalproex sodium for agitation in nursing home residents with Alzheimer's disease. Upcoming trials include the use of statins to potentially slow the progression of Alzheimer's disease and the use of high-dose supplements to reduce homocysteine and possibly slow the rate of cognitive decline in Alzheimer's disease.

The National Institute on Aging is funding several other large, multicenter, primary prevention clinical trials including the Alzheimer's Disease Anti-inflammatory Prevention Trial (ADAPT); an Alzheimer's disease endpoint (PREADVISE) was added to the Selenium and Vitamin E Chemoprevention Trial (SELECT) to prevent prostate cancer; and a trial of estrogen is ongoing.

Wyeth-Ayerst also added an Alzheimer's disease endpoint to the Women's Health Initiative. The European Union recently approved memantine for the treatment of moderate to severe Alzheimer's disease following a favorable recommendation by the Committee of Proprietary Medicinal Products (CPMP). The FDA is negotiating with the company for approval in the United States.

Several studies now are aimed at altering the underlying neurobiology of disease. A high-profile study of a vaccine trial to remove beta amyloid from the brain was started but then halted as a result of side effects. Several pharmaceutical companies are developing agents with the potential to inhibit beta or gamma secretase in an effort to retard the buildup of beta amyloid.

Alternative Treatments

One study suggested that a high-dose vitamin E supplement (2,000 IU/day) delayed overall time to one of the following outcomes: death, institutionalization, loss of the ability to perform basic activities of daily living, or severe dementia. The mechanism of this effect, and its specificity, remains to be elucidated because vitamin E did not appear to have an effect on cognitive function. Some, but not most, studies suggest that Ginkgo biloba may be of benefit in Alzheimer's disease. A trial funded by the National Center for Complementary and Alternative Medicine is ongoing.

Behavioral Management

The course of Alzheimer's disease often is punctuated by neuropsychiatric disturbances. Although psychotic symptoms may present at any time during the course of the dementing illness, they are more common in the middle and late stages. Common psychotic symptoms include delusions (theft of belongings, abandonment by family, spousal infidelity), misinterpretation of delusions (characters on television are real; others are living in the house [phantom boarders]), or hallucinations. Physical aggression that may result can have the most severe consequences for the family, eventually leading to institutionalization of the patient. Numerous studies have addressed the pharmacologic management of behavioral disturbances among patients with Alzheimer's disease. Antipsychotic medications are the only agents with proven efficacy for the psychosis of Alzheimer's disease. High-potency agents such as haloperidol and fluphenazine have predominantly extrapyramidal adverse effects and have fallen out of favor in the treatment of psychosis in patients with Alzheimer's disease. The atypical antipsychotics (risperidone, olanzapine, quetiapine, clozapine) have replaced conventional neuroleptics as firstline pharmacotherapy for psychosis associated with Alzheimer's disease. Risperidone often is used at a dose of 1 to 2 mg/day and is effective in reducing psychotic symptoms and aggression. The development of parkinsonism (a side effect of risperidone) is seen in patients taking more than 2 mg/day risperidone. Some patients benefit from as little as 0.25 to 0.5 mg/day.

Depression and alterations of sleep–wake cycles respond to pharmacologic intervention and should be treated. Few controlled studies exist from which to guide the dose and duration of pharmacotherapy. In persons with dementia and depression, agents such as sertraline, citalopram, paroxetine, and mirtazapine have been used. In persons with disturbances of sleep, a low-dose, sedating narcoleptic or trazodone may be preferable to hypnotics for the non-depressed patient with Alzheimer's disease with a significant sleep disorder. Some studies suggest that melatonin, or phototherapy, may be beneficial for sleep disorders associated with Alzheimer's disease.

Rehabilitation

There has been several studies on cognitive rehabilitation. In general, these have met with limited success. Further, many investigators believe that the stress induced on patients by being reminded of their deficits may not be offset by the possible small therapeutic gains of this intervention.

Special Considerations for Hospitalized Patients

There are three special considerations regarding hospitalized patients. First, because many persons with Alzheimer's disease are not diagnosed, hospital staff must be sensitive to the possibility of unrecognized dementia among subjects admitted to the hospital for an unrelated reason. Because the hospital setting can be very disorienting, this situation can easily unmask a mild, unrecognized dementia. Thus, in the evaluation of conditions that can cause a delirium (see later), the physician should seek detailed information regarding the patient's premorbid function. Second, patients with dementia frequently become agitated in the hospital setting, often to the point of needing physical and/or chemical sedation that can frighten patients, staff, and family.

Thus, whenever possible, one should avoid hospitalizing patients with a known dementia. When hospitalization is necessary, a geriatric psychiatry unit may be preferred over a medical floor because the nurses, staff, and setting may be better prepared to care for these problems. Family should be encouraged to stay with the patient, and the use of infusing tubes and machines, including intravenous lines and urinary catheters, should be brief.

Delirium

Delirium differs from dementia by the onset and duration of cognitive impairment and by the level of consciousness. The onset of cognitive impairment in delirium is typically hours to days, and it lasts days to weeks. In addition, patients are often either hyperalert or hypoalert. However, in older persons, altered consciousness may be less evident and, as already mentioned, a delirium may be the initial manifestation of an underlying, unrecognized dementia. Thus, data suggest that delirium in the elderly may take many months to resolve or may not resolve at all. The occurrence of delirium in the hospitalized elderly has been associated with excess mortality.

Toxic/Metabolic Conditions

Drug toxicity is a common reversible cause of delirium in the elderly. Older persons may be more susceptible than younger persons to drug side effects on cognition. This is the result of many factors, including altered drug kinetics and use of multiple medications in older persons with several illnesses or complaints ("polypharmacy"). Clinicians also should be alert to the possibility of drug side effects further impairing cognition in persons with preexisting cognitive impairment. A typical presentation is the rapid worsening of dementia following the administration of a new drug (or following the reinstitution of a previous medication that the patient has not taken for some time), with or without altered level of consciousness. Psychotropics, such as neuroleptics and sedative–hypnotics, and cardiovascular medications, especially antihypertensives, are common offending agents.

Metabolic and Hematologic Disorders

Hypothyroidism has been recognized for many years as being associated with altered mental state, although it is currently quite rare in the United States. Similar cases are seen with disorders of calcium metabolism, especially hypercalcemia, and also with an electrolyte imbalance.

Chronic liver and renal diseases frequently are associated with an altered mental state. However, it is unusual for these diseases to be present without prominent manifestations of the primary illnesses. Repeated episodes of hypoglycemia can cause dementia, although in this case, the history is usually episodic rather than gradual.

Pernicious anemia can cause altered mental state even without hematologic or other neurologic findings. Whether this is also true for folate deficiency is unclear. This deficiency syndrome, however, is not as clearly described as that of B_{12}.

Korsakoff's syndrome, as a result of thiamine deficiency, also can present with an amnestic syndrome. It classically develops in the wake of an acute Wernicke's encephalopathy with confusion, ophthalmoplegia, and ataxia. However, many patients with Korsakoff's syndrome do not present with a Wernicke's encephalopathy. Although alcoholism is the most frequent setting for this syndrome in developed countries, it also may be associated with other conditions leading to nutritional deficiency, including starvation, malnutrition, protracted vomiting, and gastric resection. It also can be precipitated by administration of carbohydrates to patients with marginal thiamine stores.

Infections

Cognitive impairment is among the most common neurologic manifestations of acquired immunodeficiency syndrome (AIDS) and may precede the development of other signs of infection with the human immunodeficiency virus (HIV). Patients with the AIDS dementia complex present with forgetfulness and poor attention, typically over several months. The memory impairment is typically less striking than that seen in Alzheimer's disease. Other signs of AIDS should be sought, and, if found, a high index of suspicion for other infections should be maintained.

Chronic meningitis, especially cryptococcal meningitis, can present as dementia, although there are almost always other associated signs and symptoms. The same can be said for neurosyphilis. Brain abscesses, like brain tumors, can present solely with dementia, although focal findings usually also are present.

When to Refer to a Neurologist

Patients and families must be assured of the likely cause of their dementia, and a neurologic referral is useful to establish that all treatable causes of dementia have been considered. Because a variety of new medications are available and more are being tested, the neurologist can outline the current treatment options so that the non-neurologist, patient, and family can make appropriate decisions. Often, regular day-to-day management of Alzheimer's disease and other dementias is directed by non-neurologists with a once-annual consultation with a neurologist.

Over the past several years, many neurologists have specialized in dementia care. Thus, most major medical centers now have a multidisciplinary, dementia referral center. These centers often are staffed with nurses and social workers with special expertise in dementia care as well as with a team of neurologists and/or geriatric psychiatrists. Referral to these centers should be considered for behavioral management, family planning, and pharmacologic treatment in the context of complicated medical illnesses. In addition, many patients and families are eager to participate in clinical trials and other kinds of research and find comfort in the fact that although available pharmacotherapies are less than ideal, they have an opportunity to work with investigators to develop treatments. Most university-based Alzheimer's disease centers have newsletters that the non-neurologists can obtain to keep informed about educational and research options for patients and families.

QUESTIONS AND DISCUSSION

1. A 75-year-old man is brought to the physician by his wife for evaluation of memory problems. She states that over the last few years he has become more forgetful and is having difficulty in doing some household tasks. Initially his wife felt this was just the result of getting older, but she became more concerned when her husband got lost driving to a store that they both go to regularly. In addition, at a recent party he had noticeable problems recalling friends' names and did not participate in conversations as much as he had in the past. Family members mentioned that the patient appears "sad" at times, but no changes in the patient's hobbies, sleep, or appetite have occurred. Medical history includes hypertension for 5 years (controlled with enalapril) and a history of angina. Physical and neurologic examinations are unremarkable except for a Mini-Mental Status Exam score of 25. Psychometric testing reveals mild short-term memory impairment. Attention and orientation are mildly impaired, and language, praxis, and visual perception are in the normal range. Mood is not suggestive of depression. A workup for reversible causes of dementia (including thyroid-stimulating hormone and vitamin B_{12} levels) is normal. An MRI of the brain reveals mild cortical atrophy with no evidence of stroke.

2. The differential diagnosis for this patient is:

A. Mild cognitive impairment
B. Depression
C. Alzheimer's disease

The answer is (C). Recent literature suggests that individuals evolving to dementia generally will go through a transitional phase of mild cognitive impairment (MCI). In its purest form, memory impairment is the most prominent feature of MCI on cognitive testing, with relatively sparing of other cognitive functions. This patient's neuropsychologic profile suggests that more than one cognitive domain is affected (in addition to memory problems), and thus a MCI diagnosis is incorrect. Because of the lack of depressive symptomatology, depression is also not thought to be a major contributor to the patient's memory problem. The patient's history and clinical and neuropsychologic examinations are consistent with the early stages of Alzheimer's disease.

3. The physician makes the diagnosis of Alzheimer's dementia. Which of the following drugs is a suitable first choice for the treatment of cognitive decline associated with Alzheimer's disease?

A. Donepezil
B. Rivastigmine
C. Galantamine
D. Memantine

The answers are (A), (B), or (C). All three medications can be used as firstline medications. There have been no head-to-head trials of these medications to warrant one medication as being the firstline drug over another. Possible drug interactions, clinical history, convenience in dosing, and ability to tolerate some of the side effects of the medication are important factors in prescribing acetyl-cholinesterase inhibitors. The clinical history suggests a possible coronary history, and thus a baseline electrocardiogram could be warranted to rule out sinus bradycardia or sick sinus syndrome. This would preclude the use of donepezil (Aricept). Presently, memantine is approved for use in moderate to severe Alzheimer's disease only.

4. Based on current evidence, which is the most appropriate add-on therapy for the treatment of Alzheimer's disease in this patient?

A. Estrogen
B. Selegiline
C. Vitamin E
D. Ginkgo

The answer is (C). There is some evidence for increased oxidative stress and free radical injury in the brain with Alzheimer's disease. One study demonstrated that two antioxidants, alpha tocopherol (vitamin E) and selegiline (a monamine oxidase inhibitor), provided similar improvements in outcomes in Alzheimer's disease. Because the safety and cost profile of vitamin E are better than that of selegiline, vitamin E can be recommended. Ginkgo is the over-the-counter herbal agent that many take as a memory aid. A review of the literature emphasizes the limited and inconsistent data in support of ginkgo. Additional research is needed before this remedy can be accepted as a valuable treatment in Alzheimer's disease. Estrogen continues to cause controversy as to its potential role in Alzheimer's disease. Plausible mechanisms for the protective role of estrogens on cognition suggest that estrogen increases release of acetylcholine in certain brain regions and protects neurons from oxidative stress and beta amyloid–induced toxicity. Some studies have suggested a decreased risk of Alzheimer's disease among estrogen users. To date, there is no evidence to support the use of estrogen in men.

5. The patient started taking donepezil 2 years ago, but on his first return visit to the clinic, his Mini-Mental Status Exam score dropped to 18. His wife reports that he has been experiencing behavior changes—mainly mild agitation, hallucinations, and delusions. On examination, he has very mild parkinsonian signs with no evidence of tremor. Which of the following neuroleptic medications is the most suitable choice for the long-term management of psychosis in this patient?

A. Clozapine
B. Risperidone
C. Haloperidol
D. Olanzapine

The answer is (A), (B), or (D). Haloperidol may be useful in the acute treatment of psychosis or agitation in patients with Alzheimer's disease but should not be used for long-term management. The risk of drug-induced parkinsonism and tardive dyskinesia is high, and this patient already is having very mild parkinsonian signs. The other medications are all atypical neuroleptics, which have a lower incidence of drug-induced parkinsonism and tardive dyskinesia. Clozapine can be used for long-term management; however, it requires weekly blood draws for 6 months and monitoring of the complete blood count. It can cause a fatal agranulocytosis, which has a prevalence of 1% during the first year of exposure. If medication compliance or the potential for loss of follow-up in the clinic is an issue, the other choices [(B), (D)] are preferable.

SUGGESTED READING

American Psychiatric Association. Practice guideline for the treatment of patients with Alzheimer's disease and other dementias of late life. *Am J Psychiatry* 1997;154(Suppl 5):1–39.

Bennett DA, Wilson RS, Schneider JA, et al. Natural history of mild cognitive impairment in older persons. *Neurology* 2002;59:198–205.

Bennett DA, Wilson RS, Schneider JA, et al. Apolipoprotein E ε4 allele, Alzheimer's disease pathology, and the clinical expression of Alzheimer's disease. *Neurology* 2003; 60:246–252.

Callahan CM, Hendrie HC, Tierney WM. Documentation and evaluation of cognitive impairment in elderly primary care patients. *Ann Intern Med* 1995;122:422.

DeKosky ST, Ikonomovic M., Styren S, et al. Upregulation of choline acetyltransferase activity in hippocampus and frontal cortex of elderly subjects with mild cognitive impairment. *Ann Neurol* 2002;51:145–155.

Doody RS, Stevens JC, Beck C, et al. Practice parameter: management of dementia (an evidence-based review). Report of the Quality Standards Subcommittee of the American Academy of Neurology. *Neurology* 2001;56:1154–1166.

Farlow MR, et al. Memantine donepezil dual therapy is superior to placebo/donepezil therapy for treatment of moderate to severe Alzheimer's disease. *Neurology* 2003;60: 4–12.

Gregg EW, Yaffe K, Cauley JA, et al. Is diabetes associated with cognitive impairment and cognitive decline among older women? Study of Osteoporotic Fractures Research Group. *Arch Intern Med* 2000;160:174–180.

Hebert LE, Scherr PA, McCann JJ, et al. Is the risk of developing Alzheimer's disease greater for women than for men? *Am J Epidemiol* 2001;153:132–136.

Inouye SK. The dilemma of delirium: clinical and research controversies regarding diagnosis and evaluation of delirium in hospitalized elderly medical patients. *Am J Med* 1994;97:278–288.

Jick H, Zornberg GL, Jick SS, et al. Statins and the risk of dementia. *Lancet* 2000;356:1627–1631.

Katz IR, Jeste DV, Mintzer JE, et al. Comparison of risperidone and placebo for psychosis and behavioral disturbances associated with dementia: a randomized double blind trial. Risperidone Study Group. *J Clin Psychiatry* 1999;60:107–115.

Knopman DS, DeKosky ST, Cummings JL, et al. Practice parameter: diagnosis of dementia (an evidence-based review). Report of the Quality Standards Subcommittee of the American Academy of Neurology. *Neurology* 2001; 56:1143–1153.

McKeith IG, Perry EK, Perry RH. Report of the second dementia with Lewy body international workshop: diagnosis and treatment. Consortium on Dementia with Lewy Bodies. *Neurology* 1999;53:902–905.

McKhann GM, Albert MS, Grossman M, et al. Clinical and pathological diagnosis of frontotemporal dementia: report of the Work Group on Frontotemporal Dementia and Pick's Disease. *Arch Neurol* 2001;58:1803–1809.

Mittelman MS, Ferris SH, Shulman E, et al. A family intervention to delay nursing home placement of patients with Alzheimer disease: a randomized controlled trial. *JAMA* 1996;276:1725.

Morris MC, Beckett LA, Scherr PA, et al. Vitamin E and vitamin C supplement use and risk of incident Alzheimer's disease. *Alzheimer Dis Assoc Disord* 1998;12:121.

Mulnard RA, Cotman CW, Kawas C, et al. Estrogen replacement therapy for treatment of mild to moderate Alzheimer disease: a randomized controlled trial. Alzheimer's Disease Cooperative Study. *JAMA* 2000;283: 1007–1015.

Nordberg A, Svensson AL. Cholinesterase inhibitors in the treatment of Alzheimer's disease: a comparison of tolerability and pharmacology. *Drug Saf* 1998;19:465–480.

Petersen RC, Stevens JC, Ganguli M, et al. Practice parameter: early detection of dementia: mild cognitive impairment (an evidence-based review). Report of the Quality Standards Subcommittee of the American Academy of Neurology. *Neurology* 2001;56:1133–1142.

Reisberg B, et al. Memantine in moderate to severe Alzheimer's disease. *N Engl J Med* 2003;348:141333.

Roman GC, Tatemichi TK, Erkinjuntti T, et al. Vascular dementia: diagnostic criteria for research studies. Report of the NINDS-AIREN International Work Group. *Neurology* 1993;43:250.

Sano M, Ernesto C, Thomas RG, et al. A controlled trial of Selegiline, alpha-tocopherol, or both as treatment for Alzheimer's disease. *N Engl J Med* 1997;336:1216.

Schneider JA, Wilson RS, Cochran EJ, et al. Relation of cerebral infarctions to dementia and cognitive function in older persons. *Neurology* 2003;60:1082–1088.

Tangalos EG, Smith GE, Ivnik RJ, et al. The Mini-Mental State Examination in general medical practice: clinical utility and acceptance. *Mayo Clin Proc* 1996;71:829.

Tanzi RE, Bertram L. New frontiers in Alzheimer's disease genetics. *Neuron* 2001;32:181–184.

Wilson RS, Mendes de Leon CF, Barnes LL, et al. Participation in cognitively stimulating activities and risk of incident Alzheimer's disease. *JAMA* 2002;287:742–748.

Wilson RS, Bienias JL, Berry-Kravis E, et al. The apolipoprotein E ε2 allele and decline in episodic memory. *J Neurol Neurosurg Psychiatry* 2002;73:672–677.

Wilson RS, Schneider JA, Beckett LA, et al. Parkinsonian-like signs and risk of incident Alzheimer's disease in older persons. *Arch Neurol* 2003;60:539–544.

Winblad B, Poritis N. Memantine in severe dementia: results of the 9M-Best Study (benefit and efficacy in severely demented patients during treatment with memantine). *Int J Geriatr Psychiatry* 1999;14:135–146.

Yaffe K, Krueger K, Sarkar S, et al. Cognitive function in postmenopausal women treated with raloxifene. *N Engl J Med* 2001;344:1207–1213.

Zhu L, Fratiglioni L, Zhenchao G, et al. Association o f stroke with dementia, cognitive impairment, and functional disability in the very old: a population based study. *Stroke* 1998;29:2094–2099.

17

Neurotoxic Effects of Drugs Prescribed by Non-Neurologists

Katie Kompoliti

Neurotoxicology is a growing field of clinical interest, and physicians increasingly are required to evaluate and treat patients with numerous complications of toxic exposure. The usual compounds discussed in a chapter on neurotoxicology would include metals (e.g., lead, mercury, and arsenic), industrial toxins (e.g., organic solvents, gases, pesticides, and other environmental toxins), and biologic toxins (e.g., bacterial exotoxins, animal poisons, venoms, and botanical poisons). Syndromes associated with these toxins, however, are not frequently encountered by the non-neurologist. Yet many drugs that are commonly prescribed by treating physicians may precipitate neurotoxic signs or exacerbate underlying neurologic disease. The neurologic complications of drugs commonly prescribed for the medical management of ambulatory adults are discussed in this chapter.

ANTIBIOTICS

Penicillins

Penicillin and related agents rarely cause nervous system toxic effects, although seizures and myoclonic jerks have been reported with high intravenous (IV) doses. Such effects appear more commonly in elderly patients with compromised renal function. Meningitic inflammation may enhance neurotoxic effects by promoting the penetration of these drugs into the central nervous system (CNS) and decreasing their egress. Polyneuritis, with paresthesias, paralysis, and loss of tendon reflexes, also has been reported.

Cephalosporins

Cephalosporins may cause a number of neurotoxic effects, especially in patients with renal dysfunction or in those receiving high doses. Symptoms can include confusion, coma, tremor, myoclonic jerks, asterixis, and hyperexcitability. Status epilepticus that did not respond to anticonvulsant therapy and subsequently resolved with discontinuation of cefepime has been described in two patients receiving this fourth-generation cephalosporin.

Aminoglycosides

The toxicities of all aminoglycoside antibiotics—neomycin, kanamycin, streptomycin, gentamycin, tobramycin, and amikacin—are similar. The two major adverse effects are (a) damage of the eighth cranial nerve and hearing apparatus and (b) a potentiation of neuromuscular blockade. Cochlear and vestibular damage is the result of direct toxicity of these drugs. Auditory toxicity is more common with the use of amikacin and kanamycin, whereas vestibular toxicity predominates following gentamycin and streptomycin therapy. Tobramycin is associated equally with vestibular and auditory damage. The incidence of clinical ototoxicity as a result of use of these drugs ranges from 5% to 25%, depending on whether audiometry is used to detect hearing deficits. Aminoglycoside hearing loss is usually irreversible and may even progress after the discontinuation of drug therapy.

A potentially fatal neurotoxic effect of all aminoglycosides is a neuromuscular blockade. The aminoglycosides act similarly to curare, blocking the neuromuscular junction. Aminoglycosides also possibly potentiate ether and other anesthetics during surgery. Sudden or prolonged respiratory paralysis resulting from aminoglycoside use may be reversed by the administration of calcium or neostigmine.

Antifungal Agents

The polymyxins are related closely to the aminoglycosides in structure and neurotoxicity. The incidence of neurotoxic reaction has been estimated at 7%, and syndromes other than neuromuscular blockade include paresthesias, peripheral neuropathy, dizziness, and seizures. Respiratory paralysis, however, is the most serious neurotoxic reaction. An underlying renal dysfunction predisposes to the neuromuscular blockade induced by this drug group. Signs of neuromuscular blockade include diplopia, dysphagia, and weakness.

Amphotericin B is widely used against systemic fungal infection. When the drug is used intrathecally, seizures, pain along the lumbar nerves, mononeuropathies (including foot drop), and chemical meningitis have occurred.

Antituberculous Drugs

Isoniazid (INH) has been associated with neurotoxic effects felt to be related to drug binding of pyridoxine and resultant excessive vitamin excretion. A prominent polyneuropathy is associated with chronic INH administration, and symptoms include paresthesias; diminished pain, touch, and temperature discrimination; and eventual weakness. Seizures, emotional irritability, euphoria, depression, headache, and psychosis rarely may occur. The neurotoxic reactions from INH use are dose related and are more common in "slow inactivators." In these patients, neurotoxic reactions can be prevented or diminished by the administration of pyridoxine at a dose of 50 mg daily. Patients who intentionally or inad-

vertently overdose acutely with INH may develop severe ataxia, generalized seizures, and coma. Supportive measures, anticonvulsants, and pyridoxine should be administered to these patients.

Rifamycin frequently is administered with INH. Neurologic side effects are uncommon but may include headache, dizziness, inability to concentrate, and confusion. Less commonly, signs of peripheral neuropathy may develop. Ethambutol precipitates a reversible optic neuritis as well as a more generalized peripheral neuropathy. A metallic taste in the oral cavity frequently is associated with ethambutol therapy and may be due to the result of an impairment of receptor activity.

Antiviral Drugs

The treatment of selected viral infections in individuals who are not positive for the human immunodeficiency virus (HIV) individuals has become possible over the past few years. The neurologic complications of HIV and the drugs used to treat it will be discussed elsewhere.

Acyclovir can be administered either intravenously or orally. Acyclovir is used orally for the treatment of localized or ophthalmic varicella zoster, treatment of minor herpes simplex virus, and reducing the severity of varicella. Neurologic side effects rarely are associated with oral acyclovir. However, seizures, encephalopathy, hallucinations, and coma have been described, as has tremor.

Amantadine has been used to prevent influenza A infections. This agent appears to have, in addition to its antiviral action, anticholinergic and dopaminergic effects, which has led to its use in mild Parkinson's disease. The neurologic side effects associated with amantadine include sedation, confusion, myoclonus, hallucinations, delirium, and seizures. As amantadine is excreted through the kidney, the presence of renal impairment may reduce its clearance, causing it to accumulate in the body and resulting in amantadine toxicity.

OTHER COMMONLY PRESCRIBED ANTIBIOTICS

Sulfonamide, pyrimethamine, and trimethoprim are used mainly in the treatment of urinary tract infections (UTIs). They generally are considered safe drugs and are not associated with marked neurotoxicity. They may cause headache, fatigue, tinnitus, and acute psychosis, however. Some signs may mimic meningitis. On the second or third day of therapy, patients may complain of difficulty in concentrating and impaired judgment. Nitrofurantoin also is used commonly in the treatment of UTIs. A polyneuropathy is the major toxic syndrome with this drug. Like the Guillain-Barré syndrome, this neuropathy is usually subacute and begins in the distal extremities, often with sensory complaints of paresthesias and numbness. The neuropathy ascends and involves the motor system, with progressive weakness and areflexia. Discontinuation of the drug is essential, and not all patients will recover. The prognosis appears to relate most significantly to the extent of the neuropathy at the time of drug withdrawal.

Tetracycline can be associated with pseudotumor cerebri or increased intracranial pressure. The syndrome is characterized by headache; papilledema; elevated spinal fluid pressure; and, in babies, bulging fontanels. Significant vestibular toxicity also has been associated with a tetracycline derivative, minocycline.

Erythromycin is probably the least toxic of the commonly used antibiotics from a neurologic perspective. An uncommon side effect is temporary hearing loss. Erythromycin interacts with carbamazepine; thus the anticonvulsant levels increase rapidly when erythromycin is introduced.

Azithromycin, a new macrolide antibiotic, also has been reported to cause hearing loss. Clarithromycin has been reported to precipitate an acute psychotic episode.

Nitrofurantoin therapy has been associated with polyneuropathy. Generally seen with prolonged therapy, neuropathy can occur as early as the first week of treatment. It is usually subacute, begins in the distal extremities with paresthesias, and tends to progressively ascend to involve the motor system with weakness and areflexia. Although this polyneuropathy clinically resembles Guillain-Barré syndrome, the spinal fluid is usually normal, except that 25% of patients have a slight increase in protein without pleocytosis. When polyneuropathy is recognized, drug withdrawal is essential, although 10% to 15% of patients will not improve and 15% will have only partial recovery. The prognosis appears to correlate with the extent of the neuropathy at the time of drug withdrawal but not to the total dose exposure or the duration of therapy.

ANTIRETROVIRAL MEDICATIONS

Patients infected with the HIV virus are living longer than before as the result of a better understanding of the disease process and newer pharmacologic agents often used in combination to control viral loads. The currently available classes of antiretrovirals for HIV infection include protease inhibitors, nucleoside reverse transcriptase inhibitors, and nonnucleoside reverse transcriptase inhibitors. New drug regimens support the use of concomitant medications from each class in HIV-positive individuals to prevent the complications of AIDS.

The major neurologic side effects of nucleoside reverse transcriptase inhibitors include peripheral neuropathy. This is typically a distal symmetric predominantly sensory neuropathy and has been described with zalcitabine, didanosine, and stavudine. Electromyography demonstrates an axonal neuropathy. It may be difficult to determine the origin of the neuropathy because HIV infection also can cause a distal sensory neuropathy. The treatment includes removal of the offending agent. Myopathy of mitochondrial origin has been reported with both the nucleoside reverse transcriptase inhibitors and the non-nucleoside reverse transcriptase inhibitors. This is a proximal symmetric myopathy with a mitochondrial pattern of ragged-red fibers. Removal of the offending agent is the best treatment.

The major neurologic side effects of the nonnucleoside reverse transcriptase inhibitors include dizziness, somnolence, diminished concentration, and confusion. The patient also may experience psychiatric disturbances including agitation, depersonalization, hallucinations, insomnia, vivid dreams, depression, and euphoria. These symptoms are most severe at initiation of therapy. They typically resolve with elimination of the offending medication.

CARDIAC DRUGS

Glycosides

Digitalis and related agents are the mainstay of treatment for congestive heart failure. Neurologic complications of digitalis therapy have been recognized for almost 200 years and are characterized by nausea, vomiting, visual disturbances, seizures, and syncope. Adverse effects on the CNS reportedly occur in 40% to 50% of patients with clinical digitalis toxicity and may occur before, simultaneously with, or after the signs of cardiac toxicity develop.

The most frequent and often the first sign of clinical intoxication is nausea, which appears to be the result of central mechanisms rather than gastrointestinal irritation. The incidence of digitalis-related visual disturbances has been estimated at 40%, and although these symptoms may occur as an isolated symptom, they usually occur concomitantly with other toxic signs. Blurred vision, reversible scotomas, diplopia, defects of color vision, and total amaurosis represent the spectrum of optic side effects.

Seizures most commonly are seen in pediatric patients. The incidence of digitalis-related seizures is difficult to estimate because other seizure etiologies (e.g., arrhythmia) are so high in cardiac patients. Transient mental aberrations felt to be caused by intermittent cerebral hypoperfusion resemble transient global amnesia. Syncope, probably the result of conduction delay or hyperactivity of baroreceptors, also has occurred in digitalis toxicity. Other neurotoxic reactions include facial neuralgia, paresthesias, headache, weakness, and fatigue. Cerebral symptoms consisting of confusion, delirium, mania, and hallucinosis have been reported in as many as 15% of patients with digitalis toxicity. Although the mechanism for the symptoms is unknown, it is felt that they are not the result of altered cardiac function.

Antianginal Agents

Nitroglycerin and nitrate therapy frequently is associated with headache. According to currently proposed mechanisms, nitric oxide is the common mediator in experimental vascular headaches. Nitroglycerin produces a throbbing or pulsating sensation in many patients and an overt headache in many others. Often, the headaches attenuate or disappear with time, but 15% to 20% of patients will not be able to tolerate long-acting nitrates because of headache. Patients should be encouraged to use analgesics during the initial days or weeks of nitrate therapy and should be educated as to the nature of this problem and its probable resolution with time.

Nitroglycerin therapy can cause dose-related increases in intracranial pressure, which in rare cases can result in a clinically overt syndrome. Furthermore, the hypotensive effects of nitroglycerin can result in dizziness and light-headedness or even syncope.

Antiarrhythmics

Quinidine is used mainly to treat auricular fibrillation. Nervous system manifestations are usually not significant, but with overdosage or in susceptible individuals the following may occur: headache, nausea, vomiting, blurring of vision, ringing of the ears, flushing, palpitations, and even convulsions. A precipitous decrease in blood pressure related to vagal influences can cause syncope, vertigo, and respiratory arrest (on rare occasions).

Lidocaine-induced CNS toxicity occurs commonly and may relate to its rapid absorption across the blood–brain barrier. The syndrome appears to relate to a diffuse excitement of neuronal systems, with an early prodrome of altered behavior. Garrulousness and loss of inhibitions may be the prominent feature, as may agitation or psychosis. Circumoral numbness, diplopia, and tinnitus also may occur, with progressive muscle twitches and tremors. Generalized myoclonic seizures and finally CNS and respiratory depression are seen with higher doses. In both cardiac and surgical patients, hypoxia and acidosis develop rapidly if the lidocaine syndrome is not reversed. Treatment focuses on adequate oxygenation and support because the half-life of bolus lidocaine given acutely is 6 to 8 minutes. Because repeated injections change the kinetics of lidocaine and prolong its half-life to approximately 90 minutes, however, more long-lasting effects can be seen.

Procainamide may cause light-headedness and even syncope because of the hypotensive action. Additionally, a lupus erythematosus syndrome can develop in patients taking procainamide, and 80% of patients receiving the drug for 6 months have antinuclear antibodies; these antibodies clear with the withdrawal of the agent. During lupuslike syndrome, encephalopathy with confusion and agitation can develop. Procainamide also has a curarelike effect at the neuromuscular junction and hence can precipitate myasthenia gravis or exacerbate it.

Tocainide hydrochloride is an antiarrhythmic agent that is structurally and pharmacologically similar to lidocaine, except that it is well absorbed when given orally. Tocainide has been proven effective in managing various ventricular arrhythmias; however, because it crosses the blood–brain barrier, it frequently causes several neurologic side effects, which include light-headedness, dizziness, tremor, twitching, paresthesias, sweating, hot flashes, blurred vision, diplopia, and mood changes. Peak plasma concentrations of tocainide oc-

cur within 1 to 2 hours of ingestion; the plasma half-life is 12 to 15 hours in patients with unimpaired renal and hepatic systems. CNS side effects appear to be linearly related to the dose.

Bretylium is a parenteral antiarrhythmic drug used in the prophylaxis and treatment of ventricular fibrillation and life-threatening ventricular arrhythmias that do not respond to firstline agents such as lidocaine. The antiarrhythmic mechanisms of bretylium in humans are not clearly defined, but in animals it increases the ventricular fibrillatory threshold and also the action potential duration and effective refractory period. It induces a state of chemical sympathectomy.

The most significant side effect of this drug is severe supine and orthostatic hypotension. Patients report dizziness, light-headedness, vertigo, and faintness. Bretylium may also rarely cause flushing, hyperthermia, confusion, paranoid psychosis, mood changes, anxiety, lethargy, and nasal stuffiness.

Amiodarone is an orally effective antiarrhythmic drug that, like bretylium, slows repolarization in various myocardial fibers and raises the threshold for ventricular fibrillation. Early reports of adverse effects include corneal microdeposits, thyroid dysfunction, and cutaneous photosensitivity. However, toxic neurologic side effects now have been described, and, in a series of 54 patients studied, these side effects were the most common reason for either altering or discontinuing amiodarone therapy.

A reversible syndrome of tremor, ataxia, and peripheral neuropathy without nystagmus, dizziness, encephalopathy, or long-tract signs developed in 54% of these patients. Tremor occurred earliest and most frequently (29%). The 6- to 10-Hz flexion–extension movements in the fingers, wrists, and elbows were indistinguishable from essential tremor. Of the patients, 37% reported ataxia associated with falls, staggering, and difficulty in dressing the lower limbs. The ability to walk was seriously impaired in 18% of the patients. None of these patients had preexisting gait problems, and none had sensory or long-tract abnormalities on examination. Peripheral neuropathy associated with this drug was first reported in 1974 and continues to account for a significant portion of the neurologic toxicity reported today. The neuropathy is sensorimotor in type and generally causes numbness and tingling of all four extremities. Proximal weakness occasionally accompanies the paresthesias. Sural nerve biopsies have been examined and have revealed demyelination with mild axonal loss in some cases. Lamellated inclusions of lysosomal origin were found in all cell types in the nerves and are a characteristic finding of this neuropathy.

Diuretics

Diuretics are divided into three principal groups: thiazide, loop, and potassium sparing. Diuretics most frequently cause extracardiac side effects as a direct result of the electrolytes lost or retained in the renal system. Each group, however, can cause adverse effects that are linked indirectly to electrolyte and water balance.

The thiazide diuretics have been reported to cause syncope, acute muscle cramps and pain, hyporeflexia, weakness, flaccid paralysis, and epileptiform movements. The deterioration of mental function, including the development of coma, can be precipitated with thiazide administration in patients being treated for cirrhosis. Thiazides given concomitantly with triamterene and amantadine can increase the likelihood of neurotoxicity from the amantadine.

If loop diuretics, particularly furosemide, are given quickly and in high doses, they can cause deafness and paresthesias. If they are given to a patient who also is receiving lithium chronically, loop diuretics can alter the renal clearance of lithium and increase the risk of lithium toxicity and fluid electrolyte abnormalities. Loop diuretics also potentially can increase the success with which succinylcholine blocks the neuromuscular junction in anesthetized patients.

Potassium-sparing diuretics, including spironolactone and triamterene, have been re-ported to cause confusion, drowsiness, muscle weakness, paresthesias, dizziness (although this may be a result of cardiac rhythm changes), and headache.

Sympatholytics

Methyldopa can cause sedation, which is usually transient in nature but may persist in as many as 5% of patients. Mood alterations including depression are not uncommon, although most patients who develop behavioral changes usually have a prior history of affective illness. The depressive state is reversible on withdrawal of the drug. Parkinsonism, resulting from dopamine antagonism, has been reported several times; however, considering the widespread use of this agent, this is probably rare. Other minor neurologic complaints associated with methyldopa include confusion, dizziness, headaches, and syncope.

Clonidine is an alpha$_2$-noradrenergic agonist, and some have suggested that this drug induces an overall decrease in norepinephrine release, possibly through a presynaptic mechanism. Sedation is the most common adverse neurologic effect of clonidine. Other less common neurotoxic reactions include depression, nightmares, and reversible dementia syndrome.

Reserpine historically was a popular drug in the treatment of hypertension, but disabling neuropsychiatric side effects have limited its current use. Drug-induced parkinsonism can occur and is felt to relate directly to the depletion of central dopaminergic stores by reserpine. This effect may occur in patients with no prior neurologic deficits or can be seen as a marked and sudden exacerbation of already present, but mild, Parkinson's disease. Psychiatric depression with early morning awakening, melancholy, loss of appetite, and diminished self-confidence also are seen with reserpine therapy and also may relate to central neurotransmitter depletion. This effect is more common with higher dosage and in patients with a history of prior affective disturbance. Drug withdrawal does not always result in immediate reversal, and early symptoms of depression should alert the physician to discontinue therapy.

Neuropsychiatric symptoms occur frequently during treatment with beta blockers. The pharmacology of CNS side effects is unclear, although presynaptic and postsynaptic adrenergic inhibition has been implicated, as has serotonergic antagonism. Nonselective beta blockers seem to cause CNS-related side effects to a greater extent than beta$_1$-selective blockers. It is unclear to what degree lipophilicity is responsible for this kind of side effect. Lassitude or insomnia and depression are the most common reactions, although vivid dreams, nightmares, hypnagogic hallucinations, and psychotic behavior have been reported with high doses (more than 500 mg/day of propranolol). Preexisting major psychiatric illness and hyperthyroidism may predispose to the previously mentioned symptoms.

Prazosin competitively blocks the vascular postsynaptic alpha-adrenergic receptors and is the first of a class of similar antagonists derived from quinazoline. The selective affinity of prazosin for alpha-receptors allows it to block the contractile response of vascular smooth muscle to norepinephrine, consequently lowering mean arterial pressure and peripheral resistance. Like other antihypertensives that cause vasodilatation, prazosin causes hypotension; dizziness and faintness have been reported in up to 50% of patients receiving this drug. These are most pronounced after the first dose(s) or in patients who have had a hiatus from the drug and are reinstituting treatment. Hypotension can be minimized if the initial dose is small and is given at bedtime. Other CNS side effects include headache, dry mouth, nasal stuffiness, lassitude, hallucinations, depression, paresthesias, nervousness, and priapism.

Vasodilators

Hydralazine is the only direct-acting vasodilator generally available for the treatment of chronic hypertension. The neurologic side effects of hydralazine are few and uncommon in clinical practice. Peripheral neuropathy characterized by diffuse numbness and tingling is the only consistent neurotoxic reaction and is felt to be the result of a direct toxic effect of the drug.

Calcium channel blockers, particularly flunarizine and cinnarizine, have been associated with dystonia, parkinsonism, akathisia, and tardive dyskinesia (TD). Theoretic explanations for these events include the inhibition of calcium influx into striatal cells and direct dopaminergic antagonistic properties. Evidence also suggests that inhibition of proton pumping and catecholamine uptake are possible mechanisms. In addition, the chemical structures of flunarizine and cinnarizine, which are related to neuroleptics, may explain the greater incidence of such side effects with these agents compared with those of calcium channel blockers available in the United States. Suggested risk factors appear to be advanced age and a family history of tremors or Parkinson's disease, or both. The onset and type of presentation are unpredictable. The long-term evolution was assessed in a prospective follow-up study of 32 patients with diagnoses of calcium channel blocker–induced parkinsonism. Eighteen months following discontinuation of the offending agent, 44% of the patients had depression, 88% had tremor, and 33% still had criteria for diagnosis of parkinsonism.

Angiotensin-Converting Enzyme Inhibitors

Angiotensin-converting enzyme inhibitors have been used in the United States to treat moderate to severe hypertension, based on its effect on the renin–angiotensin–aldosterone (RAA) axis. This cascading hormonal axis simultaneously maintains systemic arterial pressure and sodium balance by detecting and correcting even small changes in renal perfusion. Alongside the increased understanding of the RAA axis has come the discovery of drugs that specifically and selectively inhibit the RAA cascade.

Few neurologic side effects have been reported; however, in a large multinational study,

5% of the participating patients reported symptoms of hypotension, including dizziness, lightheadedness, and vertigo. These symptoms were generally transient and mild and most frequently occurred in patients who were sodium or water depleted. Dysgeusia occurred in 2% to 4% of patients participating in this small trial. The incidence of taste change or loss increased in patients with impaired renal function.

Cholesterol-Lowering Agents

Clofibrate, an aromatic monocarboxylic acid, is capable of inducing myotonia in humans and experimental animals and is clinically significant because it is widely used to reduce serum triglyceride levels. The mechanism by which it induces myotonia is believed to be through a decrease in chloride conductance.

Lovastatin and pravastatin are HMG-CoA reductase inhibitors that are effective cholesterol-lowering agents used in the treatment of hypercholesterolemia. They can induce myotonia by blocking chloride channels on the muscle membrane. Lipid-lowering agents can cause a myopathy. The risk of myopathy is highest when multiple lipid-lowering agents are used together and can be as high as 5%. Clinically, patients have myalgias, elevated creatinine kinase levels, and proximal weakness. Recovery is typical after discontinuation of the offending medications.

GASTROINTESTINAL AGENTS

Common gastrointestinal problems include the hypermotility disorders with vomiting and/or diarrhea; hypomotility disorders, with constipation; or excessive acid secretion leading to "heartburn" or ulcerations. A wide variety of drugs commonly are recommended for these disorders. Fortunately, neurologic complications from these frequently prescribed agents are infrequent.

Laxatives

There are only a few neurologic complications associated with the drugs used to treat constipation. Docusate sodium (Colace) is a stool softener that occasionally causes nausea or a bitter taste. The long-term use of nonprescription laxatives may cause neurologic complications arising secondary to depletion of electrolytes. Profound muscle weakness may occur from the potassium depletion following chronic laxative intake. The irritant purgatives, such as cascara, may damage the myenteric plexus of the colon, leading to a reduction of intestinal motility and a worsening of constipation.

Antiemetics

Of the antiemetic drugs, several commonly prescribed agents act as dopamine-receptor blockers in similar fashion to the neuroleptic drugs described later. Metoclopramide (Reglan), prochlorperazine (Compazine), and promethazine (Phenergan) are three widely used antiemetics with neuroleptic properties. Sedation may occur as an early complaint with the introduction of these agents. In addition, acute dystonia, with distressing involuntary spasms of head, neck, eyes, facial, and trunk muscles, may occur, particularly in children treated with prochlorperazine. If not recognized by the clinician, these acute, sometimes bizarre, symptoms may be inaccurately thought to have a psychogenic etiology. The treatment of the acute dystonia from the dopamine-receptor–blocking antiemetics is the administration of anticholinergic agents.

In addition to acute dystonia, these dopamine-receptor antagonist, antiemetic agents may cause a parkinsonian syndrome, clinically indistinguishable from idiopathic Parkinson's disease. Those of more advanced age appear to be more susceptible to this neurologic complication and may even be treated with antidopaminergic agents if the symptoms are not recognized as being associated with the medication. Akathisia also may occur as a side effect of these medications. If these agents are used on a long-term basis, as in the treatment of chronic esophageal reflux, the potentially irreversible symptoms of TD even may occur.

A different type of agent with predominantly anticholinergic effect, scopolamine, is prescribed for the treatment of motion-induced nausea and vomiting. Scopolamine has become available in a long-acting, transdermal patch preparation. The neurologic side effects of scopolamine are those associated with blockade of muscarinic receptors. The most frequent is xerostomia. The reduction in saliva production, if severe, can lead to mucosal ulcerations and dental problems. Other peripheral effects of scopolamine include blurred near vision resulting from alterations in accommodation, reduced sweating, and urinary retention from effects on bladder muscles. A potentially irreversible effect of the anticholinergic agents is the exacerbation of closed-angle glaucoma with the potential for causing blindness.

The CNS side effects of these drugs include sedation and confusion. Losses in recent and immediate memory can occur at high doses. Finally, with toxicity, delirium and hallucinations have been described.

Antidiarrheals

Drugs used to symptomatically alleviate diarrhea frequently contain morphine or morphine derivatives. These compounds act to reduce the propulsive contractions of the small bowel and colon. The neurologic adverse effects from these agents include sedation, respiratory depression, and coma, typically with pupillary constriction.

Anticholinergic agents also have been used to treat symptoms of diarrhea. Diphenoxylate–atropine (Lomotil) is a widely prescribed antidiarrheal agent. Overdoses of this agent most frequently cause a predominantly opioid intoxication.

Some antidiarrheal compounds (e.g., Donnatal) are combinations of morphine derivatives and from one to three different anticholinergic agents. Donnatal contains phenobarbital, hyoscyamine, atropine, and scopolamine. Although each component is present only in small amounts, patients taking several tablets a day or elderly persons may experience significant side effects.

Bismuth compounds, as found in the non-prescription bismuth subsalicylate (Pepto-Bismol), have been recommended for the treatment of "traveler's diarrhea." The neurologic sequelae of these agents are rare. There have been reports of an acute reversible psychotic reaction following excessive use of these compounds as a result of acute bismuth toxicity. More commonly, tinnitus is noted with large doses, arising from the salicylate component in this compound.

Antiacidity Agents

The magnesium and aluminum antacids, if taken in large quantities or with renal impairment, may cause neurologic symptoms secondary to alteration in electrolytes. Sucralfate is an aluminum compound that coats the gastric mucosa. Although little of this agent is absorbed directly, sucralfate may reduce the absorption of phenytoin and, in those taking this anticonvulsant, may result in a drop in phenytoin levels below the therapeutic range.

The H_2-receptor antagonists inhibit acid secretion from the parietal cells. Currently, four H_2-receptor antagonists are approved for use in the United States. Cimetidine (Tagamet) was the first to be developed. More recently developed H_2-receptor antagonists include ranitidine (Zantac), nizatidine (Axid), and famotidine (Pepcid). The neurologic complications of these medications include lethargy, confusion, depression, hallucinations, and headache. Individuals treated with these drugs who develop unexplained encephalopathic symptoms may improve with the discontinuation of these agents. Additionally, the effect of cimetidine—and, to a lesser degree, the other H_2 blockers—on the cytochrome P-450 enzymes in the liver may alter the pharmacokinetic profile of other drugs undergoing hepatic degradation, including warfarin and phenytoin.

RESPIRATORY AGENTS
Adrenergic Drugs

Of the three types of adrenergic receptors (alpha, B_1, fl_2), it is the B_2 receptor that mediates bronchodilation. The first sympathomimetics available for the treatment of asthma were not B_2 selective (metaproterenol, isoproterenol, epinephrine, ephedrine); therefore, in addition to dilating the bronchioli, they also produced significant cardiac and CNS effects. The introduction of B_2-selective agents (albuterol, terbutaline) resulted in a reduction in the number of adverse effects. These agents are administered most efficiently by inhalation, resulting in benefit with minimal side effects. When these agents are administered parenterally, there may be nausea, vomiting, headache, and a variable-amplitude postural and action tremor associated with these agents.

Xanthine Bronchodilators

The xanthine compounds include aminophylline and theophylline. These agents now are prescribed only for those patients suffering with chronic rather than intermittent symptoms of bronchoconstriction. Theophylline is metabolized primarily in the liver, and drugs that affect hepatic enzymes, including tobacco, may alter the metabolism of theophylline. Liver disease, heart failure, and pulmonary disease tend to slow the metabolism of theophylline, sometimes resulting in toxicity even at low dosages. The therapeutic serum concentration of theophylline is 10 to 20 µg/ml. The side effects from theophylline tend to be dose related. However, even in the therapeutic range, neurologic side effects may occur. These include nausea, nervousness, insomnia, and headache. Although usually associated with toxic levels of theophylline, seizures also may occur in the high therapeutic range, particularly in the elderly or those with a history of previous brain injury. This latter group is likely to develop prolonged seizures with a poor outcome. The mechanism of theophylline-induced seizures is not clearly understood. In otherwise healthy asthmatics, the seizures are typically short-lived with a good outcome. A recently described neurologic side effect observed in children is the occurrence of acquired stuttering, which resolves with the discontinuation of this drug.

PSYCHIATRIC DRUGS

Neuroleptic Agents

The neuroleptic agents or major tranquilizers exert their antipsychotic activity by blocking dopaminergic receptors at the level of the limbic system, forebrain, and basal ganglia. They also have antihistaminergic, anticholinergic, and anti–alpha$_1$-adrenergic properties. The newer, so-called atypical agents include clozapine, olanzapine, quetiapine, and risperidone. Many newer agents have some affinity for 5-HT$_2$ serotonin receptors as well (clozapine, risperidone). The atypical neuroleptic agents have become favored because of their lower side effect profile. Many newer agents have some affinity for 5-HT$_2$ serotonin receptors as well (clozapine, risperidone). Neuroleptics, as a class, are associated with a variety of important neurologic complications. These can be classified as acute, subacute, and chronic side effects.

Neuroleptics may cause a toxic confusional state, especially in the elderly, and confusion occurs more frequently with the low-potency, high-anticholinergic activity subclass (chlorpromazine, thioridazine, mesoridazine). These drugs also can produce profound sedation, especially with initiation of therapy.

Neuroleptics also lower the seizure threshold and have been associated with exacerbation of preexisting epilepsy as well as the *de novo* appearance of seizures. Clozapine has been associated with generalized and myoclonic seizures. Seizures were present during the titration phase at low dosages (<300mg/day) and at high dosages during the maintenance phase ($\geq$600mg/day).

Neuroleptic malignant syndrome (NMS) is associated with neuroleptic use. The pathogenesis of NMS is not completely understood. Alterations in dopaminergic transmission, changes in sympathetic outflow, alterations in central serotonin metabolism, and abnormalities in muscle membrane function have been implicated. NMS has been associated with all groups of neuroleptics, although high-potency agents, specifically haloperidol and fluphenazine, have been cited most frequently.

NMS has been described with the atypical neuroleptic medications, clozapine, risperidone, and olanzapine. NMS tends to occur with the initiation of treatment or increases in dose and is more common with depot forms of neuroleptics. Affective disorder, concomitant lithium carbonate administration, psychomotor agitation, dehydration, exhaustion, and mild hyperthermia seem to increase susceptibility toward this condition. The principal features of NMS are hyperthermia, muscle rigidity, autonomic dysfunction, and mental status changes. Laboratory findings include elevated creatine kinase; polymorphonuclear leukocytosis; elevated aldolase, alkaline phosphatase, lactic dehydrogenase (LDH), alanine aminotransferase (ALT), and aspartate aminotransferase (AST); hypocalcemia; hypomagnesemia; low iron; proteinuria; and myoglobinuria. Approximately 40% of patients with NMS develop medical complications that may be life threatening. NMS is a clinical diagnosis based on the presence of the proper historical setting and the characteristic constellation of signs. Disorders with similar features include malignant hyperthermia; heat stroke induced by neuroleptics; lethal catatonia; other drug reactions; and vascular, infectious, or postinfectious brain damage.

NMS is a potentially fatal disease, and a high index of suspicion is required for early recognition and intervention. Treatment includes ceasing of the offending agent, providing supportive measures, and administering dantrolene or bromocriptine or a combination of the two.

Acute neuroleptic-induced dystonia can be seen early in the course of neuroleptic therapy or with dose increases. It often is seen following a single parenteral dose of neuroleptics. The manifestations can be diverse, although the most typical clinical signs involve oculogyric crises and opisthotonic posturing. Risk factors include young age, male gender, and use of high-potency neuroleptics. Acute dystonic reactions are self-limited, and if they are left untreated, they usually subside within 24 hours. Parenteral administration of anticholinergics, such as benztropine or diphen-hydramine, offers immediate relief in the majority of cases, but oral anticholinergics should be continued for a few days until the causative neuroleptic is cleared.

Akathisia is a severe form of restlessness associated with the need to move. Typically the patient paces incessantly in place and cannot sit down without continual volitional movement of the legs or feet. The pathophysiology of the syndrome is not well understood but may relate to the development of acute imbalance between the dopaminergic and cholinergic systems. This neuroleptic side effect usually occurs within the first days of therapy or with dose increases, and it resolves with withdrawal of the neuroleptic agent. Anticholinergics, amantadine, beta blockers, clonidine, and benzodiazepines also have been used with variable success. Late-onset akathisia may be a form of TD (see later) and may be more difficult to treat.

Neuroleptic-induced parkinsonism is the result of striatal dopaminergic underactivity resulting from dopaminergic D_2 receptor blockade. Clinically, it cannot be distinguished from idiopathic Parkinson's disease, although its development occurs as a subacute syndrome within the first weeks of drug introduction or drug-dosage increase. Parkinsonian symptoms resolve over a few weeks to 6 months after stopping the causative agent or with the use of antiparkinsonian drugs. Proposed risk factors for development of neuroleptic-induced parkinsonism are female gender, older age, and the use of high-potency agents. Treatment consists of discontinuing or reducing the dose of the offending agent. A lower-potency neuroleptic or one of several novel neuroleptics that lack prominent striatal receptor blockade, such as clozapine, can be substituted. Anticholinergics, amantadine, and electroconvulsive therapy are also possible treatments.

TD usually appears after several months or years of treatment with antipsychotic medications and almost never before 3 months. No consistent neuropathologic changes have been seen in patients with TD, and the predominant hypothesis for its genesis is denervation supersensitivity of the striatal dopamine receptors following chronic blockade. Risk factors for the development of TD include old age; female gender; presence of affective disorders; history of neuroleptic-induced parkinsonism; presence of organic brain disease; high-potency neuroleptics use; sufficient duration of treatment with neuroleptics; and possibly the use of anticholinergic medications, previous electroconvulsive treatment, and drug holidays.

In addition to the well-known oral–buccal–lingual masticatory movements and generalized chorea, dystonia, akathisia, tics, and myoclonus have been described. Once TD has appeared, its peak severity is reached rapidly and often is maintained. Following neuroleptic withdrawal, TD may transiently worsen, but this exacerbation is short lived. TD resolves in up to 33% of patients within 2 years after discontinuation of the offending agent. A prospective study comparing risperidone and haloperidol in 350 neuroleptic-naive patients, however, showed that each drug had a similar incidence of dystonia, parkinsonism, akithisia, and dyskinesia.

At present, prevention is the treatment of choice for TD. Therefore, neuroleptic agents should be used only when specifically needed and at the lowest possible doses. Once TD develops, the causative agent should be discontinued, if possible. Alternatively, the patient should be switched to an atypical neuroleptic such as clozapine, which not only does not regularly cause TD but may even improve its symptoms. If neurologic impairment, disfigurement, or discomfort exists, treatment with the dopamine depleters reserpine or tetrabenazine should be considered. Noradrenergic antagonists (propranolol, clonidine); gamma-aminobutyric acid (GABA) agonists (clonazepam, diazepam, valproate, baclofen); botulinum toxin injections; and to a lesser degree, vitamin E, buspirone, and calcium channel blockers have been used with variable success.

Anxiolytics

Benzodiazepines are commonly prescribed anxiolytic agents. The therapeutic index of these agents is 10 to 30 times that of the barbiturates and, hence, their absolute toxicity is less. However, because these agents are so widely used, adverse reactions frequently are reported. The predominant toxic symptom is drowsiness or paradoxical excitation. Withdrawal seizures also have been reported. Dry mouth, tachycardia, dilated pupils, and depressed bowel sounds may occur early after the introduction of benzodiazepines because of possible anticholinergic effects. Withdrawal symptoms include excessive apprehension, anorexia, nausea, postural tremulousness, insomnia, and confusion. Withdrawal symptoms are best handled in the hospital, and barbiturates usually are substituted.

Antidepressant Agents

Tricyclic antidepressants (TCAs) induce an acute encephalopathy that is characterized by agitation, confusion, mydriasis, and sometimes convulsions. Tremor and myoclonus may be prominent motor features of this syndrome. Medical complications of these drugs include complex cardiac arrhythmias and heart block. Generalized support measures should be instituted for the patient who takes an overdose of TCAs. Physostigmine, a centrally active cholinesterase inhibitor, 1 to 2 mg given IV, often will awaken a patient from coma. This finding suggests that much of the toxic mental alteration relates directly to central anticholinergic toxicity.

TCAs also may precipitate a more chronic neurotoxic syndrome in which tremor and sedation or insomnia are the prominent features. The tremor is usually postural or intentional and resembles that seen with amphetamine intoxication or use of lithium. Currently, most TCAs can be monitored with plasma levels, so that intoxication can be detected at early stages.

Newer-generation antidepressants have been developed to be more selective for the noradrenergic or serotonergic systems. Many of these agents (e.g., trimipramine, amoxapine, or maprotiline), however, still have significant anticholinergic side effects, including blurred vision, urinary retention, and confusion. Trazodone can cause priapism.

Selective serotonin reuptake inhibitors (SSRIs) are potent and selective inhibitors of serotonin reuptake at the presynaptic terminal. They currently are considered firstline therapy for depression because of their prescribing ease and superior side effect/safety profile. SSRI-induced side effects are usually transient and rarely result in discontinuation of the medication. In addition, they appear to be safer than TCAs in overdose.

The major CNS side effects of the SSRIs include nausea, headache, dry mouth, insomnia/somnolence, agitation, nervousness, sweating, dizziness, tremor, and sexual dysfunction. Fluoxetine often is associated with anxiety, nervousness, insomnia, and anorexia. Paroxetine, fluvoxamine, and nefazodone are associated with sedation. Sexual dysfunction manifests itself as ejaculatory delay in men and anorgasmia in women. There have been reports suggesting that fluoxetine can induce or exacerbate suicidal tendencies, and several mechanisms have been proposed. However, because suicide is an important feature of depression, it is difficult to draw conclusions; however, it is difficult to exclude the possibility that suicidal ideation occurs as a rare adverse reaction with some drugs.

SSRIs have been shown *in vitro* and *in vivo* to inhibit the P-450 system and therefore to result in increased levels of drugs that are substrates of P-450 as well (e.g., TCAs). There has been debate over whether the combination of SSRIs and monoamine oxidase (MAO) inhibitors or TCAs can lead to the serotonin syndrome characterized by hyperpyrexia, myoclonus, rigidity, hyperreflexia, shivering, confusion, agitation, restlessness, coma, autonomic instability, nausea, diarrhea, diaphoresis, flushing, and (rarely) rhabdomyolysis and death. This occurrence is probably very uncommon but should be watched for and handled immediately with supportive care and drug withdrawal if it occurs. Several case reports in the literature suggest that SSRIs can produce extrapyramidal symptoms in the form of akathisia, dyskinesia, acute dystonia,

and deterioration in Parkinson's disease, but controlled clinical studies are needed to determine the validity of these observations.

MAO inhibitors are drugs that have been used for decades in the treatment of depression. The characteristic of acute MAO inhibitor intoxication is hyperpyrexia, with fevers as high as 108°F. Coma, tachycardia, tachypnea, dilated pupils, and profuse sweating occur. Rapid recovery after hemodialysis suggests that this means of therapy is effective. A second cataclysmic syndrome is the hypertensive crisis associated with combined use of MAO inhibitors and tyramine products or other centrally active agents. Cheese, chicken livers, chocolate, wine, and some forms of herring have been associated with this syndrome in patients ingesting MAO inhibitors. Much less dramatic and also more common are mild side effects, such as mild dizziness, a generalized weakness, dysarthria, and confusion, which can occur in patients receiving therapeutic doses of these agents.

Lithium carbonate is well established as an effective agent in the treatment of manic-depressive illness. Neurotoxic effects are not rare, and the most common and annoying effect is a fine postural intention tremor, which may be seen even in therapeutic doses. A reduction of the dosage usually either will eliminate the tremor or significantly reduce its intensity. The beta-adrenergic blocker propranolol may prove beneficial. Toxic confusional states also may occur with lithium, and, if this develops, lithium blood levels should be checked. Ataxia, seizures, and coma can occur in high doses (serum levels exceeding 2.0 mEq/l). There is no specific antidote for severe lithium intoxication. After severe intoxication, residual symptoms including ataxia, nystagmus, choreoathetoid movements, and hyperactive deep tendon reflexes have been reported.

Hypnosedative and Other Agents

Barbiturates usually are used to manage seizure disorders but still are used to calm patients and facilitate sleep. Drowsiness is a common complaint associated with their use, and ataxia (often without nystagmus) can develop when the plasma level rises above 50 µg/ml. In higher doses, severe ataxia, nausea, vomiting, and nystagmus predominate. A second encephalopathic syndrome occurs in children taking phenobarbital and is highly distinctive. Instead of somnolence, these children develop remarkable agitation and hyperactivity. This can give the picture of attentional deficit disorder (ADD), or childhood hyperactivity. Patients with chronic toxic exposure to barbiturates show ataxic gait, slurred speech, and periods of intermittent agitation. Tremors and confusion, as well as diplopia and nystagmus, are characteristic.

Ethchlorvynol has a rapid onset and a short duration of action. The common side effects associated with its use are a strange mintlike aftertaste, dizziness, nausea, vomiting, and facial paresthesias. Idiosyncratic reactions characterized by marked excitation and histrionic behavior also have occurred. Chronic abuse of this drug results in both tolerance and physical dependence. Withdrawal symptoms resemble those seen with delirium tremens and may be especially severe in elderly patients.

Methaqualone may induce transient and persistent paresthesias and other signs of peripheral neuropathy. Paradoxic restlessness and anxiety instead of sedation and sleep also are reported with this drug. As with many of the drugs already mentioned, methaqualone with alcohol may have addictive sedating effects. Other drug interactions include enhanced effect of MAO inhibitors and TCAs. Delirium and marked myoclonus also may occur in patients who acutely overdose with these drugs.

Disulfiram is used in the rehabilitation of alcoholics because high levels of acetaldehyde accumulate when alcohol is ingested with the drug. Chronic disulfiram therapy is associated with two distinct neurotoxic syndromes, an encephalopathy and a neuropathy. The encephalopathy is usually acute or subacute in onset, characterized by delirium and paranoid and psychotic behavior, and it often

is confused with the diagnosis of schizophrenic reaction. The behavioral response to neuroleptics or other psychotropic drugs is generally not marked, a finding that should suggest a toxic cause; withdrawal of disulfiram and mild sedation with supportive care (but without neuroleptic therapy) are recommended in the treatment of disulfiram encephalopathy.

Disulfiram also is associated with a rare, axonal distal sensory/motor polyneuropathy. The recovery after drug withdrawal both clinically and pathologically suggests a dying-back or distal axonopathy rather than new degeneration secondary to the loss of nerve cells. It is not known whether disulfiram is the responsible agent or whether a toxic metabolite induces the neuropathy. Disulfiram possibly is metabolized to carbon disulfide, a compound capable of causing an axonal neuropathy in humans and animals.

ANTIINFLAMMATORY AGENTS

Salicylate Compounds

Because of their ready availability in most households, salicylates represent a common source of intoxication, accounting for the largest yearly number of serious childhood poisonings. In acute intoxication, the prominent neurologic and respiratory signs may immediately suggest the correct diagnosis and direct prompt and appropriate intervention. The neurologic manifestations of salicylate toxicity include a rapid and dramatic alteration in consciousness and global function with convulsions and coma. Confusion and restlessness are seen early, leading within a few hours to excitability, tremor, incoherent speech, and often delirium or hallucinosis. This phase has been referred to as a "salicylate jag" to indicate its similarity to alcoholic inebriation, although euphoria and elation are conspicuously absent with salicylates. After this phase, a gradual depression in the level of consciousness occurs with a rapid lapse into coma. Seizures are especially common in children and are usually generalized. The pathophysiology of the convulsions appears to relate to combined effects of metabolic and respiratory disturbances. In infants, salicylate intoxication induces a marked hypoglycemia, and seizure activity is especially hazardous in this young age group. Diplopia, dizziness, and decreased visual acuity also can be seen with salicylate intoxication. Involvement of the audiovestibular (eighth cranial) nerve can lead to tinnitus, vertigo, and complete deafness. This complication is more common with chronic salicylate intoxication and is seen especially in elderly patients treated for arthritic or headache conditions where aspirin or salicylate compounds are ingested daily. The treatment of salicylate toxicity involves minimizing drug absorption, hastening drug elimination, correcting acid–base disturbance, and treating existing neurologic or medical complications. Induced emesis in the awake patient is the most effective means of emptying the stomach. Enhanced elimination is affected by alkalinization of the urine or by peritoneal dialysis or hemodialysis. Careful fluid and electrolyte management is tantamount and depends on the age of the patient and the stage of intoxication. The complications of hypoglycemia in infants must be anticipated and thereby prevented. Seizures usually are treated with phenytoin and phenobarbital.

There is a poor correlation between the serum salicylate levels and the clinical severity of intoxication. Despite apparently adequate treatment and progressive lowering of toxic plasma salicylate levels, sudden and unexplained deaths are not rare.

Steroids

Steroids induce three neurotoxic syndromes: increased intracranial pressure (pseudomotor cerebri), toxic encephalopathy, and myopathy. Infants are more likely than adults to develop steroid-related, increased intracranial pressure; hydrocephalus; and papilledema. This syndrome may occur while patients are receiving steroids or after withdrawal. The pathophysiology of this syndrome is unknown, although it may relate to

water intoxication. When it occurs, patients have been treated for weeks or months with steroid compounds.

In contrast, steroid-induced toxic encephalopathy may occur within days of steroid introduction. The behavior is varied and fluctuant, ranging over 24 hours from momentary euphoria to depression to fully developed psychosis. Depersonalization and motor retardation may make these patients difficult to manage during the intoxication phase. Paranoia with visual and auditory hallucination and markedly delusional thinking may predominate. Although this syndrome typically occurs early in the course of steroid therapy, cases exist where mental decline developed after more than 3 months of treatment. Doses of medication do not clearly correlate with symptoms, although the encephalopathy is generally more frequent in high-dose treatment groups. Patients with a prior history of psychiatric care or depression may be at higher risk for encephalopathy than other patients. Suicides have occurred, making this encephalopathy a significant source of potential morbidity. Treatment focuses on withdrawal of the steroid and medical and psychiatric support. Steroids sometimes can be reintroduced later without the reappearance of the problem.

Steroid myopathy, characterized by proximal weakness and atrophy, appears unrelated to the actual duration of drug treatment, and type II fibers appear to be selectively affected. Patients complain of progressive weakness that focuses primarily on the proximal muscles (shoulders and thighs).

Because the steroid compounds alter coagulation factors, secondary hypercoagulable states can occur, resulting in cerebrovascular disease. Rapid withdrawal of steroids induces the behavioral manifestations seen clinically in Addison's disease. These manifestations are secondary phenomena and are not related directly to drug neurotoxicity.

Nonsteroidal Agents

The nonsteroidal antiinflammatory agents (NSAIDs) account for approximately 4% of the prescription market. There are a variety of types currently available, and ibuprofen is available in low doses as a nonprescription drug. Despite widespread use, these agents infrequently cause significant neurologic adverse effects. The most common neurologic side effect is headache. Other rare but serious central disturbances include confusion, hallucinations, and overt psychosis. Although these agents have not been evaluated well in controlled studies, it has been suggested that there may be subtle, associated cognitive and memory changes, particularly in more elderly patients. Another infrequent yet important side effect described is the occurrence of aseptic meningitis. Initially reported in 1978, there have been subsequent case reports in which ibuprofen was the most commonly associated drug, although sulindac, naproxen, and tolmetin also have been implicated. From these case reports, it appears that young women with connective tissue disorders are the most likely to develop this side effect. The clinical picture is that of aseptic meningitis, with fever, chills, and meningismus. The cerebrospinal fluid has an elevated protein content, a pleocytosis of granulocytes, and a normal or reduced glucose level. The underlying mechanism for this syndrome is felt to be a hypersensitivity reaction to the drugs. Although an infectious source for meningitis must be sought, no communicable agent has been isolated. The meningeal syndrome resolves with the discontinuation of the nonsteroidal agent, only to recur, sometimes more rapidly and severely, if treatment is reinitiated.

Indomethacin has proved to be a potent antiinflammatory drug but appears less efficacious than salicylates in the treatment of arthritis and rheumatoid variants. Its mode of action is still uncertain, but it may act by way of inhibition of prostaglandin synthesis. CNS toxicity is one of the most frequent dose-limiting factors, precluding the use of indomethacin in 30% to 50% of patients. Neurotoxic effects consist of headaches, depression, agitation, and (rarely) hallucinations. Ataxia, clumsiness, and impaired postural reflexes also may occur, although slow increases in dosage may prevent their development.

Naproxen has been associated with adverse neurologic reactions in approximately 8% of patients. These effects include headache, drowsiness, vertigo, inability to concentrate, and depression. Because of its protein-binding affinity, naproxen can be associated with phenytoin toxicity in seizure patients. By displacing phenytoin from proteins, naproxen causes higher levels of unbound phenytoin to circulate, so that toxic signs develop although the total serum phenytoin level remains in the therapeutic range.

Sulindac is another recently marketed NSAID recommended for use in various types of arthritis. Its mode of action may be the inhibition of prostaglandin synthesis by one of its metabolites, a sulfide. The neurotoxicity of sulindac has been estimated to be between 1% and 10%, with headache and dizziness being most common. Vertigo, tinnitus, and decreased hearing occur in less than 1% of reported patients. Paresthesias, peripheral neuropathy, and transient blurring of vision are rare, but more clinical experience is needed to confirm the true incidence of these reactions.

Hormones

Female hormones in the form of oral contraceptives or postmenopausal replacement therapy have become widely prescribed. It is clear that oral contraceptives increase by three to eight times the risk of stroke in women taking them. Oral contraceptive–associated strokes can occur in any vascular distribution. Factors predisposing to cerebrovascular disease in women taking birth control pills include the use of compounds containing high levels of estrogen, multiparity, and a change in migraine headache pattern. Of probable but less certain importance are previous thrombotic or embolic disease and hypertension. Inherited resistance to activated protein C, which is caused by a single factor V gene mutation, is a frequent risk factor for thrombosis.

Activated protein C resistance was found to be highly prevalent in women with a history of thromboembolic complications during pregnancy or use of oral contraceptives. The gene defect is common in the general population, and the question is raised as to whether it would be reasonable to perform general screening for activated protein C resistance early during pregnancy or before prescription of oral contraceptives.

Chorea is another serious problem related to oral contraceptives. The involuntary movements appear days or weeks after starting birth control pills and may be more frequent in patients with a prior history of Sydenham's chorea. The chorea starts abruptly and may involve only one side of the body. A similar phenomenon occasionally occurs during pregnancy when a woman develops severe involuntary movements that spontaneously resolve when the pregnancy ends (chorea gravidarum). Birth control chorea may disappear within 48 hours of cessation of the medication, although the abatement can take longer.

Whereas pseudotumor cerebri can occur in patients taking oral contraceptives, other conditions that may cause blurring of the optic disc are papilledema related to venous sinus obstruction or retrobulbar optic neuritis, which also occurs in patients taking birth control pills. Vascular headaches also may appear for the first time or suddenly change in pattern when oral contraceptives are started. Common migraine may become classic migraine, with patients experiencing symptoms or signs of focal cerebral dysfunction at the onset of the headache. In cases in which migraines either appear for the first time, increase in frequency, or become focal, cessation of oral contraceptives is suggested. However, a subgroup of patients with headache find relief of headache pain while taking oral contraceptives. These headaches may have a close relationship to menstruation, and while taking the oral contraceptives, the patient has minimal pain.

Various other neurologic disorders occasionally are associated with the use of oral contraceptives. Seizures may change in pattern of frequency. Carpal tunnel syndrome of median nerve neuropathy or other pressure neuropathies may occur related to the increased fluid retention associated with oral contraceptives. Drug-induced and reversible myasthenia gravis also has been reported but rarely.

Vitamins and Additives

Caffeine and other xanthine derivatives, including aminophylline, are CNS stimulants that excite all levels of the CNS, the cortex being the most sensitive. Caffeine increases energy metabolism throughout the brain but decreases cerebral blood flow, inducing a relative brain hypoperfusion. The drug activates noradrenaline neurons and may act as a second messenger at dopamine receptors to affect the local release of dopamine. Mobilization of intracellular calcium and inhibition of specific phosphodiesterases occurs at high, non-physiologic concentrations of caffeine. The most likely mechanism of action of methylxanthine is the antagonism at the level of adenosine receptors.

Caffeine's psychostimulant action on humans is often subtle and difficult to detect. Its effects on learning, memory, performance, and coordination are related to methylxanthine-induced arousal, vigilance, and fatigue. An increased awareness of the environment or hyperesthesia may be an unpleasant experience for some patients. The patient becomes loquacious and restless and often complains of ringing in the ears and giddiness. In high doses, xanthines affect the spinal cord, resulting in increased reflex excitability, tremulous extremities, and tense muscles. Caffeine clearly alters sleep patterns, and if taken within 1 hour of attempted sleep, it increases sleep latency, decreases total sleep time, and worsens the subject's estimate of sleep quality. Less time is spent in stages three and four and more in stage two. Xanthine-associated seizures are seen as a complication of aminophylline therapy, especially when the drug is administered intravenously. They usually are generalized but can be focal. Cessation of the use of products containing caffeine can cause a withdrawal syndrome of headaches; drowsiness; fatigue; decreased performance; and, in some instances, nausea and vomiting. These symptoms begin within 12 to 24 hours after the last use, peak at 20 to 48 hours, and last approximately 1 week.

Nicotine increases circulating levels of norepinephrine and epinephrine and stimulates the release of striatal dopamine. It exerts stimulant effects through specific nicotinic receptors, whose activation may facilitate dopaminergic transmission centrally. Nicotine has been reported to affect a number of neurologic diseases, such as spinocerebellar degeneration, multiple system atrophy, multiple sclerosis, tic disorders, parkinsonism, and myoclonic epilepsy.

Nicotine, despite being a powerful stimulant, has no major therapeutic application. Its high toxicity and presence in tobacco smoke give nicotine a considerable medical importance, however. Clinically, tremors and convulsions are major neurologic signs of nicotine intoxication. Respiration is stimulated, and vomiting is induced. Nicotine also has marked antidiuretic activity resulting from direct hypothalamic stimulation. If acutely ingested, nicotine can be fatal at a level of approximately 60 mg of the base product. Autonomic overactivity with dilated pupils, irregular pulse, sweating, and muscle twitching are characteristic signs of nicotine toxicity. Coma may rapidly supervene, although convulsions are usually not present. If death occurs, it is caused by paralysis of respiratory muscles. Cardiac arrhythmias are significant and are other potential sources for demise. Chronic intoxication as a result of nicotine occurs among tobacco pickers, or "croppers," consisting of nausea, vomiting, dizziness, and prostration. The illness is intermittent and lasts between 12 and 14 hours; it then clears, only to recur with return to work. There are no mortalities or long-term sequelae, however. During the 1973 harvesting season, an estimated 9% of the 60,000 tobacco growers in North Carolina reported illnesses.

Vitamins are vital trace substances, and neurologic syndromes generally are associated with deficiency syndromes. However, because health enthusiasm has reached passionate proportions for many individuals, especially Americans, clinicians are encountering neurotoxic syndromes associated with these seemingly safe agents. Of the fat-soluble vitamins, vitamin A is directly associated with neurotoxicity, and vitamin D can alter bone and renal metabolism, causing secondary neurologic dysfunction. Of the water-soluble vitamins, only pyridoxine (B6) is established to provoke neurologic complications.

Vitamin A, required for normal growth, vision, reproduction, and maintenance of epithelium, in high doses accumulates and can induce the syndrome of increased intracranial pressure (pseudotumor cerebri). Foods high in vitamin A include broccoli, cabbage, and liver, although dietary hypervitaminosis A is most unusual. Medically, vitamin A is used in the treatment of acne vulgaris and other dermatologic illnesses. Whereas the generally recommended daily allowance is 5,000 IU, individual capsules can contain five times that value, with subjects often ingesting 100,000 IU daily. At these doses, intoxication will develop over several months; at 200,000 IU daily, intoxication may develop within weeks. Publicity about the cancer preventive properties of vitamin A may increase the number of people who expose themselves to this product.

Early signs of increased intracranial pressure include headaches, blurred vision, transient obscuration of vision, and sixth cranial nerve paresis. On funduscopic examination, gradual papilledema develops without further signs of focal neurologic deficit. No neurologic clue exists to establish the etiology, but the skin changes, organomegaly, and history of vitamin ingestion will establish the diagnosis. Because vitamin zealots are often "antimedication," these patients must be questioned specifically about vitamins.

Vitamin D, when given in massive amounts, mobilizes bone calcium and phosphorus. When there is bone demineralization and degeneration, nerve root and spinal cord compression can occur. Alterations in the calcium balance can produce generalized weakness, muscle aches, cramps, and mild metabolic encephalopathy. Meningeal symptoms and trigeminal neuralgia are two additional reported findings without clear pathogenesis. The latter may relate to bony foraminal alterations. When renal impairment occurs, progressive secondary encephalopathy, not directly related to the vitamin, develops, and coma may result.

Pyridoxine, or vitamin B_6, has been implicated in a highly selective toxic syndrome provoking a sensory ataxia and dorsal root gangliar dysfunction. Widely used, especially by women to treat premenstrual tension and edema, pyridoxine induces this neurotoxic syndrome in occasional patients consuming chronic daily doses of 2 g or more. Gradually, the patient notes difficulty walking, with lightning-like dysesthesias in the back. Numbness of the extremities occurs, and, importantly, facial dysesthesias, so uncommon with most toxic neuropathies other than trichloroethane, quickly develop. Areflexia, stocking-glove sensory loss, and profound sensory ataxia with preserved strength are typical. On electromyography, marked slowing of the sensory nerve conduction is seen with normal motor conduction.

Tryptophan is an amino acid that has become popular for management of insomnia and behavioral changes related to the menstrual cycle (premenstrual syndrome). Myalgia and eosinophilia have been reported in numerous patients, as well as a progressive neuropathy affecting primarily the lower extremities with aching weakness. In some instances, patients are so disabled that they are wheelchair bound and need ventilatory assistance. Cessation of exposure to tryptophan and plasma exchange have been associated with clinical improvement in some cases.

QUESTIONS AND DISCUSSION

1. Match the cardiac drug with a prominent side effect:

A. Propranolol 1. Visual disturbance in as many as 40% of patients

B. Digitalis 2. Depression and impotence

C. Alpha-methyldopa 3. Garrulous, uninhibited behavior

D. Lidocaine 4. Parkinsonism

5. Peripheral neuropathy in 25%

The correct matches are (A) and (2); (B) and (1); (C) and (4); and (D) and (3). Propranolol and other beta-antagonists can cause depression and impotency that can be obscured in the rehabilitative setting after a myocardial infarction or surgery. Digitalis has prominent visual side effects, and patients often complain of halos around everything. Alpha-methyldopa can cause or aggravate parkinsonism, and lidocaine often is associated with a bizarre and alarming change in behavior.

2. Factors that contribute to the acid–base abnormality of salicylate intoxication include the following:

A. Salicylates initially depress medullary breathing activation.

B. Salicylates are acids that displace bicarbonate and also can lead to ketosis.

C. Myoglobinuria usually precipitates renal shutdown and metabolic acidosis.

D. All of the above.

The answer is (B). Salicylates initially activate the medullary breathing center and cause respiratory alkalosis. Later, at high doses, the medullary breathing center can be inhibited. In addition, salicylates induce and enhance the chemosensitive response and are acids as described in (B). The net response is a metabolic acidosis with either a respiratory acidosis or alkalosis. Myoglobinuria is not a feature of salicylate intoxication.

3. True statements regarding birth control pills and neurologic disability include:

A. Peripheral neuropathy of the axonal type can mimic multiple sclerosis.

B. Cerebrovascular accidents usually relate to cardiac valvular vegetations.

C. Chorea often resolves within days or weeks of drug cessation and is rarely a permanent sequela of oral contraceptive ingestion.

D. Papilledema, when it occurs, is caused by the steroid-induced hypervitaminosis A.

The answer is (C). Birth control pills are not associated with a peripheral neuropathy; instead, their toxicity relates predominantly to a CNS function. Cerebrovascular accidents are an alarming complication of these drugs in young women and may be of embolic or thrombotic origin. They do not relate specifically to valvular vegetations. Chorea often occurs within days of the first ingestion of birth control pills and may stop promptly after drug cessation. Only in rare instances (usually a hemiballistic syndrome) will the chorea be longstanding after drug cessation. In such cases, a static cerebrovascular accident is hypothesized to underlie the chorea as opposed to the transient chorea, which probably relates to a hormonally induced functional alteration in dopaminergic sensitivity at the striatum. Papilledema, when it occurs in patients taking birth control pills, may have multiple etiologies, including venous thrombosis and pseudotumor cerebri. It does not appear to relate to hypervitaminosis A.

4. Five neurologic complications of neuroleptic therapy are listed in (1) through (5). Match them with their usual characteristics using the (A) through (C) list.

A. Acute, occurring minutes or hours or, at most, days after starting the drug

B. Subacute, occurring days, weeks, or a few months after starting the drug

C. Chronic, occurring after several months or years of drug treatment

1. Dystonia
2. Parkinsonism
3. Chorea
4. Tremor
5. Oculogyric crises

The correct matches for (A) are (1) and (5); for (B) are (2) and (4); and for (C) are (1) and (3). The acute neurologic side effects related to neuroleptic drugs are dystonia and akathisia. The contorted posture of dystonia is frightening to see or experience. An oculogyric crisis, with the eyes thrown back and the neck usually hyperextended, is only one example of a dystonic complication of neuroleptics. A late-onset dystonia has been described as within the realm of tardive dyskinesia, but this is probably uncommon. Tardive dyskinesia is mainly a choreic or stereotypic disorder but may be dystonic and

is the major chronic side effect of neuroleptic drugs. The subacute problem associated with neuroleptic medication is parkinsonism, which may include any of the following: tremor, bradykinesia, rigidity, or postural reflex compromise.

5. True statements regarding the use of antiemetic drugs include:

A. Metoclopramide is particularly useful in patients with Parkinson's disease with nausea secondary to their dopaminergic medication.

B. Children receiving prochlorperazine for gastrointestinal distress are least likely to have neurologic complications.

C. In a patient using a scopolamine patch who reports acute right eye pain, an emergency visit to an ophthalmologist and removal of the patch should be recommended.

D. Scopolamine may cause drug-induced parkinsonism by a mechanism similar to that of neuroleptics.

The answer is (C). Scopolamine is an anticholinergic agent that may exacerbate narrow-angle glaucoma, with painful symptoms in the eyes. If not recognized and treated emergently, this may result in blindness. Both metoclopramide and prochlorperazine are dopamine-receptor blockers, similar to the neuroleptics. Hence, both agents may cause drug-induced parkinsonism or worsen preexisting Parkinson's disease. Children treated with these drugs are at more risk for developing acute dystonic reactions. In contrast, scopolamine, being an anticholinergic agent, does not cause drug-induced parkinsonism.

6. In patients receiving theophylline, which of the following is true?

A. Seizures occur only if serum levels are in the toxic range.

B. Theophylline is a useful agent in an elderly patient with congestive heart failure and a previous stroke with a history of intermittent asthma.

C. A child receiving IV infusions of theophylline is at increased risk for developing acute dystonic reactions.

D. The pharmacokinetics of drugs metabolized in the liver may affect the metabolism and serum levels of theophylline.

The answer is (D). Theophylline is metabolized by the hepatic enzymes. Other drugs metabolized in the liver may alter theophylline metabolism, affecting the serum levels. The seizures associated with theophylline may occur in the therapeutic range. In particular, patients with previous brain injury are at increased risk. Congestive heart failure may increase theophylline levels even when the drug is administered at recommended doses. Theophylline is a xanthine compound without dopamine receptor activity, and it is not known to cause acute dystonic reactions.

7. Which of the following antibiotics is associated with a high incidence of neurotoxicity?

A. Penicillin
B. Trimethoprim
C. Minocycline
D. Erythromycin

The answer is (C). Minocycline provokes ototoxicity, and women are more susceptible to these effects than men. The remaining agents are associated with neurotoxic syndromes only on occasion, unless they are given by unusual routes or in unusual doses.

8. Which condition is associated with vitamin excess?

A. Clinical findings of Guillain-Barré syndrome
B. Increased intracranial pressure
C. Myasthenia gravis
D. Wernicke–Korsakoff syndrome

The answer is (B). Excess vitamin A and B_6 are known to cause neurotoxic syndrome. B_6 provokes a sensory neuropathy with loss of reflexes, but it should not be confused with Guillain-Barré, which predominantly affects the motor system. Vitamin A causes the syndrome of pseudotumor cerebri, with increased intracranial pressure, often associated with headache and other nonfocal neurologic findings. (Sixth-nerve paresis, unlike other cranial neuropathies, is a "false-localizing" sign. Because of the long trajectory of the nerve along bony surfaces, a sixth-nerve paresis does not locate the level or side of neurologic damage.) Vitamin D, when given in high doses chronically, affects calcium and phosphorus balance, which may clinically provoke global weakness. The classical neuromuscular fatigue typical of myasthenia and the response to edrophonium are not seen. Wernicke–Korsakoff syndrome is related to vitamin deprivation and not to intoxication.

SUGGESTED READING

Bahls FH, Ma KK, Bird TD. Theophylline-associated seizures with "therapeutic" or low toxic serum concentrations: Risk factors for serious outcome in adults. *Neurology* 1991;41:1309.

Carbone JR. The neuroleptic malignant and serotonin syndromes. Emerg Med Clin North Am 2000;18(2):317–325.

Giménez-Roldàn S, Mateo D. Cinnarizine-induced parkinsonism. *Clin Neuropharmacol* 1991;14:156.

Goetz CG, Kompoliti K, Washburn KR. Neurotoxic agents. In: Joynt RJ, Griggs RC, eds. *Clinical neurology.* Philadelphia: Lippincott-Raven, 2002;1.

Goetz CG. Neurotoxins in clinical practice. New York: SP Medical and Scientific Books, 1985.

Heiman-Patterson TD, Bird SJ, Parry GJ, et al. Peripheral neuropathy associated with eosinophilia–myalgia syndrome. *Ann Neurol* 1991;28:522.

Hoppmann RA, Peden JG, Ober SK. Central nervous system side effects of nonsteroidal anti-inflammatory drugs. *Arch Intern Med* 1991;151:1309.

Kompoliti K, Stacy S, Horn S. Drug-induced and iatrogenic neurological disorders. In: Goetz CG, ed. *Textbook of clinical neurology.* Philadelphia: WB Saunders Company, 2003;1225–1256.

Lipsy RJ, Fennerty B, Fagan TC. Clinical review of the histamine-2 receptor antagonists. *Arch Intern Med* 1990; 150:745.

Miller LG, Jankovic J. Persistent dystonia possibly induced by flecainide. *Mov Disord* 1992;7:62.

Pappert EJ. Neuroleptic-induced movement disorders: Acute and subacute syndromes. In: de Wolff FA, ed. *Intoxication of the nervous system,* Part II. Amsterdam: Elsevier Science BV, 1994.

Sacristan JA, Soto JA, de Cos MA. Erythromycin-induced hypoacusis: 11 new cases and literature review. *Ann Pharmacother* 1993; 27:950.

Silverstein A, ed. *Neurological complications of therapy: Selected Topics.* Mt. Kisco, NY: Futura, 1982.

Spencer PS, Schaumburg HH, eds. *Experimental and clinical neurotoxicology.* Baltimore: Williams & Wilkins, 1980.

Stenzel MS, Carpenter CC. The management of the clinical complications of antiretroviral therapy. *Infect Dis Clin North Am* 2000;14(4):581–578.

Vinken PJ, Bruyn GW, Cohen MM, et al, eds. Intoxications of the nervous system. *Handbook of clinical neurology,* Vols. 36 and 37. Amsterdam, North Holland, 1979.

Wald JJ. The effects of toxins on muscle. *Neurol Clin* 2000;18(3):695–718.

Yokota T, Kagamihara Y, Hayashi H, et al. Nicotine-sensitive paresis. *Neurology* 1992;42:382.

18

Traumatic Brain Injury for the Non-Neurologist

Michael J. Makley

EPIDEMIOLOGY AND OVERVIEW

The wide spectrum of possible presentations in traumatic brain injury (TBI) offers several challenges to the clinician. Often the clinician is not only asked to manage the patient medically but also to prognosticate regarding outcome and return to former activities such as school, work, or driving. Managing each of these patients is complicated additionally by various factors that will affect outcome and recovery, such as the extent and severity of injury, age, genetic factors, premorbid learning disability, or substance abuse history. This chapter briefly will discuss this wide spectrum of patient presentations with TBI. Topics covered will range from the patient in coma to guidelines for dealing with sports-related concussion. In this overview it is hoped that the reader will come away with a sense of the breadth of the disease process; an understanding of some basic terminology and pathophysiology; and finally, some fundamental concepts of managing these patients at various levels of disease severity.

The aftermath of brain injury has a huge impact not only on individuals and families but also on society at large. It has been estimated that 1.5 to 2 million people suffer a traumatic brain injury each year, with nearly a million of these being treated in an emergency room. In relative terms this outpaces the yearly incidence of stroke, spinal cord injury, and multiple sclerosis combined. The incidence of severe TBI is 14 per 100,000 people, with nearly 60% of these people dying from their injury. The incidence for moderate and mild TBI is 15 and 131 per 100,000, respectively.

There is a bimodal distribution in regard to age and TBI. The first peak, in the second and

third decade of life, is predominantly related to motor vehicle accidents (MVA); the other peak, in the sixth decade of life, is predominantly related to falls. In the younger age groups it is a predominantly male disease (2:1), whereas in the older age groups it becomes more evenly distributed between genders. TBI is the leading cause of death and disability in young adults, affecting this population in their peak income-producing and reproductive years. The economic impact in the United States has been estimated for both direct and indirect costs of lost wages and productivity at $39 billion per year.

PATHOPHYSIOLOGY AND OPERATIONAL TERMS

To understand TBI at any injury severity level it is important to understand some fundamental pathophysiology. The two main types of injury generally considered to be at work in acceleration/deceleration injury are related to impact injury or focal cortical contusion and diffuse axonal injury (DAI). As can be seen in Fig. 18.1, the point of impact is primarily the bilateral frontal poles and bilateral temporal poles, which correspond to the brain overlying the inside of the skull's orbitofrontal ridge and each wing of the sphenoid bone, which cradles the temporal lobes. These areas of damage ultimately will lead to long-term behavioral sequelae of TBI as manifested by executive dysfunction, specifically deficits in behavior modulation, attention, and memory encoding and retrieval. Other focal injuries to motor, language, and visual cortex will lead to more obvious neurologic syndromes such as spastic hemiparesis, aphasia, and hemianopsia.

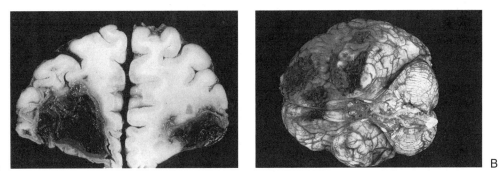

FIG. 18.1. Hemorrhagic contusion at frontal and temporal lobes after TBI.

The pathologic hallmark of DAI on a cellular level is the presence of axonal retraction balls, as seen in Fig. 18.2. Originally it was thought that these occurred with shearing forces to the axon at the moment of impact and that these "balls" were just the effect of the axon rolling up like a window shade that was wound too tightly. Postmortem studies, however, have shown that these retraction balls are not evident for 12 to 24 hours postinjury. It now is thought that impact causes a perturbation in axoplasmic transfer that, over several hours, leads to axonal swelling and finally disconnection and Wallerian degeneration. This disconnection leads to widespread deafferentation, which is thought by some to be one of the most significant factors in terms of long-term morbidity and recovery. Although DAI is a pathologic, postmortem diagnosis, patients who survive TBI are described as having had axonal injury when there is a prolonged loss of consciousness with a normal computed tomography (CT) scan or neuroimaging findings that show diffuse petechial intraparenchymal hemorrhage (Fig. 18.3).

Other factors that contribute to injury severity include extraaxial and intraparenchymal hemorrhage, anoxia, and impact depolarization with widespread release of excitatory neurotransmitters and generation of free radicals. For every level of injury this secondary cascade of events also will have an impact on outcome and recovery. Anoxic injury in addition to TBI is associated with the worst outcome, and the prognosis for a good recovery is poor. Finally, in considering outcome, it is important to keep in mind that the extent of each person's recovery from TBI may be determined by an individual's genetic makeup. There has been research suggesting that patients carrying a mutant allele of

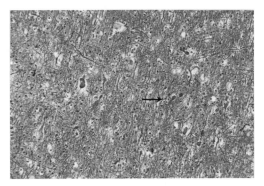

FIG. 18.2. Axonal retraction ball formation seen in diffuse axonal injury (DAI).

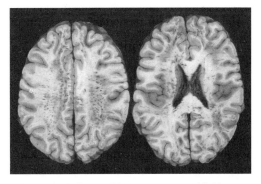

FIG. 18.3. Diffuse white matter petechial hemorrhage seen in diffuse axonal injury (DAI) on gross section.

apolipoprotein E have increased beta amyloid deposition in the brain and a significantly longer recovery following TBI.

Before discussion of patient management, it is helpful to define certain terms used in the field of treating TBI. Because of the lack of any specific functional or structural imag-ing test that can reliably define the extent of injury, the field has relied primarily on de-scriptor scales to describe brain injury sever-ity. Two of the most prevalent scales used in TBI are the Glasgow Coma Scale (GCS) (Figs. 18.4 and 18.5) and the Rancho Los Amigos Scale (RLAS). The GCS is widely

PATIENT'S RESPONSE

SCORE

EYE OPENING

- Eyes open spontaneously.............................. 4

- Eyes open when spoken to 3

- Eyes open to painful stimulation 2

- Eyes do not open 1

MOTOR

- Follows commands 6

- Localizes to pain 5

- Withdrawal to pain 4

- Flexor posturing to pain 3

- Extensor posturing to pain.............................2

- No motor response to pain...............................1

VERBAL

- Oriented to place and date..............................5

- Converses but is disoriented............................4

- Utters inappropriate words.............................3

- Incomprehensible nonverbal sounds 2

- Not vocalizing...1

                                    TOTAL_____

FIG. 18.4. The Glasgow Coma Scale Scoring Sheet.

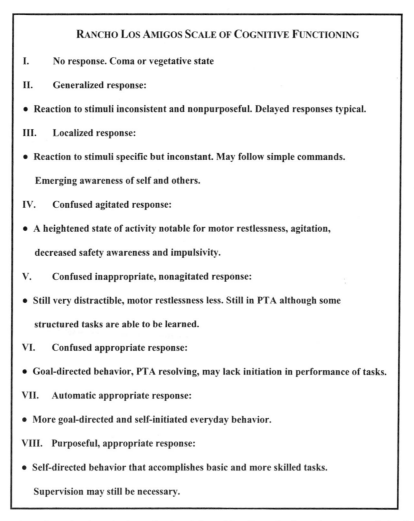

RANCHO LOS AMIGOS SCALE OF COGNITIVE FUNCTIONING

I.   No response. Coma or vegetative state

II.   Generalized response:

● Reaction to stimuli inconsistent and nonpurposeful. Delayed responses typical.

III.   Localized response:

● Reaction to stimuli specific but inconstant. May follow simple commands.

    Emerging awareness of self and others.

IV.   Confused agitated response:

● A heightened state of activity notable for motor restlessness, agitation,

    decreased safety awareness and impulsivity.

V.   Confused inappropriate, nonagitated response:

● Still very distractible, motor restlessness less. Still in PTA although some

    structured tasks are able to be learned.

VI.   Confused appropriate response:

● Goal-directed behavior, PTA resolving, may lack initiation in performance of tasks.

VII.   Automatic appropriate response:

● More goal-directed and self-initiated everyday behavior.

VIII.   Purposeful, appropriate response:

● Self-directed behavior that accomplishes basic and more skilled tasks.

    Supervision may still be necessary.

FIG. 18.5. The Rancho Los Amigos Scale of Cognitive Functioning after traumatic brain injury.

used in trauma centers to describe the level of awareness in the patient with a TBI. This scoring system occurs over three domains of motor, verbal response, and eye opening. The lower scores (3–8) are associated with coma or the minimally responsive patient, and the higher scores (13–15) describe a person who may be a little confused but is oriented and following commands. The GCS also has been used to grade severity of TBI, as shown in Fig. 18.6.

GRADE OF TBI	GLASGOW COMA SCORE
MILD	13 -15
MODERATE	9-12
SEVERE	< 9

FIG. 18.6. Severity of brain injury graded by Glasgow Coma Scale (GCS).

The RLAS is used primarily in the postacute or rehabilitation setting, in which the bottom of the scale I and II is associated with a vegetative state and the top of the scale at VIII is associated with mild cognitive deficits. This scale is a narrative description of emergence stage by stage from diffuse axonal injury where the duration of each stage on the scale is directly proportional to the severity of injury. In the least severe injury, such as concussion, passage through the first stages may be fairly rapid. In the more severe cases the passage up these stages can be months to years, and for some patients their progress can stall at any point on the Rancho scale.

TBI is unique among acquired brain disease because of the predominance of behavioral and memory deficits over motor and sensory deficits. Because of this, it is important to understand the concept of posttraumatic amnesia (PTA), a unique memory disorder of TBI. PTA is a compound amnestic syndrome in which a person has lost both previously acquired memory (retrograde amnesia) as well as the ability to lay down new memory (anterograde amnesia).

Obviously the inability to lay down memory has implications for any rehabilitation program, but the duration of PTA also has been used to describe severity of TBI as well as predict outcome in terms of disability. Harvey Levin, a neuropsychologist, developed a neuropsychologic screen to determine the duration of PTA called the Galveston Orientation and Amnesia Test (GOAT), in which a score of 75 or greater is associated with resolution of PTA. Serial scoring of this test provides the length of time spent in this amnestic state. PTA of longer than 24 hours is considered to be associated with a severe TBI. Data from Katz and Alexander showed that for those with PTA of less than 2 weeks 76% reached a level of good recovery, whereas 22% were moderately disabled and 2% were severely disabled at 1 year. For survivors with 8 to 12 weeks of PTA, only 12% had a good recovery at 1 year, whereas 75% suffered moderate disability and 13% were severely disabled. No one with PTA longer than 12 weeks had what was described as a good recovery.

ACUTE HOSPITALIZATION

Most patients who experience a brief loss of consciousness and present to the emergency department with a GCS of 13–15 will have routine evaluations that should include a complete neurologic examination, CT scan looking for evidence of extraaxial blood, and radiographic clearance of any neck injuries. Those with a normal neurologic and radiographic examination often will be sent home after a period of observation. The acute hospitalization of moderate to severe TBI typically will be managed in a trauma center and will be provided by a neurosurgeon or an experienced team of trauma specialists and intensivists.

In the acute hospitalized setting the primary focus of care often will be the management of increased intracranial pressure and intracranial hemorrhage. Patients with expanding epidural hematomas will be taken to the operating room immediately. Subdural and intraparenchymal blood will be assessed for evacuation according to the grade and severity as well as the underlying neurologic examination. The blood generally will be removed when it is associated with mass effect and shift of midline structures or a deteriorating neurologic examination.

With severe impact injury the secondary cascade of widespread depolarization can lead to an overwhelming increase in intracranial pressure from intraparenchymal edema. Even without an expanding mass lesion this type of diffuse swelling can rapidly lead to herniation and death. Typically the neurosurgeons will monitor this with an intracranial pressure monitor that is passed through the skull. Patients are given mannitol and are hyperventilated to bring their P_{CO_2} down to 25 mmHg. Pentobarbital coma is the next step when these measures fail to bring down the pressure. Even with all of these interventions, patients with severe trauma can continue to have unrelenting elevated pressures. The last measure to reverse this process is craniectomy and duraplasty. This surgery simply removes the cranium and places a duraplastic patch on the dura that allows the brain to expand unimpeded by the calvarium. The skull flap is frozen in the pathology lab and replaced after all of the swelling has subsided. Although many patients will survive the acute edema, carefully controlled studies have not been done for this dramatic intervention and long-term outcome data are unknown.

Another issue that arises in the acute care setting is the issue of seizure prophylaxis. People with closed head injury are at a greater risk of developing seizures. Various studies have found between 2% and 12% of patients with closed head injury will develop posttraumatic seizures. For those with dural-penetrating injuries, the rate may be more than 50%. A study in the early 1990s by Temkin and colleagues looked at seizure prophylaxis using a double-blind, placebo-controlled paradigm in patients presenting with TBI. Their results showed that there was no benefit to phenytoin after the first 7 days in terms of preventing the development of posttraumatic seizures. Patients with penetrating head injury, however, because of the higher risk of developing posttraumatic seizures, should be maintained on seizure prophylaxis for 6 months to 1 year, depending on the severity of injury.

POSTACUTE HOSPITALIZATION

As methods for acute resuscitation improve with the development of the acute trauma centers there has been a dramatic increase in brain-injured patients at the lowest level of responsiveness. Data from the National Traumatic Coma Data Bank have shown that nearly 10% of the patients discharged from an acute trauma center are discharged in a vegetative state, yet there is no consensus on their appropriate management. Often these patients are discharged to nursing homes poorly equipped and trained to manage the complex needs of these patients. Although functional goals clearly are limited in the minimally responsive patient, there is a role for an interdisciplinary approach to the management of these low-level patients, particularly just after acute hospitalization. In one study, 60% of patients admitted to a specialized low-level head-injury program emerged and progressed on to an acute rehabilitation program with age being the most significant predictor of successful emergence.

In these low-level patients the most important medical management issues revolve around the complications that come from an immobile, minimally responsive patient. Such a patient needs provision of aggressive pulmonary toilet, treatment of infections, prevention of decubitus ulcers, maintenance of adequate nutrition, management of spasticity, and access to comprehensive family education. The role of the interdisciplinary therapy team within a specialized low-level brain injury program is not only for passive range of motion and sensory stimulation. Trained therapists also assess the person's level of responsiveness to his or her environment using a systematic scoring tool such as the JFK Coma Recovery Score or other scoring system. The physician, in addition to treating medical issues and spasticity, often will blend in various neurostimulants, such as methylphenidate, amantadine, bromocriptine, or a levodopa/carbidopa compound. These agents are thought to augment arousal and attention and perhaps correct an underlying disturbance of sleep–wake cycle (Fig. 18.7). Although there is widespread use of these agents in this patient population, there are no large-scale, placebo-controlled trials that guide their use to date.

After emerging from coma, patients with severe TBI will progress on to RLAS III–VII behavior. At this stage they will exhibit emerging awareness and evolving communication; however, they will have severe cognitive deficits as well as deficits in attention, self-monitoring, and safety awareness. The early part of this period is also marked by motor restlessness, sleep–wake cycle disturbance, and continued anterograde amnesia. This phase of an emerging head-injured pa-

ACTIVATING AGENTS USED IN BRAIN INJURY

MEDICINE	EFFECTS	DOSING
Amantadine	Both pre- and post-synaptic dopaminergic effect	100 mg bid Max dose 300 mg/day
Bromocriptine	Dopamine agonist	1.25–2.5 mg bid
Carbidopa/levodopa	Neurotransmitter that will affect all central sites but primary target is mesial and prefrontal dopaminergic projecting pathways	Starting dose of 25/100 tid and titrate up to 1–1.5 g of levodopa
Methylphenidate	Indirect catecholamine agonist	Starting dose at 2.5 to 5 mg bid. Can titrate up to 20 mg/d. Dose at an a.m. and a noon dosing schedule
Modafinil	Exact mechanism unknown Increases extracellular dopamine	200 mg q a.m. Max dose 400 g/day

FIG. 18.7. Activating agents commonly used in low-level responsive head injury and in abulia.

tient's recovery is best managed in an acute rehabilitation setting with a dedicated staff of interdisciplinary specialists experienced in brain injury providing physical therapy, occupational therapy, and speech and language therapy. In addition, a neuropsychologist or behavioral psychologist who can address the behavioral aspects of these patients is an essential part of the multidisciplinary team.

As their working memory returns and patients move on into the RLAS VII and VIII levels, they frequently are discharged from an acute rehabilitation setting to their families with continued outpatient therapy in the community. Almost all patients, when discharged from a rehabilitation setting after a moderate to severe injury, will require 24-hour supervision, which is often a very large burden on the family and caregivers.

Once in the community patients should be connected with resources for vocational or educational reentry. There are regional advocacy groups for patients and families with TBI that offer resources and support groups to assist in this transition. Frequently school systems have programs in place to reintegrate adolescents with TBI back into the classroom. Some states have funded programs for voca-

tional evaluation and placement following head injury. In terms of motor-vehicle operation, each state has individual requirements and protocols for return to driving after a head injury, and the physician should investigate these particulars before clearing the person. In closed-head injury the biggest risk for driving is the risk of seizures. In those states without a formal medical review board determining when a person can return to driving, it may be prudent to refer the patient to a neurologist for an opinion.

SPECIAL CHALLENGES OF THE HOSPITALIZED PAITIENT

Dysautonomia

In patients with moderate to severe head injury it is not uncommon to observe tachycardia; tachypnea; hypertension; profuse neurosweats; and persistently and markedly elevated temperature, particularly in patients at low levels of responsiveness, as described by a GCS of less than 8 or a RLAS of I or II. These symptoms commonly are attributed to being centrally mediated, although it must be remembered that, for the most part, this is a diagnosis of exclusion. Prior to this clinical conclusion the patient should be evaluated thoroughly for infection, dehydration, pain, pulmonary embolus, thyroid disease, and other clinical entities. True, centrally mediated symptoms are thought to be related to hypothalamic damage and most often are treated symptomatically and observed. Typically these symptoms remit after emergence from coma. Beta blockers are often used for this condition and serendipitously may help with agitation later on as the patient emerges to the next level on the Rancho scale. In patients with neurosweats the physician should watch for dehydration, particularly in the patient who is receiving nutrition and hydration through a feeding tube because often the dietitian who is calculating the diet for the patient may overlook this.

HYPONATREMIA

Low serum sodium is a fairly common occurrence in people with TBI related to their brain injury or medications. Most often electrolyte analysis of serum and urine will show that it is related to the syndrome of inappropriate antidiuretic secretion from the anterior hypothalamus (SIADH). Also considered in the differential diagnosis is cerebral salt-wasting syndrome. It is important to distinguish the two by laboratory evidence because the treatment will be completely different (Fig. 18.8).

Drugs often are implicated in SIADH, particularly carbamazepine, so a complete review of the patient's pharmacology also should be performed. Management involves removal of potential pharmacologic etiologies such as carbamazepine, selective serotonin reuptake inhibitors (SSRIs), and non-steroidal antiinflammatory drugs (NSAIDs). For SIADH, the patient is typically fluid restricted to 1500 cc of fluid per day. In refractory cases, demeclocycline, a tetracycline that blocks the effect of vasopressin on the renal collecting duct, is used. The mainstay of treatment for cerebral salt wasting is volume replacement.

LATE-ONSET HYDROCEPHALUS

Another late complication in TBI is hydrocephalus. Subarachnoid blood blocking the egress of cerebrospinal fluid (CSF) in the arachnoid villi is thought to be the etiology. Such a diagnosis should be considered in a patient who does not progress in terms of re-

Clinical	SIADH	CSWS
HYDRATION STATUS	HYPERVOLEMIC OR EUVOLEMIC	DEHYDRATED
WEIGHT	↑	↓
URINE NA	↑	↑
SERUM K	NO CHANGE or ↓	NO CHANGE or ↑
SERUM NA	↓	↓
SERUM OSMOLALITY	↓	NORMAL or ↑
BUN	NORMAL	↑
URIC ACID	↓	NORMAL

Adapted from Zafonte and Mann, 1997.

FIG. 18.8. Hyponatremia with traumatic brain injury.

covery or who was progressing and then stops or regresses. At least one follow-up CT scan should be performed on patients in a vegetative state following their acute hospitalization or in any patient who regresses in their rehabilitation program without a clear etiology. It remains controversial as to who will benefit from a shunt procedure because it is often not clear whether the widened ventricles are ex-vacuo changes from diffuse neuronal loss and atrophy or indeed a result of a high-pressure system in need of shunting. Therapeutic spinal taps are rarely conclusive to determine whether a person needs a shunt though they often are performed. Some neurosurgeons advocate placing a temporary lumbar drain to evaluate for clinical improvement. Others will place a shunt as a trial for 4 to 6 months.

AGITATION

One of the major management problems for the clinician dealing with patients emerging at a RLAS III–V level is agitation. Typically the agitation is somewhat generalized and related to their amnestic state and their impulse dyscontrol. This type of agitation is very similar to generic delirium, and causes for delirium should be explored in each of these patients before attempting to treat agitation thought to be related to emerging head-injury behavior. Specific entities the clinician should watch out for include infection, drug or alcohol withdrawal, metabolic abnormality, or adverse drug reaction. In the low level and confused patient pain is a commonly overlooked although prevalent problem in individuals who often are involved in a multitrauma injury with concomitant orthopedic and musculoskeletal injuries.

In general, agitation should be dealt with non-pharmacologically if possible by removing all identifiable triggers for the patient's agitation. For example, limit the number of friends and family who visit and keep environmental stimuli to a minimum (i.e., turn down the lights, turn off the Jerry Springer show on the television). Part of agitation can be iatrogenic, caused by attempts to keep the patient safe because of their poor insight, memory, and poor safety awareness. Restraints and locking belts invariably escalate problems in the patient who is confused and delirious, and their use should be minimized, although at times they are unavoidable.

A number of theories have been put forth about the agitation in TBI. One behavioral theory holds that because of severe frontal lobe injury, the patient becomes stimulus bound. In other words, because of frontal injury the patient has no block or filter on their reaction to their environment or internal needs. This is compounded by several factors, including their confusional/amnestic state, the strange environment of a rehabilitation hospital, and restraint use.

Another theory of agitation in head injury holds that it is related to attentional deficits. Analogous to the child with attention-deficit hyperactivity disorder, the patient with TBI is overwhelmed with sensory stimuli, and that causes random, generalized striking out or hostile behavior. This school of thought would advocate giving stimulant medication to try to hone attention and thereby reduce agitation. Although seemingly paradoxical, for some patients with prominent attentional deficits, giving stimulants works well.

Although commonly used for agitation in this patient population, in general, it is thought that one should avoid neuroleptic medications in patients with TBI because of experimental evidence suggesting these agents have a detrimental effect on brain recovery. The exception to this rule is the patient with paranoid delusions or the violently agitated patient whose actions endanger staff or themselves. For the patient who is acutely agitated and in danger of hurting himself or others, the use of haloperidol intramuscularly or intravenously is indicated. For patients with paranoid delusions but who are not at imminent safety or health risk, one of the more selective dopaminergic blockers is preferred.

When non-pharmacologic measures fail to control symptoms, the clinician should proceed in a rational and stepwise manner through beta blockers, antiepileptic drugs,

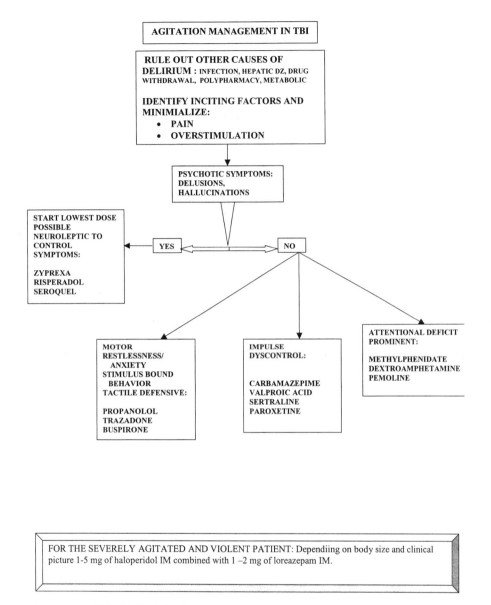

FIG. 18.9. Agitation management in traumatic brain injury.

and SSRIs (Fig. 18.9). The primary aim should be patient and staff safety, and in time most people with brain injury will pass through this phase. For the small minority whose behaviors do not improve, they often are referred to a specialty program with specific expertise and experience in dealing with the refractory behavioral sequela of TBI. In some places this might be a psychiatric hospital or a chronic neurorehabilitation center.

LACK OF INITIATION

At the other end of the spectrum from agitation is the patient with TBI without any motivation or self drive, which is described as abulia, derived from the Greek word meaning "without will." This describes a patient who is awake but wholly disconnected from his or her environment. In the most extreme cases the person is completely without motivation or initiation and, in fact, will starve to death if not fed. As in the patient who is comatose or in a vegetative state, these individuals primarily are treated with the same dopaminergic agents used for the vegetative patient or serotonergic reuptake inhibitors.

SPASTICITY

Spasticity is a frequent and difficult problem for patients, particularly those with severe head injury. With the onset of increasing tone in these patients the therapists in the acute or rehabilitation centers will begin using conservative measures to try and counteract spasticity. These measures include passive range of motion, weightbearing, and serial casting, in which the affected limb is casted into a more neutral, or functional, position in the upper or lower extremity. When conservative measures fail to control spasticity, more aggressive pharmacologic interventions will need to be used.

In patients with TBI it generally is considered that one should avoid baclofen because of its gamma-amino-butyric acid (GABA)-agonist activity as well as the significant sedation that it frequently causes. GABA is the primary inhibitory neurotransmitter in the central nervous system, and many research studies have suggested that GABA agonists may slow the recovering brain. Also, baclofen may be so sedating as to obscure a person's emergence from a low level of responsiveness. For these reasons the firstline agent generally is considered to be dantrolene sodium. This is a medication that works peripherally on the muscle by inhibiting the release of calcium from the sarcoplasmic reticulum, thereby inhibiting excitation contraction coupling between the myosin and the myosin light chain kinase. To treat areas of focal spasticity or to try and improve positioning of the upper and lower extremities, focal blocks with either botulinum toxin or phenol are useful. These are often very helpful while the therapists try measures such as serial casting. Although systemic spasmolytics such as baclofen and tizanidine are avoided in brain injury, there are times when spasticity becomes so overwhelming that these agents cannot be avoided. An intrathecal baclofen pump should be considered in cases of unrelenting spasticity when systemic spasmolytics cause intolerable sedation. This is a small programmable pump device that is implanted into the abdomen wall. A silastic catheter comes off the pump reservoir and is tunneled around the abdomen and inserted into the lumbar cistern. The pump can deliver continuous microgram amounts of baclofen directly to the spinal column capillary beds, thus providing spasticity relief at a much smaller total dose while leaving cortical neurons relatively unaffected.

MILD TBI

As stated in the introduction, mild TBI, or those patients with a presenting GCS of 13–15, composes the largest percentage of all occurrences of brain injury. It is a significant public health problem and probably the most common brain injury presentation to face the primary care physician or non-neurologist. The American Congress of Rehabilitation Medicine delineates specific components of the diagnosis of mild TBI (Fig. 18.10).

The postconcussive syndrome that follows a mild head injury has a myriad of associated symptomatology with the most common be-

Mild TBI Criteria
•   HEAD TRAUMA
WITH:
○   Confusion or
○   LOC < 30 min
•   PTA < 24 hours
•   GCS 13–15

FIG. 18.10. The American Congress of Rehabilitation Medicine's specific components of the diagnosis of mild traumatic brain injury.

ing headache, vertigo, depression, fatigue, irritability, sleep disturbance, slowed reaction time, slowed information processing, and loss of concentration and memory. Subdural or epidural blood, seizures, tremor, or dystonia are rare occurrences that also have been reported following mild TBI.

Typically these patients will present with many subjective symptoms but with a normal neurologic examination and unremarkable imaging studies. That litigation is not infrequently involved often colors the clinician's opinion in these cases. It is important to keep an objective sense of this symptomatology despite lack of hard objective findings on examination or conventional neuroimaging studies.

Headaches

Posttraumatic cephalgia is one of the most common complaints after a mild TBI. These often are described with components of both a tension-type headache and a vascular- or migraine-type headache. For instance, a patient may complain of a daily headache that is pressure in character and associated with photophobia and nausea and vomiting. These "mixed-type" headaches respond nicely to low-dose amitriptyline taken at bedtime in a dosage range of 25 to 50 mg. It is important to inform the patients that the amitriptyline is not a pain reliever *per se* and should be taken consistently at bedtime for at least 1 week before titrating up. For acute pain relief NSAIDs are often beneficial. Typical migraine headache will respond to conventional migraine interventions but perhaps would be handled better by a neurologist or headache specialist. Cases of posttraumatic cephalgia that do not respond to tricyclics and NSAIDS would be better handled by a specialist as well.

Vertigo

Vertigo, or the sensation of movement with any turn of the head, is quite common after head injury of any severity level even in minor concussive injury. It often comes to light in the outpatient clinic after the person with moderate to severe injury is discharged from the rehabilitation center. In mild TBI it often can be a presenting complaint. Symptoms are thought to be related to concussive forces knocking otolith crystals off of hair cells in the inner ear. Typically patients will report that when they are lying in bed or when they turn their head suddenly either they will have a sensation of spinning or have the sensation that the room is spinning around them. Nearly all patients will have a recovery after 6 months, and often symptoms are such that the only treatment necessary is gentle reassurance. For patients whose symptoms are interfering with function, any of the vestibular suppressants such as anticholinergics or benzodiazepines can be used; however, all of them have the side effect of drowsiness, which may worsen other symptoms associated with mild TBI such as fatigue and mental slowness. Persistent symptoms should be referred to an ENT surgeon with expertise in vestibular disorders.

Sports-Related Concussive Injury

The non-neurologist often is asked to clear an athlete following concussive injury for return to sports. That decision should be based on the severity of the concussive injury and the duration of concussive symptomatology. The clinician also should keep in mind that the effects of concussive injury are thought to be additive. Guidelines published by the American Academy of Neurology can help with these decisions. Concussive injury is described by grades. Those with transient confusion, no loss of consciousness, and concussive symptoms that last less than 15 minutes are rated as grade 1. People with transient confusion and no loss of consciousness but concussive symptoms or mental status abnormalities that last greater than 15 minutes are considered grade 2. Grade 3 concussive injury is anyone with loss of consciousness of any duration. Any athlete with grade 3 concussion should be transported to an emergency room for a full evaluation to include a CT scan of the head and neck. It should be kept in mind that under most circumstances the neck should be immobilized until this evaluation. Grade 2 concussions should eliminate the athlete from the contest or sporting activity, whereas an athlete with a grade 1 injury should be watched carefully and only permitted to return to play if all symptoms clear in less than 15 minutes. CT imaging of grade 2 concussive injuries should be done for those with persistent postconcussive symptoms.

WHEN TO REFER TO A NEUROLOGIST OR OTHER SPECIALIST

Refractory Headaches

Posttraumatic cephalgia is common in closed head injury and is usually self-limited or treatable with a combination of low-dose tricyclic antidepressants and NSAIDs. Those patients with headaches that do not respond to doses of tricyclics at 100 mg/day probably should be sent to a neurologist or a headache specialist who might use other therapeutic options such as occipital nerve block, transcutaneous electrical nerve stimulator (TENS) units, or antiepileptic medications. Also, patients who develop migraine-type symptoms following their head injury, such as pulsatile headache with photophobia, scintillating scotoma, and nausea and vomiting, also should be referred to a specialist for treatment.

Posttraumatic Epilepsy

All patients with moderate to severe head injury should be informed of their increased risk for epilepsy as a result of their injury, and family members or significant others should be counseled on basic seizure first aid. First-time seizure patients should be instructed to go for evaluation in an emergency room, including a CT scan and a general workup. At some point they should follow up with an evaluation by a neurologist that should include an electroencephalogram. Carbamazepine is the current drug of choice for

seizures that result from closed head injury because these will be, because of the nature of the injury, focal in onset with secondary generalization. Carbamazepine has the added effect of being a mood stabilizer, and for patients with impulse dyscontrol or agitation this may have a secondary benefit. One antiepileptic drug that should be avoided in this patient population, particularly in the acute recovery phase, is phenobarbital, which has the side effects of both cognitive and motoric slowing that only compounds already existing problems for the patient who is brain injured.

Neuropsychologic Testing

Formal neuropsychologic testing always is indicated in patients returning to school or any type of high-level management or professional occupation. Information from such testing may be helpful to reintegrate the student back into their academic track or help modify a work environment that allows successful return to employment or professional life. This testing is of no use in a period of ongoing PTA and is probably best utilized 4 to 6 months after injury. Sometimes it is helpful to then have the tests repeated at 1 year to see if there are improvements in any domains of intellect.

Severe Behavioral Disorder/Depression

In all levels of TBI there are patients who come out of it with severe and refractory behavioral disorders that do not resolve with time. Patients with severe impulse dyscontrol, aggression, agitation, or depression should be referred to a neurologist with experience in TBI or a neuropsychiatrist who can manage these difficult patients with appropriate pharmacology. Unfortunately, some of the most impaired of these patients will not be able to function outside of a structured institutional setting.

Depression is a fairly common occurrence among survivors at all injury levels. Depression that is complicated by psychotic features or is unresponsive to firstline agents such as the commonly used SSRIs should be referred to a psychiatrist for further evaluation and treatment.

SUMMARY

TBI is a prevalent disease process with often life-changing consequences for those affected and their families. The cost to society is equally large. Although there has been some suggestion of a decline in head injury incidence in the United States, there is still a great deal to learn on how to effectively treat survivors of TBI to return them to their highest level of functioning within their community. These patients have a number of problems at every level of severity that the physician is asked to manage—from headaches to agitation and impulse dyscontrol. Very often victims of closed head injury are relatively young and can have a normal life span while living with symptoms and the after effects of their brain injury. On the horizon are exciting new treatments in both the acute center and the outpatient arena that may change the ultimate outcome and quality of life for survivors of TBI.

QUESTIONS AND DISCUSSION

1. A 26-year-old man is discharged to a rehabilitation facility after sustaining a severe closed-head injury from wrecking his motorcycle. His blood alcohol level was elevated, and he had an open book fracture of his pelvis, a right femur fracture, and a T4 compression fracture. He is transferred, after 5 weeks at the trauma center at what the speech therapist is calling "Rancho 4 level." He exhibits a great deal of motor restlessness in bed and frequently is found by the nursing staff to be attempting to climb out of the bed. He is non-verbal. The nurses are requesting medication for agitation. The most likely cause of this agitation is:

A. An acute meningeal infection
B. Part of his brain injury
C. Alcohol withdrawal

D. Pain
E. Acute paranoid delusions

The answer is D. Part of the emergence from severe head injury does involve this generalized agitation and motor restlessness, but it is important for the physician not to overlook treating musculoskeletal pain in patients, particularly those who have multitrauma injury and who might not be able to communicate their needs. It is well past the point for him to be going through acute alcohol withdrawal at 5 weeks.

2. A 20-year-old man is involved in a severe motor-vehicle accident and is admitted to a rehabilitation center in a vegetative state. The therapists who are working with him report steady gains in the coma recovery scoring tool that they are using until week 5, which is 9 weeks after his injury. They tell you he actually is regressing in some parts of the scoring system. The most likely cause is:

A. Vasospasm and infarct
B. Drug-related encephalopathy
C. Hydrocephalus
D. Depression
E. Expanding epidural hemorrhage

The answer is C. Hydrocephalus is a late-onset complication from severe head injury and is thought to be related to subarachnoid blood blocking the egress of CSF from the arachnoid villi. Communicating hydrocephalus should be suspected in anyone with a decline in function but should be a particular concern in those at the lowest level of responsivity. Often these patients will respond to ventriculoperitoneal shunting. Expanding epidural hematoma would be a much more dramatic change in neurologic functioning and would, under most circumstances, need rapid neurosurgical intervention.

3. A 32-year-old mother of a newborn comes in with complaints of dizziness. She was involved in a motor-vehicle accident 1 week before, and she reports that she was knocked unconscious for a brief period. She was taken to a local emergency room for evaluation, where a head CT was done that was negative. She was sent home after a brief period of observation. She has little recollection

of any events before being in the hospital. She reports that when she is lying down on the sofa and turns her head a certain direction she feels as if the room is spinning. Her neurologic examination is normal. She most likely has:

A. Postpartum depression

B. Subdural hematoma that was missed on the first CT scan

C. Dislodged otolith crystals off of her hair cells

D. Complicated migraine

E. Postconcussive syndrome

The answer is C. Although it can be part of a postconcussive syndrome, this patient is describing a type of positional vertigo that is common after concussive injury.

The most appropriate treatment for this patient is:

A. Neurontin

B. Diazepam

C. Antivert

D. Gentle reassurance that the symptoms will resolve within 6 months.

The answer is D.

4. You are at your daughter's lacrosse game, which is the last game of the season against their arch rivals. One of the senior forwards, and leading scorers, takes a stick to the head (National Collegiate Athletic Association women's lacrosse rules do not mandate helmets) and for a brief moment is knocked unconscious. On the sidelines she briefly is confused, but this clears quickly (<5 minutes) and she wants to get back into the game. She denies headache, dizziness, nausea, or vomiting. She is alert and oriented. The coach looks at you standing on the sidelines and, knowing you are a physician, asks your opinion. Your opinion is:

A. Girls should really have to wear helmets in lacrosse.

B. She should not be allowed back in the game and should be taken to the emergency room immediately for evaluation.

C. She can return to play, but if she suffers another blow to the head she should be taken out of the game.

D. She should be removed from the contest and not allowed to return that day.

The correct answer is both A and B. Any loss of consciousness is considered a grade 3 or severe concussion, and an evaluation in an emergency room is warranted. One also should keep in mind that if the athlete went down there could be a spine injury, and cervical immobilization would be prudent until this can be evaluated in an emergency room. After a brief grade 3 concussion, the athlete should be withheld from play for a minimum of 2 weeks.

5. A 50-year-old dairy farmer is up early milking his cows one day and falls off his tractor, approximately 15 feet, suffering a closed head injury and a fractured right humerus. A CT scan in the emergency room shows a right temporal contusion. His posttraumatic amnesia resolves within 1 week,

TABLE 18.1. *Commonly Used Neurostimulant Agents for Low-Level Responsive Patients Following TBI*

Medicine	Effects	Dosing
Amantadine	Both presynaptic and postsynaptic dopaminergic effect	100 mg bid Max dose 300 mg/day
Bromocriptine	Dopamine agonist	1.25–2.5 mg bid
Carbidopa/levodopa	Neurotransmitter that will affect all central sites, but primary target is mesial and prefrontal dopaminergic projecting pathways	Starting dose of 25/100 tid and titrate up to 1–1.5 g of levodopa
Methylphenidate	Indirect catecholamine agonist	Starting dose at 2.5–5 mg bid. Can titrate up to 20 mg/day. Dose at a morning and a noon dosing schedule

TBI, traumatic brain injury.

and he is discharged from the acute hospital to home and outpatient therapies. His wife brings him in to your family practice for an office visit the week after his discharge and wants to know how long he needs to be taking the Dilantin. She says it makes him "foggy." She relates that to her knowledge he never had a seizure and there is no one in the family who has seizures. Your response:

A. Because of his advanced age and the location of his contusion he is at a high risk for seizures and should be maintained for 1 year.

B. He needs to see a neurologist to determine this.

C. He can stop taking Dilantin.

D. He needs to be switched to Tegretol, which works better than Dilantin.

The correct answer is C. There is fairly conclusive evidence in the literature that there is no benefit to the use of antiseizure medications beyond the first week in TBI. The patient should be reminded that they are still at risk for having a seizure because of their head injury, and the patient and family should be informed of this and counseled in what to do should their family member have a seizure.

SUGGESTED READING

Katz DI, Alexander MM. Traumatic brain injury: predicting course of recovery and outcome for patients admitted to rehabilitation. *Arch Neurol* 1994;51:661–670.

Mysiw WJ, Sandel MME. The agitated brain injured patient. Part 2: Pathophysiology and treatment. *Arch Phys Med Rehabil* 1997;78(February):213–220.

Practice parameter: Antiepileptic drug prophylaxis in severe traumatic brain injury. *Neurology* 2003;60(January): 10–16.

Practice parameter: The management of concussion in sports (summary statement). *Neurology* 1997;48(March): 581–585.

Report of the Consensus Development Conference on the Rehabilitation of Persons with Traumatic Brain Injury. Bethesda, MD: National Institutes of Health, 1998.

Ross D, Zafonte D, Mann NR. Cerebral salt wasting syndrome in brain injury patients: a potential cause of hyponatremia. *Arch Phys Med Rehabil* 1994;78(May): 540–542.

Temkin NRM, Dikmen SSP. A randomized, double-blind study of Phenytoin for the prevention of post-traumatic seizures. *N Engl J Med* 1990;323(n8):497–502.

19

Neuromuscular Diseases

Hans E. Neville, Dianna Quan, and Steven P. Ringel

Disorders that result from abnormalities of spinal cord motor neurons, the peripheral nerve, the neuromuscular junction, or muscle constitute "neuromuscular disease." Weakness is a common symptom, but unlike central nervous system (CNS) disorders, neuromuscular diseases may be accompanied by muscle atrophy, often striking, and diminished muscle tone. Patients also may develop muscle pain, stiffness, cramps, twitching, limb deformities, or myoglobinuria.

This chapter will discuss the variable clinical presentations of neuromuscular disease except for disorders of peripheral nerve, which will be covered in a separate chapter. The section is organized to include clinical presentations; diagnostic laboratory investigations; descriptions of specific neuromuscular disorders including genetics (Table 19.1); outpatient treatment principles (Table 19.2), which summarizes pharmacologic treatment; special problems in managing the hospitalized patient; and suggestions on when to refer to a neurologist.

CLINICAL PRESENTATIONS

Weakness

A useful clinical generalization for neuromuscular disorders is as follows: all motor neuron, neuromuscular junction, and muscle diseases have no sensory changes accompanying the weakness. Coexisting sensory complaints or findings strongly suggest a peripheral nerve disorder (see Chapter 13).

The rapidity of onset, location, and progression of weakness are important diagnostic features. Rapidly developing weakness (hours to several days) is characteristic of most diseases of the neuromuscular junction, the Guillain-Barré syndrome, toxic myopathies, and acute electrolyte disturbances. Acute remissions and relapses are seen with myasthenia gravis (MG), periodic paralysis, and other channelopathies. Insidious and slowly progressive weakness occurs in many diseases affecting muscle or spinal cord motor neurons. Three distribution patterns of weakness can be encountered: proximal, distal, and cranial. Each pattern is associated with typical symptoms related by the patient and with some signs easily observed even before individual muscles are tested. These distribution features usually are absent in patients with nonorganic complaints, where symptom description is characteristically vague. Such individuals often prove to have normal strength or a "give-away" pattern of weakness, which suggests lack of full voluntary effort.

Proximal weakness is characteristic of many muscle disorders, some spinal muscular atrophies, and MG. These patients report difficulty in climbing stairs or arising from low chairs. When arising from a chair, they will lean forward and "push off" with their hands on the armrests. In arising from the floor or a squatting position, they may require one or more supports with the hands on the floor, knees, and thighs (Gowers' maneuver, Fig. 19.1). The gait of a person with proximal weakness has a waddling appearance of the buttocks because of weakness of hip fixators. Knee extensor weakness may cause the leg to "give out." The knee is kept locked, gradually leading to hyperextension (back-kneeing), which in turn produces an exaggeration of the lumbar lordosis. Shoulder–girdle weakness produces difficulty in elevating the arms and may be accompanied by scapular winging (Fig. 19.2). With the arms hanging at the sides, the scapulae may slide laterally to produce a curving inward of the shoulders with the backs of the hands facing forward and an

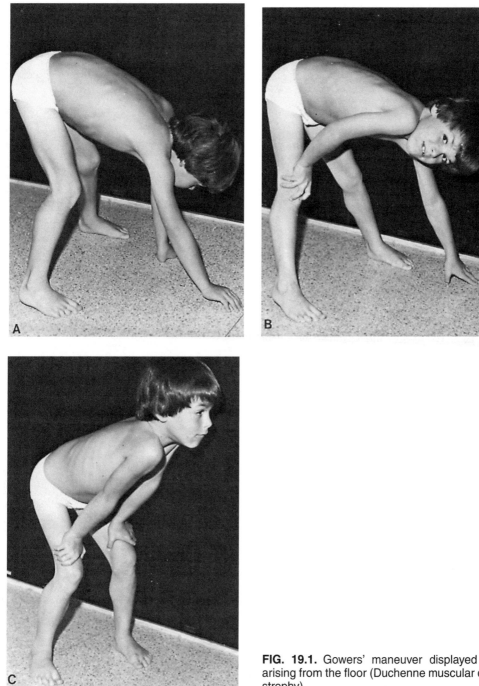

FIG. 19.1. Gowers' maneuver displayed in arising from the floor (Duchenne muscular dystrophy).

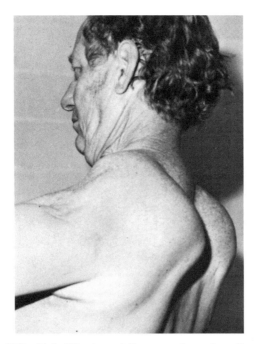

FIG. 19.2. Winging of the scapulae when the arms are elevated (fascioscapulohumeral dystrophy [FSH]).

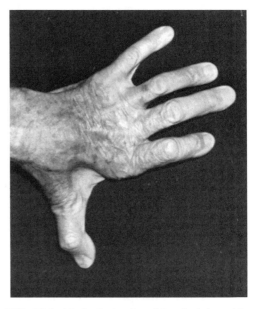

FIG. 19.4. Marked atrophy of the first dorsal interosseous muscle in motor neuron disease.

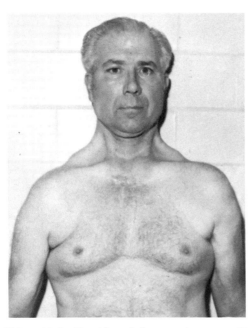

FIG. 19.3. Shoulder–girdle weakness with "trapezius hump," "step-sign" with prominent down-sloping clavicles, and an oblique anterior axillary crease (LGD).

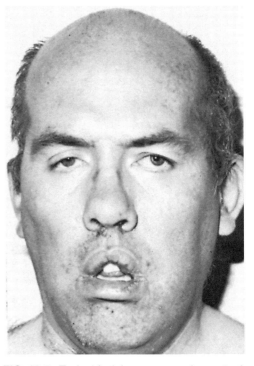

FIG. 19.5. Typical facial appearance in myotonic dystrophy with frontal balding, temporalis and masseter atrophy, ptosis, and protuberant lower lip.

associated oblique "axillary crease" (Fig. 19.3). The high-riding scapulae produce a conspicuous "trapezius hump"; the clavicles may slope downward and stand out prominently from the atrophic neck musculature (Fig. 19.3).

Distal weakness in the presence of atrophy is commonly seen in amyotrophic lateral sclerosis (ALS) (Fig. 19.4), inclusion body myositis (IBM), and myotonic dystrophy. These patients find it difficult to manipulate small objects including buttons, and they also have difficulty when eating or using writing utensils. They may complain of "dragging" their legs because of a "foot drop" or of frequent tripping, particularly on uneven ground. With each step the knees are raised high while the feet flap limply; shoe soles may show asymmetric wear.

Cranial nerve weakness affects the extraocular, facial, and oropharyngeal muscles and is an important differential feature in diagnosis of various dystrophies (Figs. 19.5 and 19.6).

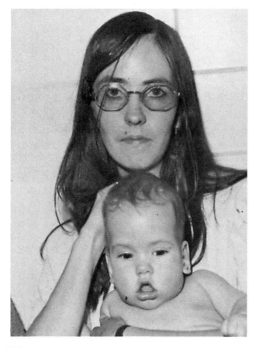

FIG. 19.6. Myotonic dystrophy in mother (note "hatchet face") and infant (note "shark mouth"). Diagnosis first made in the child suggested the same diagnosis in the mother.

Ptosis and ophthalmoparesis occur in several myopathic disorders. Swallowing and speech changes can be early signs of either ALS or MG.

Atrophy and Hypertrophy

The disuse of a limb will produce modest muscle atrophy, as is seen after only a few weeks following the casting of a bone fracture. The muscle retains much of its strength in disuse atrophy, and the apparently atrophied limbs of an elderly person may be surprisingly strong. In contrast, patients with neuromuscular disease may have striking muscular atrophy with obvious weakness.

Atrophy of the muscles around the shoulder girdle commonly reveals underlying bony prominences. Flattening of the thenar eminence and guttering of the interossei can produce a wasted, clawlike deformity of the hand (see Fig. 19.4). Several disorders produce characteristic appearances. Examples include "Popeye arms" (very atrophied biceps/triceps with a normal appearing forearm) in facioscapulohumeral dystrophy, the "hatchet face" (temporalis wasting) appearance in myotonic dystrophy (see Figs. 19.5 and 19.6), and the enlarged calves of Duchenne dystrophy (DUD; Fig 19.7). Diffuse hypertrophy of all limb muscles is commonly seen in myotonia congenita, rarely in hypothyroidism, and very rarely in amyloidosis.

Pain, Stiffness, and Cramps

Inflammatory myopathies and other collagen-vascular diseases may produce muscle pain and tenderness, but the absence of these symptoms does not exclude the diagnosis. In older patients, pain, aching, and stiffness in the shoulder and hip-girdle muscles should suggest polymyalgia rheumatica. Most patients with limb aching and pain without weakness do not have a neuromuscular disease. The diagnosis of fibromyalgia often is evoked, particularly in otherwise healthy middle-aged women who have diffuse aches and pains; however, the nature of this purported

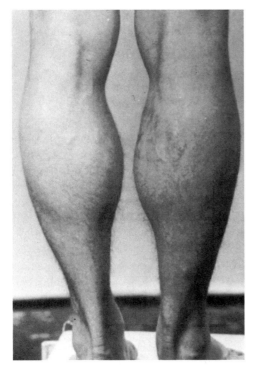

FIG. 19.7. Pseudohypertrophy of the calves (Duchenne dystrophy).

fibers in single motor units. Fasciculations appearing in a strong muscle are usually benign and are exacerbated by many factors, including fatigue and caffeine intake. When they occur in a weak muscle, they may be associated with ALS, but they also may occur in the setting of root compression or peripheral nerve injury.

Hypotonia

Various unrelated disorders present with infantile hypotonia. The most frequent abnormality in the "floppy baby" is a CNS disease, such as seen after perinatal asphyxia. The hypotonic infant may exhibit normal muscle strength, with the ability to lift its head or limbs against gravity. In the absence of other abnormalities, the prognosis for normal development may be excellent. In infants with obvious weakness, the underlying disorder may be spinal muscle atrophy or one of the congenital myopathies. Weaknesses of sucking and respiration are serious concomitant findings, which, if undiagnosed and untreated, usually are fatal.

entity is highly controversial and it has no pathologic foundation.

Stiffness may be a nonspecific symptom, or it may be a symptom of myotonia, a phenomenon consisting of a delayed relaxation of the muscle following voluntary contraction or percussion. This produces difficulty in releasing the grip or initiating movements after a period of rest.

Muscle cramp, a prolonged involuntary contraction, is a universal and generally benign symptom that occurs with increased frequency during unaccustomed exercise, "body building," pregnancy, or electrolyte disturbance. It also may occur in hypothyroidism, partial denervation (especially in ALS), tetany (with hypocalcemia, hypomagnesemia, or alkalosis), and certain metabolic myopathies.

Muscle Twitching

Fasciculations (the tiny twitches with the terrible reputation) are contractions of muscle

Deformities

Neuromuscular disorders often are associated with skeletal deformities and should be suspected in the patient with unexplained hip dislocation, scoliosis (Fig. 19.8), contracture, or malformation of the feet (e.g., club foot, equinovarus, or pes cavus deformity). Arthrogryposis or multiple congenital limb deformities may occur with various diseases affecting any part of the motor unit.

Myoglobinuria

The syndrome of myoglobinuria consists of weakness and painful swelling of affected muscles in association with headache, nausea, and vomiting. The urine turns reddish brown within 24 hours and is positive for benzidine and Hemastix. An elevation of creatine kinase peaks at 5 to 7 days after the initial muscle injury. Most episodes are related to unusual cir-

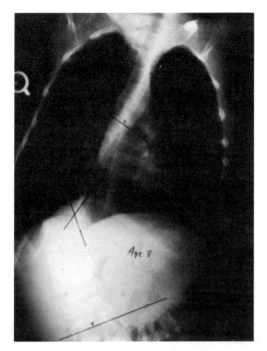

FIG. 19.8. Scoliosis in type 2 SMA. The angle of curvature is measured and followed closely (55 degrees in this patient).

cumstances that produce acute muscle necrosis, such as from vigorous exercise (particularly in someone deconditioned) and from certain myotoxic agents such as alcohol, cocaine, amphetamines, heroin, neuroleptics, and halothane in susceptible individuals.

A patient with recurrent myoglobinuria should be evaluated for an underlying metabolic neuromuscular disease.

DIAGNOSTIC LABORATORY INVESTIGATIONS

Enzyme Elevation

Muscle necrosis results in elevated levels of serum creatine kinase (CK). The highest levels occur in the syndrome of myoglobinuria, Duchenne muscular dystrophy, and polymyositis with slightly to moderately elevated values in most of the other dystrophies and motor neuron disorders. The most common causes of a modest CK elevation include

recent, vigorous exercise in an otherwise normal individual and hypothyroidism.

Electrodiagnostic Studies

Electrophysiologic investigations including nerve conduction studies (NCS), needle electromyography (EMG) examination, repetitive nerve stimulation, and single-fiber EMG provide both qualitative and quantitative information about neuromuscular disease states.

Nerve conduction studies broadly differentiate between primary demyelinating and axonal neuropathies and provide quantitative data for following the course of disease. In conditions affecting muscle, a NCS only rarely is abnormal and then only if significant loss of muscle tissue causes low-amplitude compound motor actions potential recordings.

Needle EMG almost always is performed as a complement to NCS and is useful in differentiating neuropathic from myopathic disorders (Fig. 19.9). Neuropathic disorders resulting from loss of anterior horn cells or peripheral nerve leave fewer motor units available for voluntary recruitment, especially early in the course of disease. This manifests on EMG as a decrease in the electrical interference pattern. In the acute period of neuron or axon loss, spontaneous electrical activity from denervated muscle fibers may be recorded in the form of fibrillation potentials and positive sharp waves (Fig. 19.9, item 4). Following chronic denervation, surviving motor axons develop collateral sprouts that reinnervate muscle fibers. Spontaneous electrical activity disappears, and the electrical potentials produced by these large motor units have high amplitudes and an increased number of phases (Fig. 19.9, item 3).

In myopathic disorders, the random loss of individual muscle fibers results in decreased motor unit potential amplitudes (Fig. 19.9, item 2). To generate the same amount of force as a healthy muscle, more of the smaller myopathic motor units are needed. During voluntary contraction this is seen as "early recruitment" of motor unit potentials and the

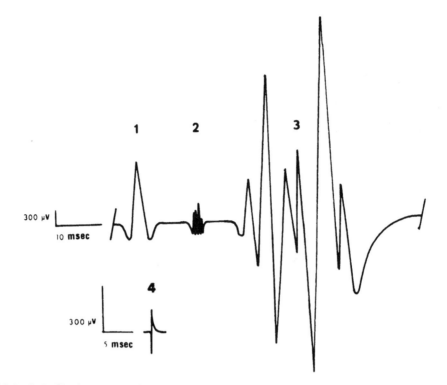

FIG. 19.9. 1–4: Single motor unit action potentials recorded by electromyography in a voluntarily contracting skeletal muscle. **1:** Normal motor unit action potential. **2:** The myopathic potential is brief, small amplitude, and polyphasic. **3:** The neuropathic potential is prolonged, high amplitude, and polyphasic. **4:** A fibrillation potential is spontaneously produced by a denervated muscle fiber at rest.

early development of a maximum interference pattern.

In disorders of the neuromuscular junction, more specialized testing such as repetitive stimulation studies or single-fiber EMG can be performed. Repetitive stimulation of a peripheral nerve in these conditions may produce a characteristic increase or decrease in the amplitude of the compound motor action potential, depending on the type of defect. Single-fiber EMG may reveal increased "jitter," a measure of the synchrony of depolarization occurring in muscle fibers from the same motor unit.

Muscle and Nerve Biopsy

Muscle biopsy is performed easily under local anesthesia as an outpatient procedure, allowing for rapid histologic and histochemical preparation to aid in diagnosis. Characteristic changes are well described for many conditions affecting the motor neuron and muscle.

Genetic Testing of Neuromuscular Diseases

Molecular biology techniques have produced a torrent of information describing gene abnormalities underlying many neuromuscular disorders. Table 19.1 summarizes known gene mutations operating to produce motor neuron diseases, dystrophies, muscle storage disorders, mitochondrial dysfunction, congenital myopathies, and channelopathies. Further genetic details are provided in subsequent descriptions of specific diseases.

TABLE 19.1. *Gene Abnormalities in Neuromuscular Disease*

Disorder	Chromosome	Recessive (R) or Dominant (D)	Gene Product	Special Features
Motor Neuron Disease				
Spinal muscular atrophy				
SMA 1, 2	5	(R)	SMN and rarely NAIP protein in SMA 1, 2, 3	SMN protein mutation in 95% of Type 1, 2, 3
SMA 3	5	(R) and (D)		
SMA 4 (adult)	Unknown	(R) and (D)	SMN defect in some	Clinical overlap with progressive muscular atrophy
Spinal and bulbar muscular atrophy (Kennedy's disease)	X	(R)	Androgen receptor	Androgen receptor gene enlarged (multiple CAG repeats)
Amyotrophic lateral sclerosis				
Sporadic (90%–95%)	No known defect		None known	See text
Familial (5%–10%)				
SOD-1 mutation	21	(D)	More than 90 known mutations	SOD-1 mutation in only 20% of familial cases
Other mutations	2, 9, 15, 18	(D) or (R)	Unknown	Mutations very rare
Peripheral Nerve (See Chapter 13)				
Neuromuscular Junction				
Acquired MG	No gene defect	—	—	—
Congenital MG	17	(R)	Subunit of acetylcholine receptor protein	No antibodies to the receptor protein, and immunosuppression is ineffective
Muscular Dystrophies				
Duchenne/Becker dystrophy	X	(R)	Dystrophin	Gene deletion (60%–70%); point mutation in rest
Facioscapulohumeral dystrophy	4	(D)	Unknown	Specific deletions in 95% on chromosome 4, but gene itself is still unknown
Limb–girdle dystrophy (recessive)	2, 4, 5, 13, 15, 17	(R)	2A Calpain	LGMD2A mildly weak
			2B Dysferlin	LGMD2B proximal and distant weakness (Myoshi)
LGMD 2A, 2B, 2C, 2D, 2E, 2F, 2G, 2H, 2I, 2J			2C, D, E, F sarcoglycan defect	LGMD 2C–J tend to have severe symptoms, some resembling Duchenne dystrophy (see text)
			2G Telethonin defect	
			2H E-3 Ubiquitin defect	
			2I Fukutin-related protein	
			2J Titan-related protein	
Limb–girdle dystrophy (dominant)				
LGMD1A	5	(D)	Myotilin	Dysarthria seen
LGMD1B	1	(D)	Laminin	Cardiac involvement
LGMD1C	3	(D)	Caveolin	"Rippling" muscle
Emery-Dreifuss muscular dystrophy	X, 6	(R)	Emerin	Elbow contractures and cardiac changes
Congenital muscular dystrophy	1, 6	(R)	Absent merosin in some	Normal mentation
	9	(R)	Fukutin defect	Severe mental and developmental retardation
Oculopharyngeal dystrophy	14	(D)	Protein regulates polyadenylation and mRNA size	Ptosis, swallowing defects
Myotonias				
Myotonia congenita	7	(D) and (R)	Muscle chloride channel	Autosomal recessive form most common; dominant forms rare (Thomsen's disease)
Myotonic dystrophy (DM1)	19	(D)	Myotonin	Gene has triplet (CCTG) repeats
Myotonic dystrophy (DM2 or PROMM)	3	(D)	An mRNA binding protein	Disease worse with increasing number of repeats
				Gene has multiple CCTG repeats

continued on next page

TABLE 19.1. Gene Abnormalities in Neuromuscular Disease

Disorder	Chromosome	Recessive (R) or Dominant (D)	Gene Product	Special Features
Inflammatory Myopathies				
Inclusion body myositis	9	(R)	Unknown	Rare autosomal dominant form (most IBM is sporadic)
Glycogen Storage Diseases				
Phosphorylase deficiency (McArdle's)	11	(R) and (D)	Muscle phosphorylase	Exercise intolerance, cramps
Acid maltase deficiency	17	(R)	Acid maltase	Fatal in infants; moderately severe in adults
PFK deficiency	1	(R)	Phosphofructokinase	Exercise intolerance
PGAM-M deficiency	7	(R)	Phosphoglycerate mutase	Exercise intolerance
PGK deficiency	X	(R)	Phosphoglycerate kinase	Myopathy rare
LDH deficiency	11	(R)	Lactic dehydrogenase	Myopathy rare
Debranching enzyme deficiency	21	(R)	Debranching enzyme	Survival to adulthood common
Branching enzyme deficiency	3	(R)	Branching enzyme	Early death common
Phosphorylase b kinase deficiency	X, 16, 7, 6	(R)	Phosphorylase b kinase	Fatal in infancy, moderately severe in adults
Lipid Storage Disorders				
CPT II deficiency	1	(R)	Carnitine palmitoyl transferase II	Diagnosis by muscle biopsy and CPT enzyme assay
Carnitine deficiency	Unknown	(R)	Unknown	Diagnosis by muscle biopsy and muscle carnitine assay
Mitochondrial Myopathies				
Kearns-Sayres syndrome (KSS)	Mitochondrial DNA	Maternal inheritance	Various mitochondrial proteins	Extraocular muscle paresis, cardiac conduction block
MELAS	" "	"	tRNA	Lactic acidosis, stroke
MERRF	" "	"	tRNA	Myoclonus epilepsy, ataxia
				Diagnosis by distinctive muscle biopsy changes
Congenital Myopathies				
Myotubular myopathy Neonatal, late infantile, adult-onset forms	X in some	(R) and (D)	Myotubularin in neonatal form	Neonatal often fatal
	Unknown	(R) and (D)	Unknown in adult form	
Central core disease	19	(D)	Ryanodine receptor	Same gene as for malignant hyperthermia
Nemaline myopathy	1, 2, 19	(R) and (D)	Mutations reported in nebulin, alpha actin, alpha and beta tropomyosin, troponin	Respiratory problems common
Channelopathies				
Hypokalemic periodic paralysis	1	(D)	Muscle calcium channel	Diaphragm never involved
Hyperkalemic periodic paralysis/ paramyotonia congenital/ potassium aggravated myotonia	17	(D)	Muscle sodium channel	Different mutations of sodium channel gene define unique clinical features of each

SMA, spinal muscular atrophy; SMN, survival motor neuron; NAIP, neuronal apoptotic inhibitory protein; CAG, cytosine-adenine-guanine; SOD, superoxide dismutase; MG, myasthenia gravis; LGMD, limb-girdle muscular dystrophy; mRNA, messenger ribonucleic acid; CTG, cytosine-thymine-guanine; DM, myotonic dystrophy; PROMM, proximal myotonic myopathy; PFK, phosphofructo kinase; PGAM-M, phosphoglycerate mutase; PGK, phosphoglycerate kinase; LDH, lactic dehydrogenase; CPT, carnitine palmitoyl transferase; MELAS, mitochondrial myopathy, encephalopathy, lactacidosis, stroke; tRNA, transfer RNA; MERFF, myoclonus epilepsy with ragged-red fibers.

SPECIFIC NEUROMUSCULAR DISORDERS

The following section will describe clinical features of specific diseases; commonly used diagnostic tests; genetics; prognosis; and, when appropriate, specific drug treatment. For the motor neuron disorders and the genetically determined muscle diseases, where effective pharmacotherapy is limited or nonexistent, we will cover general rehabilitation principles for outpatients and the hospitalized patient in a later section.

Motor Neuron Diseases

Spinal Muscular Atrophies

The spinal muscular atrophies (SMA) constitute a group of hereditary disorders characterized by a severe reduction in spinal cord and cranial motor neurons. Virtually all cases are based on autosomal recessive inheritance.

Type 1 SMA

In patients with type 1 SMA (Werdnig-Hoffmann disease), symptoms of hypotonia, poor feeding, weak cry, and respiratory distress may be present at birth or may develop by age 6 months. Examination reveals flaccid, areflexive extremities, fasciculations of the tongue, pooling of saliva in the posterior pharynx; and paradoxical respiration. Many patients die of respiratory failure by 2 years of age.

Type 2 SMA

Type 2 SMA (intermediate SMA) presents during the first 18 months of life with delay of motor milestones as a common initial observation. On examination there is limb hypotonia and weakness as well as tongue fasciculations. These children often learn to sit independently but rarely either stand or walk. Sensation is normal. Progressive limb weakness, if untreated, will lead to skeletal deformities, including contractures at the hips and knees, hip dislocation, and scoliosis (see Fig. 19.8). Many patients survive into adolescence

or adulthood but ultimately succumb to respiratory insufficiency. Symptomatic treatment for these highly intelligent and motivated children will be covered in a later section of this chapter.

Type 3 SMA

Type 3 SMA (Kugelberg-Welander disease) presents with insidious proximal weakness beginning in late childhood or early adolescence. The clinical picture often mimics that of limb–girdle dystrophy with proximal arm and leg weakness. The appearance of tongue fasciculations and severe limb atrophy should alert the clinician to the possibility of a motor neuron disorder. Progression is slow, but because of leg weakness many patients require a wheelchair by their mid 30s. The prevention of contractures and scoliosis and good respiratory care are important.

Type 4 SMA

Type 4 SMA (adult SMA) presents in patients who are normal until their 20s, when they develop slowly progressive weakness and atrophy of leg and arm muscles. The deep-tendon reflexes are hypoactive or absent, and sensation is normal. Recessive inheritance is common, but in about one-third of patients inheritance is autosomal dominant. When there is no family history, patients with developing lower motor neuron symptoms are considered to have progressive muscular atrophy (PMA). This is essentially a lower motor neuron disorder sharing many of the clinical findings of type 4 SMA.

Genetics Types 1, 2, and 3 SMA are inherited as an autosomal recessive trait as a result of variable mutations of the survival motor neuron (SMN) gene on chromosome 5. Defects in both SMN alleles are present in about 95% of patients with the SMA phenotype. Rarely, there may be mutations of a closely adjacent neuronal apoptotic inhibitory protein (NAIP) gene. Patients with type 4 SMA are rare, and of the few studied, SMN mutations are found inconsistently.

X-Linked Spinal and Bulbar Muscular Atrophy (Kennedy's Disease)

X-linked spinal and bulbar muscular atrophy (Kennedy's disease) is an unusual disorder that can be confused with ALS. Patients in their 30s and 40s present with swallowing dysfunction, slurred speech, perioral and tongue fasciculations, facial weakness, mild limb weakness, hand tremor, gynecomastia, and impotence. The disorder is very slowly progressive but, unlike ALS, rarely is fatal.

Genetics This familial disorder results from a gene abnormality on the X chromosome. Thus, only males are affected; there is never male-to-male transmission; and females, although unaffected clinically, are carriers. The disease is caused by multiple cytosine-adenine-guanine (CAG) trinucleotide repeats in the androgen receptor gene. As numbers of CAG repeats increase, the age of disease onset is earlier but there is no correlation with disease severity.

Amyotrophic Lateral Sclerosis

ALS is characterized by progressive muscle wasting and weakness resulting from degeneration of brainstem and spinal cord lower motor neurons. There is coexisting spasticity and hyperreflexia caused by degeneration of upper motor neurons. The vast majority of cases are sporadic, although between 5% and 10% are familial. Initial clinical symptoms may be limited to asymmetric limb weakness in the presence of fasciculations. A foot drop or marked hand deformity resulting from interosseus wasting (see Fig. 19.4) can be seen. In addition to hyperreflexia, there are pathologic reflexes (Hoffman's response and crossed adductor responses) and in some cases extensor plantar responses. The sensory examination is normal in about 90% of patients, but abnormalities of pin and position sense are reported. Speech may develop a slurred or spastic quality.

For many years a coexisting dementia was not considered a part of ALS, but sophisticated psychologic test batteries reveal that cognitive defects may be seen in as many as 30% of cases.

The rate of spread and involvement of different muscles in ALS is unpredictable. Although facial weakness may be seen late in the disease, eye movement is never affected. Weight loss is commonly seen in the later phases of the illness as swallowing becomes increasingly impaired. Diaphragm weakness often leads to a critical time in the disease, as vital capacity drops progressively. The average survival after diagnosis is 3 to 4 years, but 10% survival at 10 years has been reported.

The treatment of ALS is primarily symptomatic (Table 19.2). Of the many drugs and trophic factors tried, only the oral agent riluzole is of value, prolonging survival by about 2 months. Trials are under way using new classes of drugs that act to reduce CNS glial inflammation and programmed neuronal death. On a purely theoretic basis, the antioxidants vitamin E and C are recommended to patients.

A troublesome symptom in up to 30% of patients with ALS is inappropriate laughing or crying, termed "pseudobulbar affect." Amitriptyline can help this condition, or, alternatively, the combination of quinidine and dextromethorphan may be used. For cramps, baclofen or quinine have been successful. For excessive salivation, nortriptyline can help.

Genetics The vast majority of ALS cases are sporadic and have no demonstrable genetic defect. Of the 5% to 10% of patients with ALS who have a positive family history, approximately one-fourth demonstrate a gene mutation on chromosome 21. The resulting ALS phenotype, termed ALS1, is the result of any one of more than 90 mutations that produce an atypical SOD-1 (superoxide dismutase) protein (thought to remove intracellular free radicals). The associated ALS probably does not result from a loss of SOD-1 function because in some mutations the SOD-1 molecule has normal or even high enzyme activity. In fact, the very presence of a defective SOD-1 may trigger reactions that result in premature neuronal death (apoptosis).

Additional autosomal dominant families with non–SOD-1 gene mutations on chromosomes 2, 9, 15, and 18 present in adolescents

TABLE 19.2. *Pharmocologic Treatments*

Disorder	Drug Start Dose; Expected Effect	Stable Dose Range	Interactions/Side Effects
Motor Neuron Disease			
Amyotrophic Lateral Sclerosis Sporadic or familial	RILUZOLE 50 mg bid Extends life 2–3 months	50 mg bid	Abnormal hepatic enzymes in 5%—stop drug
	ANTIOXIDANTS (theoretic value—no trials)		
	Vitamin E 800 IU/day	800 IU/day	None
	Vitamin C 1000 mg/day	1000–3000 mg/day	None
	Coenzyme Q10–50 mg/day	50–300 mg/day	None
	PSEUDOBULBAR AFFECT		
	Nortriptyline 10 mg bid	Up to 50 mg tid as tolerated	Excessive sleepiness
	Dextromethorphan 25 mg and quinidine 25 mg	Recent trial using this dose (unpublished)	Nausea, dizziness, sleepiness, loose stools
	CRAMPS		
	Baclofen 10–20 mg bid	20–40 mg qid	Muscle weakness at higher doses
	Quinine 325 mg/day		Ringing in ears
	EXCESS SALIVA		
	Nortriptyline 10 mg bid	325 mg bid to tid	Sleepiness
Neuromuscular Junction			
Myasthenia gravis	Prednisone 50 mg/day	50–80 mg/day depending on patient weight. Try tapering dose after strength back to normal. Use with azathioprine.	Weight gain, mood changes, cataract, osteopenia, diabetes, hypertension
	Azathioprine 50 mg/day	Increase each week by 50 mg increments until taking 50 mg qid. Add on to stable prednisone dose and after 2–3 months, try tapering the prednisone.	May cause leukopenia and liver function abnormalities, so monitor with weekly studies until maximal dose reached. Then, can do blood safety studies every 3 months. Also may cause skin rash.
	Micophenolate mefetil (Cellcept) 0.5 g/day	Increase over 2–3 weeks to 1 g bid	Not authorized by FDA for MG. Used primarily as antirejection drug for organ transplant but occasionally of use in MG when other drugs fail. Major side effect is GI distress.
	Pyridostigmine (Mestinon) 60 mg q4hr	60–120 mg q4hr, 180 mg timespan appropriately spaced	Symptomatic only and used primarily for mild ocular symptoms when risk of immunosuppression is unacceptable. Overdosage and cholinergic crisis can occur, however.
	Plasma exchange	3–5 daily exchanges and repeat as needed	Used for acute worsening if best pharmacologic treatment fails.
	IVIG 400 mg/kg	400 mg/kg × 5 days, reassess; repeat as needed	Used in patients totally refractory to all other therapy.
Muscular Dystrophies			
Duchenne and Beckers	Prednisone 0.65 mg/kg	Maintain at this dose for months to years depending on side effects	Treatment is controversial, and there are steroid side effects, as described for MG. In addition, there is growth retardation in children.
Myotonias			
Myotonia congenita	Mexilitine 150 mg bid	Increase by 50 mg increments every week to a maximum of 200 mg tid	GI distress, lightheadedness, tremor are side effects. Drug interactions with phenytoin, phenobarbital, rifampin, cimetidine, and theophylline.
Lipid Storage Disorders			
Carnitine deficiency	L-carnitine 2–4 g/day in adults 100 mg/kg/day (children)	Maintain at starting doses	
Channelopathies			
Hypokalemic periodic paralysis	Acetazolamide 250 mg bid	Increase to 250 mg tid as needed	Interactions with various drugs. Taste change, anorexia, nausea, drowsiness, kidney stones.
Hyperkalemic periodic paralysis	Hydrochlorthiazide 25 mg/day in AM	Increase to 50 mg/day in AM, and add 12.5 mg in PM, if necessary	Interactions with various drugs. Weakness, hypotension, electrolyte disturbance.

FDA, Food and Drug Administration; MG, myasthenia gravis; GI, gastrointestinal; IVIG, intravenous immune globulin.

with prominent upper motor neuron components. These families are exceedingly rare.

Poliomyelitis and Postpolio Syndrome

Acute poliovirus infection in non-immunized individuals leads to a non-specific febrile illness, followed by paralytic symptoms in a minority. Although the widespread use of immunization has reduced the frequency of new cases in industrialized countries, many adult patients still have residual weakness.

Unpredictable, progressive weakness may develop after many years of static deficit, the so-called "post-polio syndrome." This condition is best treated with symptomatic rehabilitation measures. There is no evidence for viral reactivation.

Diagnosis of Anterior Horn Cell Diseases

The diagnostic confirmation of any of the motor neuron diseases relies heavily on accurate electrical studies, which will show acute and chronic denervation in multiple arm and leg muscles in the presence of normal motor and sensory nerve conduction velocities. In infants and children suspected of SMA, EMG and nerve conduction velocity (NCV), although challenging to perform, can provide laboratory confirmation and avoid muscle biopsy. When biopsy is carried out in suspected patients with SMA, abnormalities will include distinctive group atrophy and type grouping. In all the motor neuron disorders, serum creatine kinase is modestly elevated but rarely reaches levels greater than 1,000.

Disorders of the Peripheral Nerves

This topic is discussed in Chapter 13.

Disorders of the Neuromuscular Junction

Myasthenia Gravis

Myasthenia gravis (MG) is an autoimmune disorder associated with a postjunctional defect of the acetylcholine receptor. It may occur at any age but is most frequent in women in the third decade and men in the fifth decade of life. Fluctuating weakness and fatigue in cranial, limb, or trunk musculature are characteristic. Ocular symptoms, including alternating ptosis, diplopia, and blurred vision, are present initially in more than 50% of patients and eventually in 90%. Facial muscles are often weak, producing a snarling appearance when laughing. Speech becomes increasingly slurred, nasal, or hoarse as the patient continues to talk, and progressive dysphagia with choking and aspiration of food may occur. Neck muscle weakness may be so prominent that the patient resorts to using a hand to prop up the head. Generalized MG frequently involves the respiratory muscles, producing symptoms of shortness of breath.

The clinical course occasionally is fulminating but is characterized more commonly by a gradual progression of symptoms with frequent remissions and relapses. Sudden worsening may occur with an overdose of anticholinesterase medication, superimposed infection, electrolyte disturbance (especially hypokalemia), pregnancy, emotional stress, or the development of hyperthyroidism.

A diagnosis of MG is confirmed by the presence of acetylcholine receptor antibodies found in the serum of 85% to 90% of patients with generalized MG. In instances of negative antibodies, neurodiagnostic testing by repetitive stimulation of a peripheral nerve may produce a characteristic decremental response in the train of muscle twitches. An intravenous injection of edrophonium (Tensilon) may briefly correct ptosis, ophthalmoparesis, or limb weakness but often is misinterpreted.

The treatment of MG has changed considerably in the last two decades, with increasing recognition of the primary autoimmune disturbance. The anticholinesterase agent pyridostigmine (Mestinon) used for symptomatic relief is no longer the mainstay of treatment because progressive lack of effect and inadvertent overdosage.

Prednisone, 50 mg/day, is the initial drug of choice for MG. When given initially, a transient exacerbation of weakness may occur in the first 2 weeks with a potential for respiratory failure, but this complication is extremely rare. Prednisone is continued for 2 to 6 months until normal strength is regained.

Thymectomy is recommended for all patients with generalized MG, except the very young and very old. It generally is performed 3 to 6 weeks into prednisone therapy when the patient has become asymptomatic. Of patients, 10% harbor a thymoma, but all patients are believed to benefit from surgery.

Long-term prednisone therapy is not desirable because of the side effects of weight gain, cataracts, diabetes, hypertension, and osteopenia. Following thymectomy, prednisone can be tapered gradually and, in some instances, discontinued. For patients unable to stop taking prednisone, azathioprine can be added for several months and then the prednisone taper can be tried again or the agent mycophenolate mofetil (Cellcept) can be tried.

Plasmapheresis or intravenous immune globulin becomes necessary for patients with MG with acutely worsening weakness, problems with secretions, or respiratory distress when conventional immunosuppression is failing. These treatments are reserved for patients in myasthenic crisis in whom a rapid response to treatment is desired. Both modalities confer only transient benefit, and oral immunosuppressive therapy must be continued to achieve a sustained remission.

Other ancillary measures include the use of ephedrine and potassium and the avoidance of medications known to potentiate neuromuscular blockade, including aminoglycoside antibiotics, propranolol, procainamide, phenytoin, quinine, and curare.

Patients with isolated ocular symptoms (ocular MG) may develop generalized MG, but the risk is low after 2 years. These patients may not require surgery or intensive immunosuppression. MG in childhood differs little from the adult form but is treated conservatively because aggressive treatment may retard growth.

Neonatal Myasthenia Gravis

Of infants born to affected mothers, 15% develop transient myasthenic symptoms such as hypotonia and feeding difficulties, probably as a result of the transplacental passage of maternal acetylcholine receptor antibodies. These newborns usually respond to anticholinesterase medication with symptom resolution over 6 to 12 weeks.

Congenital Myasthenia Gravis

Congenital MG is a rare and clinically heterogeneous group of conditions marked by ptosis, extraocular eye movement restriction, and facial and limb weakness, often from birth. These patients are not helped by immunosuppressive agents or thymectomy. Some have a demonstrable defect in the acetylcholine receptor protein channel subunit from a gene mutation on chromosome 17. Very specialized diagnostic testing is required for diagnosis.

Lambert–Eaton Myasthenic Syndrome

Lambert–Eaton myasthenic syndrome (LEMs) is a rare autoimmune disease resulting from antibodies directed against presynaptic voltage-gated calcium channels at the neuromuscular junction. About 60% of patients with small-cell lung carcinoma exhibit these antibodies. In contrast to MG, muscles innervated by the cranial nerves usually are spared in LEMS. Patients may complain of weakness, fatigue, distal paresthesias, or dry mouth. Repetitive electrical stimulation studies demonstrate a decrement in compound motor unit action potentials at rest and large incremental responses after brief muscle exercise. The diagnosis mandates a search for malignancy. Symptoms may improve with the removal of the malignancy, immunosuppression, and intravenous immune globulin.

Disorders of Muscle

Muscular Dystrophies

Duchenne and Becker Dystrophy

Duchenne muscular dystrophy (DUD) is an X-linked recessive disorder in which new spontaneous mutations account for about one-third of cases. From the time they first walk, boys who are affected with this disorder have a clumsy waddling gait. An examination reveals a protuberant abdomen resulting from an accentuation of the lumbar lordosis, pseudohypertrophy of the calves (see Fig. 19.7), and tight heel cords with a tendency toward toe walking. In arising from the floor, these children demonstrate a Gower's maneuver (see Fig. 19.1). Subnormal intelligence is common, whereas eye movements, swallowing, and sensation are unaffected. By the age of 9 to 12 years, increasing proximal weakness makes independent walking progressively unsteady and unsafe. Once in a wheelchair, these children develop progressive kyphoscoliosis, contractures in all joints, and equinovarus deformity of the feet. In subsequent years, these children become virtually immobile and require comprehensive, around-the-clock care. The combination of weak respiratory muscles and kyphoscoliosis drastically reduces pulmonary reserve, and they generally succumb by the late teens or early 20s.

Becker dystrophy (BD) differs from DUD only in that onset is usually later, the course is more benign, and survival is seen into the 30s and 40s. Mental impairment is seen less often.

Diagnosis is aided by the often incidental observation that serum creatine kinase (CK) is markedly elevated (20 to 100 times normal) even before the disease is clinically evident. For diagnosis, the DNA test to detect a deletion or mutation of the dystrophin gene now is done routinely. Although it is performed less commonly now for diagnosis, muscle biopsy will show characteristic dystrophic features.

Effective drug treatment is controversial. Prednisone at a dose of 0.65 mg/kg/day, advocated by some based on well-designed trials, does slow the progression of DUD. Use is tempered by corticosteroid complications including growth retardation, weight gain, and behavioral problems.

Genetics Duchenne and Becker dystrophy are the result of a variety of deletions and point mutations in the area of the X chromosome coding for the membrane protein dystrophin. Mutations here may lead to a total absence of dystrophin (DUD) or the production of a smaller-molecular-weight dystrophin present in diminished quantity. For children suspected of having the disease, a blood specimen should be screened first because 60% to 70% of cases will demonstrate a deletion or duplication. The abnormality detected in these may be specific for either the Duchenne or Becker form of the disease. For the remaining 20% to 30% where no deletion or duplication is found, or where the differentiation between Becker and Duchenne is necessary, a small specimen of skeletal muscle can be obtained and used to determine the quantity and quality of dystrophin by immunohistochemistry.

The carrier status of females can be determined on peripheral blood to detect DNA deletions or duplications in the dystrophin gene. Prenatal diagnosis of the fetus may be achieved by using cells obtained at amniocentesis or chorionic villus biopsy.

Facioscapulohumeral Dystrophy

Facioscapulohumeral (FSH) dystrophy is an autosomal dominant disorder characterized by a slowly progressive weakness with predominant involvement of the shoulder–girdle muscles and variable degrees of facial and peroneal muscle weakness. Symptoms may begin insidiously in the first two decades of life and progress slowly, or they may not be noted until later decades. Common symptoms include difficulty whistling, blowing up a balloon, or drinking through a straw. The lips often are pouting (bouché de tapir), and the smile is transverse. During sleep the eyes may remain slightly open. The clavicles are prominent and downsloping, and the shoulders droop to produce an oblique axillary crease. The scapulae wing out when the patient attempts to elevate the arms (see Fig. 19.2), and the trapezius muscles can be pushed up prominently. Atrophy of the triceps and biceps contrasts with preserved forearm muscles, producing a "Popeye arm" appearance. Peroneal muscle weakness with foot drop occurs in some patients, but hip muscles generally are spared and patients retain the ability to walk. The characteristic clinical findings in a patient with a positive family history make diagnosis fairly straightforward. EMG and muscle biopsy usually will show mild but nonspecific myopathic changes.

Genetics A mutation of a gene localized on chromosome 4 is thought to lead to the clinical weakness seen in FSH dystrophy, but, to date, the gene has not been identified. The presence of deletions near the telomeric end of chromosome 4 occur in 85-95% of FSH cases and, thus, provide laboratory confirmation of the disease.

Limb–Girdle Muscular Dystrophy

Limb–girdle muscular dystrophy (LGMD) is an autosomal dominant or recessive, clinically heterogeneous group of disorders with symptom onset ranging from early childhood to late 20s. In the most common autosomal recessive forms, LGMD 2A and 2B, weakness usually begins in proximal leg muscles and later is seen in the arms, along with scapular winging. Facial, tongue, and pharyngeal weaknesses usually are lacking. An anterior axillary fold and neck flexor weakness is common. Respiratory muscle involvement may occur in some patients. The clinical variation of the disorder is expressed in some families, where both the proximal pattern is expressed in some and in others distal leg weakness is the first and most prominent finding. Some families consist entirely of patients with predominantly distal weakness, so-called Miyoshi myopathy. Depending on the gene mutation involved, the patient may be severely weakened at an early age and resemble DUD or simply may display scapular winging and mild proximal leg weakness. Diagnosis now rests on a search for the specific gene defect using molecular diagnostic techniques on blood and muscle biopsy samples. Treatment is similar to those for any muscle disorder and are outlined at the end of this chapter.

Genetics Research into muscle protein abnormalities underlying the limb–girdle dys-

trophies resulted in a very complex picture for what was once thought to be a single disease. It now is known that there are multiple mutations affecting 10 different gene loci in families with recessively inherited disease (LGMD 2A-2J) and three gene loci affected in families exhibiting autosomal dominant inheritance (LGMD 1A-1C). The most common seem to occur with defects in or absence of the muscle membrane protein dysferlin (LGMD 2B) or a metabolic enzyme calpain (LGMD 2A).

Congenital Muscular Dystrophy

With advances in molecular biology this rare neuromuscular disease now has been expanded into multiple overlapping phenotypes resulting from identifiable mutations of three or more gene loci (Table 19.1). All patients show hypotonia, multiple contractures, and delayed milestones. In one group mentation is normal, and in a second group (Fukuyama) severe mental deficiency is characteristic.

Genetics Transmission is by autosomal recessive inheritance in all forms, and diagnostic confirmation relies on research laboratories having a special interest in the disorder.

Emery–Dreifuss Muscular Dystrophy

Emery–Dreifuss muscular dystrophy is a rare form of muscular dystrophy characterized by onset of elbow contractures in childhood; thin habitus; weakness of biceps, triceps, and peroneal muscles; and slow or no progression. The muscle biopsy changes may be quite extensive, similar to that seen in DUD despite relatively mild degrees of weakness clinically. Cardiac conduction defects are a prominent feature and must be treated.

Genetics The disorder results from a mutation of an X chromosome gene coding for emerin, a nuclear membrane protein.

Oculopharyngeal Dystrophy

Patients with oculopharyngeal dystrophy are normal until their 40s or 50s, when symptoms begin, usually with progressive ptosis developing over several years accompanied by increasingly restricted eye movements without diplopia. Swallowing difficulties usually develop, and aspiration can be a serious problem in a minority of patients. Mild proximal limb weakness occurs frequently. Invariably, these patients will recall similarly afflicted family members and the pattern of an autosomal dominant disease will emerge. Diagnosis is confirmed by gene testing or on muscle biopsy where distinctive red rimmed vacuoles are found. Treatment is directed to the surgical correction of ptosis and the prevention of aspiration. A gastrostomy feeding tube occasionally is needed.

Genetics The disorder results from a polyalanine triplet (GCG) repeat expansion or unique exon duplication in the PABP2 gene on chromosome 14.

Myotonic Disorders

Myotonia Congenita

Impaired muscle relaxation is the cause of the prominent symptom of "stiffness" manifested primarily in the legs. Patients complain of difficulty in rapidly opening a clenched fist and slowness in initiating activity after a prolonged rest, but they also may describe reduction in stiffness after exercising a muscle ("warm-up" phenomenon). Muscle hypertrophy is frequent and occasionally produces a Herculean appearance. EMG is key to confirming the diagnosis. Muscle biopsy is not helpful, and CK levels are usually normal. Several medications are helpful in reducing myotonia, including phenytoin, mexiletine, and tocainide.

Genetics More than 50 mutations of the chromosome 7 gene coding for the skeletal muscle chloride channel now have been described for what is usually an autosomal recessive, but occasionally a dominant, disorder (Thomsen's disease). Because diagnostic DNA tests are available only in research laboratories, specific diagnosis rests primarily on clinical and EMG grounds.

Myotonic Dystrophy

Myotonic Dystrophy 1. The myotonic dystrophy 1 (DM1) form of the disease, the most common, presents in adults with finger grip and foot dorsiflexion weakness. This distal weakness is unlike most other dystrophies that begin with proximal symptomatology. Advanced cases have a characteristic facial appearance with ptosis; temporalis and masseter wasting; protuberant lower lip; and thinning of the sternocleidomastoid muscle, with a typical "hatchet face" appearance (see Figs. 19.5 and 19.6). Percussion and grip myotonia are distinctive findings. The speech is often dysarthric and nasal, and the patient may complain of dysphagia. As in other autosomal dominant disorders, mild and severe cases may appear in the same family; however, a commonly observed feature is that patients often are unaware that there are other affected family members, even in obvious cases (see Fig. 19.6). About 10% of patients present in infancy with severe hypotonia, weakness, and mental retardation.

In this disorder, other organ systems are involved, resulting in cataract formation, impairment of gastrointestinal motility, and endocrine abnormalities. Patients frequently are noted to have low intelligence, poor goal orientation, uneven work histories, and bizarre personalities. Progressive cardiac conduction block may lead to sudden death. Serial electrocardiograms (EKGs) are recommended, and a pacemaker should be considered. A reduced ventilatory drive may produce symptoms of alveolar hypoventilation including disturbed sleep. General anesthesia should be given cautiously because patients are unduly sensitive to barbiturates and other medications that depress ventilatory drive.

Diagnostic confirmation is useful with EMG where typical myotonia can be demonstrated, but gene testing is probably the most specific confirmatory test. Weakness of foot dorsiflexion may be improved with polypropylene splints. Proximal weakness is rarely severe enough to prevent walking.

Myotonic Dystrophy 2. Numerous families now have been described with some similarities to DM1. These patients, who have myotonic dystrophy 2 (DM2 or proximal myopathy syndrome), show distinctive proximal weakness as well as percussion myotonia; cataracts; and, rarely, cardiac conduction defects. Pain may be a prominent symptom. The gene mutation is on chromosome 3. Treatment is symptomatic.

Genetics Type 1 DM is an autosomal dominant disorder in which the chromosome 19 gene mutation consists of a variable length CTG trinucleotide repeats in a non-coding part of the gene. The clinical severity of the disease is worse as the number of repeats becomes larger, but the exact defect produced in the gene product, protein kinase, is uncertain.

In the DM2 the gene mutation responsible for the disorder has been shown to be on chromosome 3 and involves a CCTG repeat expansion of a section of the gene coding for a ribonucleic–acid binding protein. The DM1 gene region of chromosome 19 is normal.

Inflammatory Myopathies

An autoimmune disturbance underlies polymyositis (PM) and dermatomyositis (DM), whereas other syndromes may be caused by coxsackie virus, pyogenic bacteria, trichinosis, sarcoid, or tuberculous granuloma. In polymyalgia rheumatica, an inflammatory process may involve fascia rather than muscle, although patients complain of muscular pain and weakness.

DM and PM have similar clinical symptoms and signs, with the exception of the characteristic rash seen only in DM. The latter disorder may indicate the presence of a neoplasm in adults. In patients with an associated collagen-vascular disease (i.e., systemic lupus erythematosus, rheumatoid arthritis, Sjögren's syndrome), the inflammatory myopathy may be a minor or major manifestation of the disease. Patients with juvenile DM may have a systemic vasculitis with pulmonary fibrosis, myocarditis, gastrointestinal ulcers, cerebral vasculitis, skin ulceration, and calcification.

DM is seen in both children and adults, whereas PM is almost exclusively an adult disease, most frequently occurring in patients in the fifth and sixth decades of life. Either disease begins insidiously with systemic features such as fever, arthralgias and myalgias; Raynaud's phenomenon, when present, is seen only in DM. Weakness may begin relatively suddenly and may become profound, but more commonly there is a subacute progression of proximal weakness that is not readily distinguishable from other limb–girdle syndromes. Muscle tenderness may be absent. The rash of DM may take several forms, appearing before, after, or in association with the onset of weakness. The upper eyelids often have a lavender or heliotrope discoloration in children, and periorbital edema and flushing of the cheeks occur in advanced cases. The chest and neck may become reddened and develop telangiectasia. Gottron's papules are thickened erythematous patches that occur over the knuckles and other joint extensor surfaces. Skin nodules may break down and exude calcium.

The disease often has a variable course. Some patients have an acute episode with complete recovery, even without treatment. Other patients demonstrate a relapsing, remitting course with incomplete recovery between episodes or a chronic progressive course that responds poorly to treatment. The serum CK is elevated in most cases, particularly those with acute onset. A muscle biopsy in both DM and PM shows necrosis of muscle fibers and scattered inflammatory infiltrates. In DM, perifascicular atrophy and overt vasculitis is common.

Corticosteroids are prescribed once diagnosis is confirmed and is continued for several months. At that point, azathioprine can be added, and after 2 more months a gradual prednisone taper is tried. By reducing the prednisone to the lowest possible levels, prednisone side effects are minimized. Adult patients who have DM should be screened for an occult malignancy. Other treatment modalities include a home exercise program.

Inclusion body myositis (IBM) is a disorder predominantly seen in men older than age 50 years with asymmetric symptoms of hand-grip and shoulder–girdle weakness along with proximal leg weakness. The CK level is only modestly elevated. Electrical studies in such patients, some of whom may be suspected of having motor neuron disease, show a mixed neurogenic and myopathic pattern. On muscle biopsy there are distinctive findings of increased connective tissue, variation in fiber size, isolated patches of inflammatory cells, and small red-rimmed vacuoles containing amyloid within individual muscle fibers. No specific drug therapy is useful in these patients, and treatment is directed to rehabilitation measures discussed later.

Genetics The vast majority of IBM cases are sporadic. In recent years there have been reports of families with multiple affected siblings whose biopsies show typical IBM findings. Inheritance in most is autosomal recessive with a gene mutation on chromosome 9, but rare families have shown an autosomal dominance pattern.

Polymyalgia rheumatica (PMR) is characterized by muscle pain and stiffness, which is most severe in the morning and has a predilection for the shoulders. It rarely occurs before 55 years of age and is most frequent in women. Other constitutional symptoms may be present, including anorexia, fever, and night sweats. Temporal arteritis (TA), which is manifested by scalp tenderness, temporal headaches, or visual obscuration, is associated with PMR in 20% to 50% of cases and can produce a sudden, permanent blindness. With the exception of the erythrocyte sedimentation rate, which is markedly elevated, all tests are usually normal. PMR responds dramatically to low doses of prednisone. High doses are used if TA is suspected or documented by temporal artery biopsy.

Metabolic Myopathies

Glycogen Storage Diseases

These rare autosomal recessive disorders exhibit the common finding of excess glycogen in skeletal muscle and sometimes other organ systems. Symptoms do not arise from the presence of glycogen but, rather, from the defect of energy metabolism, specifically involving the conversion of glycogen to glucose.

McArdle's disease is the commonest of those listed in Table 19.1 and presents in childhood or early adulthood with symptoms of exercise intolerance because of cramping and myoglobinuria. Limb weakness is common in McArdle's disease and acid maltase deficiency but is rare in the other glycogen storage diseases. Fixed proximal weakness rather than exercise-induced cramping is a particular feature of acid maltase deficiency, in which early diaphragm involvement in adults may bring the patient to medical attention because of breathing difficulty. The other glycogen storage disorders are either fatal in infancy or present at any age, with exercise intolerance and varying degrees of muscle weakness (Table 19.1).

Diagnosis of these disorders can be made by muscle biopsy, which will show distinctive glycogen storage and abundant lysosomal material. Assays for specific enzyme deficits are available commercially. The serum CK is elevated in all.

Genetics Gene loci for all of these disorders are known and inheritance is autosomal recessive or X-linked basis (Table 19.1). McArdle's disease can occur as an autosomal dominant disease as well, but this is uncommon.

Disorders of Lipid Metabolism

Carnitine palmitoyl transferase deficiency (CPT II) may present at any age: Patients may show symptoms at birth with a rapidly fatal course; when onset is in childhood, there are severe but reversible metabolic crises. Both of these are quite rare. In another form, onset in adolescence mimics the glycogen storage diseases in that patients may develop stiffness and pain (although no cramping) with exercise and then myoglobinuria. The disorder is the most common inherited cause of recurrent myoglobinuria, which may be precipitated in these patients by general anesthesia, infection, or a high-fat meal. Diagnosis of this disorder is not always obvious because the muscle biopsy may be surprisingly normal (except after an episode of myoglobinuria). The specific CPT II enzyme defect can be detected in muscle specimens. Treatment is directed to prevention by avoiding extreme exercise and consuming food according to a high-carbohydrate and low-fat diet divided into frequent intervals.

Genetics The gene locus for this autosomal recessive disorder is on chromosome 1.

Carnitine Deficiency

A carnitine deficiency disorder results from reduced or absent carnitine, a carrier protein vital to the transport of fatty acids into mitochondria. The disease may present with only limb muscle weakness or as more serious systemic illness. The myopathic form usually begins in childhood or young adulthood with painless, proximal weakness; exercise intolerance; and, in rare instances, a cardiomyopathy and diaphragm weakness. In the more severe systemic form, onset is earlier, encephalopathy is common, and sometimes severe cardiomyopathy and rapid death occur. On biopsy, the major change is a massive accumulation of fat within the skeletal muscle, and biochemical assay can detect low or absent carnitine levels. Treatment of either form of the disease is by reducing dietary fat and taking supplements of oral L-carnitine.

Genetics It is likely that autosomal recessive inheritance is involved although the majority of cases appear sporadic and no gene defect has yet been identified.

Mitochondrial Myopathies

All of the mitochondrial myopathies share the common feature of excessive numbers of abnormal mitochondria in skeletal muscle and, often, in other tissues, resulting from mutations in mitochondrial and nuclear DNA. The result is an ever-increasing number of phenotypes based on faulty energy production in the respiratory chain that produces adenosine triphosphate.

Kearns-Sayre syndrome (KSS) was one of the first of the mitochondrial myopathies to be described. It is characterized by extraocular muscle weakness, pigmentary retinal degeneration, and cardiac conduction block. Although these abnormalities may define KSS, other mutations may produce additional clinical abnormalities, including ptosis, short stature, hearing loss, mental retardation/dementia, ataxia, peripheral neuropathy, elevated CSF protein, depressed ventilatory drive, delay of secondary sexual characteristics, and (rarely) hypofunctioning thyroid and parathyroid glands. Symptoms usually are noted in childhood, and characteristic EKG findings of heart block may require urgent pacemaker placement to prevent sudden death.

There are two rare mitochondrial myopathy syndromes. The first, termed myoclonus epilepsy with ragged-red fibers on muscle biopsy (MERRF), is characterized by limb weakness, myoclonus and generalized seizures, progressive dementia, ataxia, and hearing loss. A second disorder, termed mitochondrial myopathy, encephalopathy, lactic acidosis, and stroke (MELAS), begins in childhood and is characterized by retarded growth, recurrent strokes, progressive mental deterioration, and death by age 20. Neither of these disorders has any impairment of extraocular muscles or retinal abnormalities.

With the exception of KSS, where pacemaker placement may be lifesaving, treatment of these disorders is symptomatic. Muscle biopsy will demonstrate excessive numbers of mitochondria (the ragged-red fibers), and this in turn should prompt the ordering of mitochondrial DNA assays on blood and skeletal muscle.

Genetics All of these disorders are maternally inherited because individuals receive all of their mitochondria from the female gamete. The diagnosis can be confirmed by analysis of mitochondrial DNA. The KSS typically has a single mitochondrial deletion;

MERFF and MELAS result from a variety of single point mutations or duplications.

Malignant Hyperthermia

Patients with malignant hyperthermia are free of symptoms unless they are exposed to certain anesthetic agents, particularly halothane and succinylcholine. The full syndrome includes an elevation in temperature up to 43°C, muscular rigidity, tachycardia, marked lactic acidosis, myoglobinuria, and refractory cardiac arrhythmias. Untreated cases are uniformly fatal. Anesthesia and the surgical procedure must be terminated immediately, whereas dantrolene sodium is administered with cooling measures.

The disease is autosomal dominant in many patients, and there may be subtle evidence of an underlying myopathy. There is no reliable confirmatory test, so patients with a previous episode and their relatives should not receive these agents.

Genetics The latest work suggests that a genetic mutation closely associated with the gene defect for central core disease on chromosome 19 may cause malignant hyperthermia.

Toxic Myopathies

A wide variety of medications and toxic compounds can produce either acute muscle necrosis or a slowly progressive chronic myopathy. Alcohol can produce both of these syndromes in the same patient and is the most common myotoxin. The acute myopathy usually follows a binge of drinking and may be accompanied by myoglobinuria. Other drugs and toxins associated with acute myopathy include ipecac; amiodarone; clofibrate; other cholesterol-lowering agents; heroin; aminocaproic acid; chlorthalidone; vincristine (where a sensorimotor neuropathy usually is superimposed); and any substance that produces hypokalemia including diuretics, purgatives, licorice, carbenoxolone, or amphotericin B.

A chronic proximal myopathy is associated with prolonged corticosteroid therapy, particularly with dexamethasone and fluorinated steroids. A discontinuation leads to a slow recovery. The aforementioned drugs associated with acute myopathy also may produce a chronic myopathy.

Endocrine Myopathies

Hypothyroidism is associated with cramps, mild weakness, and "hung-up" reflexes. Hyperthyroidism may produce mild weakness, whereas ophthalmoplegia occurs in Graves' disease.

Hypoparathyroidism may lead to a carpopedal spasm or tetany. Hyperparathyroidism may combine weakness with brisk reflexes, which are reminiscent of ALS.

Acromegaly is associated with a chronic myopathy and the carpal tunnel syndrome. The weakness in Addison's disease and hyperaldosteronism probably is caused by electrolyte disturbances. Cushing's disease may produce the same myopathy as exogenous steroids.

Congenital Myopathies

Congenital myopathies constitute a heterogenous group of muscle disorders defined by unique structural changes easily identified in histopathologic preparations on muscle biopsy material. The three most common congenital myopathies are summarized in Table 19.1.

Myotubular myopathy, sometimes termed centronuclear myopathy, can present in three ways: (a) at birth with hypotonia, respiratory distress, extraocular muscle weakness, and early death; (b) in early childhood marked by delayed milestones, prominent limb weakness, scoliosis, a high arched palate, ptosis, and extraocular muscle weakness and (c) in adulthood with mild limb weakness. In all forms, the muscle biopsy shows typical chains of nuclei running centrally within muscle fibers.

Genetics The neonatal form is caused by a mutation on the X chromosome. Childhood and adult-onset forms are transmitted as autosomal recessive or dominant forms, but no gene is known.

Central core disease patients are hypotonic at birth and show delayed milestones but usually walk normally and show no progression of weakness. Hip dislocation, scoliosis, and pes cavus may be seen. Diagnosis is by muscle biopsy, where fibers show a single prominent area of noncontractile protein in the center of type I muscle fibers.

Genetics Inheritance is as an autosomal dominant pattern resulting from a point mutation for the ryanodine receptor gene located on chromosome 19.

Nemaline myopathy presents in childhood with delay of milestones, facial and limb muscle weakness, high arched palate, and scoliosis. In a minority of cases, diaphragm weakness may necessitate non-invasive ventilation. Diagnosis is by muscle biopsy, which shows distinctive, thin threadlike inclusions ("rods") throughout the muscle fiber.

Genetics Inheritance is as an autosomal recessive or dominant pattern as a result of gene mutations on chromosome 1, 2, or 19.

Channelopathies Affecting Skeletal Muscle

In recent years a number of skeletal muscle membrane gene mutations causing sodium, calcium, and chloride channel abnormalities have been shown to cause distinctive clinical syndromes. One of these involving the chloride channel has been described earlier in the section on myotonia. Several others characterized by episodic weakness and sometimes myotonia will be presented here, along with a brief description of their known genetic defects.

Hypokalemic periodic paralysis, the most common of these autosomal dominant disorders, is characterized by bouts of extreme weakness separated by periods of normal strength. Although limb weakness is profound, the diaphragm is spared so that weakness is never fatal. Meals high in carbohydrate or sodium may precipitate an attack that can last hours. Diagnosis is confirmed by the finding of a low serum potassium level during an attack of weakness. Fixed weakness can

develop with multiple attacks, and muscle biopsy in these cases will demonstrate prominent vacuoles within muscle fibers. Treatment is by avoidance of precipitating factors such as high-carbohydrate meals. Acetazolamide may prevent attacks, and potassium chloride is given acutely to shorten an attack. .

Genetics A mutation of the gene coding for the muscle calcium channel on chromosome 1 accounts for this autosomal dominant disorder.

Hyperkalemic periodic paralysis (HyperPP), **potassium aggravated myotonia** (PAM), and **paramyotonia congenita** (PMC) are discussed together because all involve mutations of the muscle sodium channel. In uncomplicated HyperPP, patients become weak, sometimes for hours, during a rest period after exercise or following a high potassium intake. PAM is characterized by onset in childhood of myotonia episodes (but no weakness) precipitated by potassium intake or exposure to cold. PMC presents with episodes of weakness that are provoked by cold exposure or exercise and, sometimes, associated myotonia. In any of these, normal or elevated serum potassium may be detected. Treatment of the acute weakness in HyperPP is with diuretics, but there is little to be done for the other two except general support measures. Prophylactic treatment is accomplished with oral acetazolamide for HyperPP and PAM and mexiletine for PMC.

Genetics These disorders are caused by numerous different point mutations of the muscle sodium channel gene located on chromosome 17.

OUTPATIENT TREATMENT PRINCIPLES

The initial reaction of the patient and family to the diagnosis of a neuromuscular disease is often one of despondency and hopelessness. In time, with support and understanding, they may understand that the future is less bleak and that a well-balanced rehabilitative approach will maximize their function, prolong ambulation, deter complications, and create a more optimistic environment. The treatment of patients with chronic

neuromuscular weakness is a team effort requiring expertise of the primary physician;
the neuromuscular specialist, physical, occupational, and respiratory therapists; an ortho-
tist; a podiatrist; an orthopedist; a nutritionist;
a social worker; and a psychiatrist.

Special Considerations in Children

For the patient with DUD, BD, or SMA
type 2, most clinicians will opt for working
with an experienced team of child rehabilitation specialists. The central goal is to improve
the quality of life for these patients. For children responsibly able to handle the controls, a
power-drive wheelchair gives them tremendous and welcomed autonomy. Education is a
must for all children with these neuromuscular disorders. The child with type 2 SMA is
generally of above-average intelligence and
will find school enjoyable as long as there is
sufficient intellectual challenge. Patients with
BD fall into the same category and often pos-
sess surprising levels of intelligence and insight into their illness. In contrast, the patient
with DUD commonly is of subnormal intelligence, has difficulty in school, and usually requires special education courses.

The prevention of contractures, particularly
of the Achilles tendon and iliotibial band, is
important early in all of these diseases. A surgical release of contractures along with the
use of long leg braces can prolong independent, although somewhat precarious, walking
for several years in DUD or BD but is rarely
an option in children with SMA.

A patient with severe limb weakness will
sleep more comfortably on an air or water
mattress designed to distribute weight evenly,
preventing unrelenting pressure and decubiti.

When the patient becomes confined to a
wheelchair, the development of kyphoscoliosis (Fig. 19.8) can be slowed with proper upright positioning and external chest bracing.
A great deal of mobility and comfort is possible for the patient who is confined to a wheelchair if the wheelchair is properly designed
and fitted. Detachable arm rests and swing-
away elevating leg rests facilitate transferring

and prevent lower-extremity contractures and
edema that develop if the legs are constantly
dependent. Once in the wheelchair, however,
the central aim is to prevent the development
of restrictive lung disease as pulmonary reserve drops with age. The use of assisted
cough measures, chest percussion, measurements of forced vital capacity, and blood gas
measurements are all useful and best coordinated by a pediatric pulmonologist. In some
children the scoliosis reaches a critical level
where spinal fusion must be done to sustain
life. This is not always an easy decision to
make in children for whom the risk is high but
whose life expectancy might be dramatically
increased by such a procedure.

The intake of food may present special
challenges in these children. Patients with
SMA 2 may show poor weight gain, particularly during the first 2 years; even in later
years, despite a relatively sedentary existence,
their weight can plateau despite continued
growth. In contrast the patient with DUD or
BD may exhibit substantial weight gain and
obesity, especially in the preteen age years.
Once the weight is there, it is virtually impossible to lose. Advice from dietitians is critical
to prevent extremes of weight gain or loss.
Often, however, despite everyone's best efforts, the child continues to eat and is indirectly encouraged to do so by the fact that it is
the one pleasure left in a world that increasingly is denied to him or her.

For children with other primary muscle diseases marked by stable but weak limbs or
gradual deterioration of strength or in whom
strength is stabilized by drugs (e.g., dermatomyositis), the principles of strength building
and range-of-motion maintenance are the
same as for the patients with SMA and
DUD/BD. Referral to specialists in children's
rehabilitation is key to maximizing the child's
quality of life. All the principles described
here may apply to anyone in these categories.

Special Outpatient Problems in Adults

The patient with ALS probably best exem-
plifies the individual in which multiple symp-

tomatic treatments will improve the quality of life during the inevitable progressive loss of strength. Early in the disease every patient needs detailed instruction on a home program of exercise for strengthening and maintaining range of motion. The "frozen shoulder" is a particularly painful complication that can be minimized by simple range-of-motion exercises. Use of adaptive equipment and bracing, when indicated, are also helpful. Patients initially may need a cane for balance but can be expected to move on to a walker and a standard push- or battery-powered wheelchair. In patients with hip weakness, raising the height of seats with a toilet seat elevator or electric lift chair makes standing without assistance easier. Patients rely heavily on well-anchored hand supports for getting up from the toilet, getting out of a tub, or going up stairs. Weakness of the hands impairs the fine dexterity required for eating, writing, and dressing. Various pieces of adaptive equipment are designed to splint the hand and allow easier grasping. Large-handled utensils, a buttonholer, or a pencil attached to the hand with a Velcro strap may be useful. The patient who has shoulder weakness can use a long-handled reaching device to get objects from cabinets or high shelves. Patients who have severe dysarthria can develop alternate means of communication with relatively inexpensive electronic devices available with the help of a speech therapist.

Because pharyngeal weakness is common in ALS, progressive swallowing dysfunction must be identified early. Clues to swallowing dysfunction come from continuing weight loss in the face of claims that "everything is eaten," prolonged eating time (30–60 minutes per meal), and recurrent pneumonias. If aspiration is suspected, a barium swallow can be confirmatory. A first step in addressing the swallowing problem is to get the patient "safe swallowing" counseling from a speech therapist and advice on caloric intake from a dietitian. At this point a frank discussion of the pros and cons of G-tube placement should be undertaken. G-tube is being recommended earlier and earlier in the course of the disease,

although precise guidelines for when that is to be done are still not available. As a rough rule, weight loss of more than 3 pounds per month and more than one pneumonia episode in the face of demonstrable aspiration when drinking a glass of water in the office are reasonable grounds for bringing the subject to the attention of patient and family.

Early use of non-invasive ventilation (Bi-PAP) is thought to be beneficial but will have to be evaluated in a controlled trial. The failure of breathing in patients with ALS as a result of diaphragm weakness presents specific challenges best handled by a pulmonologist working closely with the neuromuscular neurologist. Nocturnal Bi-PAP using an external face mask is readily available to and tolerated by most patients. By removing carbon dioxide buildup, nighttime sleep is facilitated, daytime sleepiness is avoided, and overall quality of life is improved. With increasing bulbar weakness and difficulty with secretions, a tracheostomy usually is needed if aspiration is to be prevented and adequate ventilation is to be ensured. The thought of prolonging life on a respirator is unacceptable for many patients, but for others considerable satisfaction still can be gained if the environment is supportive. The physician, patient, and family should discuss these options well in advance. Family counseling and end-of-life decisions are critical to the care of a patient with ALS.

Specific Issues in Other Neuromuscular Disorders

Palpitations or unexplained syncope resulting from heart block can occur with various neuromuscular disorders, particularly myotonic dystrophy and Kearns-Sayre syndrome. These patients may require periodic EKGs or Holter monitoring, and a pacemaker may be indicated. With acute generalized weakness, pulmonary and swallowing function should be monitored in an intensive care unit because respiratory failure or aspiration can develop rapidly, particularly in MG.

Apart from minimizing the physical handicap, the physician must be aware of the patient's social, emotional, and sexual needs. A severely handicapped patient who relies on others for eating, hygiene, and elimination understandably will become depressed over this extreme dependency. Active counseling of the patient and family should be directed toward solutions to the various problems in "personal space" and independence that arise.

SPECIAL CHALLENGES IN THE HOSPITALIZED PATIENT

Because neuromuscular disorders can impair such vital functions as speaking, swallowing, breathing, and cardiac output, the hospitalized patient must be carefully monitored for these life-threatening complications. For patients with end-stage weakness, treatment decisions must include patient and family wishes.

Swallowing Dysfunction

Acute onset of swallowing dysfunction can occur in botulism, organophosphate poisoning, and MG. Recurrent aspiration from chronic progressive dysphagia is a continual concern in patients with ALS, MG, oculopharyngeal dystrophy, myotonic dystrophy, adult forms of SMA, and (rarely) inflammatory myopathies. The integrity of the swallowing mechanism can be tested by asking the patient to swallow water from a small glass at the bedside. Patients who choke on this clear liquid may have a serious swallowing problem, meaning that oral food intake can lead to aspiration and pneumonia. A tailored barium swallow should be done to confirm such swallowing problems. If aspiration risk is high, a simple "chin tuck" maneuver may be all that is needed. With more frequent and persistent aspiration and symptoms, an endoscopically-placed gastrostomy tube may be needed to guard against pneumonia and to maintain proper nutrition.

Respiratory Complications

Respiratory depression is to be expected and anticipated in every hospitalized patient with neuromuscular disease. Weakness of the diaphragm and accessory intercostal muscles of respiration compromise ventilation. Symptoms of respiratory distress can be mild and nonspecific and include restlessness, irritability, and confusion. Arterial blood gases and pulmonary function tests should be monitored closely for dropping vital capacity and poor inspiratory and expiratory pressures. When the vital capacity falls below 50% of predicted and the disorder appears to be progressing BiPAP ventilatory support should be considered. Bulbar dysfunction results in a poor cough and increased risk of aspiration so that early intubation may be warranted to protect the patient's airway. A patient with limited movement of the extremities is susceptible to deep-vein thrombosis and pulmonary embolism, so that performing range-of-motion exercises, wearing compression stockings, and taking subcutaneous heparin should be considered. Infrequently, patients with neuromuscular disease have a central hypoventilation syndrome that further compromises breathing.

Cardiac Complications

In a few neuromuscular disorders such as Duchenne and Becker dystrophy, myocardial involvement leads to impaired contractility and congestive heart failure. Cardiac conduction disturbances are frequent in myotonic dystrophy, in some of the mitochondrial myopathies, and in the Emery–Dreifuss syndrome. A demand pacemaker and defibrillator can be life-sustaining.

Infectious Complications

Although pneumonia is more likely in patients with bulbar dysfunction and/or respiratory muscle weakness, patients with MG and the inflammatory myopathies are at even greater risk because they frequently are treated with chronically administered corticosteroids and other immunosuppressive medications. Common sites of infection include the urinary tract and lungs, but septicemia, peritonitis, and meningitis also may occur.

Rhabdomyolysis/Myoglobinuria

Acute muscle destruction (rhabdomyolysis) may occur from a variety of insults, including extreme physical overexertion, trauma, and toxins, and far less commonly from inherited neuromuscular disorders. Muscle breakdown produces myoglobin release, which can cause acute renal failure from tubular necrosis. The resultant electrolyte imbalance can produce life-threatening cardiac arrhythmias. Careful attention should be given to maintaining adequate blood volume, urine flow, and electrolyte balance. Renal dialysis may be needed.

End-of-Life Care

The role of the physician in the care of dying patients has been the subject of renewed interest and intense debate in recent years. Although physicians understand the importance of relieving suffering, some remain uncomfortable with a competent, terminally ill patient's right to refuse life-sustaining treatment, including ventilation, hydration, and nutrition. Similarly, a patient's request for morphine or similar agents to relieve pain or dyspnea can be disconcerting in the face of ventilatory failure. In such circumstances, physicians can benefit from consultation with experts in palliative care and end-of-life decision making.

WHEN TO REFER TO A NEUROLOGIST

Primary care physicians often ask themselves when they should refer the patient with neuromuscular symptoms to a neuromuscular specialist. There is a tendency in this day of restrictive managed care plans to simply ask the specialist for informal advice by phone or during a chance meeting over coffee in the hospital cafeteria. This can be a prescription for disaster. Usually not all of the critical information is passed to the would-be consultant who is asked to render an opinion without either direct questioning or a complete neurologic examination.

A formal consultation with an experienced neuromuscular consultant serves two important purposes. First, among patients with non-neuromuscular problems, it may stop the otherwise endless chain of self referrals, which add unnecessarily to medical care costs, and needless patient anxiety. This is a particularly important function in these times when easy access to the medical world via the Internet may compound patient anxieties and lead to "doctor shopping." Secondly, in patients with an organic neurologic disease, an appropriate consultation can shorten any diagnostic delay that might be either overtly dangerous or seriously compromise appropriate therapy.

Knowing when to refer a patient to a neuromuscular specialist is not a terribly scientific decision. Sometimes it is a reflexive action that occurs when the physician realizes that the problem is beyond his or her capabilities. Occasionally, it results from the physician's frustration with a patient who returns repeatedly with symptoms that do not respond to treatment, or it occurs as a result of complaints from unhappy relatives or caregivers. A few so-called "red flags" that provide objective signals that a patient might greatly benefit from a neuromuscular consultation, follow:

In children:

The floppy infant, the hypotonic infant—think SMA, congenital myopathy

Child with slow milestones—think SMA, congenital myopathies, metabolic myopathies

Child with frequent falls, clumsy gait, abnormal use of hands to assist self, trouble getting up from a fall–think DUD, dermatomyositis, congenital myopathies

Child with toe walking–think DUD

In adults:

Muscle pain—think "too much exercise," polymyositis, polymyalgia rheumatica

Trouble with arising from a chair, climbing stairs, lifting objects over head ("trouble with chairs, stairs and into the air")—think proximal limb weakness as in MG and polymyositis

Tripping while running/walking–think foot drop resulting from peripheral neuropathy, ALS, myotonic dystrophy

Grip weakness–think ALS, myotonic dystrophy, IBM

Slurred speech–think early ALS, MG, Kennedy's disease

Swallowing difficulties, especially with thin liquids—think ALS, MG, Kennedy's disease, IBM, oculopharyngeal dystrophy

Dark urine–think myoglobinuria resulting from excessive exercise, glycogen storage disease, CPT deficiency

Muscle atrophy and/or visible twitches–think ALS

Finally, when confronted with a patient who seems to fit the diagnostic criteria for a neuromuscular disorder, ordering one or two laboratory tests is appropriate (e.g., a CK for suspected dystrophies and inflammatory myopathies, tests of glucose metabolism in suspected neuropathies, an antiacetylcholine receptor antibody for suspected MG). More expensive or esoteric tests may be deferred until the patient is seen by the specialist. Often, patients arrive in the specialist's office bringing magnetic resonance imaging scans that have no relevance to the problem or electrodiagnostic data of poor technical quality. In this age of cost awareness, allowing the neurologic consultant to direct the focused ordering of these specialty tests can result in considerable savings, both medical and economic.

The referral of a patient is a cooperative venture designed to reach a diagnostic conclusion and offer effective treatment. Referring physicians and neuromuscular consultants must work in partnership for the good of the patient. It is hoped that these guidelines will be the first step in developing such a partnership.

QUESTIONS AND DISCUSSION

1. A 61-year-old woman is admitted to the hospital with a 4-day history of progressive weakness. Her medical history is unremarkable except for congestive heart failure that is being treated. She had been constipated for several days, and she then had diarrhea after taking laxatives. Her examination was remarkable for generalized mild weakness, hypoactive reflexes, and flexor plantar responses. Cognition, cranial nerves, and sensation were normal.

Discussion: A quadriparesis with intact cognition, a lack of sensory disturbances, and flexor plantar responses most likely are caused by a disorder of the peripheral nervous system.

The differential diagnosis includes the Guillain-Barré syndrome (reflexes are more likely to be absent than diminished), botulism poisoning (lack of cranial nerve dysfunction, especially ocular, is atypical), MG (cranial nerve involvement also would be expected), acute polymyositis, and an electrolyte disturbance.

Useful studies include an electrolyte and serum CPK determination and a sedimentation rate. An EMG–nerve conduction study would be helpful early, when the physician is looking for the characteristic electrodiagnostic changes seen in myasthenia and botulism.

This patient's potassium level was 1 mEq/dl as a result of diuretics and diarrhea, and her strength returned to normal with treatment.

2. A 19-year-old pregnant woman reports that two maternal uncles died of muscular dystrophy at the ages of 15 and 16. She wants to know if her fetus or her 1-year-old daughter may be affected.

Discussion: Some cases of muscular dystrophy actually may have been spinal muscular atrophy. This is usually an autosomal recessive disorder, and the risk of the woman developing muscular dystrophy would be low.

Death occurring in the teenage years is characteristic of Duchenne dystrophy. This illness in two male siblings would not be the result of a spontaneous mutation, and it indicates that their mother was a carrier. Genetic linkage analysis requires blood samples from the affected uncles but is not an option in this case.

Blood samples on mother and daughter as well as fetal cells obtained by amniocentesis can be screened for 70% of patients carrying the abnormal gene. If no deletion is found, linkage analysis can be carried out on all specimens to determine the probabilities of all three having the identical X chromosome. Because there is no linkage information from the two deceased brothers of the pregnant mother, no accurate probability can be given concerning her being a carrier or having passed the abnormal gene on to her fetus. The situation might be clarified if the mother's CPK is significantly elevated, which would argue for her being a carrier. Because CPK levels usually decrease during pregnancy, the finding of normal values would not be helpful. In such a complex situation the assistance of an experienced genetic counselor is advised.

3. A 51-year-old woman is admitted to the hospital with symptomatic bradycardia. She reports frequent "dizzy spells" for about 1 year, but she has never fainted. She also has had lifelong stiffness in her hands and a nasal voice, and she trips frequently.

Discussion: Myotonic dystrophy is suggested by the history of grip myotonia and systemic complaints. Recurrent abdominal pain, gallstones, chronic diarrhea, dyspepsia, and dysphagia are common symptoms. Cardiac conduction disturbances may present with dizziness or may be discovered on a routine EKG. A careful examination for clinical myotonia, as well as for the characteristic fa-

cial features, supported the diagnosis in this case. Myotonic dystrophy is a common disorder, although it frequently is overlooked.

An EKG demonstrated complete heart block, and a pacemaker was implanted during the patient's stay in the hospital. Bilateral foot drop was relieved with polypropylene ankle bracing.

All relatives of this patient should be evaluated clinically for signs and symptoms of this autosomal dominant disorder. Symptomatic relatives can be counseled and followed for the disorder. Asymptomatic individuals can be given information regarding the disease. Should they wish to know their carrier status with certainty, a DNA analysis of blood would provide definite information regarding the presence or absence of trinucleotide repeat sequences. This information would be of use particularly to unaffected individuals planning families.

SUGGESTED READING

Engel AG, Banker BQ. *Myology,* Vols. 1 and 2. New York: McGraw-Hill, 1994.

Evans RW, Baskin DS, Yatsu FM. *Prognosis of neurological disorders,* Second edition. New York: Oxford University Press, 1999.

Griggs RC, Mendell JR, Miller RG. *Evaluation and treatment of myopathies.* Philadelphia: FA Davis, 1995.

Lynch DR, Farmer JM. Neurogenetics. Introduction. *Neurol Clin* 2002;20(3):xi–xiii.

Mitsumoto H, Chad DA, Pioro EP. *Amyotrophic lateral sclerosis.* Philadelphia: FA Davis, 1998.

Pourmand R. Metabolic myopathies. A diagnostic evaluation. *Neurol Clin* 2000;18(1):1–13.

20

Neurologic Aspects of Cancer

Deborah Olin Heros

Cancer and cancer treatment may affect the peripheral and central nervous system (CNS) in many ways. Cancer is the second leading cause of death in the United States, with an incidence of more than 1 million cases of cancer each year and resulting in more than 1 million cancer-related deaths per year. More than 17,500 new cases of primary brain tumors were diagnosed in 2000 in the United States. Primary CNS tumors occur in people of all ages; they are the third leading cause of cancer deaths between the ages of 15 and 34 years. Statistical data suggest that the incidence of primary CNS tumors is increasing. Autopsy studies identify metastatic tumors to the brain in 24% of patients with systemic cancer. Each year, more than 170,000 patients with systemic cancer develop intracranial metastatic tumors, the majority of which are symptomatic. Furthermore, systemic cancer may affect the peripheral and central nervous system as a result of metastatic involvement of the dura and leptomeninges, bony metastases resulting in epidural spinal cord compression, and peripheral involvement to the brachial and lumbosacral plexuses. Cancer also may result in nonmetastatic complications to the CNS, including various vascular disorders, metabolic and nutritional disorders, infection, and neurologic complications from cancer treatment. Indirect, or paraneoplastic, syndromes have been recognized as the result of systemic cancer. More than 80% of cancer patients will develop neurologic complications, and the resultant impact on their quality of life and survival is significant.

The medical specialty of neurooncology addresses the diagnosis and treatment of primary CNS neoplasms and the metastatic and nonmetastatic neurologic complications of systemic cancer. In addition, because pain is a significant component of cancer, the neurooncologist is often actively involved with cancer pain management. Neurologic complications of cancer are common and often serious. Unfortunately, the incidence of neurologic complications is increasing as a result of improved survival of cancer patients. Identification and treatment of neurologic complications may improve the quality of life and survival of the cancer patient. Often the problems associated with these neurologic complications are unique and even may present clinically before the systemic cancer has been identified. Therefore, it is very important for the physician involved in the care of cancer patients to be aware of the neurologic aspects of cancer.

This chapter addresses some of the more common problems in neurooncology. It is divided into four sections to address primary CNS tumors, CNS complications of systemic cancer from direct involvement, indirect neurologic complications of systemic cancer (paraneoplastic syndromes), and complications of cancer therapy.

PRIMARY CENTRAL NERVOUS SYSTEM TUMORS

Primary CNS tumors are classified by the cell of origin. The incidence of primary intracranial tumors is between 2 and 19 per 100,000 persons per year and is dependent on age. In adults, supratentorial tumors are more common, whereas the majority of primary intracranial tumors of childhood occur in the posterior fossa. The most common primary brain tumors are glial in origin and include astrocytomas, oligodendrogliomas, and ependymomas.

ASTROCYTOMA

The most common glial tumor is the astrocytoma, which stains positive for glial fibrillary acidic protein and is classified or graded according to histologic characteristics reflecting aggressiveness and survival. The classic classification system is the Kernohan grading system of astrocytoma, based on the pathologic characteristics of cellularity, pleomorphism, proliferation, and necrosis. Kernohan grades I and II represent the "well-differentiated astrocytoma," Kernohan grade III represents the intermediate or anaplastic astrocytoma, and grade IV astrocytoma is synonymous with a glioblastoma multiforme. In an attempt to improve the correlation between prognosis and grade of the tumor, the World Health Organization (WHO) in 1993 suggested a descriptive, three-tiered system that includes the well-differentiated astrocytoma, anaplastic astrocytoma, and glioblastoma multiforme. Because there is a slight difference between the pathologic characteristics described by the two systems, the physician must know which system is being used. The three-tiered system emphasizes cellular pleomorphism and vascular proliferation. Necrosis, the pathologic hallmark of the glioblastoma in the Kernohan system, is not necessary for the diagnosis of glioblastoma in the WHO classification system. The physician also must be aware that there are several subtypes of gliomas, with different treatment and prognostic implications. Treatment decisions for the subtypes must be appropriate to avoid causing iatrogenic complications. Furthermore, subtypes vary in their sensitivities to treatment modalities (e.g., oligodendrogliomas are sensitive to chemotherapy).

The pilocytic astrocytoma, often located in the cerebellum, is a low-grade neoplasm often occurring in a younger population. Surgical resection may offer a complete cure. The majority of astrocytomas are of the fibrillary type. The pleomorphic xanthoplasmic astrocytoma may appear histologically bizarre and similar to a glioblastoma, but, like a low-grade tumor, it actually may carry a more favorable prognosis. It is thought that this particular subtype of glioma may have been previously misdiagnosed as a glioblastoma multiforme and may account for some of the long-term survivors of glioblastoma in the literature. More recently, the pathologic entity of dysembryoplastic neuroepithelial tumor (DNT) has been recognized as a very well-circumscribed, often cortical, lesion causing seizure activity. The DNT may behave in a very "benign" manner and may represent a hamartoma rather than a true neoplasm. Often, this is treatable by surgery alone. A high-grade gemistocytic astrocytoma may portend a particularly poor prognosis.

The most important factors that determine the prognosis of a patient with an astrocytoma include histology, age of the patient, and the Karnofsky Performance Status (KPS) of the patient. Age appears to be very important. Patients younger than age 40 years with a glioblastoma have a 50% chance of surviving 18 months, whereas those between the ages of 40 and 60 years have a 20% chance, and those patients older than 60 years have a 10% chance. Patients with an anaplastic astrocytoma have a significantly better prognosis than patients with a glioblastoma, with median survivals of 36 months and 10 months, respectively. Patients with a KPS of greater than 70 have a 34% survival at 18 months compared to 13% for those patients with a KPS less than 60. Less significant prognostic factors may include a long duration of symptoms prior to diagnosis, presence of seizures, location of tumor, and degree of surgical resection. In general, younger patients have a higher chance of responding to chemotherapy than older patients. Furthermore, the extremes of age tolerate radiation therapy less well.

Risk factors for the development of an astrocytoma are poorly understood. This tumor most often occurs sporadically. Previous epidemiologic studies have suggested a slight increase in risk of developing astrocytomas with exposure to certain industrial chemicals. Recent developments in molecular biology have allowed researchers to identify various abnormalities of growth factors that play a role in tumor oncogenesis. Autocrine stimulation of growth factors and their receptors have been identified in glioblastomas. The oncogene c-sis, which encodes for part of the platelet-derived growth factor (PDGF), has been found in the glioblastoma, and the level of autostimulation has been correlated with the degree of malignancy in tumor cells. The degree of expression of PDGF and its receptor has been associated with the transformation of cells from benign to malignant. Experimental therapy using biotherapeutic agents for the treatment of malignant gliomas is addressing this observation by utilizing inhibitors of growth factors and their receptors that regulate cell growth and differentiation. The epidermal growth factor receptor (EGFR) gene is located at chromosome 7P11-P13 and is amplified in almost one-half of glioblastomas. New therapies targeting this abnormality are currently under investigation.

Chromosomal analysis of glioblastoma cells has identified multiple gene abnormalities involving chromosomes 10, 17, and 22. Chromosome 17 abnormalities have been found in all grades of astrocytoma and therefore may be an early change in tumorigenesis. Abnormalities of chromosome 10 are seen in the more anaplastic tumors. It is interesting that the hereditary neurofibromatosis syndrome type I has been associated with abnormalities of chromosome 17, and neurofibromatosis syndrome type II has been associated with abnormalities of chromosome 22. The heterogeneity of the glioblastoma multiforme and the array of abnormalities of the chromosomes observed makes it difficult to simplify the key abnormality that induces tumorigenesis in the astrocytoma. Abnormalities of the tumor suppressor gene p53 are found in tumors of the familial Li-Fraumeni syndrome. Patients with this syndrome are at risk for developing malignant astrocytomas as well as a variety of systemic malignancies. The presence of p53 mutations in glioma has been identified in a younger patient population and may be predictive of treatment response and prognosis. In the future, genetic markers may offer a new dimension to the classification system of brain tumors.

Clinical Presentation

The clinical presentation of astrocytoma is determined by tumor location, pathology, and age of the patient. The majority of astrocytomas in adults occur in the supratentorial compartment. Presenting symptoms may include headache, seizure, focal neurologic deficits, and personality change. The increasing availability of neuroimaging studies with improved resolution has resulted in earlier discovery of brain tumors. Unexplained first seizures in adults, atypical neurologic symptoms, or an unexplained change in personality or mood should be investigated by either computed tomography (CT) or magnetic resonance imaging (MRI). Contrast for the appropriate neuroimaging studies is important if a primary brain tumor is in the differential diagnosis. A brainstem glioma is less common and may present with sensorimotor abnormalities, coordination difficulties, or cranial nerve dysfunction. The tumor grade correlates somewhat with the abnormalities on the neuroimaging study. Low-grade tumors usually do not enhance, and they appear hypodense on a CT scan and have abnormalities on MRI T2-weighted images. Increasing tumor grade results in increasing contrast enhancement. Central necrosis, with surrounding enhancement and peritumoral edema, is typical for a glioblastoma.

Treatment

Treatment options for astrocytoma are determined by pathology, location, clinical presentation, and age of the patient. Often, the patient is clinically symptomatic from cerebral edema; therefore, corticosteroids (usually dexamethasone) are started prior to surgery, and they often improve symptoms. Caution should be used if a primary CNS lymphoma is in the differential diagnosis because the use of corticosteroid therapy prior to biopsy may decrease the chance of obtaining a positive biopsy. An anticonvulsant to prevent seizures for supratentorial lesions is also often started prior to surgery.

A definitive diagnosis is obtained by pathologic examination of the surgical specimen. The primary goals of tumor surgery for astrocytoma include (a) to determine pathology, (b) to identify tumor grade, (c) to identify any subtype of glioma that may affect prognosis and treatment options, and (d) to directly reduce pressure of tumor burden when debulking is possible. Surgical debulking is preferred over a biopsy, when possible, to reduce the tumor burden, provide an adequate pathology specimen, and improve symptomatic relief from mass effect. Theoretically, tumor debulking also may improve the chance to respond to adjuvant therapy. Stereotactic biopsy most often is reserved for patients whose poor medical condition precludes a craniotomy and for those with deep-seated lesions or lesions in neurologically eloquent locations. The use of neuronavigational systems and intraoperative neuroimaging studies have improved the ability of the neurosurgeon to attain maximal resection with minimal morbidity. Survival benefit has been correlated with good tumor resection, but the infiltrative nature of astrocytomas prohibits a complete resection.

Postoperative radiation therapy has been shown to increase the median survival of patients with an anaplastic astrocytoma and glioblastoma. Limited-field brain irradiation with a "radiation boost" to the most active central portion of the tumor generally is performed over a course of 5 to 6 weeks. Recently developed techniques to deliver radiation therapy to astrocytomas include radiosurgery, three-dimensional conformal radiation therapy, boron neutron capture therapy, and the use of radiosensitizers. The role of these techniques for the treatment of high-grade astrocytomas has yet to be defined.

The role of radiation therapy for low-grade astrocytomas is even less clear. Statistically, patients with low-grade astrocytomas who have received radiation therapy have improved survival over those patients not so treated. However, the timing is controversial. It is not clear whether radiation therapy

should be administered at the time of diagnosis (e.g., when the neoplasm has been identified after a single seizure or perhaps as an incidental finding by a neuroimaging study) or delayed until the tumor is more symptomatic from tumor transformation. Recent studies suggest that the timing is not a major prognostic determiner.

Various techniques of administering radiation therapy have been used in an attempt to increase its effectiveness and reduce its toxicity. Hyperfractionation (delivering radiation in more frequent but smaller doses) has been used for various primary brain tumors but without consistent benefit. Neurologic toxicity from radiation therapy may be a significant problem for patients with gliomas, in particular when additional forms of radiation therapy such as brachytherapy or radiosurgery are used. The role of radioprotective agents is being explored to reduce the risk of radiation toxicity.

Chemotherapy has not been a primary treatment for malignant astrocytomas. Its benefit is thought to be limited by the blood–brain barrier: the glial foot processes and the endothelial cells prevent the passage of systemically administered hydrophilic chemotherapeutic agents. The most commonly used agents are the lipid-soluble nitrosoureas carmustine (BCNU) and lomustine (CCNU). The recognition that some subtypes of glial tumors are chemosensitive has increased enthusiasm for chemotherapy for primary brain tumors. The anaplastic astrocytoma, especially in younger patients, is considered to be chemosensitive. The preferred combination of therapeutic agents for this tumor is procarbazine, CCNU, and vincristine (the PCV regimen). Oligodendrogliomas and mixed oligoastrocytomas are also chemosensitive, and most experience has been with the PCV regimen. Unfortunately, survival benefit of chemotherapy for glioblastoma is limited, although clinical trials suggest that some patients receiving chemotherapy have an increased chance for long-term survival at 18 months. BCNU has been the most widely used single agent for glioblastoma. The development of temozolomide, an oral alkylating agent, has demonstrated significant activity against malignant gliomas.

To circumvent the limitations of the blood–brain barrier, alternative methods of administering chemotherapy have been used for malignant astrocytomas. Intraarterial chemotherapy utilizes a first-pass benefit to increase the concentration delivered to the area of perfusion, with diminished risk of systemic toxicity. Chemotherapeutic agents including BCNU and cisplatin have been administered by this route. Unfortunately, intraarterial administration of chemotherapy appears to increase the risk of neurotoxicity. The procedure, involving repeated arterial catheterizations, is cumbersome. Tumors that involve multiple vascular territories require injections into multiple vessels.

Constant systemic infusional chemotherapy alters the pharmacokinetics of chemotherapy and may offer benefit over conventional chemotherapy. The combination of BCNU and cisplatin has been administered by constant systemic infusion. Intratumoral

chemotherapy has been attempted in various ways over the past several years using various agents including bleomycin, methotrexate, and BCNU. The recent development and availability of a biodegradable drug delivery system containing BCNU has made the concept of intratumoral chemotherapy more practical (Fig. 20.1). This treatment modality has demonstrated modest benefit for the treatment of recurrent glioblastoma in patients eligible for reoperation. More recently, intratumoral BCNU chemotherapy demonstrated efficacy in patients undergoing surgical resection for newly diagnosed high-grade malignant gliomas by extending the median survival and increasing the chance of living 2 years. Investigations using this new drug delivery system with other agents, as well as in combination with other treatment modalities, are under way. Agents to modify the blood–brain barrier, such as mannitol and RMP7, have been explored to enhance the effectiveness of chemotherapy. Unfortunately, the combination of autologous bone marrow

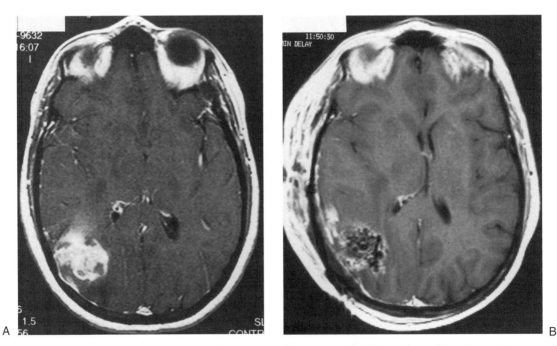

FIG. 20.1. A: Gadolinium MRI scan of a woman who presented with a seizure. The diagnosis was glioblastoma multiforme. **B:** Gadolinium MRI following resection of glioblastoma multiforme and intratumoral implantation of biodegradable chemotherapy disks containing carmustine (Gliadel).

transplantation and high-dose chemotherapy has not offered benefit for the treatment of malignant glioma.

Newer experimental agents to treat malignant glioma by inhibiting angiogenesis include thalidomide. Other agents inhibit the activity of tumor growth factors and their receptors. As we better understand the mechanism of tumorigenesis, we hope to find newer agents to specifically target and inhibit tumorigenesis. Chemotherapeutic agents such as paclitaxel have demonstrated activity against glioma. Given the limited prognosis and the predictable outcome for patients with high-grade glioma, it is important for the physician caring for these patients to be aware of the clinical protocols available and to make the appropriate referral for patients interested in investigational treatment. Ethical decisions involving the appropriateness of participation in experimental protocols for astrocytoma are very difficult when the survival rate using known treatment modalities is limited and the investigational treatments are yet unproven and potentially hazardous. In a national survey, less than 8% of patients with astrocytoma were enrolled in treatment protocols. As participation in investigational protocols by patients with other malignancies has resulted in improved treatment modalities, it is important to encourage participation.

Given the availability of radiosurgery and the frequency of its use for various CNS malignancies including astrocytoma, it is important to be aware of its potential complications. Radiosurgery has for the most part replaced brachytherapy or interstitial radiation therapy. Brachytherapy uses surgically implanted catheters loaded with radioactive seeds, usually iodine-125 or iridium-131, for local administration of irradiation with limited exposure to surrounding normal tissue. This treatment approach has been used in conjunction with external-beam radiation therapy, and it also has been used for recurrences. A national brain tumor study group did demonstrate a benefit of brachytherapy in younger patients with small, well-circumscribed tumors in which catheters could be surgically

implanted. However, the procedure has been shown to be quite cumbersome and associated with risks such as hemorrhage, infection, and radiation necrosis. Local recurrence, usually within 2 cm of the original tumor, is the pattern for the majority of patients receiving conventional treatment. In long-term survivors treated with brachytherapy, distant tumor recurrence, including leptomeningeal disease as well as systemic metastases, was seen with increased frequency. The development of radiation necrosis increases the need for dexamethasone and the possibility of reoperation.

Radiosurgery allows controlled delivery of localized radiation without the invasiveness of brachytherapy. It currently is being used both as initial therapy, usually in combination with conventional external-beam radiation therapy, and at the time of recurrence. Radiation injury and radiation necrosis remain its main limitations (Fig. 20.2).

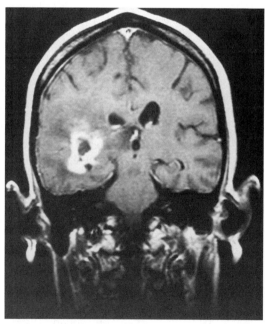

FIG. 20.2. Gadolinium MRI scan demonstrating contrast-enhancing radiation necrosis mimicking tumor recurrence. The patient had a history of glioblastoma multiforme and had been treated with combined conventional radiotherapy and radiosurgery.

Various forms of immunotherapy have been used for the treatment of malignant glioma. Interferon-alpha and interferon-beta have been of limited use. The benefit of interleukin-2-activated lymphocytes (LAK cells) appears limited, possibly because of the concomitant use of dexamethasone necessary to control the tumor-associated edema.

Neurologic Deterioration and Tumor Progression

A decline in neurologic function usually marks the recurrence or progression of an astrocytoma. However, other medical and neurologic problems may mimic tumor progression, and the physician should be aware of the differential diagnoses for neurologic deterioration in patients with an astrocytoma. Complications from radiation therapy may mimic tumor progression or recurrence. In general, radiation therapy for an astrocytoma is initially well tolerated. However, an acute encephalopathy may develop, particularly if large radiation fractions are delivered to a large volume of brain in patients with increased intracranial pressure. The patients may complain of increased headaches, somnolence, lethargy, nausea, or worsening of focal neurologic symptoms. The symptoms of acute radiation toxicity are the result of disruption of the blood–brain barrier resulting in cerebral edema, and they usually improve with corticosteroid therapy. If the symptoms are not responsive to corticosteroid therapy, the radiation therapy may need to be postponed temporarily.

Subacute or "early delayed" complications from radiation therapy usually begin within 2 weeks of completing radiation therapy and may persist up to 4 months after completion of radiation therapy. This disorder is thought to be a reversible injury to the oligodendroglial cells resulting in demyelination, and it is responsive to corticosteroid therapy. During this phase, the neuroimaging study may demonstrate an increased mass effect and increased contrast enhancement, suggesting tumor progression. However, symptoms may be controlled with dexamethasone, and the clinical situation may stabilize over time. This phase of radiation injury often is mistaken for tumor progression.

The late or "delayed" effect of radiation therapy for astrocytoma usually consists of a process known as radiation necrosis. This process cannot be distinguished from tumor recurrence by contrast-enhanced CT or MRI studies. Attempts have been made to differentiate between the two processes by various metabolic neuroimaging studies, such as positron emission tomography and single photon emission computed tomography; radiation necrosis results in a hypometabolic abnormality, whereas recurrent tumor results in a hypermetabolic area. Often, both radiation necrosis and recurrent tumor are present simultaneously. If treatment options are available, a biopsy may be necessary. Reoperation with attempted resection and debulking may reduce chronic corticosteroid needs and improve neurologic symptoms. Reoperation for a recurrent astrocytoma usually is considered when additional treatment modalities are also available. Reoperation alone offers very limited benefit.

Late effects of radiation therapy also may result in a diffuse leukoencephalopathy, manifested by gait disturbance, urinary incontinence, and dementia. Unfortunately, the symptoms do not respond to shunting, although the ventricles appear large on CT scan. Central endocrinopathies, including central hypothyroidism and adrenal insufficiency, also may occur as a late complication of radiation therapy. An elevated prolactin level may be seen as the result of radiation injury to the hypothalamus.

The possibility of anticonvulsant toxicity should be excluded in a patient with progressive neurologic deficits. Chronic corticosteroid therapy may result in hyperglycemia. Hyperosmolar coma, the extreme of this condition, has been seen in these patients. This patient population is also at increased risk for systemic infections as a result of chronic corticosteroid therapy or chemotherapy. Intracranial infections (i.e., a brain abscess) may mimic recurrent tumor. Cerebrovascular accidents have been reported in patients with astrocytomas treated with radiotherapy or intraarterial chemotherapy. A steroid myopathy resulting in proximal weakness may be mistaken for tumor progression. The patient with an astrocytoma has a particularly high risk for developing thrombophlebitis and pulmonary embolism. This risk, which appears to be the result of a generalized hypercoagulable state from the brain tumor, is added to the risks associated with a postoperative state or a nonambulatory patient with hemiparesis. This medical complication occurs with such a high frequency that any patient with astrocytoma who complains of shortness of breath, atypical chest pain, leg pain, asymmetric peripheral edema, or atypical syncope should be evaluated. There is no consensus as to whether filter or umbrella placement in the inferior vena cava or anticoagulation is the preferred therapy. Clinical judgment is important, but there does not appear to be a significantly increased risk for intracranial hemorrhage using anticoagulation, and, therefore, an astrocytoma is not an absolute contraindication to anticoagulation.

Tumor progression or recurrence usually occurs locally within 2 cm of the original tumor margin. Tumor growth occurs via the white matter; therefore, contralateral spread with deep midline tumors is not unusual. Multifocal gliomas are uncommon, occurring in 5% of patients at the time of presentation and 10% to 15% of patients at the time of tumor recurrence. Leptomeningeal or distant tumor spread is quite rare. Similarly, systemic metastases are extremely rare. Usually, the patient becomes progressively more dysfunctional with increasing somnolence that no longer responds to increasing dexamethasone doses. For the most part, pain is not a major complication of this type of malignancy.

PRIMARY CNS LYMPHOMA

Primary CNS lymphoma (PCNSL) is a non-Hodgkin's lymphoma usually of B-cell origin that arises within the brain, spinal cord, or leptomeninges. This tumor may occur in otherwise healthy patients with normal immune systems, usually in older men, but it more often occurs in patients with immune compromise. It is seen with increasing frequency as a result of the growing population with human immunodeficiency virus. This tumor does not tend to metastasize systemically and is a separate entity from systemic lymphoma with CNS metastasis. Patients with inherited, acquired, or iatrogenically induced immune-deficient states are at an increased risk for developing this tumor, particularly transplant patients and up to 10% of patients with acquired immune deficiency syndrome (AIDS). The clinical presentation may include headache, personality changes, seizures, and focal neurologic symptoms. Often the lesions are multifocal, frequently involving deep midline structures with contrast enhancement and minimal surrounding edema on neuroimaging studies. The diagnosis usually is established by biopsy, and surgical resection is usually not an option. The use of corticosteroid steroid therapy prior to biopsy may decrease the opportunity to obtain positive pathology and therefore should be avoided if possible.

The management of the immune-compromised patient may be somewhat different from that of the immunocompetent patient. The presentation may resemble CNS toxoplasmosis clinically. Therefore, it is common to treat a patient with known immune deficiency empirically for toxoplasmosis for a limited period and to follow him clinically and radiographically. If the lesions improve, the assumption is that the patient has toxoplasmosis, whereas if the lesions progress or do not improve, then the possibility of CNS lymphoma increases and a biopsy may be performed. Occasionally, an immune-compromised patient may have simultaneous toxoplasmosis and CNS lymphoma, complicating the interpretation of the empiric trial. A lumbar puncture with cytologic examination may be helpful if the tumor is in the midline or if the leptomeninges are involved. Proper studies of the cerebrospinal fluid (CSF) may demonstrate a neoplastic monoclonal lymphocytosis as opposed to an inflammatory process. Intraocular involvement does occur, and a slit-lamp examination or vitreous biopsy may be helpful to establish the diagnosis. A systemic evaluation including a bone marrow biopsy may help to exclude the possibility of systemic lymphoma or other small-cell malignancies. Most often, a brain biopsy is indicated.

Once the diagnosis of PCNSL has been established, corticosteroid therapy may offer improvement of neurologic symptoms. For many years, radiation therapy has been the mainstay of treatment, but the prognosis was limited. The median survival of immunocompetent patients with primary CNS lymphoma is approximately 14 months, and it is much less in patients with immune deficiency. A recent approach using combined modalities with chemotherapy and radiation therapy has resulted in improved survival. Unfortunately, relapse remains common, and late neurologic toxicity from combined therapy is a significant complication resulting in a progressive dementing leukoencephalopathy. Chemotherapy has generally not been used in patients with CNS lymphoma associated with immunodeficiency because of the overall poor prognosis and response rate. PCNSL has been associated with the presence of Epstein-Barr virus in patients with AIDS. As the result of this observation, antiviral therapy has been used with benefit for treatment of PCNSL. Future directions for treatment of primary CNS lymphoma include the use of various combinations of chemotherapy at the time of diagnosis, reserving radiation therapy for recurrence.

OLIGODENDROGLIOMA

The oligodendroglioma is a type of glial tumor derived from the oligodendrocyte, the myelin-producing cell within the CNS. Histologically, this tumor is identified by its characteristic "fried-egg" appearance and a positive stain for myelin basic protein. The tumor tends to be slow growing; therefore, it is most often considered to be a low-grade tumor.

However, varying degrees of anaplasia, and therefore aggressiveness, do occur. Most often, the tumor presents as a nonenhancing hypodense lesion on CT scan or abnormalities on T1 images on MRI scan. The tumor may be calcified. Enhancement may suggest a more aggressive tumor or the presence of a mixed oligoastrocytoma. Occasionally, the onset may be abrupt as the result of hemorrhage. The pluripotential glial cell may differentiate into either an astrocyte or an oligodendrocyte, which may explain the development of the mixed oligoastrocytoma.

Management of the oligodendroglioma depends on location, clinical presentation, and neuroimaging appearance. Surgical resection generally is attempted if possible. The oligodendroglioma has been identified as a chemosensitive tumor; therefore, chemotherapy has played a major role in its treatment in recent years. The use of chemotherapy for low-grade oligodendroglioma is being studied. However, in anaplastic oligodendrogliomas, chemotherapy has been found to be beneficial. The chemotherapy most commonly used for this tumor has been the PCV regimen. Although radiation therapy has been shown to improve survival of patients with oligodendroglioma, the role of radiation therapy remains controversial, especially if total resection has been accomplished. However, if subtotal resection or biopsy has been performed, radiation therapy has some survival advantage. Survival benefits of treatment are difficult to assess because of the slow-growing nature of this tumor.

EPENDYMOMA

The ependymoma is a glial tumor arising from the ependymal cells lining the ventricles and the CSF-filled spaces. This tumor usually occurs during childhood in the posterior fossa arising from the floor of the fourth ventricle, but it may present in the supratentorial cerebral hemispheres in the lining of the lateral ventricles or spinal cord. When the tumor occurs in the posterior fossa, it usually presents with symptoms of increased intracranial pressure, including headache, nausea, and vomiting, and it often causes obstructive hydrocephalus. The treatment of choice is surgical resection, and the prognosis depends on the degree of resection. A 45% overall 5-year survival is reported in the literature, with an increased chance of long-term survival after complete resection. This tumor lines the CSF pathways and may seed the neuraxis, although the majority of tumor recurrence is local within the posterior fossa. Local radiation therapy usually is recommended for supratentorial and spinal lesions. Local or craniospinal radiation therapy may be appropriate for ependymomas of the posterior fossa.

MENINGIOMA

Meningiomas are tumors derived from the arachnoid lining of the nervous system and therefore are extrinsic to the neuraxis. The tumors are most often histologically benign and are found more frequently with increasing age as the result of the slow growth rate. Often a meningioma is found as an incidental finding, and observation may be appropriate, especially in the elderly patient.

The incidence increases with age starting in the sixth decade. Women are affected two to three times more than men. Symptoms are dependent on location, size, and rate of growth. Symptoms may include seizures from cortical irritation over the convexity of the cerebral hemisphere, headache from pressure within the cranium, or symptoms of cranial nerve or brainstem dysfunction from direct compression of neural structures.

The meningioma is usually isodense with respect to brain tissue on an unenhanced CT or MR study and demonstrates homogenous enhancement following administration of contrast. Often the dural attachment is seen to help identify the tumor as a meningioma radiographically. Significant edema surrounding the mass is not typically seen and its presence should raise the suspicion for either an atypical, malignant meningioma or another type of tumor such as a metastatic tumor, especially from breast or prostate origin. Meningiomas

are also more common in women with breast cancer.

The treatment for meningioma is most often surgical resection with the goal of complete removal because the risk of recurrence is directly related to the completeness of the resection. This in turn mainly is determined by the location of the tumor; tumors that are not amenable to complete resection have a much greater risk for recurrence. For example, tumors over the cerebral convexities are more accessible surgically as compared to tumors at the base of the skull, and therefore cerebral convexity tumors are less likely to recur.

Radiotherapy by conventional fractionated radiation, stereotactic radiosurgery, or fractionated radiosurgery may play an important role for incompletely resected or recurrent tumors.

The role of traditional chemotherapy is limited, but agents such as hydroxyurea and interferon alpha 2-beta have been described as having some activity. Meningiomas may contain progesterone and, less frequently, estrogen receptors. Clinically the tumors also may enlarge during elevated hormonal exposure such as pregnancy. Treatment with antiestrogen or antiprogesterone agents such as tamoxifen or mifepristone (RU-486), respectively, have been used.

Although the majority of meningiomas are histologically benign, infrequently atypical or malignant variants with more aggressive behavior may occur. A subtype of meningeal tumor, the hemangiopericytoma, may present with similar clinical presentation, but it has a high rate of recurrence and a propensity to seed the leptomeninges and metastasize outside of the CNS.

CENTRAL NERVOUS SYSTEM COMPLICATIONS OF SYSTEMIC CANCER

Intracranial Metastases

Systemic cancer may spread to the CNS to involve the skull, dura, parenchyma, or leptomeninges. Specific tumors may metastasize in predictable patterns, and understanding these trends is important to correctly diagnose metastases and offer palliative therapy. Tumors of the breast, prostate, and lung; malignant melanoma; and cancers of the head and neck region have a propensity to metastasize to the skull. Symptoms are most common if the tumor involves the base of the skull, resulting in localized pain, headache, or cranial nerve dysfunction (Fig. 20.3). Special views

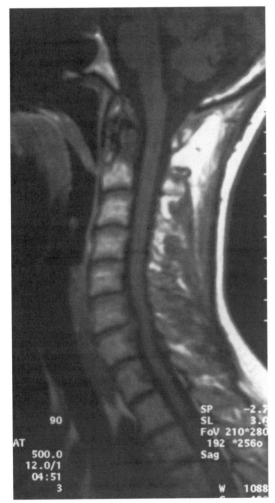

FIG. 20.3. MRI scan demonstrating metastatic cancer to the upper cervical spine in a man with lung cancer and severe, localized occipital pain. Metastasis to the base of the skull was clinically suspected from the location of the pain. However, it is interesting that the pain was aggravated by neck movement.

on a CT or an MRI scan may be necessary to identify base-of-the-skull metastases. Standard screening studies may not image this region well, giving the false impression of a negative study; thus the opportunity to offer effective palliative therapy may be missed. The nuclear bone scan is not a very sensitive study (despite the fact that the symptoms are the result of bony metastases) because of the overlapping nuclear isotope uptake by the venous sinuses in this region. Localized radiation often offers effective palliation of symptoms, especially pain.

Intraparenchymal brain metastases occur in nearly 25% of patients with systemic cancer. Patients with tumors of the breast and lung and malignant melanoma have a propensity to develop brain metastases. Less commonly, tumors of the gastrointestinal tract, kidney, or genitourinary system spread to the brain. The majority of tumors metastasize to the cerebral hemispheres and less commonly to the brainstem and cerebellum in the posterior fossa. Metastases to the pituitary region, often from tumors of breast origin, have been described.

The risk of developing brain metastases from lung cancer varies with the pathology of the primary lung tumor. Small-cell lung cancer has the highest risk (60%), adenocarcinoma has an intermediate risk (40%), and squamous cell carcinoma is the least likely to spread to the brain (20%). From 25% to 30% of patients present with neurologic symptoms and do not have a known primary cancer. Nearly one-half of these patients have a tumor of lung origin. Although brain metastases occur with high frequency in both lung and breast tumors, brain metastases often occur early in lung cancer (within months), whereas brain metastases are more likely to occur much later in breast cancer (i.e., in years). Although malignant melanoma is a relatively uncommon tumor, it has a very high propensity (80%) to spread to the CNS, often with multiple metastases.

Brain metastases originate from hematogenous spread, and therefore the majority of patients develop multiple lesions. Approximately 20% to 30% of patients have a single metastatic tumor. Treatment options often are determined by whether the lesion is single or multiple.

The signs and symptoms are determined by the size, number, and location of the tumors. Metastatic tumors of the cerebral hemispheres may cause progressive hemiparesis, language disturbance, confusion, seizures, sensory symptoms, visual field abnormalities, or personality changes. The development of depression in a patient with cancer should raise the suspicion of brain metastases, in particular if he has never been previously prone to depression. Tumors in the cerebellum may result in dizziness, unsteadiness of gait, dysarthria, clumsiness of an extremity, or headaches from obstructive hydrocephalus. Cranial nerve dysfunction, motor and sensory signs, unsteadiness, and incoordination result from brainstem involvement. Hemorrhage into a metastasis may result in the abrupt onset of neurologic symptoms. Metastatic tumors with a tendency for hemorrhage include melanoma, renal cell carcinoma, choriocarcinoma, and various lung tumors.

The diagnosis of metastatic brain tumor is established by a neuroimaging study, either CT or MRI. A CT scan without contrast is the diagnostic study to assess for a hemorrhage. A contrast-enhanced CT scan then may demonstrate an enhancing tumor, usually with surrounding vasogenic edema. An MRI with gadolinium is the most sensitive test for detecting metastatic disease and often is performed to search for small, multiple tumors, especially when surgery is being considered to remove a presumably single brain metastasis.

When a patient presents with brain metastases without a known primary tumor, diagnostic studies are performed to identify the primary tumor, with special attention to imaging of the chest, remembering that approximately one-half of these patients subsequently will be found to have a primary lung cancer.

TREATMENT

Corticosteroids, usually dexamethasone, are very effective in treating patients with symptoms that result from vasogenic edema. The appropriate dosing is determined by the number, size, and location of lesions and by the severity of the symptoms. The most common initial dosage of dexamethasone is 4 mg four times daily. It often is used in conjunction with an H_2-receptor antagonist to reduce the risk of gastric complications from the corticosteroid therapy.

An anticonvulsant medication is indicated if the patient has experienced a seizure. The role of prophylactic use of an anticonvulsant is less clear, and many physicians prefer to avoid the risk of side effects from the medication in patients who have not experienced a seizure. Perhaps this approach is appropriate for patients with lesions in the deep white matter, cerebellum, or brainstem. It may be prudent to consider the use of a prophylactic anticonvulsant medication for lesions in potentially epileptogenic areas of the cerebral hemispheres such as near the motor cortex. Serum drug levels should be monitored appropriately.

Conventional treatment of brain metastases includes whole brain radiation therapy (3,000 cGy over 10 fractions). The whole brain is treated because of the high likelihood of multiple lesions and the chance of multiple microscopic foci of metastatic tumor from hematogenous dissemination. Advances in neuroimaging and neurosurgical techniques and the development of radiosurgery have increased the options for treatment of metastatic tumors. In general, surgery is reserved for removal of a single lesion in a surgically accessible area (e.g., a tumor in the posterior fossa causing hydrocephalus or a large tumor in the cerebral hemispheres) (Fig. 20.4). Shunting also is considered for treatment of hydrocephalus if the cause of the hydrocephalus cannot be surgically excised. Stereotactic biopsy may be considered in patients presenting with neurologic symptoms without a known primary tumor or in patients in whom the specific tumor type cannot be established otherwise. Current recommendations regarding the role of whole brain radiation therapy are being reviewed now that radiosurgery is available. The current trend is to use radiosurgery (a) to boost the effect of whole brain radiation therapy or (b) to treat recurrences of metastatic tumors after whole brain radiation therapy. Some clinicians are using ra-

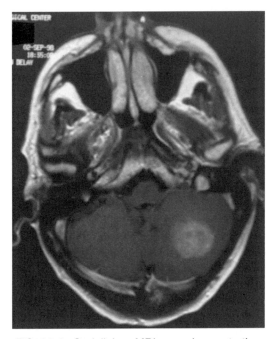

FIG. 20.4. Gadolinium MRI scan demonstrating contrast-enhancing single metastasis of the cerebellum in a patient with gastric carcinoma. His headaches, nausea, and unsteadiness improved after surgical resection.

diosurgery alone for the treatment of metastatic tumors. The maximal number of tumors that may be treated with radiosurgery is under investigation. The experience of using chemotherapy for brain metastases is limited as the result of the blood–brain barriers and the inability for most chemotherapeutic agents to penetrate the blood–brain barrier. The development of temozolomide, an oral alkylating agent, readily crosses the blood–brain barrier and is being used for treatment of primary brain tumors but, more recently, for metastatic brain tumors. Clinical trials using temozolomide and other agents, such as thalidomide, are being done. Metastatic tumors including melanoma, non–small-cell lung cancer, and breast cancer appear to benefit from this agent.

Untreated, the median survival for patients with brain metastases is 4 to 6 weeks. Appropriate therapy offers an improved quality of life and prolongation of survival. The overall median survival of patients treated for metastatic brain tumors is 6 months. Long-term survival usually is described in patients

treated with surgery. The cause of death in patients with brain metastases is most often progression of systemic disease.

LEPTOMENINGEAL METASTASES

Systemic tumors may diffusely seed the leptomeninges, resulting in a condition known as neoplastic meningitis. Terms used in the literature to describe this condition (carcinomatous meningitis, carcinomatosis of the meninges, and lymphomatous meningitis) reflect the tumor of origin. The incidence of this serious complication is thought to be increasing as control of systemic disease improves. The CNS, including the leptomeninges, serves as a sanctuary site from systemic therapy as a result of the blood–brain barrier. Neoplastic meningitis may occur as the only CNS involvement or in combination with other sites of CNS involvement, such as intraparenchymal brain metastases. Most commonly, the solid tumors causing neoplastic meningitis include tumors of the breast and lung and malignant melanoma. Less commonly, tumors of the gastrointestinal tract, ovary, prostate, uterus, and bladder spread to the leptomeninges. Various types of lymphoma and leukemia have a tendency for leptomeningeal spread. The clinical presentation of neoplastic meningitis is variable and often subtle. Symptoms and signs reflect the diffuse involvement of the neuraxis at three levels: (a) the cerebral cortex, resulting in confusion, headache, and seizures; (b) cranial nerves, resulting in diplopia, facial numbness, hearing loss, visual loss, and tongue weakness; and (c) spinal and nerve roots, with a propensity for the lumbosacral spine region, resulting in low back pain, leg numbness and weakness, and sphincter dysfunction. Communicating hydrocephalus develops in 15% to 20% of patients with neoplastic meningitis. The diagnosis should be suspected in a patient with cancer with neurologic symptoms and signs at various levels of the neuraxis. Often the findings on clinical examination are multiple and out of proportion to the symptoms described by the patient. The diagnosis of neoplastic meningitis is established by positive cytology of the CSF. The literature stresses the importance of repeated CSF examinations to establish the diagnosis. The CSF examination also may demonstrate elevation of opening pressure, mild pleocytosis with a lymphocytic predominance, a depressed glucose level, or protein elevation. Elevated biochemical markers may be used to diagnose the condition as well as to follow the response of treatment. Such markers include carcinoembryonic antigen, beta human chorionic gonadotropin, and alpha-fetoprotein. If a sufficient number of lymphocytes are present, specific immunohistochemical studies may help differentiate reactive inflammatory lymphocytes from neoplastic lymphocytes in patients with lymphoma and leukemia.

Gadolinium MRI of the brain and spinal cord may demonstrate leptomeningeal enhancement, excluding the possibility of intracranial brain metastases that would contraindicate a lumbar puncture. Bulky disease that may be treated with localized radiation therapy also may be identified. In general, MRI with gadolinium is more sensitive than CT with contrast (Figs. 20.5 and 20.6).

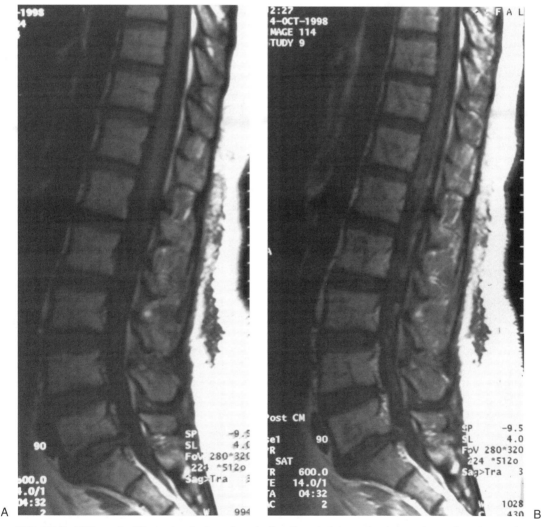

FIG. 20.5. MRI scan of the spine before **A** and after **B** gadolinium, demonstrating enhancing nodular defects in the leptomeninges of a woman with metastatic breast cancer, who presented with paraparesis and urinary retention. Cerebrospinal fluid examination from an Ommaya reservoir confirmed the diagnosis of neoplastic meningitis.

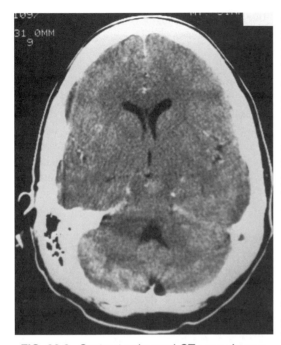

FIG. 20.6. Contrast-enhanced CT scan demonstrating multiple metastatic tumors in the woman (with metastatic breast cancer) seen in Fig. 20.5. The patient required focal radiotherapy to the cauda equina, whole brain radiotherapy, and intrathecal chemotherapy.

Treatment

Treatment of neoplastic meningitis includes the use of intrathecal chemotherapy by lumbar puncture or through an Ommaya reservoir into the lateral ventricles. A limited number of chemotherapeutic agents are available for intrathecal use, including methotrexate, cytosine arabinoside, and thiotepa. Liposome-encased cytarabine arabinoside administered intrathecally allows for treatment every 2 weeks, in contrast to twice weekly with standard chemotherapy, and has been beneficial for lymphoma and some solid tumors causing neoplastic meningitis. Systemic chemotherapy is not thought to be effective. Radiotherapy is reserved for localized treatment of bulky disease. Patients with sphincter dysfunction may benefit from local radiotherapy to the conus medullaris and cauda equina. In patients with cranial nerve dysfunction, radiotherapy to the basal cisterns may be beneficial. Dexamethasone may improve symptoms. Untreated, the median survival of neoplastic meningitis is 6 weeks. The overall median survival with treatment is 4 to 6 months. A chance for longer survival in select patients has been described in patients with chemosensitive tumors such as breast cancer. Patients with neoplastic meningitis from malignant melanoma have a particularly poor prognosis. Often, a patient with neoplastic meningitis will have concomitant progression of systemic cancer.

SPINAL METASTASES

Spinal cord dysfunction from metastatic cancer may be the result of tumor metastasis to vertebral bodies, extension of a paravertebral mass, or intramedullary metastases from hematogenous spread to the spinal cord (5%). The most common cause of spinal cord compression is metastasis to the vertebral body from tumors with a tendency to spread to bone, such as multiple myeloma and tumors of breast, lung, or prostate origin. Pain is present in the majority of patients, and the presence of back or neck pain in a patient with known cancer should raise the suspicion of a spinal metastasis and prompt appropriate investigation. Pain may be localized or radicular and often directs the clinician to the appropriate spinal level. The absence of pain in a patient with spinal cord dysfunction should suggest the possibility of another etiology for the patient's symptoms such as radiation myelopathy, intramedullary spinal cord metastases, or a paraneoplastic syndrome. The neurologic examination is very important to determine the level of spinal cord involvement. Symptoms may include motor and sensory abnormalities and sphincter dysfunction. The neurologic examination may demonstrate hyperreflexia and dorsal column signs, with impairment of position sense and vibration. Spinothalamic dysfunction may result in abnormalities of pain and temperature sensitivities. A knowledge of the anatomy of the spinal cord is important in interpreting the neurologic examination.

Spinal cord compression from metastatic tumor represents one of the true neurologic emergencies in the patient with cancer. The rate of progression is variable, and failure to diagnose and treat spinal cord compression may result in irreversible neurologic injury, thus limiting the quality of life as well as potentially the survival of the patient with cancer. In general, the neurologic outcome is determined by the neurologic status at the time treatment is initiated. A patient who is ambulatory at the time of treatment has a good chance of remaining ambulatory, whereas it is unlikely that the nonambulatory patient will regain significant function. Sphincter involvement is considered to be a poor prognostic sign and often occurs later in spinal cord compression. Early involvement should alert the clinician to consider conus medullaris or cauda equina involvement.

Spinal MRI with gadolinium is the neuroimaging study of choice for evaluation of spinal cord dysfunction because 15% to 30% of patients with spinal cord compression may have involvement at multiple levels. The entire length of the spine should be imaged for optimal planning of radiotherapy. A gadolinium MRI also may identify leptomeningeal involvement or intramedullary metastasis.

Treatment

Corticosteroids, usually dexamethasone, are administered when the diagnosis of spinal cord compression is made. Initial doses range between 20 and 100 mg. The subsequent dosing is determined on symptoms, rate of progression, and extent of disease. Radiotherapy and surgery are the main therapeutic options. Radiotherapy usually is initiated urgently in a patient with known cancer. Surgery is appropriate for patients without a known cancer or in the setting of deterioration despite radiotherapy. Newer approaches to surgical decompression using anterior and anterolateral approaches address the location of tumor involvement and may be preferred to the more traditional posterior surgical decompression. However, often the cancer patient in this situation has extensive systemic disease with a limited life expectancy and surgery is not well tolerated.

NONMETASTATIC COMPLICATIONS

Cerebrovascular Complications

Patients with cancer are at increased risk for a variety of cerebrovascular complications resulting either from the effects of malignancy or from treatment. The cerebrovascular complications may be either ischemic or hemorrhagic. Accelerated atheromatous disease resulting in thrombotic strokes may occur following radiation therapy to the head and neck region. Systemic cancer may cause a hypercoagulable state, resulting in arterial or venous sinus occlusion. Patients with mucin-producing adenocarcinomas, in particular, have been described to be at risk for the development of a hypercoagulable state and suffer subsequent cerebral infarction. Mucin deposits have been found in the venous walls at the sight of the infarct. Nonbacterial thrombotic endocarditis is a well-recognized complication of cancer and may result in cerebral embolism.

Bacterial endocarditis may occur as a complication of tumor therapy, because of neutropenia, and it may cause septic emboli resulting in stroke. Less commonly, a mycotic aneurysm may develop with the risk of subarachnoid hemorrhage.

Thrombocytopenia, either as a direct result of the malignancy (usually one of a hematologic origin) or a consequence of tumor therapy, may cause hemorrhagic complications including subdural hematoma, spinal epidural hematoma, or intracerebral hemorrhage. Lumbar puncture should be performed with a sufficient platelet count and appropriate coagulation parameters to avoid an iatrogenic spinal epidural hematoma with spinal cord compression. The cancer patient may be receiving warfarin for thrombotic complications related to the cancer-induced hypercoagulable state. In such a situation, the warfarin needs to be discontinued and the coagulation parameters needs to be corrected prior to performing a lumbar puncture.

A non-contrast CT scan is performed in patients in whom a hemorrhage is suspected. MRI is more sensitive than CT for identifying non-hemorrhagic cerebrovascular insults. A magnetic resonance angiogram provides a noninvasive means to visualize the extracranial and intracranial circulation to evaluate a thrombotic stroke. The treatment depends on the type of cerebrovascular complication and the underlying cause.

Metabolic and Nutritional Complications

Metabolic abnormalities may develop as a direct result of systemic cancer or secondary to cancer treatment, and they affect both the peripheral and central nervous system. Metabolic derangements may cause a diffuse encephalopathy, resulting in generalized confusion, personality changes, alteration of alertness, seizures, and coma. The physical and neurologic examination may suggest a metabolic etiology by the presence of tremor, myoclonus, asterixis, and fluctuation of symptoms. The cancer patient is often taking multiple medications, including narcotics for pain management. A thorough review of the medication list is essential in evaluating the cancer patient with neurologic symptoms. Although narcotics and pain medications most commonly are implicated to cause neurologic symptoms in the cancer patient, the clinician needs to be aware of the potential neurologic side effects of all medications the patient is receiving. The author has been impressed with the spectrum of neurologic symptoms caused by a drug such as metoclopramide including gait disturbance (initially thought to be spinal cord compression by a medical oncologist), tremor, rigidity resembling Parkinson's disease, physical and mental restlessness (akathisia), and confusion.

Corticosteroids are used for a variety of reasons in the patient with cancer. Systemic and neurologic complications are common (Table 20.1). Anxiety, somnolence, and emo-

TABLE 20.1. *Complications of Corticosteroids*

Medical
  Weight gain, striae
  Diabetes mellitus
  Skin fragility
  Insomnia
  Infection susceptibility
  Candidiasis (oral thrush, esophagitis)
Neurologic
  Anxiety, emotional lability
  Psychosis, confusion
  Proximal myopathy
  Spinal lipomatosis (rare)

tional lability, also common, may be managed either by altering the schedule (e.g., to avoid a late-night dose that causes insomnia) or by the administration of an antianxiety medication such as a benzodiazepine. Chemotherapeutic agents can affect the peripheral and

TABLE 20.2. *Neurotoxicity of Chemotherapy*

Cerebral Hemispheres
  Acute encephalopathy
    Procarbazine
    Interferon
    Interleukin-1,2
    Ifosfamide
    Methotrexate (high-dose intravenous or intrathecal)
    Asparaginase
    Vincristine
  Chronic encephalopathy
    Methotrexate (high-dose intravenous or intrathecal)
    Fludarabine
  Leukoencephalopathy
    Methotrexate
    5-fluorouracil + levamisole
    Carmustine (intraarterial)
Cerebellum
  5-fluorouracil
  Cytarabine
Visual System
  Tamoxifen (reversible retinopathy)
  Fludarabine (cortical blindness)
  Cisplatin (cortical blindness)
  Intraarterial chemotherapy (optic neuropathy)
Myelopathy
  Methotrexate (intrathecal)
  Cytarabine (intrathecal)
  Thiotepa (intrathecal)
Peripheral Nerves
  Vincristine
  Cisplatin
  Paclitaxel
  Suramin
  Etoposide

central nervous system in a variety of ways (Table 20.2). Toxicity depends on the age, specific agent, drug dosage, and associated therapies. It is imperative that the clinician caring for a patient with cancer be aware of the neurotoxicity associated with each chemotherapeutic regimen.

Nutritional status, often poor in the patient with cancer, should be addressed if there are neurologic symptoms. Neurologic syndromes from deficiencies of thiamine, folate, and B_{12} are well recognized.

PARANEOPLASTIC SYNDROMES

Several distinct syndromes have been recognized in patients with systemic cancer that are not related directly to metastatic disease or treatment toxicity. These syndromes are considered to be remote effects of the cancer and are known as paraneoplastic syndromes. The paraneoplastic syndromes are of clinical significance for two reasons:

1. The neurologic symptoms may cause significant morbidity and therefore have a significant impact on the quality and survival of life of the cancer patient.
2. The neurologic symptoms may develop prior to the actual diagnosis of the systemic cancer; therefore, if the clinician is familiar with the various paraneoplastic syndromes, an earlier diagnosis of the systemic malignancy is potentially possible.

The disorders have been thought to be related to an autoimmune process, and various antineuronal-specific antibodies have been identified (Table 20.3).

SPECIAL CHALLENGES FOR HOSPITALIZED PATIENTS

The general oncology patient may require intermittent hospitalization during the course of illness as the result of severe nausea and vomiting, dehydration, sepsis, pain, or new neurologic symptoms. The various medical problems often cause secondary somnolence, weakness, and alternation of mental status. The oncology patient often is receiving multiple medications that may cause somnolence, confusion, or weakness. Physicians need to be alert and sensitive to metabolic abnormalities, nutritional and hydration needs, the possibility of infection, and unusual medication schedules that may contribute to any of these problems. The toxicity profile of cancer therapy, including radiotherapy and chemotherapy, also needs to be considered. If metastatic disease is a consideration, MRI with gadolinium is overall superior to CT imaging.

Appropriate localization of the neurologic symptoms is important to request the appropriate imaging study. A base-of-skull MR study or CT of the base of the skull, using appropriate contrast enhancement, may be helpful for evaluation of cranial nerve dysfunction. A neuroimaging study ordered as a "brain" study may not be adequate and therefore may not identify the cause of the symptoms.

The patient with a primary brain tumor may require hospitalization for management of seizures, increased intracranial pressure, or neurologic deterioration with disease progression.

TABLE 20.3. *Paraneoplastic Syndromes*

Syndrome Associated	Autoantibodies	Associated Tumors
Cerebellar degeneration	Anti-yo (Anti-Purkinje cell)	Ovarian, breast
Encephalomyelitis	Anti-Hu	Lung
Opsoclonus—myoclonus	Anti-Ri	Breast, bladder, lung
Subacute sensory neuropathy	Anti-Hu	Lung
Lambert–Eaton syndrome	Anti-VGCC (antisynaptotagmin)	Lung (small-cell)

WHEN TO REFER A PATIENT TO A NEUROLOGIST

Neurologic symptoms may develop in a patient with known cancer or may be the presenting symptoms in a patient with no previous diagnosis of cancer. The symptoms may be the direct or indirect result of the malignancy or may develop as the result of treatment for the cancer. The patient with known cancer should be referred to a neurologist for evaluation of neurologic symptoms to determine if the central or peripheral nervous system is being affected by the malignancy directly as the result of metastases or as a secondary result of treatment. If the symptoms are treatment related, the patient then may be monitored during subsequent treatment.

Treatment-related symptoms often affect quality of life. The neurologist may work in conjunction with a physiatrist to examine the level of function for patients with problems such as steroid myopathy (strengthening exercises), leg paresis (bracing the knee or ankle), pain, or general deconditioning. Referral to a pain specialist may assist in management of cancer-related pain. A neuropsychologist may assist in managing the patient with cognitive deficits and emotional changes related to a brain tumor, primary or secondary, and treatment.

In a patient with known malignancy, increasing tumor markers, new depression, lethargy, or personality changes should be screened for neurologic involvement. Because a patient without a known malignancy may develop neurologic findings first, a patient with unexplained neurologic symptoms, new onset of lethargy, depression, or personality changes may be referred to a neurologist to consider evaluation for an underlying malignancy.

QUESTIONS AND DISCUSSION

1. A 50-year-old woman enters a walk-in clinic. She had an unexplained episode of loss of consciousness while home alone. She was aware of being incontinent of urine and complained of a very sore tongue. You determine that she probably had a seizure. She does not have a history of seizures. As the physician, you:

A. Send her home and tell her to see her doctor if it happens again.

B. Start her taking phenytoin and tell her to see her doctor if it happens again.

C. Order a CT scan of the brain and tell her to see her doctor.

D. Perform a complete neurologic examination, order appropriate tests for toxic and metabolic causes of a seizure, order a CT or MRI scan of the brain, and arrange for hospital admission or appropriate follow-up.

The answer is (D). An underlying cause for this seizure needs to be investigated. The onset of idiopathic epilepsy at this age is quite unusual. This patient should not be sent home if she is alone. She should not be allowed to drive. Hospitalization for observation and evaluation is preferred, although each situation should be reviewed individually.

2. The patient's MRI with gadolinium contrast demonstrates multiple ring-enhancing lesions in various parts of the cerebral hemispheres. She is neurologically intact. You then:

A. Start her taking dexamethasone and an H_2-blocker.

B. Request an oncology consult.

C. Start her taking an anticonvulsant medication.

D. All of the above.

The answer is (D). If she has no evidence to suggest these lesions may be infectious, then metastatic tumor is the most likely diagnosis. Dexamethasone is very effective at reducing the vasogenic edema. In view of the abnormalities on the MRI and the fact that she already has experienced a seizure, prescribing an anticonvulsant medication is prudent.

3. An evaluation to establish a diagnosis and identify the primary site of tumor may include:

A. Chest X-ray and chest CT scan

B. Mammogram

C. Abdominal CT scan

D. Complete blood count, urinalysis, and liver function tests

E. Serum tumor markers

F. All of the above

The answer is (F). About one-half of patients presenting with metastatic brain tumors, without a known primary tumor, subsequently will be found to have a primary lung cancer. Unfortunately, although metastatic brain tumors most often present later in patients with breast cancer, synchronous presentation may occur in the most aggressive forms of breast cancer. Renal cell carcinoma, tumors of the gastrointestinal tract, and lymphoreticular neoplasms also should be considered. The various scans also will assist in establishing the extent of metastatic disease.

4. The chest CT scan is abnormal, and a diagnosis of adenocarcinoma of the lung is confirmed histologically by bronchoscopy. The patient is treated with whole brain radiation therapy in 10 fractions. She returns to the clinic 1 month after therapy with headache, fatigue, and mental slowness. Your evaluation should include:

A. Carbamazepine level

B. Serum electrolytes, including sodium, potassium, and calcium

C. Serum glucose

D. All of the above

The answer is (D). Carbamazepine was chosen as the anticonvulsant medication because of the risk of dermatologic toxicity from the combination of phenytoin and whole brain radiotherapy. However, phenytoin is still the most commonly used anticonvulsant in this situation. Carbamazepine may cause the syndrome of inappropriate antidiuretic hormone (SIADH), as may the underlying lung cancer. Dexamethasone may cause significant hyperglycemia. The increasing symptoms also may be related to tapering the dexamethasone, so increasing the dose may treat the symptoms effectively.

5. The lung tumor also was treated with radiotherapy because it was thought to be blocking a bronchus. Four months later, the patient returns with urinary frequency and bilateral leg weakness. You then:

A. Assume it is a side effect from the chest radiotherapy.

B. Order a contrast MRI of the spine, using the neurologic examination to guide localization

C. Consider a lumbar puncture

D. Assume the patient has a steroid myopathy

The answer is (B) and (C). The major clinical concerns are epidural spinal cord compression from bony metastases and neoplastic meningitis. Epidural spinal cord compression most often causes pain. The MRI of the spine should be performed with gadolinium. Neoplastic meningitis may produce leptomeningeal enhancement. Lumbar puncture with cytologic examination should be considered to confirm the diagnosis of neoplastic meningitis. Steroid myopathy does not cause urinary frequency. Radiation-induced myelopathy is a rare diagnosis usually occurring later, and it should be considered only if the other direct metastatic complications have been excluded.

6. A 62-year-old man complains of a 2-month history of burning numbness in his legs and feet. He has lost 10 pounds and describes decreased appetite. As his physician, you:

A. Order serum glucose, thyroid functions, B_{12} level

B. Obtain a chest x-ray

C. Obtain an anti-Hu antibody test

D. Order electromyography and nerve conduction velocity studies

E. Determine toxic exposure by history

F. All of the above

The answer is (F). The symptoms suggest a polyneuropathy. The subacute onset, painful quality, and weight loss are concerning. Diabetes, hypothyroidism, and B_{12} deficiency should be excluded. This may represent a paraneoplastic syndrome and may be the first symptom for lung cancer. Excessive alcohol use or toxic exposure should be reviewed in the history.

SUGGESTED READING

Antonadou D, Paraskevaides M, Coliarakis N, et al. Temozolomide enhances radiation treatment efficacy in brain metastases: a randomized phase II study [abstract]. *Proc Am Soc Clin Oncol* 2001;20P57a:Abstract 224.

Bindal AK, Bindal RK, Hess KR, et al. Surgery versus radiosurgery in the treatment of brain metastasis. *J Neurosurg* 1996;84:748.

Cairncross JG, MacDonald DR, Ramsay DA. Aggressive oligodendroglioma: A chemosensitive tumor. *Neurosurgery* 1992;31:78.

Chamberlain MC. Current concepts in leptomeningeal metastasis. *Curr Opin Oncol* 1992;4:533.

Dardoufas C, Miliadou A, Skarleas C, et al. Concomitant temozolomide (TMZ) and radiotherapy (RT) followed by adjuvant treatment with temozolomide in patients with brain metastases from solid tumours [abstract]. *Proc Am Soc Clin Oncol* 2001;20:75b:Abstract 2048.

Heros DO. Neuro-oncology. In: Weiner WJ, Shulman LM, eds. *Emergent and urgent neurology.* New York: Lippincott Williams and Wilkins, 1999.

Hochberg FH, Miller DC. Primary central nervous system lymphoma. *J Neurosurg* 1988;68:835.

Hwu WJ, Raizer J, Panageas KS, et al. Treatment of metastatic melanoma in the brain with temozolomide and thalidomide. *Lancet Oncol* 2001;2:634–635.

Kori SH, Foley KM, Posner JB. Brachial plexus lesions in patients with cancer: 100 cases. *Neurology* 1985;35:8.

Moll JWB, Antoine JC, Brashear HR, et al. Guidelines on the detection of paraneoplastic anti-neuronal-specific antibodies. *Neurology* 1995;45:1937.

Patchell RA, Tibbs PA, Walsh JW, et al. Surgery versus radiosurgery in the treatment of brain metastasis. *J Neurosurg* 996;84:748.

Perrin RG, McBroom RJ. Metastatic tumors of the spine. In: Rengachary SS, Wilkins RH, eds. *Principles of neurology.* St. Louis: Wolfe, 1994.

Posner JB. *Neurologic complications of cancer.* Philadelphia: FA Davis, 1995.

Raez L, Cabral L, Cai JP, et al. Treatment of AIDS-related primary central nervous system lymphoma with zidovudine, ganciclovir, and interleukin 2. *AIDS Res Hum Retroviruses* 1999;15:713–719.

Smalley SR, Laws ER, O'Fallon JR, et al. Resection for solitary brain metastasis: Role of adjuvant radiation and prognostic variables in 229 patients. *J Neurosurg* 1992;77:531.

Stupp R, Dietrich PY, Ostermann Kraljevic S, et al. Promising survival for patients with newly diagnosed glioblastoma multiforme treated with concomitant radiation plus temozolomide followed by adjuvant temozolomide. *J Clin Oncol* 2002;20:1375–1382.

Thomas JE, Cascino TL, Earie JD. Differential diagnosis between radiation and tumor plexopathy of the pelvis. *Neurology* 1985;35:1.

Westphal M, Hilt DC, Bortey E, et al. A phase 3 trial of local chemotherapy with biodegradable carmustine (BCNU) wafers (Gliadel wafers) in patients with primary malignant glioma. *Neuro-oncol* 2003;5(2):79–88.

21

Neurologic Evaluation of Low Back Pain

Russell H. Glantz

The purpose of this chapter is to distinguish non-neurologic from neurologic causes of back pain. The physician frequently must determine whether back pain from disease of the spine and its surrounding structures has involved the nervous system by spinal cord or spinal root compression. Neurologic involvement has specific prognostic and management implications.

The most common form of back pain is spondylogenic. This pain originates in the vertebral spinal column and associated soft-tissue structures. These soft tissues most frequently are incriminated in the causes of back pain and include diseases of the associated tendons; muscles; joints; and, most importantly, intervertebral discs.

Vascular back pain may result from abdominal aneurysms and is often a deep-seated, boring lumbar pain. In addition, vascular insufficiency of the superior gluteal artery may give rise to buttock pain of a claudicant nature. These symptoms may even radiate down the leg. The pain of vascular insufficiency is, however, not aggravated by other stresses on the lumbar spine, such as bending, twisting, or stooping.

Viscerogenic back pain may result from retroperitoneal tumors or diseases of the kidneys or pelvic viscera. Backache, however, is rarely the sole symptom of a visceral disease. Furthermore, this pain is neither aggravated by activity nor relieved by rest. Patients with severe visceral pain frequently writhe around to obtain relief.

Primary neurogenic pain is caused by a disease of the nervous system, which is reflected as back pain. Some causes are neurofibromas, ependymomas, astrocytomas, and other lesions within the dural contents but outside the spinal cord itself. These conditions are uncommon, however, and it is beyond the scope of this chapter to discuss the differential diagnosis of all primary neurogenic back pains. The emphasis is placed instead on accurate diagnosis of the more common causes of nerve root compression in the lumbar spine. A physician most frequently sees nerve root compression as a result of acute or chronic intervertebral disc degeneration.

ANATOMY AND PHYSIOLOGY

Each vertebra has three functional components: (1) the vertebral bodies, (2) the neural arches, and (3) the bony processes (spinous and transverse). The vertebral bodies are connected by the intervertebral discs, and the neural arches are joined by the zygapophyseal joints. The vertebral bodies are braced front and back by the anterior and posterior longitudinal ligaments (Fig. 21.1). The stability of the spine depends on two types of supporting structures: the ligamentous (passive) structures and the muscular (active) structures. Although the ligaments are strong, they alone cannot resist the enormous forces on the spinal column. Most of the stability is dependent on the reflex contractions of the sacrospinalis, abdominal, glutei, and hamstring muscles.

One of the most important anatomic features of the lumbar spine is the relationship that the neural elements bear to the bony skeleton and the intervertebral discs. The spinal cord ends at L1. From this point, all the lumbar, sacral, and coccygeal nerve roots run as distinct entities within the dural sac and exit through the lumbar, sacral, and coccygeal intervertebral foramina. The nerve roots course downward and outward. They cross the

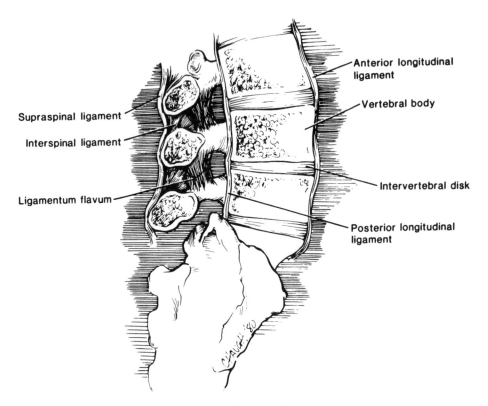

FIG. 21.1. Anatomic landmarks of lumbosacral spine.

intervertebral disc and pass anterior to the superior articular facet, hugging the medial aspect of the pedicle before emerging into the intervertebral foramen. The nerve root, therefore, is vulnerable to compression by pathologic changes occurring at several points during its course down the spinal canal. The L4 root emerges between L4 and L5—in other words, below the vertebra that is numerically similar (Fig. 21.2). In the same way, the L5 root emerges between L5 and S1. However, in syndromes caused by disc protrusion, an L4–L5 disc protrusion usually will compress the L5 root. This is because the more usual protrusion is posterolateral, and it catches the more medially placed downcoming root from a higher segment (Fig. 21.3). If a protrusion is far lateral, the L4 root is compressed in an L4–L5 syndrome; however, this situation is

unusual. An L5–S1 protrusion generally implies an S1 root compressive syndrome. Similarly, an L3–L4 protrusion would give rise to an L4 root compressive syndrome, and an L2–L3 protrusion will cause an L3 root compressive syndrome.

The anatomy is different in the cervical region: The root emerges above the vertebra from which it takes its name. The C6 root emerges between C5 and C6; the C7 root emerges between C6 and C7; the C8 root emerges between C7 and T1 (see Fig. 21.2). The root, from this level downward, emerges below the vertebra from which it takes its name. As a general rule, for both cervical and lumbar compressive syndromes, the clinical lesion corresponds to the lower vertebral segment (C5–C6 = C6 syndrome, L5–S1 = S1 syndrome).

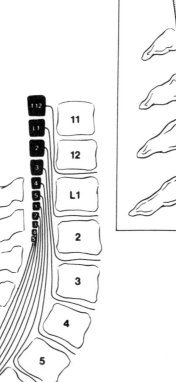
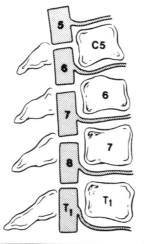

FIG. 21.2. Cervical *(upper right)* and lumbosacral *(lower left)* spine, showing the emergence of spinal roots.

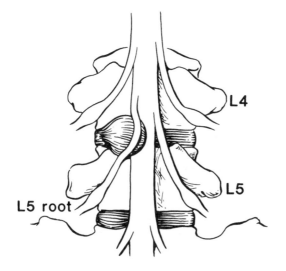

FIG. 21.3. Herniated disc at L4–L5 compressing the L5 rootlet.

DIAGNOSIS

Back pain of non-neurogenic or neurogenic origin may be (1) local, (2) referred, or (3) radicular (or root). Once a diagnosis is made in terms of these simple guidelines, the physician may focus on the differentiation between non-neurogenic causes (e.g., spondylogenic, viscerogenic, or vascular) and neurogenic causes.

Local pain is caused by any pathologic process that irritates sensory endings in the back. The fact that nerve endings are irritated does not necessarily mean that the cause is primarily neurogenic. The final expression of any pain, whatever the cause, has to be through nerve endings. Local pain may be the result of the involvement of bone, muscle, ligaments, or periosteum. The pain is usually steady; it may be sharp or dull; and it is always felt in or near the affected part of the spine. The pain may change with a variation in position or activity. Firm tissue pressure in the region involved usually evokes tenderness and thus helps in localization. Most local pains fit generally into the spondylogenic category.

Referred pain may be projected from the spine into viscera and other structures lying within the area of the lumbar and upper-sacral dermatomes. Referred pain also may be projected from the pelvic and abdominal viscera to the spine. Pain resulting from upper lumbar spine disease usually is referred to the anterior aspects of the thighs and legs. This pain may have to be distinguished from L3 radicular pain, which has a similar distribution. Pain from the lower lumbar spine usually is referred to the lower buttock; it is caused by an irritation of lower spinal nerves that activate the same pool of neurons that also serve the posterior thighs and calves. The referred pain often parallels in intensity the local pain in the back, thus maneuvers that alter local pain have a similar affect on referred pain. This is not the case with lancinating radicular pain, which may shoot suddenly and may be unassociated with a maneuver that causes aggravation of local pain. Furthermore, referred pain rarely is felt below the knees, whereas pain from root irritation may spread into the calf or even the foot.

Radicular or root pain relates to an irritation or damage of neural structures by primary neurologic diseases or non-neurologic disease (e.g., discs) and hence must be specifically distinguished from local or referred pain. The misdiagnosis of local or referred pain as radicular pain often results in unnecessary investigations and unwarranted treatment. Root pain has some of the characteristics of referred pain but differs in its greater intensity; distal radiation; circumscription to the territory of a root; and, very importantly, the factors that induce it. Typically, any maneuver that increases the pressure of the spinal fluid (with secondary pressure on nerve roots) usually aggravates radicular pain. Hence, coughing, sneezing, and straining at stool characteristically evoke this sharp radiating pain.

Most root pain is the result of nerve root compression by a herniated intervertebral disc. True neurologic causes of the same syndrome include neurofibromas, ependymomas, and cysts, and these may give rise to similar symptoms and signs. Furthermore, the root entrapment may be bony in etiology, as in spinal stenosis, but here the problem is asymmetric and bilateral.

The symptoms of nerve root compression may present in three ways: (1) backache only, (2) pain resulting from radiation only (sciatica), or (3) pain and backache together. The onset is frequently dramatic in the fully developed syndrome. There is a severe knifelike pain that is aggravated by any movement or Valsalva maneuver (e.g., sneezing or coughing). Most patients lie still in bed with legs flexed at the knees and hips. Some patients find a lateral decubitus position more comfortable. Not infrequently, patients will contort themselves into strange postures to alleviate their pain. A sitting position often is painful. Some patients with nerve root tumors, simulating radicular disc compression symptoms, find relief by walking around.

When examined, the patient's posture is characteristic. The lumbar spine is flattened and slightly flexed. The patient usually leans toward the side of his pain, and this action becomes more obvious when he is trying to bend forward. Symptoms may be improved by standing with the hip and knee slightly flexed and with the forced scoliosis to the sound side. This posturing diminishes any stretch on the sciatic nerve. Pain typically may be provoked by pressure over the involved vertebral spines and along the course of the sciatic nerve (sciatic notch, retrotrochanteric gutter, posterior surface of thigh, head of fibula). Pressure at one point may cause pain and tingling to radiate down the leg. It would be unusual not to find local vertebral spine pain when direct pressure is applied in a disc syndrome. Its lack, or the presence of symptoms with more lateral pressure, should cast some doubt on the diagnosis.

On further assessment of the degree of root involvement, it is important to test specifically for root tension. The two most useful tests are the straight-leg-raising and bowstring signs (Figs. 21.4 and 21.5). The patient should be lying on a flat surface, and the leg should be raised slowly. The knee must be fully extended. If the test is positive, pain will be produced in the back or the leg. Pain in the popliteal fossa produced by simple stretching of the legs does not signify a positive test. Two additional maneuvers add significance to straight-leg raising: (1) aggravation of pain by forced dorsiflexion of the ankle at the limit of straight-leg raising, and (2) relief of pain by knee flexion. Sciatic pain almost always is relieved by flexing the knee. The bowstring sign can be another important indication of root compression. The straight-leg-raising test is carried out to the point at which the patient experiences some discomfort. At this level, the knees are allowed to flex and the examiner allows the patient's foot to rest on his shoulder. The test demands sudden firm pressure applied to the popliteal nerve behind the knee. The reproduction of pain in the leg or in the back is irrefutable evidence of nerve root compression. As in the case of straight-leg raising, local popliteal fossa pain does not indicate a positive result. These maneuvers aim to diagnose radicular pain but do not distin-

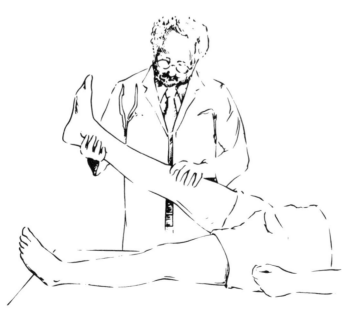

FIG. 21.4. Straight-leg-raising sign. Note that the examiner maintains the knee in the extended position.

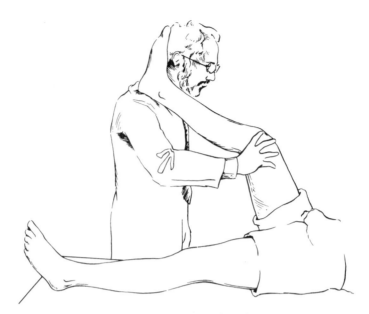

FIG. 21.5. The bowstring sign.

guish the specific causes of such pain (e.g., disc or tumors).

Lesions of the fifth lumbar and first sacral roots are the most common. The former lesions usually give symptoms of pain in the hip, groin, posterior lateral thigh, lateral calf, and dorsum of the foot including the first to third toes. Paresthesias in this distribution may be of great diagnostic aid. There may be a weakness of dorsiflexion of the foot and great toe. The extensor hallucis (great toe extensor) is a powerful muscle and should not be overcome even in a slightly built or generally weakened patient. A weakness in this muscle is, therefore, very significant in the diagnosis of an L5 lesion. No reflex change will be present, the knee and ankle jerks being subserved by L2–L4 and S1, respectively.

Lesions of the first sacral root give rise to pain in the midgluteal region, the posterior thigh, the posterior calf to the heel, and the sole of the foot extending over to the dorsum and involving the fourth and fifth toes. Weakness, if present, involves the flexors of the foot and toes, the abductors of the toes, and the hamstring muscles. The ankle reflex invariably is decreased or lacking, and this finding forms an important diagnostic criterion in S1 root compression.

Symptoms of nerve root compression may be confined to back pain. In patients who have recurrent episodes, the presentations may be difficult on each occasion. For example, the patient initially may present with the complete syndrome and, subsequently, with back pain only. The physician, therefore, must take an accurate history when trying to formulate the anatomy of any particular pain complex. Root entrapment resulting from disc protrusion has been mentioned. It is certainly the most common and frequently the most dramatic type of pain. Chronic lumbar spondylosis (which is more insidious than disc degeneration) and osseous overgrowth also may cause nerve entrapment. Pain resulting from these latter causes is usually chronic and has a local and referred component. Typical back and radicular pain are lacking. There, however, may be appropriate neurologic signs (e.g., loss of ankle reflex) indicating nerve root dysfunction.

Special Diagnostic Investigations

Spinal Radiography

Spine x-ray films will not diagnose disc disease, but they are still useful in the initial workup of all acute and chronic low back pain syndromes. This noninvasive test may reveal a tumor deposit, marked osteophytosis, or even inherent bony anomalies such as lumbarization or sacralization.

Magnetic Resonance Imaging, Computed Tomography, and Myelography

Magnetic resonance imaging (MRI) is the imaging technique of choice in the evaluation of low back disorders when the clinical situation or plain x-ray films suggest the need for further evaluation. MRI is particularly good at producing a detailed picture of soft tissues, and it is an excellent way to visualize the state of the intervertebral disc (Fig. 21.6). The computed tomography (CT) scan is also a powerful tool in the diagnosis of low back disease. Unlike MRI, which does not involve ionizing radiation, the CT scan involves significant radiographic exposure. However, the CT scan gives information not only about the state of the disc but also about bony structures (Figs. 21.7 and 21.8).

Magnetic resonance imaging is useful for diagnosis not only of lumbar disc herniation but also of spinal tumors, spinal trauma, and sometimes even failed low back surgery because the paramagnetic contrast medium gadolinium produces images that can distinguish between scar and disc. In cases of suspected spinal stenosis, MRI imaging is still an excellent tool, but CT may be preferred because of its ability to evaluate bony abnormality to a greater degree.

The role of myelography (Fig. 21.9) has changed since the advent of MRI and CT scanning. Although water-soluble dyes now are used in the performance of myelography, it is not a benign procedure: complications occur in 10% to 20% of patients undergoing this examination, which is used to identify the cause of headache and, more rarely, seizures.

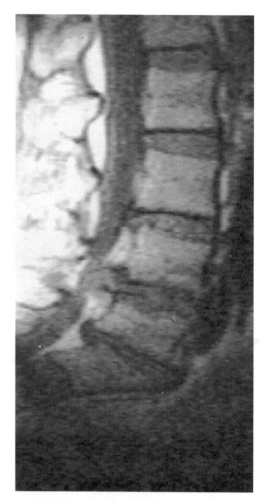

FIG. 21.6. Sagittal spinal cord magnetic resonance imaging showing evidence of extruded disc material between L4 and L5.

Myelography is used today in situations where the MRI or CT scan give an equivocal result. When the myelogram is followed by a CT scan, smaller, previously missed lesions may be visualized.

Electromyography

Electromyography (EMG) is the only test that may reveal functional impairment. The aim of this test is to localize the level of root or nerve involvement and also to help distinguish nerve damage from non-neurogenic disease, which may be the source of back pain. A

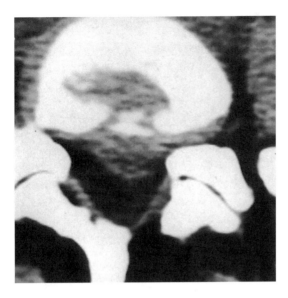

FIG. 21.7. Computed tomography scan of the lumbar spine showing prominent disc protrusion into the spinal canal.

normal muscle is silent at rest, but a denervated muscle gives rise to involuntary electrical discharges. These discharges take the form of fibrillation potentials or altered wave forms (positive waves). On voluntary contraction of a normal muscle, the motor unit potentials are biphasic or triphasic in form. With partial denervation, the quantity of motor units recorded is diminished and polyphasic potentials are seen (see Chapters 3 and 13).

The paraspinal muscles are supplied by the posterior primary rami of the emerging lumbosacral roots. No electrical activity is seen in the paraspinal muscles in a normal person

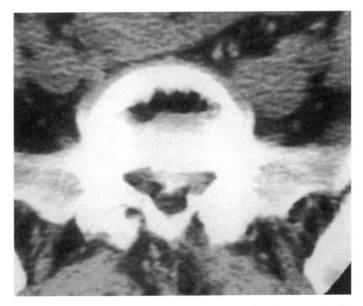

FIG. 21.8. Computed tomography evaluation of lumbar spine showing a markedly narrowed spinal canal as a result of protrusion of disc material as well as encroachment by bony hypertrophy and spurring. The vacuum disc phenomenon caused by disc degeneration is noted in the upper half of the picture.

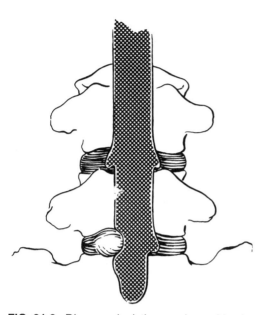

FIG. 21.9. Diagram depicting myelographic sign of indentation from extradural defect (speckled area represents dye column).

who is completely relaxed. The physician may sample the high lumbar, mid lumbar, and low lumbar areas, thereby gaining a fairly accurate localization of proximal nerve damage. These findings can be corroborated with the results of needle studies on other muscles. For example, the gluteus medius and tibialis posterior muscles are almost purely innervated by L5. Conversely, the soleus muscle has almost a pure S1 innervation; therefore, finding denervation in the gluteus medius, tibialis posterior, and low lumbar paraspinals without soleus denervation is strong evidence for L5 denervation. Similar inferences can be made with S1, L3, L4, and so forth.

The H reflex is a subtle electrical test of S1 function. The physician stimulates the afferent limb of S1 in the popliteal fossa and measures the time it takes to travel up the dorsal root, through the reflex arc, and back down the lower limb, eventually producing a contraction of the gastrocnemius. This is equivalent to the ankle jerk, except that the stretching of the Achilles tendon is bypassed. The H reflex may elicit minor degrees of S1 root involvement before clear evidence of motor, re-

flex, and sensory dysfunction is seen clinically.

The EMG also may reveal root lesions at many levels, such as may be seen in lumbar spondylosis and stenosis with multilevel nerve root encroachment.

Other Diagnostic Techniques

Other techniques can be used in special cases when the previously mentioned procedures have not led to a satisfactory diagnosis. Discography combined with CT may demonstrate disruption of the disc and tracking of the dye toward the side of symptoms. Functional testing with somatosensory evoked responses also has been used in the evaluation of lower back pain. Although this type of testing has become fairly widely used for the diagnosis of spinal cord lesions, there is controversy as to whether these tests are more or less sensitive than EMG in diagnosing radiculopathies. When their results are clearly abnormal, these tests may be the only way of documenting a purely sensory radiculopathy; in those instances, they may be better than EMG. Overall, however, EMG is the preferred test to evaluate suspected radiculopathy.

TREATMENT

The hallmark of conservative management is rest. The degree and length of time of rest is patient dependent. In situations where there is an acute radiculopathy, there is self-imposed rest because motion of any kind is extremely painful. In past times, patients were admitted to a hospital facility and given bed rest for weeks, often with traction. Today, such treatment is impractical and not economically feasible. However, there may be rare instances in which hospitalization is required. For the most part, an individual would be advised to remain at home, off work, for a few days, up to approximately 10 days. During this time, the patient will be taking antiinflammatory medications, as discussed later in this chapter. The patient should lie on a firm mattress, if available. A bed board is unnecessary, and, in some instances, may even increase the level of discomfort the patient experiences. While in bed, the patient should be placed in a position such that the hips and knees are flexed to a moderate and comfortable degree. During this period of rest, the patient also can use simple modalities, such as ice or heat. In individuals in which there is no neurologic component to the back pain—in which the back pain is mechanical—bed rest of this nature is not generally recommended.

The intelligent use of drug therapy is an important adjunct during the period of conservative therapy (Table 21.1). Because diminution of inflammation around the degenerated disc is the primary aim of therapy, an antiinflammatory drug should be used. At this point, the choices are between a steroidal medication versus a non-steroidal antiinflammatory drug (NSAID). The author prefers a short treatment with steroidal medication in acute radiculopathic back pain. Dexamethasone (Medrol), available in a Dosepak, is recommended. Alternatively, or if steroids are contraindicated, an NSAID may be used. Of the NSAID drugs, no one drug has been clearly shown to be better than another with respect to treatment of low back pain. The newer NSAIDs, selective for the cyclooxygenase-2 receptor, have a more limited adverse effect profile, but they cost more. These medications are appropriate in patients with a specific history of peptic ulcer disease, although there still needs to be caution, even with newer NSAIDs. Whether the patient is placed on systemic steroids or a NSAID, the stomach should be coated with food to prevent gastric irritation. Depending on the particular situation, an antacid or H_2 blocker may be used.

If there is a prominent amount of paravertebral muscle spasm, which may be present, especially in the acute phase, a muscle relaxant may be therapeutically effective. A drug such as cyclobenzaprine hydrochloride (Flexeril) may be tried. This medication is sedating, and the author prefers to prescribe this drug, mainly for nighttime use, starting with 5 mg and increasing the dose as tolerated.

Although the antiinflammatory drugs also have an analgesic action, this latter effect may not be sufficient, and additional pure analgesia may be required, especially in patients with severe pain. In patients with severe pain, hydrocodone, or equivalent analgesia, is necessary. This medication often will be necessary for the first week to 10 days, and as symptoms wane, this drug may be replaced with non-narcotic analgesia.

In the subacute phase of the disease, as the patient is recovering and the pain is disappearing, lumbar flexion exercises should be started. The overall aim of these exercises is to reduce the lumbar lordosis and strengthen the lumbosacral area of the spine. In practice, they should not be started sooner than about 3 weeks after the initiation of conservative therapy. The exercises should be started gently and should be discontinued immediately if a flare-up of symptoms appears. In the very acute phase of the condition, physical therapy modalities such as massage and ultrasound

TABLE 21.1. *Drugs Used in Treatment of Acute-Subacute Radicular Pain*

Drug Name	Mg/Dose	Standard Daily Administration	Side Effects
Dexamethasone	4	24 mg first day, then 20 mg, 16 mg, 12 mg, 8 mg, 4 mg, then 0 mg	Increased glucose, hypertension, gastrointestinal
NSAIDs			
Celecoxib	200–400	400 mg first day, then 200 mg daily	Gastrointestinal
Rofecoxib	25–50	50 mg first day, then 25 mg daily	Gastrointestinal
Hydrocodone (or equivalent)		One or two every 4–6 h	Sedation, confusion, constipation
Cyclobenzaprine	5–10	5 mg qhs up to 10 mg tid	Sedation
Amitriptyline	10–25	10–50 mg qhs or divided doses	Sedation
Gabapentin	100–300	Begin at 100 mg tid and increase to 600 mg tid	Lethargy, dizziness

are not contraindicated, but it is the author's experience that it is difficult for a given patient to travel to and from a physical therapy location two to three times weekly when the pain is so acute. The previously described regimen of rest and medication, along with the application of ice/heat, is preferred until the subacute phase of the disease.

If the response to conservative treatment is not adequate and surgery is not contemplated at that particular time, lumbar epidural steroid injections are used. This has become a popular method of treatment and involves up to three injections, given over a period of weeks.

Anticonvulsant medications have been used in chronic neuropathic pain with success. In some patients, in the subacute phase there may be a role for an anticonvulsant, such as gabapentin. The dosage of gabapentin is dependent on age because of its propensity to cause tiredness or dizziness. The usual starting dose is 100 to 200 mg three times daily, building up to 1,200 to 1,500 mg daily for radiculopathic pain. Tricyclic antidepressant drugs also may be useful in the subacute phase. Amitriptyline, 10 mg to 50 mg, at night may be useful. The newer antidepressant drugs, such as the SSRIs, are more expensive than amitriptyline but may be useful adjunctive agents in certain individuals.

REHABILITATION AND USE OF ALTERNATIVE THERAPIES

The issue of exercise and physical therapy has been discussed earlier. However, once the acute or subacute phase has passed, it is important to stress the value of lifelong stabilization exercises for proper rehabilitation. This is especially important in the patient who has had prior episodes of radiculopathy with repeated episodes of low back pain. There are different ways to accomplish this; the author prefers referring the individual to a physical therapist experienced in low back rehabilitation. The patient should be given a program of exercises under the guidance of the therapist. After about 3 weeks, the patient would continue such exercises independently and continue this for the remainder of his or her life.

Some physicians also additionally use alternative therapies. Muscle massage, as part of the acute or more chronic therapy is used by some physicians. Such therapy may help to alleviate the acute muscle spasm, which can accompany an acute radicular process. If used, this method would be in concert with pharmacologic therapies. As stated earlier, it is difficult for an individual with hyperacute lumbar radiculopathy to travel to and from a therapist or massage therapist, and the use of ice/heat may suffice. Acupuncture has been tried, but its usefulness has not been documented in the literature.

SPECIAL CONSIDERATION FOR THE HOSPITALIZED PATIENT

Hospitalization today for acute lumbar radiculopathy is unusual. Most insurance companies would not reimburse such an admission. Of course, there are exceptions. In the circumstances in which an individual's pain is so severe and uncontrollable by the usual means discussed earlier, hospitalization may be necessary for the use of parental narcotics. For example, a patient-controlled analgesia morphine pump would be useful in such an individual. Also, if the pain is severe an epidural steroid injection during hospitalization may be considered. Usually such an injection would be used only after the usual oral medications have been tried. If the pain was so severe as to require hospitalization, that individual would need to be prescribed bed rest, without any shower privileges. The individual would be allowed only bathroom privileges. Also, physical therapy modalities, in terms of heat, ultrasound, and massage, may be useful in the acute phase in an individual with such severe pain. Although traction was popular in years past, it seldom is used in hospitalized patients with acute lumbar radiculopathy.

Besides strict bed rest, special positioning does not have an added advantage in terms of speedier recovery. The patient needs to lie in the position of greatest comfort to that individual. There are no special beds or mattresses to recommend.

WHEN TO REFER THE PATIENT TO A NEUROLOGIST

Patients with lower back pain and radiculopathy who do not improve with conservative treatment including physical therapy and rehabilitation outlined previously, will require referral to a physician who specializes in spine care. This would include a neurologist, orthopedic surgeon, neurosurgeon, physiatrist, rheumatologist, or occupational medicine expert. The most important symptom/signs necessitating referral would be progressive neurologic deficits including numbness, weakness, or bladder symptoms. In these cases, expeditious evaluation and appropriate treatment are needed by a specialist. The neurologist will specialize in defining the area of neurologic impairment and designing a medically based referral treatment plan. Considerations of surgical referral for intervention would depend on the neurologic findings and patient response to medical treatments.

QUESTIONS AND DISCUSSION

Answer true or false to each of the following statements.

1. The most common cause of low back pain is nerve root compression from disc protrusion.

The answer is false. The most common cause of low back pain is spondylogenic; this includes bone, muscle, tendon, and disc abnormalities. Thus, although disc abnormalities are frequent, secondary nerve root compression is less common. The neurologist, however, frequently is consulted about whether nerve compression exists.

2. The L1 nerve root emerges between L1 and L2.

The answer is true. The nerve root exits below the vertebra from which it takes its name in the thoracic, lumbar, and sacral regions. In the cervical region, the root emerges above the vertebra with which it is associated numerically. For example, the C2 root emerges between C1 and C2. However, disc lesions that compress roots clinically follow the lower vertebrae for both cervical and lumbar areas.

3. Tingling or numbness on the lateral aspect of the leg extending to the great toe signifies an S1 root lesion.

The answer is false. This sensory distribution strongly suggests an L5 lesion. Supportive evidence would be weakness of the great toe extensor. An S1 lesion usually causes numbness of the posterior calf and sole and also a diminution of the ankle jerk.

4. The H reflex is an electrically obtained equivalent of the ankle reflex.

The answer is true. The H reflex tests the same reflex as the ankle jerk. However, stimulation of the Achilles tendon is bypassed in this case. When ankle reflex diminution is equivocal, the prolongation of the electrical H reflex may be useful, especially in the diagnosis of S1 root lesions.

5. In a patient with clinical symptoms and signs of nerve root compression unresponsive to conservative therapy, MRI is the radiologic investigation of choice for further evaluation.

The answer is true. MRI is the preferred imaging technique and is best for evaluation of a protruded disc.

SUGGESTED READING

Dugan SA, Frost DA, Sullivan KP. An active cost-conserving approach to the management of low back pain. *Hospital Physician* 2002(38(10).

Faas A, Van Eijk J, Chavannes A, et al. A randomized trial of exercise therapy in patients with acute low back pain. *Spine* 1995;20:941–947.

Frymoyer JW. *The adult spine: principles in practice,* 2nd ed. New York: Lippincott-Raven, 1977:663–670.

Herniated disc. In: *North American Spine Society Phase III Clinical Guidelines for Multi-Disciplinary Spine Care Specialists.* LaGrange, IL: North American Spine Society, 2000.

Levin KH, et al. Neck and back pain. In: *Continuum: lifelong learning in neurology,* Vol. 7, No. 1, Philadelphia: Lippincott Williams and Wilkins, 2001.

Long DM. Effectiveness of therapies currently employed for persistent low back pain and leg pain. *Pain Forum* 1995;4 (2):122–125.

Ropper A, Victor M. *Adams and Victor's principles of neurology.* New York: McGraw-Hill, 2000.

Van Tulder MW, Koes BW, Bouter LM. Conservative treatment of acute and chronic non-specific low back pain. A systematic review of randomized control trials of the most common interventions. *Spine* 1997; 22:2128–156.

22

Sleep Disorders

Ružica Kovačević-Ristanović

Sleep is a subject that has fascinated physicians and the public since antiquity. A search for a "sleep center" in the brain has demonstrated the complexity of the sleep process, the multiplicity of structures involved in sleep, and the reciprocal interactions necessary for the initiation and maintenance of this behavior.

The structures found to facilitate sleep are the basal forebrain (i.e., the preoptic area of the hypothalamus, specifically the ventrolateral preoptic nucleus [VLPO], promoting sleep via gamma-amino-butyric acid [GABA]/galanin activity), the area surrounding the solitary tract in the medulla, and the midline thalamus. It has been proposed that the sleep-promoting role of the anterior hypothalamus results from its inhibitory action on the posterior hypothalamic awakening neurons nuclei (mainly tuberomammillary histaminergic neurons [TMN] projecting widely to the cortex). Structures found to facilitate waking are newly discovered wake-promoting hypocretin (orexin) system and the ascending reticular activating system of the pons and midbrain and posterior hypothalamus. The role of the hypothalamus has been revised recently since the discoveries of sleep-promoting GABA/galanin activity in the VLPO and wake-promoting hypocretin (orexin) system activity in the dorsolateral hypothalamus around the perifornical nucleus. Although no direct interaction between the VPLO and hypocretin systems is reported, both systems innervate the main components of ascending arousal systems such as adrenergic locus coeruleus (LC), serotonergic dorsal raphe (DR), dopaminergic ventrotegmental area (VTA) and histaminergic TMN. The VPLO (GABA/galanin) system inhibits and the dorsolateral hypothalamic (hypocretin [orexin])

system activates these "arousal" systems. Destruction of the VPLO system results in insomnia, whereas destruction of the hypocretin system results in narcolepsy (hypersomnolence/sleep attacks and cataplexy). The control of alternating sleep stages (NREM [nonrapid eye movement]/REM [rapid eye movement] cycling) is attributed to interaction between antagonistic aminergic and cholinergic systems in the brainstem. The aminergic and cholinergic systems also are involved in the process of cortical activation of arousal. In addition to the previously mentioned systems, the dopaminergic system is involved in control of alertness as well, especially the ventral tegmental area (A10). Dopaminergic neurons of the VTA but not substantia nigra (SN) are excited by hypocretins, and there is a greater hypocretin innervation of the VTA than SN. Dopaminergic neurons in the ventral periaqueductal grey (PAG) also are activated during wakefulness. The dopaminergic system, including the descending A11 projection, may be particularly important for sleep disorders accompanied by anomalies of sleep-related motor control (cataplexy and periodic limb movement [PLM] disorder). Circadian sleep rhythm is modulated by the hypothalamic suprachiasmatic nucleus (SCN). The SCN sets the body clock period to approximately 25 hours, with the light and schedule cues ("time givers") entraining it to 24 hours. The retinohypothalamic tract conveys light stimuli to the SCN that directly influence its activity. Melatonin has been implicated as a modulator of light entrainment because it is secreted maximally during the night by the pineal gland ("hormone of darkness"). Thus, the anterior hypothalamus may serve as a center for "sleep switch" under the influence of the circadian clock.

Understanding the neurochemistry of sleep is important for practical reasons. The discovery of the involvement of different neurotransmitters and neuromodulators in control of arousal and sleep has raised the possibility of more specific treatments of sleep disorders (e.g., hypocretin agonists and/or GABA/galanin antagonists for treatment of excessive sleepiness). Most current treatments for sleep disorders do not relate to the known neurochemical substrates for sleep. Even more important, the myriad effects on sleep of currently used medications (both those used to alter sleep and those used for an unrelated purpose) should be understood.

The important clinical, diagnostic, and therapeutic features of some sleep disorders are described in this chapter. Useful guidelines for diagnosis and therapy also are presented, although there are few universally accepted treatments for common sleep complaints.

SLEEP ARCHITECTURE

Because the workup of many patients with sleep disorders involves the use of a sleep laboratory, it is important to understand the tests available and the parameters measured. A portion of the sleep recording, referred to as a polysomnogram (PSMG) of a normal subject, is shown in Fig. 22.1. Three basic parameters are needed to define the stage of sleep: an electroencephalogram (EEG), an electrooculogram (EOG), and an electromyogram (EMG). The normal EEG of an alert, resting subject with closed eyes shows an 8- to 12-Hz posterior activity known as alpha. Two major sleep stages are distinguished: NREM and REM sleep. Electroencephalographically, NREM sleep is composed of four stages. Stage 1 sleep is the stage of NREM sleep that directly follows the awake state. An EEG shows a low-voltage tracing of mixed frequencies predominantly in the theta band with alpha activity less than 50%, vertex sharp activity, and slow eye movements. Stage 2 sleep is the stage of NREM sleep that is characterized by the presence of sleep spindles (12 to 14 Hz) and K-complexes against a relatively low-voltage, mixed-frequency background. High-voltage delta waves may constitute up to 20% of Stage 2 sleep. In Stage 3 of NREM sleep, at least 20% but not more than 50% of the period consists of EEG waves less than 2 Hz; if more than 50% of the period contains such slow waves, the stage is Stage 4 NREM sleep. Stages 3 and 4 often are combined into a Stage delta NREM sleep because of the lack of documented physiologic differences between the two stages. This sleep occurs predominantly in the first third of the sleep period (Fig. 22.2).

REM sleep alternates with the NREM sleep at about 90-minute intervals in adults and 60-minute intervals in infants. The EEG pattern during REM sleep resembles Stage 1 sleep but is accompanied by rapid eye movements. In addition, EMG activity is low. There is a general activation of the autonomic system, with a higher average respiratory rate, heart rate, and blood pressure, and, more importantly, much more pronounced variability throughout the REM period. In about 80% of awakenings from REM sleep, people recall vivid dreams, compared to only 5% of awakenings from NREM sleep. However, in about 60% to 80% of awakenings from NREM sleep, people may recall thoughtlike fragments. Population studies have shown that the percentage of time spent in each stage varies with age and sex. Figures 22.1 and 22.2 represent a sleep PSMG and architecture plot from a normal adult.

CLASSIFICATION OF SLEEP ABNORMALITIES

The new International Classification of Sleep Disorders divides the primary sleep disorders into (a) the dyssomnias, or disorders that produce a complaint of either insomnia or excessive daytime sleepiness, and (b) the parasomnias, or disorders that intrude or occur during sleep but do not produce a primary complaint of insomnia or excessive daytime

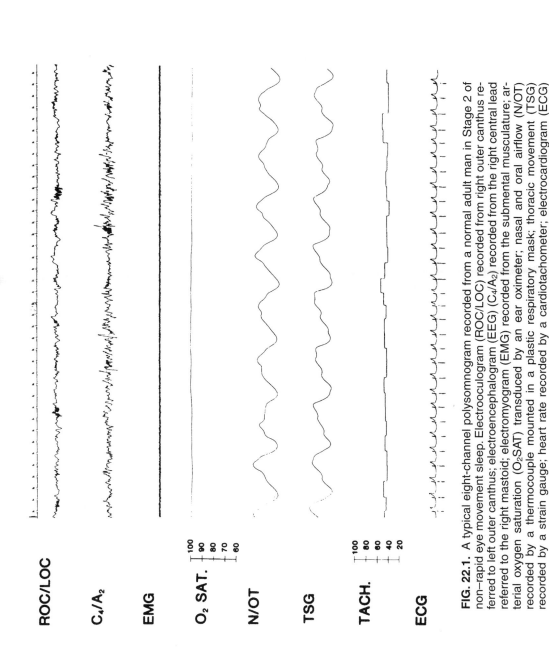

FIG. 22.1. A typical eight-channel polysomnogram recorded from a normal adult man in Stage 2 of non–rapid eye movement sleep. Electrooculogram (ROC/LOC) recorded from right outer canthus referred to left outer canthus; electroencephalogram (EEG) (C_4/A_2) recorded from the right central lead referred to the right mastoid; electromyogram (EMG) recorded from the submental musculature; arterial oxygen saturation (O_2SAT) transduced by an ear oximeter; nasal and oral airflow (N/OT) recorded by a thermocouple mounted in a plastic respiratory mask; thoracic movement (TSG) recorded by a strain gauge; heart rate recorded by a cardiotachometer; electrocardiogram (ECG) recorded from V_5 referred to the left mastoid.

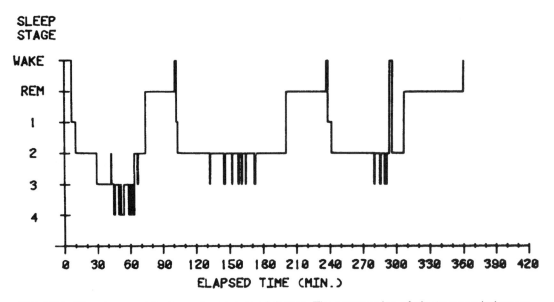

FIG. 22.2. The sleep architecture of a normal adult man. The progression of electroencephalogram (EEG) stages of sleep demonstrates a concentration of Stages 3 and 4 within the first half of the sleep period. Episodes of rapid eye movement (REM) sleep occur at approximately 90-minutes intervals, and the majority of REM appears within the latter half of the sleep period. Waking arousals are few.

sleepiness. The dyssomnias are subdivided further into extrinsic, intrinsic, and circadian sleep disorders. Thus, the causes of insomnia and hypersomnolence may be either within the body (intrinsic) or outside the body (extrinsic). These definitions of both types of primary sleep disorders differ from the medical–psychiatric definitions of sleep disorders. Future advances in the understanding of the pathophysiology of sleep disorders will result in improved classification along the lines of pathology.

SLEEP DISORDERS ASSOCIATED WITH INSOMNIA

Insomnia is a perception of inadequate, disturbed, insufficient, or non-restorative sleep despite an adequate opportunity to sleep, accompanied by daytime consequences of inadequate sleep. A 2002 Gallup phone survey found that 35% of respondents report experiencing at least one of the symptoms of insomnia every night or almost every night in the past year.

Among the intrinsic sleep disorders are psychophysiologic insomnia, sleep-state misperception, restless legs syndrome (RLS), and idiopathic insomnia, all of which produce the complaint of insomnia. Similarly, many extrinsic sleep disorders, such as inadequate sleep hygiene, environmental sleep disorder, altitude insomnia, adjustment sleep disorder, limit-setting sleep disorder, food allergy insomnia, hypnotic-dependent sleep disorder, and alcohol-dependent sleep disorder, are likely to be accompanied by insomnia. Among circadian rhythm sleep disorders, delayed sleep-phase syndrome is associated with a complaint of sleep-onset delay, whereas advanced sleep-phase syndrome is accompanied by a complaint of early awakening. In general, the pattern of insomnia may be primarily (a) difficulty falling asleep (sleep-onset delay), (b) early morning arousal (premature awakening with inability to fall asleep again), or (c) sleep fragmentation (repeated awakenings).

Insomnias can be transient (lasting less than 3 to 4 weeks) or chronic (lasting longer than that). Multiple factors can trigger transient insomnia, including life stress, brief illness, rapid change of time zones, drug withdrawal, use of central nervous system (CNS) stimulants, and pain. Transient insomnia is experienced by everyone, and recovery usually is rapid.

Chronic insomnia may be lifelong. It usually is related to chronic psychophysiologic arousal; psychiatric disorders; use of drugs and alcohol; and other medical, toxic, and environmental conditions. However, it also may represent a primary sleep disorder in the form of sleep apnea syndrome, alveolar hypoventilation syndrome, sleep-related (nocturnal) PLMs, and "restless legs."

SLEEP-ONSET DELAY

Sleep-onset delay is a common problem and probably accounts for most patients who present with a complaint of insomnia. It usually has psychogenic causes. Sleeplessness may develop from a continued association with stimulating practices and objects at bedtime. Such patients sleep better away from their bedrooms and usual routines. A conditioned internal factor also may develop in the form of apprehension about unsuccessful and excessive efforts to sleep. Conscious efforts to fall asleep result in CNS arousal. These patients consider themselves "light sleepers." They often have multiple somatic complaints such as back pains, headaches, and palpitations that lead to occasional abuse of alcohol, barbiturates, and minor tranquilizers. The sleep of such patients in the sleep laboratory is usually good because the conditioning factors that are active at home are reduced in the laboratory. Multiple specific psychiatric illnesses associated with anxiety, such as personality disorders (e.g., anxiety and panic disorders, hypochondriasis, obsessive–compulsive disorders), and schizophrenia also can be associated with sleep-onset difficulty.

Drugs also can compromise the initiation of sleep. When obtaining a history, the physician should inquire specifically about possible precipitants of drug-induced insomnia. In addition to steroids and dopaminergic agents, xanthine derivatives (e.g., caffeine and theophylline) may cause sleep disruption. A frequently overlooked class of agents is the beta-adrenergic agonists, such as terbutaline and phenylethylamine derivatives (used as stimulants, appetite suppressants, and decongestants). If such medications are taken late in the day, and in increasing amounts because of the development of tolerance, they easily can cause sleep-onset delay as well as sleep fragmentation and "lightening" of sleep. Such inadequate sleep provokes daytime symptoms such as sleepiness, which is responsible for a further increase of ingestion of the drug to promote alertness.

In addition to the psychologic and drug-induced causes of sleep-onset delay, patients who have a disturbed circadian rhythm may have the same sleep complaint. In delayed sleep-phase syndrome, patients naturally fall asleep at 2 or 3 AM or later. They cannot fall asleep if they go to bed at conventional times. If they must get up for a job or school at 6 AM, they will be sleepy in the morning. However, they have no trouble going to sleep and getting full rest if they can go to bed late and sleep until midday. A change in lifestyle and a course of chronotherapy at a sleep disorder center can correct this problem. Chronotherapy, an individually designed sleep schedule consisting of a gradual sleep-onset time delay until a desired time is reached, also may help patients with irregular sleep–wake patterns, who sleep for short and variable periods throughout the 24 hours. These people have difficulty falling asleep at conventional times because they have napped recently. Shift workers and those who travel frequently across time zones often experience sleep-onset delay (in addition to jet lag). Most patients affected by sleep-onset delay do not require drug treatment for therapy.

Treatment

The treatment of chronic insomnia is a significant challenge. The physician first should identify any underlying conditions, which may include psychiatric disorders such as depression, alcohol or substance abuse, chronic medical disorders, sleep apnea, aging, and alteration in the circadian rhythm. Treatment then should be based on concurrent problems, age, and hepatic and renal function. Whereas the non-pharmacologic interventions listed later could be considered alternative treatments in other neurologic diagnoses, they are standard for insomnia. Pharmacologic treatment should be used judiciously and should be combined with non-pharmacologic treatments.

Counseling appears to play an important role in the therapy of sleep disorders. If the physician spends time talking with these patients, he or she may find that they actually are attempting to discuss problems that they find difficult to raise, such as impotence, marital discord, or alcoholism in a family member. The complaint may be resolved if attention is given to these problems, regardless of whether sleep behavior actually is altered.

Sleep hygiene includes setting a fixed hour for retiring each night; eliminating daytime naps; avoiding drinking caffeine-containing beverages and engaging in anxiety-producing activities at night; and ensuring that the bedroom is quiet, dark, and comfortable. Because patients may not think of over-the-counter preparations as drugs, mentioning the need to avoid sympathomimetic substances may prove fruitful.

Only a few practical points concerning behavioral therapies need to be reviewed here. Techniques that attempt to increase relaxation, either through biofeedback or more conventional learning paradigms, may be valuable if they are aimed at a specific physiologic disturbance. For example, a patient whose PSMG indicates a large amount of muscle activity prior to falling asleep might benefit from EMG biofeedback. These techniques generally will require the facilities of a sleep laboratory. Attempts at operant and classic conditioning as aids in treating insomnia also have had some limited success. A widely accepted behavioral modification technique—stimulus control—is especially useful in correcting maladaptive association of arousal with bedtime routine. Other techniques aimed at reducing tension include progressive muscular relaxation and autogenic training.

Sleep restriction relies on restricting time spent in bed to the estimated sleep time the patient accumulates during the night, as documented by sleep logs, and then gradually increasing it until an optimal sleep time is achieved. This treatment is based on the observation that insomniacs spend too much time in bed in an attempt to obtain more sleep. Reduction of time spent in bed leads to a state of mild sleep deprivation, which is likely to result in faster sleep onset, improved sleep continuity, and deeper sleep.

Cognitive therapy focuses on maladaptive thoughts that produce an emotional arousal, such as unrealistic expectations about sleep requirements, negative consequences of insomnia, and misattributions of daytime difficulties to poor sleep.

Pharmacologic treatment can be used in the management of insomnia; however, the use of medications must be considered carefully. These medications are most helpful when their use is self-limited, such as during acute hospitalization or as part of a more comprehensive program of sleep hygiene. In the latter case, they may allow the physician time to explore the roots of the sleep disturbance more thoroughly.

The choice of a sedative agent is dictated primarily by the duration of clinical sedation; ideally, the hypnosedative effect should cease by the time the patient arises. An effective hypnotic drug should decrease sleep latency and increase the total sleep time. The value of a hypnotic depends on the balance of its efficacy and side effects. The efficacy is defined by its ability to induce and maintain sleep, and it directly depends on the drug's dose, absorption, and duration of action. Thus, an efficacious hypnotic is absorbed rapidly and has duration of action consistent with the sleep period (usually around 8 hours). Ideally, such a hypnotic has no adverse effects. However, hypnotics with a duration of action that exceeds the sleep period usually lead to residual sedation during daytime. In contrast, use of short-acting hypnotics in doses higher than required often is associated with major adverse effects such as rebound insomnia and anterograde amnesia. Dependence is also an undesirable possibility with the use of hypnotics. This possibility can be minimized by the intermittent use of low doses, together with limited duration of drug intake and gradual withdrawal if treatment has been continuous for more than a month. The available drugs have a surprisingly heterogeneous set of effects on sleep architecture.

Although almost all agents used as hypnosedatives will suppress REM sleep when given in sufficiently large quantities, two patterns of effects are seen at lower doses. Barbiturates, chloral hydrate, anticholinergics, tricyclics, and ethanol demonstrate REM suppression, whereas most benzodiazepines decrease Stages 3 and 4. They all appear to decrease sleep latency and reduce the number of spontaneous awakenings. Although the drugs that have the least effect on sleep architecture may offer a theoretic advantage in the therapy of insomnia, there is no clear demonstration that they induce "better" sleep. Data on commonly used sleep-promoting medications and some miscellaneous agents are summarized in Table 22.1.

Sleep latency usually is decreased with these agents, and there is seldom a reason to use more than a single agent in the treatment of insomnia. A failure to obtain an adequate response on the first night does not imply a need to increase the dosage immediately; a trial of at least two or three nights is indicated. Sleep induction is related to the rate of drug absorption. Sleep maintenance is related to dosage and half-life. The timing of the intake of the medications is, therefore, important. Hypnotics with longer half-lives (lasting more than 24 hours) show increased efficacy with two or three nights of administration, but they also show increased residual daytime effects. Some benzodiazepines, such as flurazepam (Dalmane), produce persistent long-

acting metabolites and cause definite impairment in alertness, motor performance, and cognitive function in the morning.

When the initial therapy is unsuccessful, changing classes of medications may be useful.

Because of the intrinsic "tapering" effect of compounds with long half-lives, rebound and/or withdrawal phenomena appear to be unlikely; when they do occur, such effects are delayed in onset and are relatively mild. However, there is a much higher likelihood of rebound or withdrawal effect after abrupt discontinuation of short-half-life hypnotics, for which dose tapering is appropriate.

In the last decade, benzodiazepines have almost completely replaced barbiturates. Only five benzodiazepines are marketed for hypnotic purposes in the United States: triazolam, (Halcion), temazepam (Restoril), quazepam (Doral), flurazepam, and estazolam (Prosom). Various benzodiazepine anxiolytics (e.g., diazepam [Valium], alprazolam [Xanax], lorazepam [Ativan], or oxazepam [Serax]) also are prescribed for insomnia associated with anxiety disorders. Unfortunately, there is limited evidence to support their efficacy for these disorders. The drug of choice for sleep-onset insomnia differs from that for sleep-maintenance insomnia (i.e., triazolam for the former, and temazepam for the latter).

Onset of action after an oral dose depends on rapidity of absorption from the gastrointestinal tract. Duration of action of a single dose of a benzodiazepine hypnotic depends on its distribution (e.g., it may concentrate in sites such as adipose tissue, where it exerts no pharmacologic activity) and on elimination and clearance. With repeated administration at a fixed dosing rate, a drug will accumulate in plasma and brain until a steady state is reached. Time necessary to reach a steady-state condition depends only on the drug's elimination half-life. For a drug such as triazolam with a very short elimination half-life, accumulation will be complete within 1 day; that is, the mean plasma concentration will be no higher after multiple days of therapy than after the first day. At the other extreme is a

TABLE 22.1. *Commonly Used Sleep-Promoting Medications*

Drug Name	Initial Dose (mg)	Maintenance Dose (mg)	Drug Interactions
Temazepam[a]	7.5–15	15–30	Combination contraceptives may stimulate glucuronide conjugation of temazepam
Estazolam[a]	1	1–2	Cimetidine decreases the clearance, ketoconazole inhibits CYP 450 3A and 2C family of enzymes
Triazolam[a]	0.125	Usually 0.25	Drugs inhibiting cytochrome P450 CYP 3A such as ketoconazole, itraconazole and nefazodone, erythromycine, cimetidine
Lorazepam[a]	1	1–2	Combination contraceptives may increase glucuronidation; quetiapine reduces the clearance
Alprazolam	0.25	0.5	Drugs that inhibit alprazolam's metabolism via CYP 450 3A including fluoxetine, propoxyphene, diltiazem, isoniazid, macrolide antibiotics; cimetidine
Clonazepam	0.5–1.0	1–2	Cytochrome P450 inducers such as phenytoin, carbamazepine, and phenobarbital cause a 30% decrease in plasma clonazepam levels; inhibitors of P450 family of enzymes, such as oral antifungal agents, should be used cautiously
Chlordiazepoxide[a]	5–10	10–25	Antacids slow absorption; disulfiram inhibits its hepatic metabolism (hydroxylation and dealkylation); ketoconazole reduces its clearance
Zolpidem[a]	5–10	10–20	Potent inducers of CYP 450 3A4 (carbamazepine, phenytoin, rifampicin) reduce its hypnotic effect; ketoconazole causes increased plasma concentrations, SSRIs and zolpidem may lead to delirium
Zaleplon[a]	10	10–20	Drugs that are potent CYP 450 3A4 inducers (rifampin, phenytoin, carbamazepine, phenobarbital) may cause its ineffectiveness, drugs that inhibit both aldehyde oxidase and CYP 3A4 (cimetidine) increase Cmax and AUC by 85%
Amitryptiline[b]	10–25	50	Other antidepressants: SSRIs, type 1C antiarrhythmics
Desipramine[b]	25	50	Anticholinergic and sympathomimetic drugs
Imipramine[b]	25	50	Anticholinergic drugs (excessive anticholinergic effects); MAO inhibitors contraindicated; cimetidine
Nortriptyline[b]	25	25–75	Balcofen—short-term memory loss; barbiturates can increase metabolism of TCAs; TCAs may inhibit the uptake of bethanidine into NE neuron and reduce antiHTN effect; concurrent administration w/ drugs capable of prolonging QT interval is contraindicated; beladonna—potentiation of anticholinergic activity
Doxepin[b]	25	25–50	MAO inhibitors, cimetidine, alcohol, tolazamide (hypoglycemia)
Chloralhydrate[a]	500	500–1000	Increased free levels of phenytoin, initial enhancement of anticoagulation by coumarins b/c of increased free levels; furosemide
Diphenhydramine	25–50	50–100	Enhanced risk for adynamic ileus, urinary retention, chronic glaucoma with tricyclics and other antihistamines

CYP, cytochrome P enzyme; SSRI, selective serotonin reuptake inhibitor; AUC, area under the curve; MAO, monoamine oxidase; TCA, tricyclic antidepressant; HTN, hypertension.

[a]Additive effect of other central nervous system depressants and centrally acting muscle relaxants.

[b]Drugs that inhibit cytochrome P450 2D6 (quinidine, cimetidine, phenothiazines, bupropion and phenothiazines) may inhibit metabolism of TCAs via inhibition of CYP 450 2D6.

Other antidepressants: SSRIs, anticholinergic and sympathomimetic drugs; some TCAs may increase half-life and bioavailability of oral anticoagulants; with amphetamine-like agents-enhanced amphetamine effects; amprenavir may increase serum concentration of TCAs and lead to arrhythmias, due to inhibition of CYP 450 3A4 isoenzyme.

drug such as flurazepam, with its principal active metabolite desalkylflurazepam. This compound has a very long elimination half-life; 2 weeks or more of long-term treatment will be necessary for a steady state to be attained. The rate of drug disappearance following discontinuation after long-term treatment will mirror the rate of accumulation (i.e., the longer the elimination half-life, the more time will be needed for the drug to disappear). A potential benefit of accumulating a benzodiazepine is that persistence of drug at the receptor sites throughout each 24-hour dosing interval increases the likelihood of a daytime anxiolytic effect, a potential benefit for patients with both anxiety and insomnia. For short half-life hypnotics such as triazolam, however, increased daytime anxiety has been reported in some studies, possibly attributable to wide fluctuations in plasma and receptor-site concentrations between doses. Estazolam, a relatively new benzodiazepine, remains effective as a hypnotic for at least 6 weeks of continuous administration at a dosage of 2 mg at bedtime, with no evidence of clinically significant tolerance. It improves sleep latency and total sleep time, reduces the number of nocturnal awakenings, and improves both depth of sleep and sleep quality in adults with chronic insomnia.

Zolpidem is another hypnotic, a benzodiazepine receptor ligand structurally unrelated to benzodiazepines (an omega 1-selective nonbenzodiazepine hypnotic). It has an elimination half-life of 3.5 to 5.1 hours (mean, 4 hours). In young adults, zolpidem leads to a marked increase in slow-wave sleep, with reduction of Stage 2 and no change in REM sleep. In middle-aged patients, there is a reduction of awake time and increase of Stage 2 NREM sleep, without changes in REM sleep.

Zaleplon is a nonbenzodiazepine hypnotic from the pyrazolopyrimidine class. It interacts with the GABA-BZ receptor complex, selectively on omega-1 receptor on the alpha subunit of the GABA A receptor complex. In controlled trials it shortened sleep latency. It is metabolized by aldehyde oxidase and to a lesser degree by CYP450 3A4. Inhibitors of these enzymes may decrease its clearance and enhance sedative/hypnotic effect. Zopiclone, a cyclopyrrolone compound, is another hypnotic that is chemically unrelated to benzodiazepines but is not available in the United States.

Precautions

Patients who are pregnant, who are alcoholic, or who have sleep apnea should not be given hypnotics, except in low doses and only in special circumstances. Preference for benzodiazepines over barbiturates is based on the former's lower toxicity (less respiratory and cardiac depression) and less marked tolerance, rather than on its superior hypnotic effect. The prescribing of hypnotics to children is not recommended, except for rare use in the treatment of night terrors or severe somnambulism. Benzodiazepine metabolism varies and is largely age dependent. The elimination half-life of diazepam in healthy men may increase threefold to fourfold from 20 years of age to 80 years of age. The elimination of hypnotics is decreased in elderly people who might have a low renal glomerular filtration rate, a reduced hepatic blood flow, and a decreased activity of hepatic drug-metabolizing enzymes. The choice of hypnosedatives for elderly patients with sleep-onset delay, especially when they are acutely hospitalized, is complicated by the risk of a paradoxical excitation at nighttime ("sun-downing"), which may be precipitated or exacerbated by medication. Although diphenhydramine has been useful in many of these patients, there is a risk of increasing their confusion because of its anticholinergic effect. These problems can be minimized by adjunctive measures, such as leaving a light on in the patient's room, and by frequently reorienting the patient to the unfamiliar surroundings. A family member occasionally may be required to stay with the patient.

Because of the intrinsic "tapering" effect of long-half-life compounds, rebound and withdrawal phenomena appear to be unlikely; when they do occur, such effects are delayed in onset and are relatively mild. However, there is a much higher likelihood of rebound or withdrawal effect after abrupt discontinuation of short-half-life hypnotics, so dose tapering is appropriate.

Although many of these drugs, especially the benzodiazepines, have been marketed with emphasis on their short duration of action, many have long-acting active metabolites. This is often a problem in the patient who experiences a decrement in liver function. Sedative effects are additive and may convert what would have been a mild metabolic encephalopathy into a coma days after the initiation of treatment.

Alternative Therapies

The most popular and well-studied herbal treatment of depression is St. John's wort (Hypericum perforatum), a remedy used for wound healing, sedation, and pain relief. Its use as a hypnotic has not been studied systematically, but it may promote "deep sleep" and prolong REM latency.

Valerian root (Valeriana officinalis) has been used widely for its hypnotic properties. A limited number of human studies suggest that valerian could be used as a mild hypnotic with minimal side effects. It seems to affect GABA metabolism and reuptake, mainly GABA A receptors, 5HT 1a, and adenosine receptors. Numerous herbs are used in combinations by traditional Chinese medicine. However, there are no well-designed studies to document their effectiveness and safety.

Anxiety disorders often are linked to insomnia. Anxiety may respond to kava kava (Piper methysticum). Its mechanism of action is thought to involve GABA A receptors.

Melatonin is used to reset the clock and help proper positioning of the sleep cycle within a 24-hour period, but it also has a direct sedative–hypnotic effect (the most common doses are 2–10 mg 30 minutes to 2 hours before bedtime). Caution should be exercised in patients with known cardiovascular disease because melatonin reportedly causes vasoconstriction in coronary and cerebral arteries

of rats. Other possible side effects are inhibition of fertility, increased depression or induced depression, suppression of male libido, retinal damage, and hypothermia. Melatonin's interactions with other drugs are not fully understood, which is of particular concern in the elderly population. As with other dietary supplements, there is a concern about purity of the product. Catnip (Nepeta cataria) is used as a "tonic" for sleep, as is chamomile (Marticaria recutita). Several other herbs are used as sleep aids because of their reported sedative effects: gotu cola (Centella asiatica), hops (Humulus lupulus), lavender (Lavandula angustifolia and others), passionflower (Passiflora incarnata), and scullcap (Scutellaria lateriflora). Hepatoxicity was described for scullcap when used in combination with valerian root, but this may have resulted from substitution of a particular herb with species of germander (Teucrium).

The U.S. Food and Drug Administration (FDA) recalled all products of L-tryptophan in the United States, but it still is manufactured worldwide. It has resurfaced in the form of 5-hydroxytryptamine. It was found that the new product contains the same impurities previously found in L-tryptophan responsible for eosinophilia-myalgia syndrome. L-tryptophan also is found in some protein supplements.

RESTLESS LEGS SYNDROME

Insomnia characterized by marked sleep-onset delay may result from RLS because of increasing severity of unpleasant sensations in the limbs when at rest at night. The patient experiences disagreeable deep sensations of creeping inside the calves whenever at rest (sitting or lying down). These dysesthesias cause an almost irresistible urge to move the limbs and thus interfere with the sleep onset. Almost all patients with RLS also have sleep-related PLMs. Coincident PLMs are not required for the diagnosis of RLS. Diagnosis of RLS relies entirely on the patient's symptoms. Revised criteria emphasize the onset of symptoms with rest and a clear circadian pattern to the symptoms. The four essential criteria for the diagnosis have been published and widely accepted:

1. A sensation of an urge to move the limbs (usually legs)
2. Motor restlessness to reduce sensations
3. Onset or worsening of the symptoms when at rest
4. Marked circadian variation in occurrence or severity of symptoms.

Once asleep, approximately 85% of patients with RLS experience PLMs causing numerous arousals and poor quality of sleep. Many patients with RLS experience PLMs while awake (PLMW), especially in sedentary situations. Although total sleep time may be markedly reduced and sleep efficiency is very low, patients with RLS generally do not report sleepiness and/or sleep attacks, but they usually complain of tiredness and not feeling fully alert.

The large majority of patients afflicted by RLS appear to represent idiopathic cases, unrelated to any other medical condition as a possible cause.

Several secondary causes of RLS have been well documented: pregnancy, iron deficiency, and end-stage renal disease. Neuropathies and radiculopathies have been accepted as possible secondary causes of RLS, specifically neuropathy associated with rheumatoid arthritis and diabetes mellitus. Some studies suggest other causes of secondary RLS, including peripheral vascular disease, chronic obstructive pulmonary disease, asthma, and fibromyalgia. RLS prevalence is 5% to 10%. The prevalence increases with age and may be higher in women.

The exact pathophysiology of RLS is unknown. However, several studies suggest subcortical dopamine system's dysfunction, which results in reduction of the spinal and possibly cortical inhibition that may be state dependent. The positron emission tomography and single-photon emission computed tomography studies showed small decreases in dopaminergic function in the striatum of patients with RLS compared to control subjects.

All the clinical conditions (end-stage renal disease, pregnancy) associated with iron deficiency also are associated with RLS. Low brain iron may lead to dopaminergic dysfunction, as documented by decreased D2r, decreased dopamine transporter, and increased extracellular dopamine in rats deprived of iron in early life.

In some cases, restless legs and PLMs are caused or exacerbated by dietary substances (e.g., caffeine) or medications (e.g., neuroleptics and tricyclic antidepressants).

Drug Treatment

Accepted and fairly successful treatments for restless legs and PLMs include dopaminergic drugs, opioids, and some miscellaneous drugs. Treatment choices are the same for primary and secondary RLS. Dopaminergic medications are usually the treatment of first choice (Table 22.2). The dopaminergic agent carbidopa/levodopa (Sinemet) improves all of the features of both RLS and PLM disorder, including discomfort in the legs, involuntary movements during the waking state (dyskinesias while awake), PLMs during sleep, and sleep fragmentation. Side effects include gastrointestinal discomfort, nausea, and vomiting. The phenomenon of augmentation if a higher dose is used consists of increasing intensity of the symptoms, earlier onset of the symptoms in the day, reduced time at rest before symptoms start, and in some cases more widespread dysesthesias and restlessness. The dopaminergic agonists bromocriptine (Parlodel) and pergolide (Permax) have been used successfully. Nasal stuffiness, gastrointestinal discomfort, and especially hypotension are adverse effects of concern. Pergolide also has been reported to cause augmentation, but only in 17% to 25% of patients.

Direct dopamine agonists are very effective therapeutic agents in the treatment of RLS. Pramipexole (Mirapex) and ropinirole (Requip) currently are used as a treatment of choice. Numerous opioids have been used, such as codeine, propoxyphene (Darvon), oxycodone (Percodan), pentazocine (Talwin),

TABLE 22.2. *Medications for Treatment of Restless Leg Syndrome*

Drug Name	Initial Dose	Maintenance Dose (mg)	Drug Interactions
Levodopa[a]	25/100	Up to 300 mg max	MAOI, tricyclics especially in elderly with cardiac disease (reduced L-dopa response, arrhythmias, hypertension); isoniazid; pergolide (dyskinesias); phenytoin (reduced effectiveness)
Bromocriptine[a]	2.5	2.5–10 mg up to 20 mg max	With cyclosporine bromocriptine inhibits CYP 450 3A and increases cyclosporine levels; macrolide antibiotics, clarihomycin, erythromycin inhibit bromocriptine's metabolism; droperidol reduces its therapeutic efficacy
Pergolide[a]	0.05	0.1–0.75 mg up to 1–2 mg max	Other drugs bound to proteins
Pramipexole	0.25	0.25–1.5 mg up to 3.0 mg max	Cimetidine (an inhibitor of renal tubular secretion of organic bases via cationic transport system) caused increased AUC and (half life), other drugs secreted by the cationic transport metabolism, may decrease its oral clearance
Ropinirole	0.25	0.5–3 mg up to 3–6 mg max	Ropinirole is a substrate for CYP 450 1A2, any inhibitor (ciprofloxacin) or inducer of this enzyme may require dose adjustment; estrogens also reduce its oral clearance; dopamine antagonists may reduce its effect
Codeine[b]	15	15–60 mg	Quinidine inhibits CYP 450 2D6 (stops production of morphine); rifampin induces CYP 450 isoenzymes and reduces the effectiveness
Hydrocodone[b]	5–10	Up to max 30 mg	Same as codeine
Hydromorphone[b]	2	3–4 mg	
Morphine[b]	10–30	Up to 60 mg	Somatostatin (?antagonizes analgesic effect); yohimbine enhances analgesic effect; metformin (increased risk for lactic acidosis); MAOIs contraindicated
Oxycodone[b]	10	Up to max 30 mg	Same as codeine
Methadone[b]	5–10	Up to 20–40 mg	Phenytoin, carbamazepine, Rifampin (inducers of CYP 450 3A4 isoenzyme), reduce its levels and even cause withdrawal symptoms; non-nucleoside reverse transcriptase inhibitors (inhibit or induce CYP 450 isoenzymes); fluconazole, fluvoxamine (inhibitors of CYP 3A4 isoenzyme)
Propoxyphene	65	Usually 130 mg	Carbamazepine (CBZ), (propxyphene reduces CBZ's hepatic metabolism), CBZ toxicity metoprolol, propanolol levels rise (inhibition of hepatic metabolism); ritonavir (inhibits propxyphene's metabolism)
Iron (Fe sulphate, Fe gluconate) w/vitamin C	150	150–300 mg	Aluminum-, calcium-, or magnesium-containing products may reduce iron absorption; cholestyramine (reduced iron absorption b/c it binds to iron); ciprofloxacin, levofloxacin (reduced absorption due to chelation); generally decreased bioavailability of quinolone antibiotics due to chelation; levothyroxine (reduced absorption); decreased levodopa absorption

MAOI, monoamine oxidase inhibitor; CYP, cytochrome P enzyme; AUC, area under the curve.
[a]Dopamine antagonists (neuroleptics) are likely to diminish their effectiveness.
[b]Other CNS depressants and centrally acting muscle relaxants; opioid agonist/antagonists (withdrawal symptoms); inducers of CYP 450 isoenzymes may reduce their effectiveness.

levorphanol (Levo-Dromoran), and methadone. Their effectiveness has been tested formally by only a few studies. Open-label trials using gabapentin (Neurontin) demonstrated subjective improvements in many patients with RLS, especially those with pain and/or neuropathy. Although widely prescribed for the treatment of PLMs, clonazepam was not shown to reduce symptoms of RLS, and even reduction of PLMs seems to be small. Ensuring that the patient has adequate body iron stores (to reach a ferritin level of more than 45–50 µg/l) may require oral iron supplementation. Absorption is increased if it is taken on an empty stomach and 60 minutes before a meal.

Alternative Treatments

The behavioral manipulations of avoidance of smoking, certain drugs, and alcohol almost routinely are recommended to patients complaining of insomnia. Avoidance of over-the-counter stimulants such as decongestants with pseudoephedrine, phenylephrine, and appetite suppressants such as phenylpropanolamine are discouraged, especially at bedtime.

Moderate exercise prior to bedtime, vigorous enough to cause release of beta-endorphin, is suggested, preferably before 7 PM. Light calisthenics or stretching for 5 to 10 minutes at bedtime supplements the exercise regimen. Stress reduction (meditation, yoga, and relaxation response) combined with sleep hygiene complements other behavioral techniques.

Distraction or counterstimulation of the legs is another approach. It includes hot foot socks or ice packs; rubbing feet, pounding thighs, or wearing socks to bed. Massage, electrical stimulation, acupuncture, hypnosis, and cognitive therapy add to the repertoire of these approaches. Sclerotherapy, once thought to represent a promising option in patients with varicose veins, is unlikely to alleviate the symptoms, as shown in the Edinburgh vein study. Magnesium is noted to improve PLMs and RLS. Iron supplementation, vitamin E, B_{12}, folate, and B_6 are useful, especially in cases with documented deficiencies. Valerian root and kava kava may be helpful as mild hypnotic–sedative agents.

EARLY MORNING AWAKENING

Early morning awakening can be seen in numerous clinical settings, including depression, use of some drugs, and advanced sleep-phase syndrome. Endogenous depression is characterized by a typical premature awakening and an inability to fall asleep again, with variable sleep-onset disturbance depending on the individual's component of agitation. A key polysomnographic finding is shortened REM sleep latency, which is considered by some experts to be a biologic marker of depression, in addition to an increased intensity of REM sleep. Deep (delta) NREM sleep also is reduced; this is a relatively non-specific feature. In contrast, bipolar depression frequently is associated with hypersomnia; however, this state again is accompanied by a shortened REM latency and reduced Stages 3 or 4 NREM sleep. The onset of sleep is delayed and sleep is short in mania and hypomania. Insomnia may precede all other symptoms of depression, and restoration of sleep may be the first sign of recovery.

In patients with early morning awakening, sedative therapy usually is accompanied by an unacceptable degree of morning sedation. Antidepressants appear to offer the best results and should be the initial form of therapy. Tricyclic antidepressants with sedative properties, such as amitriptyline (Elavil) and trimipramine (Surmontil), reduce sleep latency and improve sleep continuity. Trazodone, a non-tricyclic, also is used widely for treatment of insomnia in patients who are depressed. Although an improvement in sleep often precedes an improvement in mood, changes of affect should determine the endpoint in therapy.

Drug-induced early morning awakening may occur with the use of some short-acting benzodiazepines, such as oxazepam or lorazepam. They are almost completely inactivated by a conjugation in the liver, and they have few residual morning aftereffects. Patients who drink alcoholic beverages prior to sleep may develop early morning awakening, apparently related to an increase in REM sleep ("REM rebound") after the alcohol is metabolized. An underlying psychiatric problem should be considered, as in any patient with an alcohol-related problem. Therapy involves a slow withdrawal of the causative agent.

Advanced-sleep-phase syndrome may mimic a pattern of early morning awakening typical of depression. It is seen most frequently in elderly people. There are no established treatments for this condition, although reverse chronotherapy or exposure to light in the evening accompanied by light deprivation in the morning may be helpful. Either treatment requires the skills of experts in sleep disorders centers.

SLEEP FRAGMENTATION

A major complaint of frequent awakenings at night often signals the presence of a primary sleep disorder, specifically sleep apnea or PLMs. Multiple medical conditions also can interfere with sleep maintenance, whereas psychiatric etiology is a less likely explanation.

In sleep apnea, sleep disruption is caused by cessation of breathing during apneic periods and subsequent frequent awakenings associated with occasional gasping for air or a choking sensation. In most cases, it is predominantly central sleep apnea occurring during sleep. Patients usually report daytime "tiredness," but they do not take naps.

PLM disorder is a condition in which insomnia is associated with the occurrence of periodic episodes of repetitive and highly stereotypical leg jerks during sleep. These are followed consistently by a partial arousal. Patients are often unaware of the movements at night; rather, they report frequent nocturnal awakenings and unrefreshing sleep. A bed partner usually can provide an accurate description of the movements.

Medical conditions that sometimes lead to insomnia include alveolar hypoventilation, which in adults could be secondary to massive obesity; chronic obstructive pulmonary disease; myopathy; cordotomy; or lesions involving structures that control sleep and breathing. Primary alveolar hypoventilation usually is reported in infants and is associated with a further worsening of hypercapnia and hypoxemia in sleep. Gastroesophageal reflux with regurgitation, heartburn, and dyspepsia; nocturnal angina; sleep-related asthma; nightmares; and cluster headaches all may cause a serious insomnia as a result of severe sleep fragmentation. Other medical and neurologic conditions can be associated with this form of insomnia, including CNS infections, head traumas, nocturnal epilepsy, fibrositis syndrome, cardiovascular disorders, pulmonary disease, any painful condition, toxic conditions, and endocrine diseases such as hyperthyroidism and Addison's disease. In these patients, treatment of the underlying disorder can be expected to alleviate the sleep disturbance and thus obviate the need for hypnotics. Hypercortisolism (especially iatrogenic) should be considered if sleep fragmentation is prominent. Parkinsonian patients receiving therapy with levodopa (or carbidopa/levodopa) also are subject to this complaint. Daytime napping frequently is reported. The response to hypnosedatives and tricyclics is unpredictable. Not taking dopaminergic drugs after eating supper is helpful for many patients. Another cause of sleep fragmentation is bruxism (teeth grinding).

WHEN TO REFER THE INSOMNIAC TO A SLEEP SPECIALIST

Primary care physicians and other non-specialists may attempt to treat an acute insomnia, especially if the trigger or the etiology is easily identifiable. The treatments include a short course of hypnotics or simple behavioral interventions (sleep hygiene). When patients present with chronic (more than 6 months) insomnia, it is advisable to refer the patient to the sleep specialist.

SPECIAL CHALLENGES FOR HOSPITALIZED PATIENTS

Anesthesiologists have to be aware of the reactions some of the patients with RLS may develop if given antidopaminergics. The reaction can be severe and look as a "forme fruste" neuroleptic malignant syndrome (crampy stiffness without fever). This is especially likely to occur when patients awaken after they were given droperidol (a potent, long-acting dopamine antagonist) while withdrawing from fentanyl (a potent, short-acting mu-opiate agonist). The timing of this emergency coincides with circadian enhancement of RLS (late afternoon). Recommended substitutes to treat nausea include ondansetron (5HT-3 blocker) and domperidone (large molecule dopamine antagonist, which does not penetrate the blood–brain barrier, but area postrema has none).

Patients with RLS may tolerate the following antipsychotic medications: quetiapine and clozapine. Although many patients have trouble sleeping in the hospital, during hospitalization special attention must be given to subjects with RLS.

SLEEP DISORDERS ASSOCIATED WITH HYPERSOMNOLENCE

Included in this category of sleep disorders associated with hypersomnolence are intrinsic and extrinsic sleep disorders as well as parasomnias and disorders associated with medical/psychiatric disorders. The chief symptoms include an inappropriate and undesirable sleepiness during waking hours, decreased cognitive and motor performance, an excessive tendency to sleep, unavoidable napping, an increase in total sleep over 24 hours ("true" hypersomnia), and a difficulty in achieving full arousal on awakening. The term "hypersomnolence" in a strict sense should be reserved for patients who have a demonstrable tendency to fall asleep in the waking state when sedentary or who have sleep "attacks." There also may be diminished alertness in the waking state, described by the term subwakefulness. In all patients presenting with these symptoms, it is important to separate excessive daytime somnolence from less specific symptoms of fatigue, malaise, or depression.

The major causes of excessive daytime sleepiness are sleep apnea syndrome (43%), narcolepsy (25%), and insufficient sleep.

SLEEP APNEA

A potentially lethal condition, sleep apnea is an abnormal breathing pattern during sleep defined as a cessation of airflow at the level of the nostrils and the mouth, lasting for at least 10 seconds. The estimated prevalence of sleep apnea syndrome ranges from 2% to 4% of the adult population. It is the most frequent diagnosis in sleep disorder centers and the most frequent cause of daytime sleepiness. Apneas are subdivided by type: obstructive or upper airway apnea secondary to a sleep-induced obstruction of the airway (Fig. 22.3); central or diaphragmatic apnea secondary to decreased respiratory muscle activity; and mixed apnea combining both phenomena. Mixed apnea usually starts as a central apnea (with no respiratory effort) and develops into an obstruction later. Either obstructive or central apnea predominates in each patient.

Obstructive sleep apnea (OSA) seems to be caused by a concentric pharyngeal collapse during inspiration and not by an active musculature contraction. Contributing factors may include abnormal anatomic relationships among the muscular or bony structures of the nasopharynx, oropharynx, or hypopharynx (e.g., a short thick neck, macroglossia, a relatively small and low-positioned hyoid bone, or a narrow pharynx). Alternatively, inappropriate involuntary respiratory control of the pharyngeal and diaphragmatic muscle tone may be responsible. Occasionally patients demonstrate increased compliance of their pharyngeal walls, especially when they have fatty or redundant pharyngeal and submucosal folds. Finally, patients may develop OSA because of abnormal amounts of inspi-

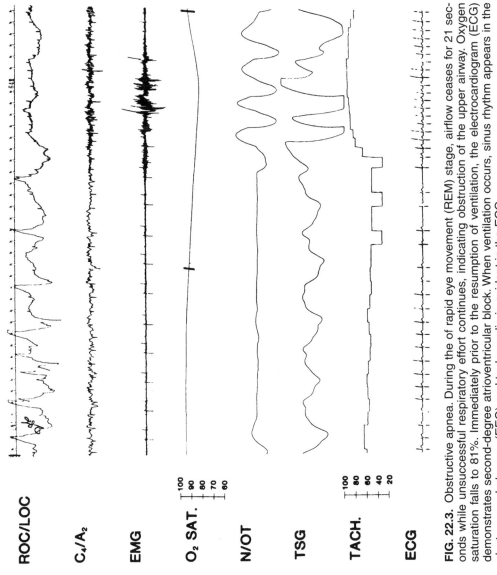

ROC/LOC

C₄/A₂

EMG

O₂ SAT.
- 100
- 90
- 80
- 70
- 60

N/OT

TSG

TACH.
- 100
- 80
- 60
- 40
- 20

ECG

FIG. 22.3. Obstructive apnea. During the of rapid eye movement (REM) stage, airflow ceases for 21 seconds while unsuccessful respiratory effort continues, indicating obstruction of the upper airway. Oxygen saturation falls to 81%. Immediately prior to the resumption of ventilation, the electrocardiogram (ECG) demonstrates second-degree atrioventricular block. When ventilation occurs, sinus rhythm appears in the electroencephalogram (EEG) and tachycardia is evident in the ECG.

ratory intraluminal negative pressure. Although many patients with OSA are moderately overweight, morbid obesity is present only in a minority. These apneas are more prevalent with increasing age and worsen after alcohol or sedative drug intake. Important features in the clinical history often best confirmed by interviewing the bed partner are loud snoring and observed respiratory pauses, excessive daytime sleepiness, and restless sleep with frequent awakenings. On examination, a large neck circumference (>17" in males and >16" in females) and micrognathia and retrognathia should suggest the diagnosis of OSA. Objective confirmation of the diagnosis is made with a sleep study that records oxymetry, breathing effort, and airflow.

Waking respiratory functions are usually within normal limits. Hypertension has been reported in 48% to 96% of patients with OSA. Alveolar hypoventilation, associated with an elevated waking $PaCO_2$, occasionally accompanies OSA. Increased $PaCO_2$ of 45 mm Hg or higher has been reported in 23% of obese patients with OSA. Marked cyclic sinus arrhythmia appears during sleep apnea. This rhythm pattern is characterized by progressive sinus bradycardia during apnea (heart rates of less than 30 beats/minute are not uncommon) with an abrupt reversal and sinus acceleration at the onset of ventilation. Second-degree atrioventricular block, prolonged sinus pauses, limited runs of ventricular tachycardia, and paroxysmal atrial tachycardia episodes also occur. Furthermore, systemic and pulmonary artery pressures increase in association with obstructive apneas. About 22% to 30% of patients with systemic hypertension were found to suffer from OSA. Although both conditions are also more frequent in men and obese people, the association of hypertension and OSA seems to be independent of obesity. When episodes of apnea occur in rapid succession, pressures do not return to baseline but show a stepwise increase. Apneas are more prevalent with increasing age and worsen following alcohol or sedative drug intake.

Central sleep apnea is not a single disease entity but results from any one of a number of processes that produce instability of respiratory control. In contrast to patients with OSA, these patients are older (i.e., their mean age is 63 years as opposed to 46 years); they complain mainly of sleep fragmentation; they are not overweight; and they have less pronounced oxygen desaturation and a more moderate hemodynamic impact. There is no definite sex distribution.

Upper airway patency does not need to be fully compromised for symptoms of daytime sleepiness to develop. The upper airway resistance syndrome is accompanied by subjective and objective evidence of pathologic sleepiness. In some individuals, even a minor reduction of airway patency with sleep onset may lead to a modest increase in upper airway resistance and a slight decrease of tidal volume without hypoxemia. In response to increased resistance, inspiratory muscles increase their effort to maintain normal tidal volume. This compensatory increase in respiratory effort usually triggers a brief alpha EEG arousal (3 to 14 seconds in duration), interrupting further development of obstruction before oxygen desaturation occurs. If the alpha EEG arousals are frequent, clinically significant daytime sleepiness may arise. Snoring is noted in most, but not all, of these individuals.

Both central and OSA can be a complication of another medical or neurologic disorder, including brainstem infarction, lateral medullary syndrome, bulbar poliomyelitis, medullary neoplasms, syringomyelia and syringobulbia, olivopontocerebellar atrophy, Alzheimer's disease, encephalitides, Creutzfeldt–Jakob disease, postencephalitic parkinsonism, cervical cordotomy, neuromuscular disorders affecting intercostal muscles and the diaphragm (such as myasthenia gravis), higher cervical spinal poliomyelitis, Guillain–Barré syndrome, limb–girdle dystrophies, and especially myotonic dystrophy. Hypoventilation and daytime drowsiness are prominent in all of these disorders. Predominantly OSA may result from enlarged tonsils (an especially important factor in the etiology of sleep apnea and snoring in children), myxedema, micrognathia and other facial and mandibular abnormalities, platybasia, neck infiltration secondary to Hodgkin's disease and lymphoma, acromegaly, and familial or acquired dysautonomia (usually mixed central and OSA).

Of special interest is the development of postpolio syndrome years after the acute stage of poliomyelitis. It starts with fatigue, new muscular weakness, musculoskeletal pain, and dysphagia. During sleep, patients experience central and obstructive sleep apnea, which is worse during REM sleep because of the combined REM sleep–induced atonia and abnormal motor (phrenic) output caused by medullary dysfunction. Poliomyelitis also can cause atrophy of respiratory accessory muscles and thoracoabdominal muscles, leading to severe chest deformity such as kyphoscoliosis. Furthermore, impairment of cranial motor nerves (hypoglossal, facial, and trigeminal) may adversely affect tongue and other upper airway muscles. As a consequence, all types of apneas may occur. These patients are vulnerable to develop respiratory failure with acute respiratory infection and may require

assisted ventilation in intensive care units until the infection is controlled.

The evaluation of patients suspected of having sleep apnea syndrome includes a history obtained not only from them but also (and most important) from their bed partner. A physical examination should concentrate on blood pressure, evidence of right heart failure, and abnormal skeletal and muscle configurations of the face and neck. The ear, nose, and throat examination is of primary importance. Chest radiographs and electrocardiograms are useful for evaluating pulmonary hypertension, determining the status of the right and left ventricles, and establishing possible coexistence of other cardiopulmonary disorders. A hemogram documents the presence of polycythemia. Pulmonary function studies may be necessary to investigate for primary hypoventilation during the waking state and responsiveness to CO_2 stimulation. These studies should be followed by an all-night polysomnographic study, which is essential for an accurate diagnosis and an estimation of the severity of oxygen desatura-

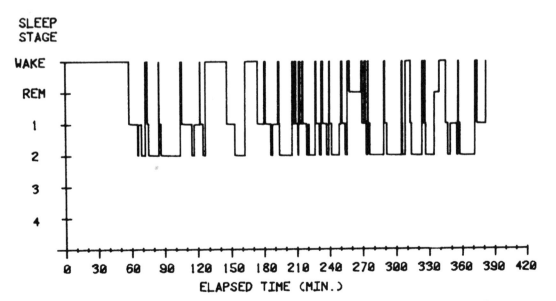

FIG. 22.4. The sleep architecture of an adult man with obstructive sleep apnea syndrome. Stages 3 and 4 are lacking; frequent arousals occur, which fragment the sleep cycle; rapid eye movement (REM) sleep is much reduced as a proportion of the sleep period; and REM periodicity is abolished. The majority of the sleep period consists of non–rapid eye movement (NREM) Stages 1 and 2.

tions. The severity of sleep apnea, defined by the so-called apnea-hypopnea index (i.e., the number of episodes per hour of sleep), the degree of oxygen desaturation, and the presence of significant arrhythmias will be derived from sleep study and will guide future treatment (Fig. 22.4).

Treatment of Sleep Apnea

The treatment of sleep apnea syndromes depends on its cause (Table 22.3). An important general treatment is weight loss, the only potentially curative measure for overweight apneics, provided the loss of weight is not only achieved but also maintained. Similarly, abstinence from alcohol and avoidance of hypnosedative drugs and beta blockers are advocated.

Pharmacologic approaches including acetazolamide, theophylline, naloxone, medroxy-

TABLE 22.3. *Treatment Options for Sleep Apnea*

Continuous Positive Airway Pressure Treatments
Nasal or Oral Positive Airway Pressure
  (NCPAP or OPAP)
Bi-Level Positive Airway Pressure (BIPAP)
Self-adjusting Positive Airway Pressure (Auto-PAP)
Oral Appliances
Pharmacologic agents (medroxyprogesterone, decongestants, nasal steroids, antihistamines, protryptiline, and serotonergic agents: fluoxetine and other selective serotonin reuptake inhibitors, L-tryptophane)
Behavioral interventions (weight loss, avoidance of alcohol and sedatives, avoidance of supine sleep position, discontinuation of smoking)
Surgical Procedures
Bypass surgery: tracheostomy
Upper airway reconstructions:
  Soft-tissue modifications
  (Uvulopalatopharyngoplasty [UPPP], laser-assisted UPPP [LAUP], somnoplasty, radiofrequency volumetric reduction of the tongue, laser lingual resection—lingualplasty, tongue base suspension, tonsillectomy)
  Skeletal modifications (mandibular osteotomy with genioglossal advancement and hyoid suspension, maxillomandibular osteotomy and advancement, hyoid myotomy and suspension to mandible, hyoid myotomy and suspension to thyroid cartilage, anterior hyoid advancement, transpalatal advancement pharyngoplasty, nasal surgery)

progesterone, and clomipramine have not been studied systematically on large numbers of subjects. The only widely used drug is protriptyline, which may exert a beneficial effect in an occasional patient with OSA. Its effect may be the result of a reported direct action on the muscle tone of the upper airway. A recent crossover unblinded trial of protriptyline and fluoxetine suggests equal effectiveness of either drug, with about 30% to 50% of patients showing improved oxygenation during sleep.

A number of studies suggest that the administration of oxygen may be a useful method of treating central sleep apnea, although the mechanism by which it reduces central apneic events has not been established. It is hypothesized that the potential destabilizing influence of the hypoxic ventilatory response on respiratory control may be counteracted by the administration of oxygen. However, in some cases, hypercapnia and the frequency of OSA may increase.

The most widely used treatment of OSA is nasal continuous positive airway pressure (CPAP), which acts by establishing a "pneumatic splint" to the upper airway. The key element of its effect is that it causes elevation of the pressure in the oropharynx, thus reversing the transmural pressure gradient across the oropharyngeal airway.

Nasal CPAP is the only treatment as effective as tracheostomy. The major reasons for CPAP failure are poor compliance for social or cosmetic reasons and nasal obstruction. Some patients whose apneas are eliminated with CPAP continue to have non-apneic desaturations, especially during REM sleep. Usually, these patients are obese, with chronic obstructive pulmonary disease in addition to sleep apnea. In such situations, supplemental oxygen may be beneficial. The benefits derived from oxygen treatment should be polysomnographically verified.

Bilevel positive airway pressure (BiPAP) offers an effective alternative for patients who are uncomfortable while expiring against the high pressures delivered by CPAP. This device allows independent titration of expiratory and inspiratory airway pressure and has been very helpful in cases of comorbid obesity, intrinsic lung disease, and chest deformity, conditions associated with hypoventilation.

Sometimes, correction of nasal obstruction can result in significant reduction of sleep apneas. Adenoidectomy, tonsillectomy, and surgical correction of the maxillofacial anomalies will abolish apneas. Patients with serious mandibular deformities can undergo surgical procedures such as maxillary, mandibular, and hyoid bone advancement, but a significant number of failures occur, primarily in patients with the most severe mandibular deficiencies.

Attempts to promote uvulopalatopharyngoplasty (UPPP) as an alternative surgical treatment of sleep apnea have not been successful. Multiple studies indicate at best a variable success rate, ranging from 33% to 70%. The success rate may improve somewhat, provided selection of patients is based on the determination of the level of obstruction prior to the surgery. More encouraging are results of UPPP in the treatment of snoring. A 75% to 100% success rate for the elimination of snoring has been reported, which is not unexpected because structures generating the sounds of snoring are surgically removed. This may be misinterpreted as a sign of apnea cure, but the apneas may persist despite the disappearance of snoring. Laser-assisted uvulopalatoplasty, involving partial resection of the uvula and soft palate using a laser, is a simple surgical procedure that can be done on an outpatient basis in two to seven sessions without general anesthesia. It seems highly effective in eliminating habitual snoring, with success rates from 70% to 84%. The American Sleep Disorders Association, however, does not recommend this procedure for treatment of sleep apnea. Prosthetic devices focus on the nasopharyngeal inlet and position of the base of the tongue. The only two devices tested in a sleep lab for their effectiveness are a tongue-retaining device (TRD) and Snore-Guard (Hayes & Meade, Inc., Albuquerque, NM). TRDs are most effective in patients demonstrating positional apnea who are not excessively obese (BMI >35 kg/m^2). For some positional apneics, just being trained to sleep on their sides may be an effective cure.

An association between OSA and cardiovascular disease was recognized early. Several groups have reported a significant relation between blood pressure and the frequency of apneas and hypopneas. Hla and colleagues found that OSA was a risk factor, independent of concomitant obesity, for the development of hypertension. In contrast to a decrease in blood pressure during non-REM sleep in nonapneic individuals, in patients with OSA, blood pressure increases during non-REM sleep. OSA can aggravate or precipitate myocardial ischemia in patients with coexisting coronary artery disease. Abolition of OSA by CPAP led to dramatic improvements in the left-ventricular ejection fraction and cardiac functional status in patients with idiopathic dilated cardiomyopathy and congestive heart failure using the CPAP for more than 1 month. Nocturnal CPAP treatment of Cheyne–Stokes respiration in patients with congestive heart failure led to significant improvements in cardiac function and quality of life. PSMG should be considered an integral part of the diagnostic evaluation of patients with cardiovascular disease because treatment of concomitant sleep-disordered breathing with CPAP can lead to an improvement in cardiovascular function, particularly in patients with congestive heart failure.

In summary, although significant progress in evaluation and treatment of sleep-disordered breathing has been made, the exact etiology and pathophysiologic mechanism(s) currently are unknown. Sleep-disordered breathing has a profound effect on health. The range of sequelae varies from sudden death or cor pulmonale to failure to thrive or to perform at work and school. If unrecognized, lifelong problems may arise.

NARCOLEPSY

Narcolepsy is a syndrome consisting of excessive daytime sleepiness and abnormal manifestations of REM sleep. The latter includes frequent sleep-onset REM periods, which may be subjectively appreciated as hypnagogic hallucinations, and dissociated REM sleep-inhibitory processes (i.e., cataplexy and sleep paralysis). The appearance of REM sleep within 10 minutes of sleep onset is considered evidence for narcolepsy. In narcolepsy, the patient falls asleep in the midst of activities, although most people will stay awake during animated conversation, walking, eating, or coitus.

The cardinal symptoms are excessive daytime sleepiness, sleep attacks, and cataplexy. Although sleep attacks are characteristic of this disease, excessive sleepiness is equally disturbing (i.e., a permanent, sometimes profound, impairment of vigilance or wakefulness between attacks). Sleep attacks usually last about 15 minutes. The patient awakens refreshed, and there is a definite refractory period of 1 to 5 hours before the next attack. Cataplexy is a sudden decrease in, or abrupt loss of, muscle tone that either is generalized or limited to particular muscle groups. Cataplexy ranges from weakness in the muscles supporting the jaw, or a sense of weakness in the knees, to a complete muscular weakness causing the patient to slump to the floor, unable to move. Cataplectic attacks characteristically are initiated by laughter, surprise, outbursts of anger, or a feeling of exaltation. These attacks generally last for only a few seconds or for as long as 30 minutes.

An auxiliary symptom of narcolepsy includes sleep paralysis, which occurs while the patient is falling asleep or waking from sleep. Consciousness is preserved, and it is accompanied by an intense feeling of fear. Hypnagogic hallucinations also occur at the onset of sleep or on awakening, and they are usually frightening. Automatic behavior, sometimes reported as a "blackout," is a reflection of severe sleepiness. Nocturnal sleep also is disturbed with frequent awakenings, frequent sleep-onset REM periods, and vivid dreams. The combination of excessive daytime sleepiness and cataplexy is pathognomonic for narcolepsy.

The diagnosis of narcolepsy is based on the following:

1. History of excessive daytime sleepiness, sleep attacks, cataplexy, and other auxiliary symptoms
2. Objective documentation of pathologic sleepiness by the Multiple Sleep Latency test (MSLT), showing a mean sleep latency of 5 minutes or less
3. Two or more sleep-onset REM periods
4. Nocturnal REM latency shorter than 20 minutes and nocturnal sleep latency shorter than 10 minutes

Nocturnal polysomnography is used mainly to rule out other etiologies of excessive daytime sleepiness (sleep apnea, PLMs).

More than 85% of all narcoleptics with definite cataplexy share a specific human leukocyte antigen (HLA) allele, HLA DQB1-0602 (most often in combination with HLA DR2), compared to 12% to 38% of the general population in various ethnic groups. DQB1-0602 may represent a genetic marker for the disorder, indicating the presence of the possible narcolepsy-susceptibility gene on chromosome 6. A negative test for DQB1-0602 does not rule out diagnosis of narcolepsy because a rare narcoleptic patient with cataplexy may be DQB1-0602 negative. Only 8% to 10% of narcoleptics are aware of another member of the family with narcolepsy/cataplexy. Prevalence studies have shown that the risk for a first-degree relative of a patient having narcolepsy with cataplexy is 1% to 2%. Usually, patients with narcolepsy can be reassured that the illness will not develop in their relatives. However, a 1% to 2% risk is 10 to 40 times higher than the prevalence observed in the general population, suggesting the existence of genetic predisposing factors. Twin studies demonstrated only a 25% to 31% concordance rate for narcolepsy in monozygotic twins. Genetic factors are defining susceptibility, but other (environmental) factors may trigger the onset of the disease. Although almost all diseases associated with the specific HLA allele are autoimmune in nature, an extensive search for known general markers (cerebrospinal fluid [CSF] oligoclonal bands, serum immunoglobulin levels, lymphocyte subset ratios) of autoimmune activation was negative.

However, as postulated by Mignot in 1995, the possibility of autoimmune cell destruction in a small part of the brain has become more likely in light of the discovery of the hypocretin system and its crucial role in the development of narcolepsy.

Genetic canine narcolepsy has been shown to be caused by mutations in the hypocretin-2 receptor gene. Almost simultaneously another group reported on the phenotype of the pre-prohypocretin (the precursor to two peptides: hypocretin-1 and hypocretin-2) knockout mice. The homozygous mice were observed to have numerous periods of "behavioral arrests." Twenty-four hour EEG recordings revealed an increased amount of sleep during the dark period, reduced REM latency, and sleep-onset REM periods. Thus, a mouse model of narcolepsy with cataplexy was discovered.

Both discoveries prompted intense research in humans. Hypocretin-containing neurons are localized in the dorsolateral hypothalamus around the perifornical nucleus. In humans, the number of hypocretin-containing neurons is estimated to range from 15,000 to 20,000 to 50,000 to 80,000. These cells project widely to the entire brain: cerebral cortex, basal forebrain structures, such as the diagonal band of Broca; the amygdala; and the brainstem areas such as reticular formation, raphe nuclei, and locus coeruleus. Human narcolepsy is believed generally not to be the result of gene mutations, but hypocretin neurotransmission is impaired. CSF content of hypocretin-1 (hcrt-1) was evaluated in patients with classical MSLT results and cataplexy. Very low hcrt-1 levels were found in the CSF of patients with narcolepsy, predominantly those with cataplexy. The results suggest that a hypocretin deficiency is involved in the pathogenesis of narcolepsy. A neuropathologic study was completed on six brains from narcoleptic patients and eight from control subjects. Hcrt-1 and hcrt-2 levels were mea-

sured. Both hcrt-1 and hcrt-2 were absent in the brains of narcoleptic patients, even in the pons, where hypocretin concentrations are very high in control subjects. Another study confirmed the results on four narcoleptic patients and documented increased number of astrocytes in the hypothalamus, indicating neuronal degeneration there. These neuropathologic studies document a loss of hypocretin production in the brains of patients with narcolepsy.

Treatment of Narcolepsy

Treatment of narcolepsy comprises treatment of the two most disabling symptoms of narcolepsy: excessive daytime sleepiness/sleep attacks and cataplexy (Tables 22.4 and 22.5).

In the rare patient, successful treatment involves only improved sleep hygiene, as previously described. Most patients, however, will need stimulants, primarily dextroamphetamine (Dexedrine) or methylphenidate (Ritalin). Stimulants enhance the release and inhibit the reuptake of catecholamines and, to a lesser extent, serotonin in the CNS. Stimulants are likely to reduce but not eliminate excessive daytime sleepiness and performance deficits. Methamphetamine (Desoxyn) in doses higher than those recommended for treatment of obesity was found to normalize sleepiness and performance in eight subjects studied, but it rarely is used because of concerns about abuse and related adverse behaviors.

Side effects often limit the use of stimulants. The dose-related clinically significant side effects include irritability, agitation, headache, and peripheral sympathetic stimulation. Stimulants may be associated with dependence. A novel wake-promoting agent, modafinil (Provigil) usually is grouped with stimulants but seems to have a different mechanism of action that is not fully understood at present time. Unlike amphetamines and methylphenidate, modafinil does not appear to significantly alter the release of dopamine or norepinephrine. Although it does

TABLE 22.4. *Wake-Promoting Drugs for Treatment of Excessive Daytime Sleepiness*

Drug Name	Initial Dose	Maintenance Dose	Drug Interactions
Dextroamphetamine	5 mg	5–60 mg	Because it is an indirect-acting sympathomimetic, may precipitate HTN crisis if taken with MAOI; with beta blockers may produce severe HTN, arrhythmias with tricyclics; may diminish the effectiveness of the antiHTN drugs; may delay absorption of phenobarbital, ethosuximide, phenytoin.
Methylphenidate	5–10 mg	10–60 mg	May decrease hypotensive effect of guamethidine. May inhibit metabolism of coumarin anticoagulants, some anticonvulsants, phenylbuthazone, and tricyclic drugs. Safe use with clonidine and other alpha-2-agonists has not been systematically evaluated.
Methamphetamine	10 mg	10–50 mg	MAOIs contraindicated; may decrease hypotensive effect of guanethidine; insulin requirement may be changed; phenothiazines antagonize stimulant effect of the amphetamines.
Modafinil	100–200 mg	200–400 mg	Coadministration of potent CYP 450 3A4 inducers (carbamazepine, phenobarbital, rifampin) or inhibitors of CYP 450 3A4 inhibitors (ketoconazole, itraconazole) could alter modafinil's levels. It is a very modest CYP 3A4 inducer (cyclosporine, steroidal contraceptive clearance may increase). Because it is a reversible inhibitor of CYP 2C19 (used for alternative metabolism of tricyclics) in patients deficient in CYP 2D6 the levels may rise.
Selegiline	10 mg	10–40 mg	Stupor, muscle rigidity, hyperpyrexia with meperidine, and MAOIs (severe agitation, hallucinations, and death). Severe toxicity w/tricyclics and SSRIs.
Sodium oxybate	4.5 g in 2 doses	3–9 g	Other CNS depressants and centrally acting muscle relaxants (benzodiazepines, opioids, barbiturates, ethanol, etc.)

HTN, hypertension; MAOI, monoamine oxidase inhibitor; CYP, cytochrome P enzyme; SSRI, selective serotonin reuptake inhibitors.

not stimulate release of norepinephrine directly, it does require an intact alpha-adrenergic system for its stimulant effect to occur. The advantage of modafinil over other stimulants is lower frequency and severity of side effects, especially less irritability and agitation; however, if it is titrated rapidly, headache may emerge. Selegiline (monoamine oxidase [MAO] B inhibitor), combined with a low tyramine diet, also improves daytime sleepiness. Sodium oxybate (Xyrem), a drug recently (2002) FDA-approved for treatment of cataplexy in patients with narcolepsy, seems to have a beneficial effect on daytime sleepiness as well.

Tricyclic antidepressants are very effective treatment for cataplexy. Cataplectic attacks respond to imipramine (Tofranil), nortriptyline (Pamelor), and protriptyline (Vivactil). One of the most effective drugs for treatment of cataplexy is clomipramine (Anafranil), a triglyceric with a potent serotonin-uptake inhibitor. Side effects, mainly resulting from their anticholinergic properties, may limit the use of tricyclics. The most frequently reported side effects are dry mouth, increased sweat-

TABLE 22.5. *Anticataplectic Medications*

Drug Name	Initial Dose	Maintenance Dose	Drug Interactions
Imipramine	10 mg	10–100 mg	See Table 22.1.
Nortriptyline	25 mg	25–75 mg	See Table 22.1.
Protriptyline	5 mg	5–40 mg	See Table 22.1.
Clomipramine	25 mg	50–150 mg	Interactions same as for other TCAs; combination with tranylcypromine is particularly hazardous and the serotonin syndrome developed with concurrent use of moclobemide.
Fluoxetine	20 mg	20–80 mg	It inhibits CYP 450 2D6 isoenzyme; this may require reduction of the dose of concomitant medication; thioridazine is contraindicated b/c of potential fatal arrhythmias; elevations of carbamazepine, phenytoin, tricyclics, clozapine levels were observed; also some benzodiazepine levels rose; sumatriptan—weakness, incoordination, hyperreflexia; other tightly protein-bound drugs (warfarin, digitoxin).
Paroxetine			Weakness and hyperreflexia if used with almotriptan; inhibition of TCA metabolism in some people—it is an inhibitor of CYP 450 2D6 and may inhibit other P450 isoenzymes including CYP 3A4; its metabolism can be inhibited by bupropion; cimetidine may increase serum concentrations of paroxetine via inhibition of CYP 450 metabolism of paroxetine; serotonin syndrome with MAOI—concurrent use contraindicated; increased serum concentration of clozapine with SSRIs; cyproheptadine reduces its effectiveness by antagonizing postsynaptic serotonin
Sertraline	25 mg	Usually 50–100 mg	Combination with other CNS drugs was not studied systematically; potential interaction with other drugs tightly bound to proteins (warfarin, digoxin) may result in increased levels; cimetidine led to significant increases in AUC and prolonged half life
Citalopram	20 mg	20–60 mg	Substrate for CYP 450 3A4 and 2C19, is expected to interact with potent inhibitors of CYP 450 3A4 (ketoconazole, itraconazole, and macrolide antibiotics), and potent inhibitors of CYP P450 2C19 (omeprazole), but no clinically significant interactions observed; increased metoprolol levels; sumatriptan in combination resulted in weakness, hyperreflexia and incoordination
Sodium oxybate	4.5 g in 2 divided doses	3–9 g	See Table 22.3.

TCA, tricyclic antidepressant; CYP, cytochrome P enzyme; MAOI, monoamine oxidase inhibitors; SSRIs, selective serotonin reuptake inhibitors; AUC, area under the curve.

ing, sexual dysfunction (impotence, delayed orgasm, erectile dysfunction, and ejaculation dysfunction) weight gain, tachycardia, constipation, blurred vision, and urinary retention and xerostomia. Sudden discontinuation of tricyclics is likely to result in severe worsening of cataplexy and even status cataplecticus. Newer antidepressants with more exclusive inhibition of serotonin uptake (e.g., fluoxetine [Prozac], paroxetine [Paxil], and sertraline [Zoloft]) are useful alternatives in the man-

agement of cataplexy, with fewer anticholinergic side effects. The anticataplectic effects of these drugs are most likely related to their desmethyl metabolites, which are potent adrenergic uptake inhibitors. An FDA-approved drug for treatment of cataplexy is sodium oxybate (Xyrem). Published and reported data indicate its powerful effect in control of cataplexy, improvement of sleep quality, and reduction of daytime sleepiness. Side effects are mild (nausea, vomiting, dizziness, enuresis, dream abnormality, headache), and the drug is generally well tolerated. Patients refractory to other treatments sometimes may require the use of MAO inhibitors.

Improvements observed with the use of L-tyrosine, codeine, or propranolol have not been documented in controlled trials. When sleep fragmentation is a major complaint, judicious use of short-acting hypnotics once or twice per week may be helpful. Significant improvement of nocturnal sleep with sodium oxybate (Xyrem) was reported in double-blind, placebo-controlled trials.

Pharmacologic approaches are generally not entirely satisfactory, and many patients benefit from social support provided by Narcolepsy Network and other similar organizations.

Alternative Wake-Promoting Agents

Caffeine is a mild stimulant derived from the seeds, leaves, or fruits of 60 plant species. These plants are sources of caffeine for beverages such as coffee (Coffea arabica, Coffea canephora) or black or green tea (Camellia sinensis). Kola (Kola acuminata), guarana (Paullinia cupana), and mate (Ilex paraguariensis) are sources of caffeine for cola and other citrus beverages.

Herbal medicinal products containing caffeine include herbal teas, antioxidant green tea preparations, and weight loss formulations. Weight loss preparations often combine caffeine with ephedrine-containing products. Caffeine enhances alertness presumably via antagonism of the adenosine receptors. Ephedra is the source of ephedrine, an over-the-counter compound used for treatment of asthma. Ephedrine also is used and abused for energy, weight loss, and body building. Lesser known sources of ephedrine or related compounds are Indian sida (Sida cordifolia) and bitter orange (Citrus aurantium), sometimes found in energy or weight loss preparations. Ginseng (Panax ginseng–Korean ginseng) is a substance used to counteract fatigue (mild stimulant) or enhance performance. Siberian ginseng (Eleutherococcus senticosus) is used

to enhance physical endurance and work capacity. There is no known herbal treatment for cataplexy.

INSUFFICIENT SLEEP

Insufficient sleep is a frequent cause of daytime somnolence. The individual is voluntarily, but often unwittingly, chronically sleep deprived. Although this relationship may seem self-evident, most patients are unaware that their chronic sleep deprivation is responsible for their continuous excessive sleepiness. When these individuals obtain adequate sleep, their complaint of somnolence during the day disappears.

Various other medical and medicinal causes of excessive daytime somnolence deserve mention. Hypnosedatives, anticonvulsants, antihypertensives, antihistamines, and antidepressants are common causes. A withdrawal from stimulants also may give rise to severe sleepiness. Multiple medical and toxic conditions may be associated with drowsiness: hyperglycemia (prior to ketoacidosis or nonketotic coma), hypocortisolism, hypoglycemia, hypothyroidism, panhypopituitarism, hepatic encephalopathy, hypercalcemia, renal insufficiency, vitamin B_{12} deficiency, chronic subdural hematoma, encephalitis, intracranial neoplasm (primary or secondary), meningitis, or the aftereffects of trauma. Hypersomnolence is a misnomer in many of these conditions because more often a state of obtundation occurs. There are also two rare periodic disorders of excessive sleepiness: (a) Kleine–Levin syndrome, characterized by recurrent periods of extended sleep, megaphagia, sexual disinhibitions, and social withdrawal if awake, and (b) menstruation-associated hypersomnia, a period of sleepiness during a patient's menstrual period (without observed changes in behavior).

When to Refer the Patient with Hypersomnia to the Sleep Specialist

Excessive daytime sleepiness is most frequently the result of sleep deprivation, poor sleep hygiene, and prescribed or non-prescribed drugs. However, it is often a life-threatening symptom in situations requiring full vigilance (driving, operating machinery, combat, etc.). Primary care physicians are advised to use short (one-page) screening questionnaires in their outpatient offices because the patients often do not volunteer the information. If the screening is positive, the patient should be referred for the evaluation and workup in the Sleep Center. Of particular importance is quick and proper diagnosis and treatment of the sleep disorders accompanied by severe sleepiness (OSA, narcolepsy) in professional drivers.

Special Challenges for Hospitalized Patients

Of all types of hypersomnolence, sleep apnea poses prominent challenges to hospital personnel who may not be familiar with patients carrying this diagnosis. No consensus exists regarding perioperative care and monitoring of patients with sleep apnea. For a patient with diagnosed sleep apnea, useful guidelines include optimizing all associated medical conditions before elective surgery and using local or required anesthesia without sedation or narcotic use whenever possible. When "light" monitored anesthesia care is used (versed, propofol, fentanyl), prolonged observation in postanesthesia care units should be used. When "heavy" generalized anesthesia is used, the CPAP/BiPAP used at home should be contained perioperatively. Patients should be monitored postoperatively with telemetry/pulse oximetry, and often intensive care admission is advised. Patients with the following are especially at risk and require extreme vigilance: heavy narcotic requirement, severe sleep apnea (based on sleep study/clinical suspicion), and severe systemic manifestations. These patients should be observed in the intensive care unit.

PARASOMNIAS

Parasomnias, which include a heterogeneous group of behavioral disturbances that occur only during sleep or are exacerbated by sleep, do not have a common pathophysiologic mechanism. They represent disorders of arousal, partial arousal, and sleep-stage transitions. Disorders of arousal (confusional arousals, sleep walking, and sleep terrors) all arise from NREM sleep, usually delta sleep; can be triggered by forced arousal from delta sleep; and are prevalent in childhood. Arousals from delta sleep are characterized by confusion, disorientation in time and space, and slow speech and mentation. These confusional arousals usually occur in children and may progress into sleepwalking (somnambulism) or sleep terror (pavor nocturnus, incubus). Typically there is very little if any recall for the event the following morning and minimal if any recall of dreamlike mentation. Most somnambulistic episodes last a few seconds to a few minutes. A sleep terror is an arousal from NREM sleep accompanied by a piercing scream or cry and behavioral manifestations of intense anxiety indicating autonomic arousal. Autonomic manifestations include mydriasis, perspiration, piloerection, rapid breathing, and tachycardia. Morning amnesia for the episode is the rule. There are several groups of factors contributing to the occurrence of disorders of arousal. They include predisposing factors (genetic factors), factors causing increased amount of delta sleep or difficulty awakening (age, recovery from prior sleep deprivation, fever, CNS depressant drugs, etc.), and factors causing sleep fragmentation (pain, environmental stimuli, stimulants, stress, etc.).

There is often a concurrence of more than one of these disorders in the same child, and a hereditary predisposition to parasomnias has been noted. Somnambulism in children is not considered to be caused by psychologic factors, although its persistence into adulthood may represent a serious problem and occasionally may be associated with diverse forms of personality disturbance and psychopathology. Most children grow out of this condition between the ages of 7 and 14 years. It is important to protect patients against injury by, for example, installing safety rails at the head of stairways and placing locks on windows. If predisposing and triggering factors are identified, every effort should be made to minimize or avoid them. Many patients respond to benzodiazepines: triazolam, clonazepam (0.5–2.0 mg) and diazepam (5–10 mg) in the usual evening doses. Tricyclic drugs, such as imipramine, desipramine, and clomipramine in the doses of 10 to 50 mg, also may be effective.

Sleep-related enuresis is involuntary micturition beginning usually during deep NREM sleep in an individual who has or should have voluntary waking control of the bladder. In contrast to this idiopathic nocturnal enuresis, symptomatic enuresis is the result of urogenital or other diseases and is generally less benign. Idiopathic enuresis and somnambulism tend to disappear by late childhood or adolescence, probably representing a phenomenon of delayed maturation. At 5 years of age, 15% of boys and 10% of girls are enuretic. Recommended treatment includes tricyclic antidepressants (e.g., imipramine, 25–75 mg at bedtime [approximately 1.0–1.5 mg/kg/day]) and daytime bladder exercises aimed at increasing bladder capacity. Oxybutynin chloride (Ditropan) has been used with variable success. Intranasal desamino-D-arginine vasopressin (Desmopressin) at low doses has been shown to have a definite effect, especially in children older than age 9 years and adults. Conditioning with a buzzer and pad is the most successful treatment for enuresis, but success may depend on continued use of the buzzer.

A nightmare is an arousal from REM sleep with the recall of a disturbing dream, accompanied by anxiety and much less prominent autonomic arousal. The awakened patient instantly is oriented and alert. Vocalization, fear, and motor activity are less intense than in sleep terrors. Nightmares are more likely to occur in the second half of the night, when more prolonged REM episodes are likely to occur. Withdrawal from alcohol, amphetamines, or hypnotics may lead to REM sleep rebound and cause nightmares.

REM sleep behavior disorder (RBD) is a parasomnia characterized by vigorous motor activity, instead of atonia, in response to dream content, often resulting in an injury. Manifestations of acting out dreams include laughing, talking, chanting, singing, yelling, swearing, gesturing, reaching, grabbing, arm flailing, punching, kicking, sitting up, jumping out of bed, crawling, and running movements. One-third of people with RBD have a demonstrable underlying neurologic disorder:

Degenerative: amyotrophic lateral sclerosis, dementia, demyelinating disorder, Parkinson's disease, progressive supranuclear palsy, multiple system atrophy, olivopontocerebellar degeneration, etc.
Developmental/congenital/familial: narcolepsy, Tourette's syndrome, etc.
Vascular: subarachnoid hemorrhage, vasculitis, ischemia, etc.
Tumor: acoustic neuroma, pontine neoplasm
Postinfectious: Guillain-Barré syndrome

Most of the cases, however, are idiopathic and tend to occur in the elderly. Transient RBD has been seen in association with acute drug intoxications and withdrawal states. Clonazepam (initial dose 0.5–1.0 mg) is the drug of choice for treatment of RBD. Anecdotal reports suggest effectiveness of desipramine, levodopa, clonidine, L-tryptophan, gabapentin, MAO inhibitors, and melatonin.

Parasomnias also include a cluster headache and the related (but more chronic) condition of paroxysmal hemicrania. Cluster headaches occur in REM sleep and may be related to an increased cerebral blood flow during REM sleep. About 45% of patients with seizure disorders have seizures mainly during sleep. Generalized seizures are markedly activated by NREM sleep; specifically, generalized tonic–clonic seizures are most common during Stages 1 and 2 NREM sleep. Partial seizures may occur during NREM and REM sleep. Prolonged EEG monitoring may be necessary in some difficult cases when a diagnosis of epileptic (as opposed to nonepileptic) episodic behavior is needed.

Sleep-related eating disorder may occur in association with OSA, somnambulism, daytime eating disorders, medication abuse; it may occur in isolation. A sleep-related eating disorder is characterized by almost nightly eating and weight gain that patients attribute to the nocturnal eating. Most patients are only partially conscious during the eating episode. Two-thirds of patients with this condition are women who generally are concerned about the weight gain. Daytime binge eating or obsessive–compulsive disorder is absent. Treatments include clonazepam (Klonopin), carbidopa/levodopa (Sinemet), and fluoxetine (Prozac).

Other parasomnias that may occur in childhood as well as in adulthood include bruxism, head banging (jactatio capitis nocturna), abnormal swallowing, and painful penile erections. Whether these conditions require a polysomnographic evaluation and treatment depends entirely on the persistence of the symptoms and the degree of the patient's disability.

Alternative Treatments

There are no alternative treatments, other than anecdotal reports of alarms triggered by assumption of an erect posture, presumably accomplishing an awakening. If fully awake the patient is less likely to be exposed to injury, consume undesirable food, or the like.

When to Refer the Patient with Parasomnia to the Sleep Specialist

Age, frequency, and the type of parasomnia should guide the non-specialist to refer the patient. In childhood usually the parents are initiating the referral because the events could be dramatic and the parents are overconcerned about the safety of their child.

USE OF SLEEP LABORATORIES AND EVALUATION OF IMPOTENCE

The examination of nocturnal penile tumescence during sleep represents a useful tool for the evaluation of impotence. Sleep-related erections are inconsistent with organic impotence—impotence is more likely to be psychogenic in nature if sleep-related erections are normal. Attention should be paid to a careful drug history because many drugs have the potential to cause an impairment of erectile mechanisms.

QUESTIONS AND DISCUSSION

1. A 23-year-old man presents with a chief complaint of "narcolepsy." His history indicates the presence of sleep attacks, cataplexy, sleep paralysis, and hypnagogic hallucinations for the last 4 years. He states he has never been treated for the disorder and recognized his problem from reading about narcolepsy in a magazine. The neurologic examination is normal. The physical examination reveals a nervous man with a heart rate of 102 beats/minute but otherwise normal vital signs. The remainder of the physical examination is normal. A routine complete blood count, SMA-25, electrocardiogram (ECG), and chest x-ray film are normal. A thyroid battery is within normal limits. Management at this point would consist of:
   A. Prescription of D-amphetamine, 5 mg three times daily
   B. Administration of D-amphetamine in combination with a tricyclic antidepressant
   C. Routine all-night PSMG
   D. Urine screening for amphetamine metabolites
   E. Scheduling for a series of daytime naps in the sleep laboratory

The answer is (D). The usual practice is to screen the urine for amphetamine metabolites before doing a more involved study. It is usually a bad sign to have a patient who knows the classic symptoms of narcolepsy and maintains he has never been diagnosed or treated. In most cases of narcolepsy, excessive daytime sleepiness and sleep attacks are initial symptoms of the disease, whereas associated symptoms develop later. A patient with all components of the syndrome early in the course of the disorder is subject to suspicion. Once urine samples are known to be "clean," all-night PSMG and nap studies are useful to establish the diagnosis. If a patient is suspected of covert stimulant use, a prolonged period of abstinence should be documented before assuming that an REM-onset sleep episode is narcolepsy (because the same pattern may appear as part of stimulant withdrawal). Empiric therapy with stimulants is a practice that should be avoided.

2. A 36-year-old schoolteacher is referred for an evaluation of excessive somnolence. The patient states that he feels extremely drowsy unless he is actively involved in a novel behavior. The problem has been present for at least 3 years but seems to be getting worse. He has fallen asleep at the wheel of his car twice in the last 6 months. He denies a significant history of alcohol ingestion and is not taking medications. The physical examination reveals a large (1.6-m, 82-kg) individual with normal vital signs. The physical and neurologic examinations are normal. After leaving the room to answer a call, you return to find the patient sleeping. A routine blood count reveals a hemoglobin of 17 g/dl, with normal indices and white blood cell count. Biochemical screening is normal. A routine ECG is normal. Thyroid hormone levels and cortisol determinations are unremarkable. A reasonable differential diagnosis at this point would include:

A. Sedative drug abuse
B. Narcolepsy
C. Sleep apnea
D. Depression
E. Idiopathic hypersomnia

Which of the following studies might be of value in evaluating these possibilities?

A. EEG
B. CT of the head
C. MRI of the brain
D. All-night PSMG study, with respiratory and cardiac monitoring
E. Urine drug screen
F. Diagnostic psychiatric interview
G. A series of daytime naps in the sleep laboratory
H. An empiric trial of D-amphetamine without additional testing

First part: all of the above.
Second part: D, E, F, G.

This is a fairly typical history—it lacks the important details that would help clarify the diagnostic possibilities: history of snoring, cataplectic episodes or episodes of sleep paralysis, episodic amnesia, morning headache, or a family history of a similar problem. Any of the possibilities could be entertained from this history. The patient's weight and sex make sleep apnea statistically more likely, but sedative drug abuse is too frequently a cause of this symptom to overlook it as a possibility. Our usual approach is to screen for sedatives, then to proceed with an all-night PSMG, with respiratory and cardiac monitoring. If the results are negative, daytime naps are studied the following day to exclude narcolepsy. The studies in answers (A), (B), and (C) are rarely of any value in evaluating these patients. In this particular case, an all-night PSMG documented the presence of a severe OSA with associated cardiac arrhythmias. The elevated red blood cell count appeared to be a secondary complication of nocturnal apnea.

3. A 71-year-old man is receiving carbidopa/levodopa for Parkinson's disease. After 2 years of therapy, he complains of severe insomnia and daytime somnolence. By history he awakens at 2 AM each night and cannot return to sleep before 4 AM. He falls asleep at 11 PM with no difficulty. Each day he finds it necessary to take one or two 1-hour naps. His wife complains that he often awakens the household during the night with loud screams. The patient is not aware of this behavior and denies any abnormal dreams. This history reflects:

A. Probable dementia in association with Parkinson's disease
B. Psychotic depression
C. A side effect of chronic dopaminergic therapy
D. An unrelated sleep disorder

Management would include:

A. Administration of a hypnosedative before retiring
B. Antidepressant therapy
C. All-night sleep study
D. Discontinuation of antiparkinsonian medications

E. Restriction of antiparkinsonian medications, avoiding administration in the evening

The answer to the first part is (C). Although there is some debate on the relationship of dementia to sleep disruption in this patient group, symptoms usually clear when dopaminergic therapy is stopped. In most cases, continued therapy is necessary, and in these patients, avoiding drug administration after 6 PM often improves the insomnia and daytime napping. Nightmares in patients receiving levodopa appear to arise out of Stage 2 sleep, and patients are frequently amnestic for the episodes. Furthermore, REM sleep behavior disorder may have developed. Hypnosedatives and antidepressants are unpredictable in their response in these patients and frequently exacerbate the complaint. In most cases, answer (E) seems to be the most appropriate management.

4. You are consulted by a 23-year-old man who described episodes of "amnesia." On several occasions, he has found himself at various locations with no recollection of having traveled to them. He recollects being at another location hours before; his memory for previous events is good, and he denies any other symptoms preceding the attack. Observers have seen him during an episode, and he appeared distracted but carried on social conversations appropriately and on one occasion drove a car without incident. He appears relatively stable, and attacks occur in situations that seem devoid of any emotional importance. The patient does not drink alcohol. The neurologic examination is normal. A sleep-deprived EEG without sedation is read as normal, although it is noted that drowsiness is followed quickly by the onset of low-voltage fast activity. Biochemical studies including a 6-hour glucose tolerance test are all normal. An MRI of the brain is normal. Empiric therapy with phenytoin (100 mg three times daily) leads to worsening of the symptoms. Your differential diagnosis at this point should include:

A. A pseudoseizure

B. Narcolepsy–cataplexy syndrome

C. Somnambulism

D. Recurrent transient global amnesia

E. Sleep apnea syndrome

F. Complex partial seizure

G. Amnestic migraine

The appropriate answers are (B) and (E). The episodes described are typical of "automatic behavior" syndrome. This behavioral abnormality is associated with the appearance of "microsleep" episodes, which electroencephalographically are Stage 1 sleep. Sleep apnea and narcolepsy are associated with this disorder. Although the diagnosis of complex partial seizures is difficult to rule out on the basis of a normal EEG, the adverse response to empiric anticonvulsants is more typical of an "automatic behavior" syndrome. Transient global amnesia presents a similar clinical picture but is an entity restricted to late middle life; frequent recurrences are unusual in this syndrome. Somnambulism is a similar phenomenon but is more frequent in childhood and arises from a period of normal sleep; it is usually a Stage 4 sleep event. Psychiatric disorders frequently are present in adults with somnambulistic disorders.

Amnestic migraine may produce recurrent amnestic episodes but usually does so in the presence of more typical migrainous episodes. There is some question of whether this is a sui generis disorder or this represents the coexistence of two phenomena in a single individual.

Pseudoseizures rarely are characterized by global amnesia and are usually situationally related.

Appropriate management in this case would include an all-night PSMG followed by the Multiple Sleep Latency test the next day as well as a routine 16-channel EEG. A careful history-taking directed specifically toward cataplexy, daytime napping, nocturnal apnea, and snoring would help in a differentiation of the underlying condition. Treatment with amphetamine is usually not entirely successful. Hypnosedatives, anticonvulsants, and diazepam usually cause worsening of the symptoms. In patients with sleep apnea of any cause, proper medical or surgical management has been reported to alleviate this symptom complex.

SUGGESTED READING

Ancoli-Israel S, Roth T. Characteristics of insomnia in the United States: results of the 1991 National Sleep Foundation survey. I. *Sleep* 1999;22 (Suppl.2):S347–S353.

Bootzin RR, Perlis ML. Nonpharmacologic treatment of insomnia. *J Clin Psychiatry* 1992;53(6)(Suppl):37–41.

Bradley TD, Hall MJ, Ando S, et al. Hemodynamic effects of simulated obstructive apneas in humans with and without heart failure. *Chest* 2001;119:1827–1835.

Chemelli RM, Willie JT, Sinton CM, et al. Narcolepsy in orexin knockout mice: molecular genetics of sleep regulation. *Cell* 1999;98:437–451.

Diagnostic Classification Steering Committee. *International Classification of Sleep Disorders: Diagnostic and Coding Manual.*Rochester, MN: American Sleep Disorders Association, 1990.

Edinger JD, Fins AI. Sullivan RJ, et al. Comparison of cognitive-behavioral therapy and clonazepam for treating periodic limb movement disorder. *Sleep* 1996;19:442–444.

Findley L, Unverzagt M, Guchu R, et al. Vigilance and automobile accidents in patients with sleep apnea or narcolepsy. *Chest* 1995;108 (3):619–624.

Fletcher EC. Invited review: physiological consequences of intermittent hypoxia: systemic blood pressure. *J Appl Physiol* 2001;90:1600–1605.

Friedman M, Tanyeri H, La Rosa M, et al. Clinical predictors of obstructive sleep apnea. *Laryngoscope* 1999;109:1901–1907.

Guilleminault C, Stoohs R, Quera-Salva MA. Sleep-related obstructive and nonobstructive apneas and neurologic disorders. *Neurology* 1992;42(Suppl 6):53–60.

Guilleminault C, Chowdhury S. Upper airway resistance syndrome is a distinct syndrome. *Am J Respir Crit Care Med* 2000;161:1412–1413.

Hanly PJ. Mechanisms and management of central sleep apnea. *Lung* 1992;170(1):1–17.

Hla KM, Young TB, Bidwell T, et al. Sleep apnea and hypertension: A population-based study. *Ann Intern Med* 1994;120:15–19.

Hornyak M, Voderholzer U, Hohagen F, et al. Magnesium therapy for periodic leg movements-related insomnia and restless legs syndrome: an open pilot study. *Sleep* 1998; 21:501–505.

Hudgel DW. Treatment of obstructive sleep apnea: A review. *Chest* 1996;109(5):1346–1358.

Kales A, ed. *The pharmacology of sleep.* New York: Springer-Verlag, 1995.

Lin L, Faraco J, Li R, et al. The sleep disorder canine narcolepsy is caused by a mutation in the hypocretin (orexin) receptor 2 gene. *Cell* 1999;98:365–376.

Montplaisir J, Boucher S, Poirier G, et al. Clinical, polysomnographic, and genetic characteristics of restless legs syndrome: A study of 133 patients diagnosed with new standard criteria. *Mov Disord* 1997;12:61–65.

Montplaisir J, Nicolas A, Denesle R, et al. Restless legs syndrome improved by pramipexole. *Neurology* 1999;52: 938–943.

Morin CM. *Insomnia: psychological assessment and management.* New York: Guilford Press, 1993.

Morin CM, Hauri PJ, Espie CA, et al. Nonpharmacologic treatment of chronic insomnia. An American Academy of Sleep Medicine review. *Sleep* 1999;22:1134–1156.

Ondo W. Ropinirole for restless legs syndrome. *Mov Disord* 1999;14:138–140.

Phillips B, Ancoli-Israel S. Sleep disorders in the elderly. Review. *Sleep Med* 2001;2:99–114.

Pierce MW, Shu VS. Efficacy of estazolam: The United States clinical experience. *Am J Med* 1990;88(Suppl 3A):6S–11S.

Powell NB, Riley RW, Robinson A. Surgical management of obstructive sleep apnea syndrome. *Clin Chest Med* 1998; 19:77–86.

Shahar E, Whitney CW, Redline S, et al. Sleep-disordered breathing and cardiovascular disease: cross-sectional results of the Sleep Heart Health Study. *Am J Respir Crit Care Med* 2001;163:19–25.

Sherin JE, Shiromani PJ, McCarley RW, et al. Activation of ventrolateral preoptic neurons during sleep. *Science* 1996;271:216–219.

Strollo PJ Jr, Sanders MH, Atwood CW. Positive pressure therapy. *Clin Chest Med* 1998;19:55–68.

Thase M. Depression, sleep and antidepressants. *J Clin Psychiatry* 1998;59(Suppl 4):55–65.

The U.S. Xyrem Multicenter Study Group. A randomized, double-blind, placebo-controlled, multicenter trial comparing the effects of three doses of orally administered sodium oxybate with placebo for the treatment of narcolepsy. *Sleep* 2002;25:42–49.

U.S. Modafinil in Narcolepsy Multicenter Study Group. Randomized trial of modafinil for the treatment of pathological somnolence in narcolepsy. *Ann Neurol* 1998;43:88–97.

U.S. Xyrem Multicenter Study Group. A 12-month, open-label, multicenter extension trial of orally administered sodium oxybate for the treatment of narcolepsy. *Sleep* 2003;1:31–35.

Walters AS. Toward a better definition of the restless legs syndrome. The International Restless Legs Syndrome Study Group. *Mov Disord* 1995;10:634–642.

Wing YK. Herbal treatment of insomnia. *HKMJ* 2001;7; 392–402.

Winkelman JW. Clinical and polysomnographic features of sleep-related eating disorder. *J Clin Psychiatry* 1998;59: 14–19.

Young T, Palta M, Dempsey J, et al. The occurrence of sleep-disordered breathing among middle-aged adults. *N Engl J Med* 1993;328:1230–1235.

23

Eye Signs in Neurologic Diagnosis

James A. Goodwin

This chapter is intended as a survey of visual signs and symptoms that are of use for localization and etiologic diagnosis in neurologic disease. The organization of the chapter reflects both anatomic and functional classifications, and in all cases the close relation between anatomic and physiologic details and a practical clinical diagnosis is drawn. This chapter includes a discussion of the afferent or sensory visual system, the pupillomotor system, and the oculomotor system. The localizing value of examining the visual systems for lesions of the cerebral hemispheres, brainstem, spinal cord, and peripheral anatomic pathways is emphasized.

AFFERENT (SENSORY) VISUAL SYSTEM: SENSORY OR MOTOR?

It seems so simple to refer to one part of the visual system as afferent and another as efferent or oculomotor, but the two parts must function together to such an extent that the separation is artificial, although it is useful in a practical sense.

Man is a foveate animal, which means that retinal morphology and function are not uniform throughout—they are specialized for high-resolution vision in a small central area called the fovea, or pit. The special architecture of the retina at the fovea and the immediate surrounding region, the macula lutea (so-called because of its concentration of yellow pigment), underlies its capacity to resolve fine detail in the visual scene.

The general structure of the retina is such that groups of photoreceptors are connected by bipolar cells to a ganglion cell that provides input to the central nervous system (CNS) by way of its axon. This basic arrangement is complicated by a host of horizontal interactions mediated by other cells in the retina.

A roughly circular array of photoreceptors that send input to a ganglion cell is referred to as the receptive field of that ganglion cell. Light captured by one of the photoreceptors within a receptive field can signal to the ganglion cell only that a visual event has occurred within its receptive field, not where in the field the photon has been captured. In areas of the retina where receptive fields are large and many hundreds of photoreceptors are connected to a single ganglion cell, the capacity for fine spatial resolution is poor. At the fovea, where there are only a few photoreceptors in the receptive field of a ganglion cell, the spatial resolution is very fine.

For example, consider two points of light near the foveal representation of the visual field (called the fixation area). These are likely to activate two photoreceptors that are connected to different ganglion cells, thus signaling the presence of two separate lights. The same two points of light at a peripheral position in the visual field would likely activate two photoreceptors connected to the same ganglion cell. The only information provided to the CNS is that light is on somewhere within that receptive field. Because there are two spots of light, the encoded brightness is greater than if only one spot were present, but information on the spatial distribution of the spots is lost.

For us to see an object clearly, the image of the object must be positioned on the fovea (an act that involves the oculomotor system interacting intimately with the afferent visual system). The afferent system must perceive that a potentially interesting object exists in the peripheral visual field and then must provide coordinates for the motor system to turn the eye so the image of that object is on the fovea. There are stages in this process that are neither clearly visual (afferent) nor motor (efferent)—they are in between. Our concepts of sensory and motor are inadequate in this grey zone between taking information in and putting it out in the form of executive or motor commands. This activity possibly takes place somewhere in the higher-order visual centers of the occipitoparietal convexity. Bilateral lesions in this region produce a clinical syndrome in which there is an unraveling of the afferent and the efferent command structure. Balint called it optic ataxia, and the syndrome now bears his name. Patients who have Balint's syndrome have special difficulty in directing their gaze in an orderly manner to scan or palpate an extended visual scene. The world for them is a fragmentary and disordered array of images, none organically articulated in a meaningful way. This perceptual difficulty can be shown to accompany a disorder of motor scanning behavior. The patient acts as though the coordinates by which to direct his gaze have been scrambled. As an example, these patients lose the highly learned and orderly scan path used by normal viewers to investigate a human face, using many fixations on areas of high information such as the eyes, nose, mouth, and brows. Instead, these patients shift their line of gaze aimlessly, often fixing on low-information areas such as an ear or a bit of hair. They fail to conceive of the object as a human face in the course of this random scanning. It can be shown that the basic afferent function, including visual acuity and visual field, are normal when tested in the usual way. Although large scenes are synthesized improperly, small objects that can be encompassed in a single fixation are recognized correctly. These patients should be tested with pictures of objects that can be shown in both small and large versions to demonstrate this special difficulty of spatial synthesis with preserved visual acuity and visual field. Visual field testing may be particularly difficult in these patients because of their inability to simultaneously perceive two points in the field. When they are aware of the central fixation

point, they fail to respond to the peripheral target; however, when they lose the fixation point, they can see the peripheral target with near-normal sensitivity. This facet of the disease has been called simultanagnosia or amorphosynthesis. Some review articles provide a broader treatment of these disorders of higher cortical visual function (Caplan, 1980).

These brief introductory remarks on the shady limits of the sensory and motor visual systems serve to promote a sense of mystery about vision. This is certainly appropriate at these limits and at every stage of visual processing. Even the retina is poorly understood in all its physiologic aspects. The neural signal that is conducted to the lateral geniculate body is highly processed even at this early stage. We are only beginning to learn the complexity of visual disorders that originate from retinal disease.

The more usual disorders of the afferent visual system and the standard office methods for testing them now will be examined. The following discussion is aimed at the practicalities of office or bedside testing without further discussion of the controversies that might be involved. The information can be considered "safe" in that it has been in common clinical usage for a long time and has proved its reliability for localizing and etiologic diagnosis.

TESTING VISUAL ACUITY

Visual acuity as tested with Snellen's optotypes is probably the best-known and most widely used visual examination. It is important to realize, however, that some conditions are poorly characterized by visual acuity testing. These conditions are diseases in which the early manifestations involve loss of the peripheral visual field. Glaucoma and papilledema are notable examples. Even total hemifield defects do not degrade the visual acuity unless they are bilateral; thus all the hemianopic disorders from lesions behind the optic chiasm cannot be characterized adequately by acuity testing.

In neuroophthalmology, reduction of central visual acuity is an important sign of optic nerve disease. The fact that visual acuity also is degraded by several other conditions unrelated to nerve function is unfortunate for diagnostic purposes. Optical blur from improper refraction is a common one, but clouding of the ocular media by corneal opacity, by cataract, or by blood or other debris in the vitreous is also a consideration. In addition, visual acuity is reduced by amblyopia ex anopsia, which is the practically permanent visual defect that accompanies childhood strabismus or early-life anisometropia (unequal refractive error in the two eyes). The differential diagnosis of poor visual acuity also includes retinal disorders that affect the macula (another broad category of diseases).

All the clinical features of a case are important to establish a diagnosis of optic nerve disease as the cause of reduced visual acuity. Once the diagnosis is established, visual acuity is the most useful and the most universally used test for following the course of optic nerve disease. Visual field examination also is required in this regard and must be used as a complement to acuity determination in the follow-up of optic neuropathies.

The ophthalmologist usually measures acuity in an examination lane, a long testing room in which letters of calibrated size are projected on a screen that the patient views. The original letters were made to be viewed at a distance of 20 feet, but the economics of office building construction have led to modifications. The commercially available projection devices can be made to project the letters small enough to make a valid test at viewing distances as short as 10 feet, and mirrors can be used to test a patient in even more cramped conditions.

An optical supply company representative should be consulted for instructions on how to set up a regular eye lane in an office. Non-ophthalmologists will probably not wish to purchase an expensive projection system for occasional use; however, inexpensive wall-mounted reading charts are available for use at various reading distances from 10 to 20 feet. Adequate lighting must be provided, and standard ceiling fluorescent lights are usually sufficient.

THE NEAR CARD

Most non-ophthalmologists, including neurologists, internists, and family physicians, test visual acuity on a near card, which is intended for viewing at 14 inches (a comfortable reading distance). The distance from eye to card should be measured if the near card is the only acuity measurement used. Once the examiner gets used to the distance, he or she usually can judge it without measuring.

Some other features need attention to make the near card approximately equivalent to a formal testing lane. The light must be sufficient and should be provided either by good fluorescent lights from the ceiling or by a bright lamp that can be positioned to illuminate the card without shining into the patient's eyes. This is not difficult to provide in the office, but hospital beds are seldom well lighted. It is best to carry a bright handlight that provides illumination even for bedside testing. The best handlights are the Finoff heads, which are angled bulb carriers that attach to the battery handle of the ophthalmoscope. Penlights seldom stay bright, and most have uneven zones of illumination. The handlight is especially useful for testing near-card acuity because the beam can be positioned to indicate which set of letters you want the patient to read. The handlight should not be held too close, however, because the diminished contrast of the spotlighted letter makes it difficult to see. It is best to create an elliptical zone that illuminates one entire line of letters by shining the handlight onto the card from one side. Oblique illumination also eliminates glare from the surface of the card.

Proper refraction is mandatory regardless of the method used to test visual acuity. Reduced acuity from needing glasses is of no neurologic interest and creates a great deal of confusion on hospital charts. A brief discussion of lenses and refraction follows. A basic understanding of these optical principles is useful for anyone planning to do visual acuity testing or a field examination, although the non-ophthalmologist will not actually be doing refraction.

LENSES AND REFRACTION

Light travels in a straight line through a homogeneous refractive medium such as air, glass, transparent plastic, or water. When light encounters an interface between refractive media of different density, its path is bent. A sheet of plate glass with flat parallel surfaces, however, does not alter the path of entering light. Light rays are bent as they enter the glass from air, but they are bent back to an equal degree as they go from the glass into air on the other side (Fig. 23.1A). Flat (plano) glass does not, therefore, alter the vergence of light.

A glass wedge bends light rays toward the base (Fig. 23.1B, C), but parallel entering rays remain parallel on exit. These pyramids are useful optical devices called prisms that often are used to measure eye deviation by shifting images to meet the line of sight of a deviated eye. Wide-based prisms bend light more than narrow-based ones (Fig. 23.1B, C), and quantitative units called prism diopters can be used to measure this degree of deviation. The patient views a small light while the examiner introduces prisms of increasing power in front of one eye. The patient specifies the amount of eye deviation by telling the examiner when the false image from the deviating eye overlies the centered (foveated) image from the other eye (the power of the prism needed to do this provides the measure of deviation).

Lenses are defined as refractive objects that change the vergence of light—light rays that enter parallel will be non-parallel when they emerge at the other side. A convex lens causes convergence of light rays and is called a positive or plus (+) lens; an upright image is created at the focal plane behind the lens, or on the side opposite the object, and is called a real image (Fig. 23.2A). A concave lens produces a divergence of light rays and is called a negative or minus (−) lens; the object is imaged inverted at the focal plane in front of the lens, or on the same side as the object, and is termed a virtual image (Fig. 23.2B). Figures 23.A and B illustrate parallel rays of light from an infinitely distant point source of light rather than rays emanating from an object with dimensions. They do not illustrate the upright or inverted quality of images. Cylin-

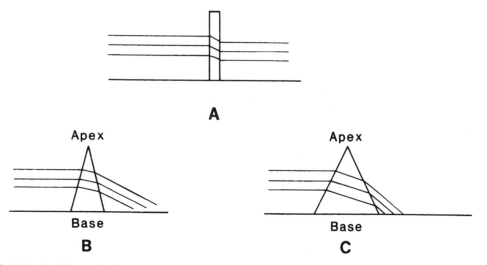

FIG. 23.1. A: The path of light through flat (plano) glass. Parallel rays enter from the left, exit parallel to the right, and the *vergence* of light is not changed. **B:** A *prism* bends light toward its base (*down* in the figure). Parallel rays remain parallel, and the vergence of light is not changed. **C:** A "stronger" prism has a broader base and a less acute angle at the apex. It bends light more drastically than the "weaker" prism in **B.**

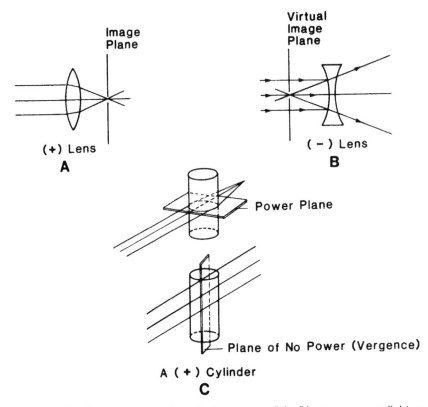

Image Plane

(+) Lens

A

Virtual Image Plane

(–) Lens

B

Power Plane

Plane of No Power (Vergence)

A (+) Cylinder

C

FIG. 23.2. Lenses alter the vergence of light. **A:** A convex or "plus" lens converges light rays to a focal point in the *image plane* on the side opposite the light source, which is the *object plane*. **B:** A concave or "minus" lens causes *divergence* of light rays. A "virtual" image is formed on the same side of the lens as the source of light rays in the object plane. **C:** Light rays converge through a "plus" or convex cylinder in the *power plane (upper figure)* and remain parallel as they pass through the cylinder in a plane orthogonal to the power plane *(lower figure)*.

drical lenses act as lenses in one plane and as plano or flat non-lenses in a plane orthogonal to the first plane (Fig. 23.2C). A plus (+) cylinder converges light rays in its plane of power and a minus (−) cylinder diverges rays in this plane. A person whose natural optical system—the cornea, aqueous humor, crystalline lens, and vitreous humor—creates a focused image of an infinitely distant point on the fovea is emmetropic (Fig. 23.3A).

Ametropia refers to a significant deviation from emmetropia. A nearsighted person, or myope, brings the image of a distant point to focus in front of the retina (Fig. 23.3B) and needs a concave or diverging lens to move the focal point of an infinitely distant point back to the retina (Fig. 23.3D). A hyperope, or far-

sighted person, creates a focused image of an infinitely distant point behind the retina (Fig. 23.3C) and needs a convex or converging lens to move the focal plane forward to the surface of the retina (Fig. 23.3E). The natural optical system of a person with astigmatism has varying power in different planes and requires a cylindrical lens to correct the aberration (not illustrated in Fig. 23.3).

Once a person has achieved the focus of distant objects, either naturally or through spectacles or contact lenses, he or she must alter the power of the crystalline lens of the eye to maintain focus for objects nearer than infinity. Specifically, the plus (+) power of the eye's crystalline lens must be increased to focus on objects near the eye. Contracting

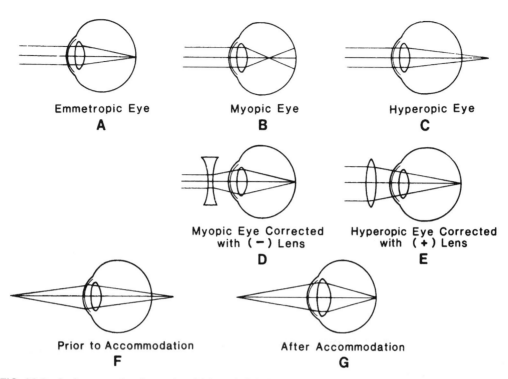

Emmetropic Eye **A** **Myopic Eye** **B** **Hyperopic Eye** **C**

Myopic Eye Corrected with (−) Lens **D** **Hyperopic Eye Corrected with (+) Lens** **E**

Prior to Accommodation **F** **After Accommodation** **G**

FIG. 23.3. A: An emmetropic eye in which an infinitely distant point source of light is imaged on the retina by the natural refractive media of the eye (cornea, aqueous, lens, vitreous). **B:** A myopic eye in which an infinitely distant point source of light is imaged in front of the retina. **C:** A hyperopic eye in which an infinitely distant point source of light is imaged behind the retina. **D:** A myopic eye corrected with a minus lens. The lens superimposes divergence on the overconverged light rays and moves the focal plane back to the retina. **E:** A hyperopic eye corrected with a plus lens. The lens superimposes convergence on the overdivergent light rays and moves the focal plane forward to the retina. **F:** A point source of light near the eye produces divergent rays entering an emmetropic eye as in **A.** Without the act of accommodation, the refractive power of the eye is unchanged and the rays are brought to a focal plane behind the retina. In **G**, the crystalline lens has become more convex or has increased its plus power by virtue of ciliary muscle contraction. The near source of divergent rays now is imaged on the retina because of the added convergent power that results from the act of *accommodation.*

the ciliary muscle, which increases the convexity of the lens, does this. This process is called accommodation. The power of accommodation is lost progressively with age: when a person reaches his mid 40s, he or she needs an additional plus lens to correct for this normal condition, which is called presbyopia. Emmetropes (normal focus for distant objects), as they become presbyopes, usually require reading glasses that they take off for distant viewing (the images of distant objects are blurred to the emmetrope wearing his reading glasses). Those individuals who constantly must look from near to far in the course of daily activities require half eyes (i.e., those narrow glasses that ride low on the nose) or bifocals with no correction in the upper segment. Moderately nearsighted (minus distance refraction) presbyopes may simply take off their distance glasses to read at 14 inches—this is what nearsighted means. Highly nearsighted people have their natural focus at distances shorter than 14 inches. Although they can see clearly at such a distance, they usually find it too close for comfortable reading. These people may have bifocals in which the lower segment is still minus but less minus than the upper segment. The relative plus power needed for near vision is added arithmetically to the distance refraction.

This information will help the non-ophthalmologist ensure that the patient is optimally corrected for an assessment of visual acuity, either in a distance lane or on the near card. The presbyopic patient always should use reading glasses or the bifocal segment when testing is done on the near card. The poor acuity that results from uncorrected presbyopia is not interesting in a neurologic assessment and creates great confusion when it is noted in the patient's chart without regard to the state of refraction. Visual acuity tested at a distance of 10 to 20 feet will require the distance correction for an ametrope. Patients should be asked to put on their distance correction or, if they have bifocals, to be sure that they are looking through the top part. The lower segment of the bifocal generally contains the near add, which refers to the additional plus power for reading distance.

PINHOLE

Those not wishing to trust themselves with the vagaries and complexities of optics can depend on the pinhole. The pinhole, known since the earliest days of the camera obscura, was the earliest focusing device. The hole is small enough to admit only the central rays from the object, eliminating the divergent rays that would not reach focus in the image plane. This has the disadvantage of admitting only a fraction of the light and thus creating a dim image. Most significant refractive errors can be bypassed, however, by having the patient read through a pinhole placed in front of the eye, approximately where a spectacle lens would sit. The hole should measure about 2 mm in diameter and can be punched in a card with a pin or purchased as a manufactured item made of plastic with numerous holes in an array. This arrangement makes it easier for the patient to find the chart through one of the holes.

TECHNIQUE OF TESTING AND RECORDING VISUAL ACUITY

Most of the technique issues have been covered. Near-card acuity is done at 14 inches for most printed cards, but the card should be checked for this information. As mentioned, the light should be good, and a standardized lighting condition in the office is preferable if the near card is to be the only method of testing. The best refraction for a near card must be used. This usually means reading glasses or the bottom segment of bifocals for the presbyope.

Ophthalmologists have a convention in which they record near-card acuity using Jaeger, which is a printer's notation system (e.g., J_1 print is equivalent to 20/25). The near cards usually show both Jaeger and Snellen fractions. Notation should be made of the reading distance chosen, so that the test conditions can be reproduced, and of the optical conditions used (e.g., "patient's bifocal segment" if the exact refractive correction is not known, or "with pinhole" if that is how the test was performed).

The Snellen fraction is not really an arithmetic fraction, although it sometimes is expressed as a decimal equivalent. For instance, 20/40 can be written as 0.5, and 20/20 would be 1.0. An acuity of 20/40 means that the patient reads at 20 feet (the numerator) that which a normal person could read at a viewing distance of 40 feet (the denominator). The definition of 20/20 as normal visual acuity was determined by doing population studies; however, this definition is too liberal. The 20/20 figures are calibrated so that at the retina, the image of each letter measures (subtends) 5 minutes of arc and the width of each stroke is 1 minute of arc. Because the retina is on the back surface of a sphere, angular measure (degrees, minutes, and seconds of arc) is more convenient than linear or tangent measure (e.g., millimeters of height or width).

OPTIC NERVE DISEASE AND VISUAL ACUITY

It was mentioned earlier that hemianopia does not degrade visual acuity. Any disorder that is constrained to affect only one-half of the visual field will leave the patient with 20/15 vision on the eye chart as long as there is no coexisting condition that diminishes visual acuity. A more inclusive corollary is that if any half of the fovea is functionally intact, then the resolving power of the fovea is not disturbed. This extends the rule to altitudinal visual field defects, in which either the upper or lower half of the visual field is selectively affected. Let us examine the anatomic underpinnings of this axiom and of the contrary rule that optic nerve diseases commonly affect visual acuity.

The functional midline in the retina is an imaginary vertical line drawn through the center of the fovea (the vertical hemianopic midline). Ganglion cells to either side of this line send axons through the optic nerve in an intermingled array without any systematic segregation of axons that arise from nasal or temporal ganglion cells. It is not until the axons reach the chiasm that there is a systematic separation of nasal fibers that cross the chiasm and temporal fibers that go through the chiasm uncrossed. Because of this, optic nerve diseases most often affect afferent units on both sides of midline and thereby degrade visual acuity. Measuring visual acuity is an important aspect of assessing either the response to treatment or the natural course of an optic nerve disease.

VISUAL FIELDS

Analysis of visual fields provides another key to localizing a diagnosis in the CNS. The principles in the following paragraphs deserve emphasis because they pertain to field defects that accompany lesions at all locations. Some particulars that relate to lesions at specific locations then will be outlined.

General Features

Monocular Versus Binocular Defects

Field defects limited to one eye suggest a lesion anterior to the optic chiasm, whereas binocular defects, when caused by a single lesion, localize to the visual pathways at or behind the optic chiasm. Of course, bilateral multiple lesions anterior to the chiasm can give binocular field defects; however, for this discussion we are concerned primarily with signs of localizing value for single lesions.

Location in the Visual Field

The location of defects in the visual field provides at least broad information regarding the responsible lesion. Central scotomas are associated with a wide variety of optic nerve lesions but are especially characteristic of optic neuritis, compressive optic neuropathy, and toxic-metabolic optic neuropathy. Nasal quadrant defects are associated commonly with glaucoma, a degenerative condition of the optic nerve head in which ganglion cell axons at the upper and lower poles of the nerve head are preferentially lost. Temporal defects, usually binocular, are characteristic of chiasmal compression. Homonymous hemianopic defects, which are on the same side in both eyes, characterize lesions anywhere from the optic tract to the calcarine cortex.

These broad principles relating lesion location with shape and locus of visual field can be used for analysis of confrontation fields. Confrontation field data usually lack precision as to the shape and density of the defect, but one generally can determine which quadrants are involved and whether a central or paracentral defect is present. The technique of confrontational visual field testing will be presented after a description of field defects.

Shape of the Visual Field Defect

The shape of the defect corresponds to the morphology of the fiber bundles in the afferent pathways. This morphology is unique for each part of the CNS, and the details for each part are discussed in the particular sections on each locus. The shape of the defect is thus one of the most important features of the visual field.

Density of the Field Defect

The density or severity of light sensitivity loss in the field defect gives some indication of the etiology. This is not as fine a distinction as some of the other features; however, vascular lesions, especially infarctions, generally produce dense or severe defects. Tumors, in particular the slowly growing ones, tend, however, to produce field defects of lesser severity because the tissue is more likely to be affected in a graded manner.

Congruity of the Visual Field Defect

For a single lesion behind the chiasm, congruity refers to the degree to which both the density and extent of the defects are similar in the two eyes. This has practical meaning only for subtotal homonymous field defects. Total hemianopia often is associated with complete tract lesions as well as with complete calcarine infarctions; total hemianopia, therefore, has no localizing value apart from placing the lesion behind the chiasm.

To understand congruity, it is necessary to imagine the overlapping fields of the two eyes, a condition affected by the binocular fusion of the foveal representations of the two eyes (Fig. 23.4). Within the binocular field, every point in visual space is registered by a particular ganglion cell in each eye (an example is point AB in Fig. 23.4).

Lesions of the optic tract characteristically produce incongruous field defects; a monocular hemianopia is one extreme case. In the optic tract, the ganglion cell axons serving receptive fields for the homologous points in visual space are not necessarily adjacent to one another. Hence, a disease process may affect the axon from one eye serving a particular point in binocular visual space without affecting the axon for the homologous point in visual space from the other eye. Axons A and B are shown separate from one another in the left optic tract in the midportion of Fig. 23.4.

The calcarine cortex, area 17 of Brodmann, is organized so that the axons from homologous points in space (here the axons are those of lateral geniculate cells) project to the same column of cortical cells. A cortical disease, therefore, will affect the visual fields of the two eyes in exactly the same way, producing congruous defects.

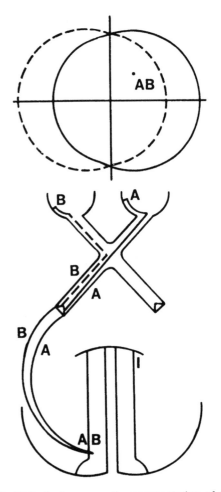

FIG. 23.4. A diagrammatic representation of the binocular visual fields and the afferent fibers serving a point in binocular visual space, point *AB* in the upper figure. A hypothetical photoreceptor, *A* in the right eye and *B* in the left eye, connects with the CNS by way of a ganglion cell axon from each eye, also labeled *A* and *B*, respectively. The ganglion cell axon from the right eye crosses in the chiasm (point *AB* is in the temporal field of that eye), while that from the left passes through to the ipsilateral optic tract (point *AB* is in the nasal field of that eye). Each ganglion cell axon synapses in the left lateral geniculate body and second-order neuron axons continue in the geniculocalcarine radiations to the occipital cortex, area 17 in the bottom figure (see text for further explanation).

Lesions in the geniculocalcarine pathways produce an intermediate degree of congruity; thus this feature is much less reliable in determining the anteroposterior position of lesions than is the case with tract and cortex lesions.

The geniculocalcarine projections A and B are shown in Fig. 23.4 as being separate anteriorly, near the geniculate body. They converge progressively as they near their point of entry into the calcarine cortex.

Slope of the Visual Field Defect

The slope of a visual field defect refers to the amount of lateral increase in the defect's size with a reduction of stimulus visibility. A steeply sloping region changes little in horizontal dimension with a major reduction in stimulus visibility. A gently sloping area of defect becomes much larger with reduced visibility. A gentle slope thus denotes a region of transition between a severe dysfunction and a milder dysfunction in the visual pathways. The marginal area of field, which is sensitive enough to see the more visible target but which is reduced in sensitivity and unable to see the less visible target, is what constitutes the sloping region.

Gentle slope denotes change. Vascular lesions that are healing and tumors that are advancing will have a dense core of total dysfunction surrounded by an area of relative dysfunction, probably related to tissue compression and edema. This gradual transition to normal function in afferent pathways brings about the gentle slope to the visual field defect. Old vascular lesions in which the dense core of infarcted tissue remains, but in which the surrounding pathways have returned to normal sensitivity, are characterized by a steeply sloped transition from defective to normal field. The defect in Fig. 23.5A is gently sloping in the right lower quadrant, typical of a fresh infarct or hemorrhage with surrounding edema. The defect in Fig. 23.5B is steeply

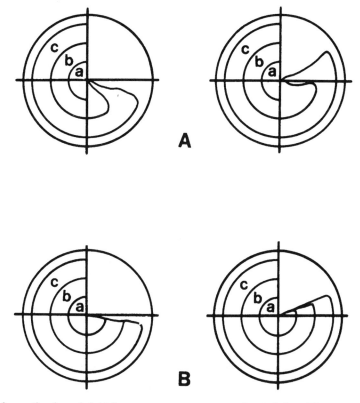

FIG. 23.5. A: A *gently sloped* right homonymous upper-quadrant defect. The extent of field defect for isopters *a* and *b* is greater than for *c* in the right lower quadrant. **B:** A *steeply sloped* defect. The extent of all isopters is the same. The defects in *A* and *B* are also *incongruous.*

sloping in the same region, as would be expected of an old infarct in which the necrotic zone leaves a field defect of absolute density but in which the transition to normal function is abrupt. The slope is readable only in subtotal hemianopia in which there is some sparing of either upper or lower sectors. The slope also should be analyzed only along the margin of the defect, where there is the opportunity of transition to normal across a gradient (i.e., adjacent to the spared sector). There is almost always an abrupt transition at the vertical hemianopic midline because here the lesion has produced maximal effects in the involved half field and has no opportunity of causing any defect in the other half field because the other half is served by the opposite cerebral hemisphere. The transition at the vertical midline is always steep, and here no information is provided on the temporal course of the lesion.

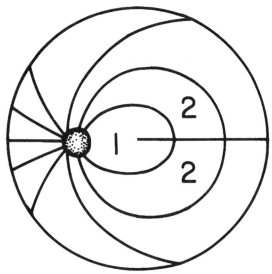

FIG. 23.6. The arrangement of retinal ganglion cell axons in a left eye fundus. Region 1 is the *papillomacular bundle* serving foveal function. Region 2 is the *arcuate bundle* or *Bjerrum region,* where ganglion cell axons from the temporal retinal periphery arch over the massive papillomacular bundle.

TOPICAL FEATURES OF THE VISUAL FIELDS

Retina and Optic Nerve

Figure 23.6 indicates the arrangement of ganglion cell axons in the retina and optic nerve. Bundles of axons coming into the optic nerve from all sides follow a converging course from ganglion cells widely distributed in the retina. On the nasal side of the optic disc (left side in the figure), the bundles have a straight trajectory in the form of a wedge whose apex is at the optic nerve head. Accordingly, interruption of a nasal retinal bundle gives rise to a wedge-shaped visual field defect with the apex at the physiologic blind spot. This normal blind spot in the visual field corresponds to the optic nerve head, where there are no photoreceptors. The papillomacular bundle (region 1 in Fig. 23.6) occupies most of the temporal side of the optic nerve head. Because of this, ganglion cells in the periphery of the retina on the temporal side of the fovea must send their axons in an arcuate course (region 2 in the figure) around the papillomacular bundle to gain access to the optic nerve at the upper and lower poles.

Embryologically, the fovea began at the margin of the retina. With development, invagination carried the fovea toward its adult position near the optic nerve with final fusion of the upper and lower halves of the retinal margin that formed the invagination. The embryonic discontinuity between the upper and lower halves in the temporal retina is reflected in the adult distribution of retinal ganglion cell axons. The term temporal raphe is used to denote the imaginary line separating the upper and lower halves of the temporal retina.

All the ganglion cells immediately above the raphe must send their axons into the upper pole of the disc via the upper arcuate region, while all the ganglion cells below the raphe are constrained to send their axons into the lower pole via the inferior arcuate region.

This forced discontinuity provides for arcuate visual field defects with an abrupt transition to normal at the nasal horizontal midline (the famous nasal step). It is typical of glaucoma to produce these arcuate defects with nasal steps; they were described long ago by Bjerrum and still are referred to by his name.

The location and shape of visual field defects are potent indicators of the site of an optic nerve lesion but also give some indication of etiology. Ischemia of either the retina or the optic nerve tends to produce upper– or lower–half field defects that "respect" or have a sharp border along the horizontal midline of the visual field. These are called altitudinal field defects and can be thought of as extended arcuate bundle defects in which the temporal quadrant is affected as well as the nasal quadrant. Because there is no retinal raphe serving the temporal quadrant, the reason for the sharp border at the horizontal midline must be sought in the patterns of vascular supply.

The reason for altitudinal-type field defects is intuitive for the case of inner retinal infarction because the retina is supplied by an upper and a lower primary branch of the central retinal artery and selective branch occlusion may occur (branch retinal artery occlusion). The altitudinal quality of visual field defects in ischemia of the optic nerve (acute anterior ischemic optic neuropathy, or AION) is more difficult to understand, however, since the anterior optic nerve is supplied by an array of arterioles that stem from an anastomotic vascular circle just behind the globe (the circle of Zinn and Haller). This arterial circle is in turn supplied by a variable number (two to five) of short posterior ciliary arteries that supply the nerve head and the adjacent vascular choroid layer of the eyeball. It has been suggested that sector infarction of the optic nerve head occurs when there is critically low perfusion in the ciliary distribution and a watershed zone between adjacent posterior ciliary artery choroidal vascular territories cuts across the optic nerve head. The orientation of these watershed zones does not always conform to an upper- or lower-half distribution, and this seems to leave the stereotyped altitudinal character of the resulting visual field defects unexplained.

Another common optic neuropathy is optic neuritis of the demyelinating type, which is strongly associated with multiple sclerosis. We used to teach that the most common type of visual field defect in optic neuritis is the central scotoma, a roughly circular area of low visual sensitivity centered on the fixation point. The scotoma may be large enough to engulf the physiologic blind spot, and then it is called a centrocecal scotoma. The Optic Neuritis Treatment Trial (ONTT), in which 448 patients with optic neuritis were randomly assigned to different treatment groups, provided a unique opportunity to study the visual field and other clinical characteristics of the disease. Among affected eyes at onset, 48.2% had diffuse field loss, but among those with focal defects (the remaining 51.8%), the most common pattern was altitudinal in 15%. The investigators concluded that the morphology of field loss is an unreliable criterion for differentiating optic neuritis from ischemic optic neuropathy. Differentiating features include pain exacerbated by eye movement, subacute evolution, and visual field abnormalities in the fellow eye, all of which are frequent in patients with optic neuritis. Features suggestive of AION include more acute onset, lack of pain, and upper- or lower-half swelling of the optic disc with flame hemorrhages.

Optic Chiasm

Axons from ganglion cells on either side of the retinal hemianopic midline, which run a mingled course in the optic nerve, separate at the optic chiasm (Fig. 23.7A). This divergence of pathways is the anatomic feature that creates the hemianopic midline and determines the existence of field defects that respect the midline (i.e., the lateral half-field defects that denote lesions at and behind the optic chiasm).

Fibers from the inferior retina (i.e., the upper temporal visual field) loop forward in the opposite optic nerve as they cross the midline. A lesion at the posterior end of one optic nerve first will encounter these inferonasal fibers of the other eye at the chiasm junction, which creates a distinctive combination of field defects in the two eyes (Fig. 23.7B1).

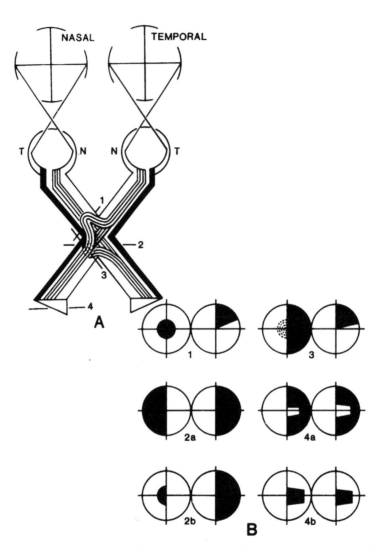

FIG. 23.7. The optic chiasm region. **A:** The arrangement of crossing and non-crossing fibers. Inferior nasal fibers from the right eye loop forward into the left optic nerve before continuing back in the left optic tract. Papillomacular bundle fibers from the left eye loop backward into the ipsilateral optic tract before decussating into the right optic tract. Lesions at levels 1, 2, and 3 produce characteristic field defects that are illustrated in **B.** *B1* is the anterior chiasm junctional syndrome; *B2a* is a typical midchiasm bitemporal field defect; *B2b* is a variation with a scotomatous temporal field defect in the left eye and a peripheral temporal defect in the right; *B3* is a posterior chiasm–tract junctional syndrome; and *B4a* is an anterior choroidal artery–geniculate infarct.

The field defect ipsilateral to the lesion is any of those typical for optic nerve disease (a central scotoma or other nerve fiber bundle defect). In the opposite eye there will be a midline respecting upper temporal defect, or "pie in the sky" defect according to J. Lawton Smith. This is the anterior junctional syndrome of the chiasm.

Some fibers from the nasal retina, especially papillomacular bundle fibers, loop backward in the ipsilateral optic tract before crossing. Thus, a lesion at the junction of the posterior chiasm and optic tract will produce a characteristic posterior junctional syndrome of the chiasm (Fig. 23.7B3). The basic defect is a homonymous hemianopia contralateral to the lesion. Homonymous means that the hemifield defect is on the same side in both eyes. A left tract lesion, for instance, gives rise to a right-sided field defect in either eye (the defect is in the nasal half field of the left eye and is also in the temporal half field of the right eye). As the tract lesion spreads anteriorly and encounters the posterior chiasm, the first chiasmal fibers affected are those from the ipsilateral nasal retina that loop back into the tract before crossing. These fibers serve central vision because the papillomacular bundle crosses in the posterior chiasm. Thus, in the ipsilateral eye there is the nasal hemifield defect that is part of the homonymous pair, plus some loss of central temporal field secondary to the involvement of the posterior looping nasal retinal fibers. The field defect thus involves both sides of the foveal field in the ipsilateral eye and reduces the visual acuity, whereas the purely hemianopic defect in the temporal field of the opposite eye leaves acuity normal, in accord with the axioms previously described.

The typical central chiasmal defects now will be considered. Most symptomatic lesions of the chiasm are tumors, and most of these encounter the chiasm from below. Chiasmal compression most often is accompanied by bitemporal visual field defects. The crossing fibers are apparently least able to tolerate mass effects, probably because they are tethered across the middle, whereas the uncrossed fibers are free to splay out over the mass. Whatever the mechanism, nine times out of ten, compression of the chiasm first will cause midline-respecting temporal field defects in both eyes. This can involve any combination of central (scotomatous) defects and peripheral defects in the two eyes. The most common variations for chiasmal field defects are demonstrated in Fig. 23.7B2a,b.

Lateral Geniculate Body

Two highly characteristic field defects caused by vascular lesions of the lateral geniculate body are shown in Fig. 23.7B. Frisén has provided elaborate detail on the dual vascular

supply of the geniculate by the anterior choroidal and the lateral (posterior) choroidal arteries. Anterior choroidal artery occlusion can be associated with upper- and lower-quadrant homonymous defects that spare a rectangular area along the horizontal midline (Fig. 23.7B4a). Lateral choroidal artery occlusion has been associated with a rectangular homonymous scotoma along the horizontal midline, sparing the upper and lower quadrants (Fig. 23.7B4b)—the exact complement of the other geniculate syndrome.

Geniculocalcarine Radiations

Figure 23.8 illustrates how the axonal outflow from the lateral geniculate radiates within the deep white matter of the cerebral hemispheres. These radiations form a thin band just external to the lateral ventricle. They take the form of a ribbon that is broad in the vertical plane but very thin in the horizontal plane (Fig. 23.8A,B). Thus, lesions must extend deep into the white matter to encounter the geniculocalcarine radiations.

Parietal lobe lesions encounter the upper radiations on the way to the upper bank of the calcarine cortex (area 1 in Fig. 23.8B) and cause inferior quadrantic homonymous visual field defects. Temporal lobe lesions interfere with the anterior looping fibers that are destined for the lower bank of the calcarine cortex (area 3 in Fig. 23.8B) and produce upper-quadrantic homonymous field defects. The anterior temporal contingent of fibers in the geniculocalcarine radiations is called Meyer's loop, after Adolph Meyer who described them.

Calcarine Cortex

A semifinal way station in the afferent system is the primary visual cortex, area 17 of Brodmann on the mesial surface of the occipital lobe. The localization of lesions can be very precise here because of the sometimes-restricted nature of the lesions. Small infarcts from branch occlusions of the calcarine artery may produce exceedingly localized, but always congruous, homonymous field defects.

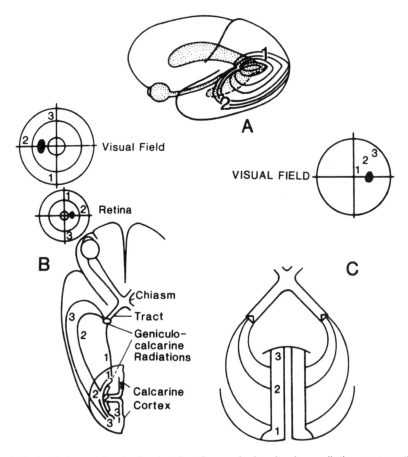

FIG. 23.8. A: Lateral view of the brain showing the geniculocalcarine radiations emanating from a focal point deep to the lateral ventricle (the location of the lateral geniculate body) and fanning out to occupy the parietal and temporal lobes on the way to the calcarine cortex. The anterior looping contingent in the temporal lobe is called *Meyer's loop.* **B:** Diagram of the geniculocalcarine radiations in a mixed horizontal and coronal section of the brain *(lower figure)* together with a diagram of the left eye retina *(middle figure)* and corresponding left eye visual field *(upper figure).* The numbers correlate with lesion locations in the lower figure with affected retinal and visual fields in the middle and upper figures, respectively. **C:** A horizontal section through the calcarine cortex is depicted in the lower figure, with successive zones from the left occipital pole to the anterior end of the left calcarine cortex numbered 1 through 3. Corresponding zones in the right visual field are shown in the *upper figure.* The fixation area is represented at the occipital pole, and the periphery of the visual field is represented at the anterior end of the calcarine cortex (see text and Fig. 23.9 for further details).

There are two basic axes of localization: from anterior to posterior in the calcarine cortex and from lip to depth of the calcarine fissure (Figs. 23.8, 23.9). The anteroposterior dimension translates to an axis from center (fixation point) to periphery in the visual fields (Fig. 23.8C). The fixation area is represented at the posterior end of the calcarine cortex, a portion of which wraps around onto the convexity of the occipital pole. The periphery of the visual field is represented at the anterior end of the calcarine fissure, near the splenium of the corpus callosum.

Sparing of the visual field, either at the center or at the far periphery, is a useful sign that localizes a homonymous hemianopia to the occipital cortex.

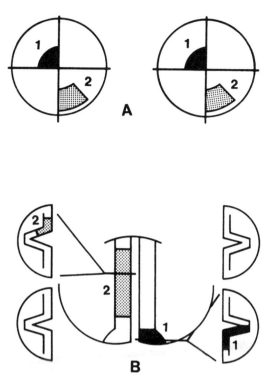

FIG. 23.9. Two practice field defects are depicted in **A**. The corresponding localization in the calcarine cortex is shown in **B** both in the horizontal plane *(central figure)* and in the coronal plane *(lateral figures)*.

Central Sparing, or Sparing of Fixation

Many cases of hemianopia result from infarction of calcarine cortex with occlusion or stenosis of the posterior cerebral artery. The occipital pole receives a collateral blood supply from the middle cerebral artery and may be spared when the flow in the posterior cerebral artery reaches a critical status and infarction occurs in the more anterior portions of the calcarine cortex.

Testing for this spared circle around fixation can best be done at the tangent screen or even on a wall as long as a vertical line through the fixation point can be drawn or imagined. The problem with eliciting fixation sparing is the fact that patients often shift their gaze a few degrees to either side of fixation and the examiner cannot always see these little eye movements. Of course, the whole hemianopic midline will shift with the angle of gaze, and the patient then may seem capable of perceiving test objects a little way into his hemianopic field.

The examiner should use two vertically aligned test spots to avoid mistaking these ocular refixations for central sparing. Most instances of "central sparing" from occipital lobe lesions involve an area no larger than 5 to 15 degrees in diameter, so the examiner should present the two stimulus spots vertically aligned, bringing one inward along the horizontal midline and the other one 20 degrees above or below the central one. The patient is asked to call out "one" or "two" when he or she first sees any test spot, depending on how many spots he or she sees. Under these test conditions, if the patient says "two," there has been a shift of the whole hemianopic midline; if the patient says "one," then the central target has fallen into a circular area of real central sparing, whereas the other (above or below) is still in a hemianopic field.

Sparing of the Unpaired Temporal Crescent

The nasal field (with a maximal extent of 60 degrees) is smaller than the temporal field (with a maximal extent of 75 to 80 degrees) in both eyes. Therefore, with binocular fusion, there is a large area of binocular field, beyond which is a crescent of 20 degrees or so in which the temporal field of one eye has no corresponding nasal field of the other—this is the unpaired temporal crescent. Posterior cerebral lesions, basically those in the occipital lobe, may spare the anterior fibers of the geniculocalcarine radiations and the anterior calcarine cortex, leaving some preserved peripheral field in an otherwise dense and complete homonymous hemianopia. If the extent of preserved periphery is all beyond 60 degrees of eccentricity, there will be no corresponding nasal field spared in one eye, and the spared crescent of field will exist only in the eye with the temporal field on the side of the hemianopia.

Imagine a right occipital lesion and a dense left homonymous hemianopia. There is some sparing of the unpaired crescent. This means that the left eye, which has its temporal field on the left (the side of the hemianopia), will perceive objects in the far periphery, but the right eye (with nasal field toward the hemianopic side) will have no peripheral sparing.

This sparing of the unpaired crescent is an important sign of occipital localization in hemianopia. It can be detected most consistently with confrontation techniques. I have seen several patients with total homonymous hemianopia by perimetry who can perceive hand motion in the far temporal periphery of the one eye but not in the nasal periphery of the other. When testing for this, the patient should cover one eye at a time and the examiner should extend his arm beside and just behind the patient's head on the side of the patient's hemianopia. The examiner should bring his hand forward, wave it up and down, or wiggle his or her fingers. This motion can be a more potent stimulus for the far visual periphery than light.

Rarely, lesions can selectively affect only the most anterior portions of the calcarine cortex, producing a visual field defect that is limited to the peripheral portion of the temporal field in one eye—the nasal field of the other eye is normal because the involvement does not extend into the binocular part of the visual field.

The other important dimension for occipital localization is a series of sectors extending from the lip of the calcarine fissure, which faces the opposite occipital cortex across the interhemispheric fissure, to the depth of the calcarine fissure. The corresponding visual field dimension is a series of pie-shaped sectors extending from an apex at fixation to a broader base at the periphery. The sector abutting the vertical hemianopic midline corresponds to the lip of the calcarine cortex, and the sector abutting the horizontal midline corresponds to the depth of the calcarine cortex. Intermediate field and tissue sectors lie between these limits. The upper bank (lip to depth) serves the inferior homonymous field quadrant, and the lower bank (lip to depth) serves the superior quadrant. Thus, we have a

dimension that extends all the way around one-half of the visual field from the upper vertical midline through the horizontal midline to the lower vertical midline in a series of pie-shaped sectors. The more sectors the pie is divided into, the more pieces there are and the finer the localization. At the cortex, this dimension flows from the inferior lip of one (right or left) calcarine cortex by way of the depth of the calcarine fissure to the upper lip.

Once the location of the pie-shaped sector has been established, localization within the sector should be established along the dimension from fixation to periphery, which is from occipital pole to anterior calcarine cortex.

An exercise in calcarine cortex localization is shown in Fig. 23.9. Two small field defects—one in the left upper quadrant and the other in the right lower quadrant—are depicted. A horizontal section through the calcarine cortex is flanked on either side by coronal sections in Fig. 23.9B. Consider first lesion 1. It extends to fixation but not far into the periphery; thus, in the horizontal section, it is represented at the pole with little anterior extension. It occupies a series of pie-shaped sectors all the way from the vertical midline to the horizontal midline. In the coronal section to the right, the lesion extends all the way from the inferior lip to the depth of the calcarine cortex. The lesion must be in the inferior bank because the field defect is in the upper quadrant.

The reader should try to map the lesion that would accompany field defect 2 in Fig. 23.9A before reading on or looking at the answer in Fig. 23.9B. Set up the cortical diagrams as in Fig. 23.9B and draw in the lesion.

The field defect caused by lesion 2 does not extend to fixation or to the periphery; hence, the lesion is in the middle of the calcarine cortex in the horizontal section, extending neither to the pole nor to the anterior end. The field defect occupies pie-shaped sectors abutting the inferior vertical midline but not extending all the way to the horizontal midline. The lesion, therefore, is in the upper bank of the left calcarine cortex; it involves the lip but does not extend all the way to the depth of the calcarine fissure.

It is fun to draw these diagrams and take them to the radiologist as you read the computed tomography (CT) scan or the magnetic resonance imaging (MRI) results. Small cortical lesions often can be identified that were radiographically questionable without the ironclad visual field correlation.

CONFRONTATION VISUAL FIELD EXAMINATION

Many patients must be tested with confrontation techniques because their overall condition and lack of mobility preclude formal testing. Bedside methods are most practical for physicians other than ophthalmologists.

Confrontation test results must be used in a special way, however, because they do not have the specificity or the quantitative detail of well-done perimetry. Nonetheless, confrontation results can indicate the proper direction for a further workup and thereby may save a great deal of time and expense.

This method is called confrontation because the examiner faces the patient and presents targets while he or she watches the patient's eyes. Eye movement during examination is a problem, as with all visual field testing, and the examiner must be able to monitor fixation. It is best always to start with the right eye because it will be easier to remember the sequence of findings and to relate them to the correct side when recording the results.

Ask the patient to cover his or her left eye with the palm of his or her left hand, and be sure that the fingers are all the way up onto the forehead so that no peeking is possible between them. To peek is human. The examiner faces the patient and closes his right eye so his open left eye is directly in front of the patient's right eye (being tested). The patient is asked to fix his gaze on the examiner's open eye. In this configuration, the examiner can watch for small eye movements and monitor fixation. Also, the patient's and examiner's hemianopic midlines are aligned, so the examiner can determine if a visual field defect "respects" that midline. The setup is reversed to test the patient's left eye.

The presentation of targets follows. The best initial test is finger counting. Although form resolution is the key function of the fovea, motion detection is performed with great sensitivity by the peripheral visual system. A waving motion of the hand or a wiggling of the fingers is, therefore, the grossest stimulus one can present to the periphery. This means that peripheral field function must be almost gone before there is failure to detect motion. Motion, then, is too gross a stimulus to be sensitive, and thus it is not the ideal screening test. Form discrimination, however, is poorly done in the peripheral parts of the visual field. Thus, finger counting, which requires spatial analysis of a stationary form, is a sensitive test for peripheral dysfunction—it will be abnormal with only minor reduction of field function.

Fingers should be presented *en face* to the patient. Obviously, the patient must be able to see all the fingers to make it a valid test, and if you orient your hand so that all the fingers are lined up one behind the other from the patient's perspective, he or she will be unable to count them.

The test can be done quickly. All that is necessary is to present enough combinations of fingers to be sure the patient is not succeeding by guesswork. Combinations should include all fingers, one, two, or none—it is difficult to present three fingers because of the way the tendons in our hands are arranged. Present the combination once in each of the four quadrants and then go around again in a random sequence of quadrants. Two presentations for each quadrant should be sufficient. If errors are made, then more presentations may be required to ensure an apparent defect is real.

Some quantitation of confrontation fields is possible, although it will never match formal quantitative perimetry. If the fingers are counted correctly in all quadrants, there still may be a field defect. First, some defects are scotomas occupying only the central 10- to 20-degree field. Finger counting often will miss these defects. Second, the degree of peripheral defect may be so minor that fingers are still adequately counted.

Color perception is an extremely sensitive, although subjective, measure of visual field dysfunction. It is common for patients to report that colors are less vivid in defective field areas—they seldom mention this, but they will agree to it when specifically asked. Present a fairly large bright red object in the four quadrants and ask the patient if there is any difference in the redness of the object in any field. Desaturation is the term applied to a subjective loss of color intensity in the defective field. Patients may report that the reds are shifted to a darker amber color or bleached toward a lighter, pinkish, or yellowish color; however, in either case, the stimulus is perceived as less red. Try to avoid the term brightness because it is a separate parameter of visual function and should be inquired about separately.

If color saturation is lost in a quadrant, the boundaries should be explored by moving the test red object and by asking the patient to indicate quickly if it becomes redder. The most important area to screen is the vertical midline. To do this, two red spots, one on either side of the midline, may be presented either above or below the examiner's eye (i.e., the fixation point), and the patient should be invited to compare the redness of the two spots. This may bring out a difference across the midline that the patient was unable to describe by viewing the spot sequentially in different quadrants. The examiner then should present one red spot as a stationary target in the normal quadrant and he or she should move the other spot horizontally from the defective field. The patient is told to indicate immediately when the two spots become equal in redness, and the examiner determines if this transition corresponds to the vertical hemianopic midline. The examiner easily senses the location of the midline—it is an imaginary vertical line through the examiner's line of sight to the patient's eye.

If the patient has trouble counting fingers in a defective field, then other stimuli can be presented to determine the relative density of the defect. Moving fingers or a waving hand is a grosser stimulus than stationary fingers. If motion is not detected, a bright light may be moved within the defect and its margins may be plotted to light.

Thus, a hierarchy of stimuli by which to grade the density of a visual field defect can be developed. From most intense to least, this hierarchy of stimuli is ordered as follows:

1. Moving light
2. Moving hand or fingers
3. Finger counting
4. Subjective judgment of color saturation

Using the hierarchy, one can even derive information on the relative slope of the defect. Consider a patient who is unable to perceive light or hand motion in the upper right field, who is able to see movement, but who is unable to count fingers in the lower right field. This finding would indicate a hemianopia that is denser in the upper than in the lower quadrant; in other words, there is a sloping defect with a transition from an upper to a lower field.

PUPILLARY SYSTEM

Irene Loewenfeld has published an encyclopedic work covering all aspects of the ocular pupil including its anatomy, physiology, neurologic control systems, and clinical disorders.

The eye has many structures and functions that are analogous to those of a camera, and the eye shares some common optical requirements with the latter. Among them is the capacity to limit the amount of light entering the optical system; this is a function of the adjustable camera diaphragm. The iris of the eye is essentially an opaque diaphragm with an adjustable central opening (i.e., the pupil). Diameter adjustments are accomplished by coordinated action of the concentrically arranged sphincter muscle together with a set of radially oriented dilator fibers. The sphincter is a 1-mm–wide band of smooth muscle surrounding the pupillary margin. The radial fibers, also smooth muscle, originate at the iris root near the limbus of the cornea and insert within the collagenous substance of the iris near the pupil and the sphincter muscle. Although the sphincter is innervated by the parasympathetic nervous system and the dilators are innervated by the sympathetic system, the two muscle groups function together as an organized unit; that is, when the sphincter is activated, the dilators are concomitantly inhibited at the CNS level. There is always a resting tonus in both systems—they are in a state of mutual opposition when the pupil is at rest. Of the two groups, however, the sphincter is stronger and tends to dominate the equilibrium determining pupil size at average levels of illumination. This is in accordance with the common observation that anticholinergic sphincter inhibitors, such as tropicamide (Mydriacyl), are much stronger pupil dilators than are sympathomimetics such as phenylephrine.

EXAMINATION OF THE PUPILS

Pupil Shape

Under normal circumstances, the entire sphincter/dilator network functions in a coordinated manner and the pupil margin remains round as diameter changes occur. There are pathologic states, however, in which an altered function in the CNS brings about unequal contraction and dilatation of the pupil in various sectors. Wilson called this condition corectopia pupillae or ectopic pupil. This condition might involve either unequal segmental sphincter contraction or independent activation of a small sector of the dilator fibers. Irregular pupils are, however, more commonly the result of direct iris muscle damage, as in trauma or infection in the eye.

Pupil Size and Reactivity

The diameter of the pupil at any particular time reflects the coordinated activity of the sphincter and the dilator systems. As already mentioned, the former is the stronger of the two but can be overcome in the presence of a massive increase in dilator tone caused by activation of the sympathetic system. The adequate sensory stimulus for activating the sphincter is light falling on the retina, whereas "psychosensory" inputs cause dilator activation by way of the sympathetic nervous system. Pupil size tends to be small in infants, with progressive enlargement through early childhood and eventual return to a smaller diameter in the elderly.

In a fixed ambient light, the pupils constrict as the subject becomes drowsy, and they dilate with arousal or startle. Fear and anxiety are thus commonly associated with larger-than-average pupils for a particular light level. Dilator system activation resulting from anxiety can even inhibit the pupil's contraction in response to light. When testing pupil function, it is common to obtain only a small response to the first series of light stimuli. The amplitude of contraction usually increases as the patient becomes less fearful and more relaxed with the situation. One should never conclude that the pupils are non-reactive or sluggish until several stimuli have been delivered and the patient has been put at ease, if possible. This anxiety-related fixity of the pupil seldom lasts more than 20 or 30 seconds under usual conditions.

Pharmacologic agents can cause prominent effects on the size of the pupil. This subject is too vast for review, but some examples are worthy of mention. Glutethimide (Doriden) is a sedative/hypnotic drug that is sometimes the causative agent in drug-overdose cases. In toxic doses, it characteristically causes widely dilated pupils that do not react to light or near effort. Opiates generally cause small pupils, as do sedative drugs. Therefore, in coma resulting from an overdose with opiates, barbiturates, and other sedative/hypnotic drugs (except glutethimide), pupils that are widely dilated should raise suspicion of anoxic damage to the CNS secondary to ventilatory suppression. The effects of atropinic substances introduced directly into the eye are discussed later. Systematically administered sympathomimetics can cause widely dilated pupils, but this seldom is observed clinically. Such a finding occasionally has been described among patients taking levodopa for treatment of Parkinson's disease. Pupillary dilatation occurs with the systemic administration of amphetamines, most commonly in the setting of drug abuse. The size of pupils in all of these situations, however, may reflect the psychic state of the patient as a result of factors other than the presence of pharmacologically active substances in the system. Furthermore, the examiner must have considerable experience to know the range of expected pupil sizes among normal persons in the usually varying sorts of illumination in which patients are examined. The light intensity in the examination area is uncontrolled in most cases; thus judgments about pupil size are often unreliable. Fortunately, in most cases, anisocoria or asymmetry of pupil diameter is more important for a diagnosis than is absolute pupil size.

Technique of Pupil Examination

Every physician should take time to define a certain reproducible type of lighting in which he or she always will perform his pupil examination. As his experience increases, he or she will better be able to assess whether a patient's pupils are abnormally large or small. The ideal area is one that can be both brightly and dimly illuminated in a standard way. Bright light causes relative activation of the sphincter system and can enhance anisocoria resulting from parasympathetic (i.e., third cranial nerve) system lesions. Similarly, dim light shifts the balance of tone to the sympathetically innervated dilator systems and may serve to uncover anisocoria caused by Horner's (oculosympathetic) syndrome. The pupils in Horner's syndrome may even be equal in bright light.

Thus, the degree of anisocoria, or the difference between diameters of the pupils in defined dim and bright light, is important in pupil diagnosis. Approximately 15% of normal individuals have anisocoria of up to 1 mm

without any lesion in either the sympathetic or parasympathetic systems. The difference in size remains the same in bright and dim lighting, which serves to distinguish this physiologic anisocoria from pathologic states. Irene Loewenfeld calls this "simple central or seesaw anisocoria" and notes that the degree of difference may vary or the smaller pupil may even reverse sides over the course of minutes, days, or weeks.

The light reaction usually is observed with the patient in a dim room. Contraction of the sphincter is evoked by shining a bright light into each eye for 0.5 to 2 seconds at a time. The most commonly used light source is a penlight, but any bright light that can be directed into one eye at a time will do. Penlights tend to become dim rapidly and also to flicker because of cheap on/off switches. The Finoff head is an angled carrier that attaches a halogen bulb to the battery handle of the ophthalmoscope. It provides a bright, steady light source that is ideal for testing the pupil. It is a small accessory that is easy to carry in the examining bag along with the ophthalmoscope and otoscope.

Light delivered to one eye causes equal contraction of both pupils. The direct light response refers to pupil constriction in the eye stimulated, and the consensual response is that which occurs when the eye opposite the observed pupil is illuminated.

The contraction of the pupils to near stimulation should be approximately as brisk and extensive as that to light. This contraction is best elicited by having the patient attempt to focus on his or her own thumb held about 2 or 3 cm from the nose. The resulting proprioceptive cues, together with common narcissistic tendencies, make this a more compelling target for near effort than any external object, even the examiner's finger. Simple awareness of near is said to be an effective stimulus for activation of the neurally linked near triad. This triad consists of (a) pupillary constriction, (b) (crystalline) lens accommodation (increase of plus lens power to focus at close range), and (c) convergence of the optic axes

TABLE 23.1. *Brief Form for Pupil Examination*

Pupil	Size in Dim Light (mm)	Light Reaction	Relative Afferent Pupillary Defect
Right	5	Brisk	None
Left	5	Brisk	None

(to maintain binocular fusion on a near object). There is often pupil constriction even if the patient does not make any convergent eye movements or accommodative changes in the lens of the eye.

Format for Reporting the Pupil Examination

The notation "pupils equal, round, regular, and reactive to light and accommodation (PERRLA)" is best avoided except under battlefield conditions, when the main distinction to be drawn is between the living and the dead. Many cases do not demand an intense, systematic examination of the pupil, so abbreviated formats sometimes are warranted. A good brief form is presented in Table 23.1. The near reaction is not included in the brief examination because it is generally unimportant if the light response is normal. The important light/near dissociated pupils, which will be discussed later, involve a failure of the light reaction with preservation of the near response (never the reverse). When the pupil is the central issue for a clinical case, extended notation can be used, as shown in Table 23.2.

OVERVIEW OF CENTRAL PUPILLARY PATHWAYS

The importance of the pupil in neurologic diagnosis rests on the fact that structures determining pupil size and motility occupy extensive portions of the CNS in addition to the circuitous pathways of the peripheral ocular sympathetic innervation in the head and neck. Lesions in widely separated portions of the body thus will lead to specific disorders of pupil function.

The cerebral hemispheres probably contribute to pupil tone, although (for practical purposes) the hemispheres do not have localizing pupillary significance because lesions and irritative states at this level do not produce any reliable changes in the pupils. It is useful to envision the pupillary motor systems as reflex arcs analogous to those in the spinal cord. Each system (parasympathetic and sympathetic) has an afferent side and a motor side to its reflex arc, which is similar to the organization at the segmental level. The optimal afferent stimuli, however, are different in the two systems. This is discussed later in more detail, but stated briefly, the parasympathetic system operates the pupillary reaction to light falling on the retinas, whereas the dilator system functions in response to psychosensory inputs.

The afferent arc of the parasympathetic reflex is mediated by way of inputs from the retina to the midbrain, where connections exist with the Edinger-Westphal subnucleus of the third cranial nerve nucleus. The motor side is mediated by way of axons of the Edinger-Westphal nucleus passing in the third cranial nerve to the ciliary ganglion, where

TABLE 23.2. *Complete Form for Pupil Examination*

Pupil	Size in Dim Light (mm)	Size in Bright Light (mm)	Light RX (D/C)	Near RX	Relative Afferent Pupillary Defect
Right	5	3	3+/3+	3+	None
Left	5	3	3+/3+	3+	0.6 log[a]

D, direct; C, consensual.

[a]Quantitation of relative afferent pupillary defect (RAPD) using neutral density (gracy) filters over the better-seeing eye.

synapses with the postganglionic fibers are found. These postganglionic fibers form neuromuscular junctions with the pupillary sphincter muscle.

Within the sympathetic system, the afferent arcs come from ascending sensory pathways, with collateral branches to the brainstem and diencephalic reticular formation. Inputs from the cerebral hemisphere are not anatomically well defined, but they probably feed into the descending reticular system, perhaps at the hypothalamic level along with other limbic–diencephalic interfaces. The efferent side is mediated by way of descending polysynaptic pathways within the brainstem and spinal cord, which then make contact with preganglionic neurons, the cell bodies of which are in the intermediolateral cell column of the spinal cord. The preganglionic and postganglionic fibers for the sympathetic system follow a complex pathway through the head and neck to reach the iris dilator fibers.

This brief overview will serve to emphasize that there is tremendous diversity of sensory inputs to the pupil systems. These afferent pathways, together with pupillomotor efferent pathways, occupy an extensive and functionally critical portion of the nervous system.

PARASYMPATHETIC PUPIL SYSTEM (LIGHT REFLEX)

The parasympathetic system provides a mechanism for reflex adjustment of pupil size in response to the amount of light entering the eye. This serves to maintain the image quality by limiting excessive quantities of light, and it also increases the depth of focus by reducing spherical aberration of the eye's optics. The same optical phenomena occur in a camera when the aperture (f-stop) of the diaphragm is reduced.

Figure 23.10 is a diagrammatic representation of the afferent and efferent sides of the reflex pupillary pathway for light. Changes of luminous intensity in the environment normally enter the system through both eyes simultaneously. However, for purposes of clar-

ity, we have chosen to illustrate the more usual mode of clinical testing, in which a light is introduced selectively into one eye. In this diagram, the flashlight is directed at the right eye, and the photoreceptors of the right retina are activated. Through several intermediate neurons in the retina, excitation is conveyed to the retinal ganglion cells, the axons of which constitute the optic nerves. An important aspect of this system is the fact that when light is introduced into one eye, both pupils constrict to an equal degree. The extent of pupillary constriction once was considered to be greater on the side of the light stimulus, but pupillographic studies have disproved this contention. The anatomic substrate for a bilateral symmetric pupil constriction with monocular stimulation will become clear on inspection of this diagram. When the right eye is stimulated (Fig. 23.10), the optic nerve carries impulses to the optic chiasm, where the fibers originating nasal to the macula (serving temporal fields) cross into the opposite optic tract, and the fibers originating temporal to the macula (nasal fields) pass undecussated in the ipsilateral optic tract. At some point anterior to the termination of these fibers in the lateral geniculate nuclei, a collateral pathway leads to the pretectal region of the midbrain just ventral to the collicular plate. Neurons in this pretectal nuclear (PTN) region are depicted in Fig. 23.10 by triangle symbols (open arrows, PTN). Right eye stimulation produces bilateral activation of pretectal nuclei because of the hemidecussation at the chiasm. Some of the pretectal neurons send axons across the midline to the opposite Edinger-Westphal nucleus, whereas others send fibers to the ipsilateral nucleus (Fig. 23.10). Thus, there are crossing fibers at two levels in the afferent system to explain the observed symmetric pupillary contraction when light stimulates one eye.

The efferent arm of the light reflex generally is considered to begin with cell bodies in the Edinger-Westphal nucleus, a subunit of the third cranial nerve (oculomotor) nuclear group. The third cranial nerve innervates

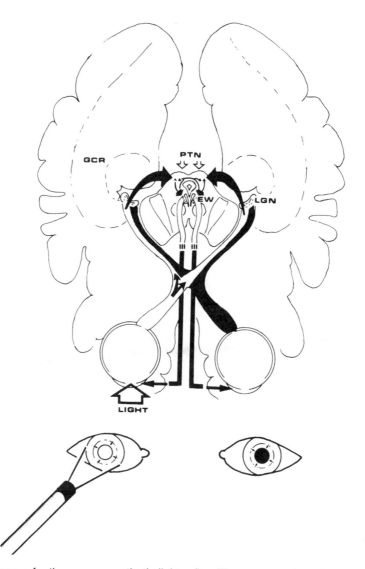

FIG. 23.10. Pathways for the parasympathetic light reflex. The upper portion of the figure illustrates afferent pathways from the retina of the right eye to both sides of the midbrain by way of the hemidecussation at the chiasm. Afferent fibers of retinal ganglion cells leave the optic tracts anterior to the lateral geniculate bodies and innervate pretectal nuclei (PTN, *open arrows*). *Closed triangles* just below the superior colliculi in the midbrain section indicate neurons of the *pretectal nuclei.* Pathways from either PTN innervate the Edinger–Westphal (EW) nuclei bilaterally, constituting a second hemidecussation in the afferent side of the reflex arc. The outflow pathways from the Edinger–Westphal nuclei are in the third cranial nerves to the ciliary ganglion, where a synapse occurs with postganglionic neurons (not shown) that innervate the iris sphincter muscle. The *inset* below illustrates that both pupils constrict to an equal degree when light is applied to one eye as a consequence of the twin hemidecussations in the afferent pathways.

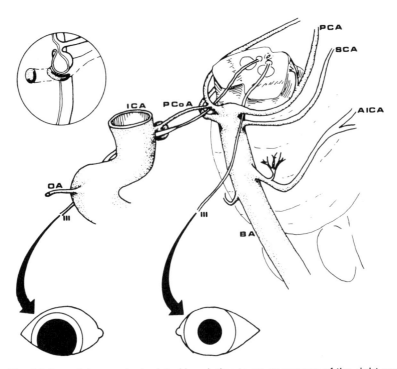

FIG. 23.11. The third cranial nerve is depicted in relation to an aneurysm of the right posterior communicating artery (PCoA). The main body of the figure illustrates the anatomic relationship of the right third cranial nerve to the posterior cerebral artery (PCA) and the superior cerebellar artery (SCA) as the nerve exits from the brainstem and crosses the subarachnoid space. It also illustrates the close relationship between the nerve and the internal carotid artery (ICA) at its junction with the PCoA more anteriorly. The figure shows that an aneurysm of the PCoA at its origin from the ICA is in an ideal position to compress the third nerve. The *upper-left-hand inset* shows the relationship of an aneurysm to the passing third nerve. Note that the pupillary parasympathetic fibers, indicated by a *solid black band,* are peripherally placed and especially vulnerable to sudden enlargement of the aneurysm or to breach of the nerve surface by localized hemorrhage. The *lower inset* indicates a typical aneurysm-type right third nerve palsy. The right eye is abducted and depressed with maximum pupillary dilatation. BA, basilar artery; OA, ophthalmic artery; AICA, anterior inferior cerebellar artery.

quite a number of extraocular muscles as well as the pupils, and the architecture of its nucleus is complex (Fig. 23.11). For the moment, we will consider only the pupillomotor fibers that exit from the midbrain within the third cranial nerve, bound for the orbit. The upper-left-hand inset of Fig. 23.11 shows the location of pupillary fibers within the nerve—they are depicted as the black band at the periphery of the nerve trunk. This is important in the diagnosis of third cranial nerve lesions because the peripheral pupillomotor fibers are vulnerable to the effects of external compression by aneurysms (Fig. 23.11).

Within the orbit, the parasympathetic fibers synapse with postganglionic cell bodies in the ciliary ganglion. The postganglionic fibers enter the anterior segments of the eyes as the long posterior ciliary nerves and form neuromuscular junctions with the pupillary sphincter muscle. The synaptic neurotransmitter at the ciliary ganglion level and at the neuromuscular junction is acetylcholine. The transmitter at the pretectal level and at the Edinger-Westphal nucleus is unknown. Pharmacologic manipulation of the cholinergic neuromuscular junction at the eye is important in the diagnosis of pupil sphincter paralysis.

CLINICAL DISORDERS OF THE PARASYMPATHETIC PUPILLARY SYSTEM

Relative Afferent Pupillary Defect (Marcus Gunn)

A neural signal that varies with the amount of light entering the eyes is conveyed by retinal ganglion cell axons to the pretectal nuclei, where it is translated into a motor command for the appropriate pupil size. The signal is relayed by way of the third cranial nerve to the iris sphincters of both eyes. The system functions as if there were a fixed relationship between the amount of light entering the two eyes and the neural code for the resultant pupil size. Anything that reduces the amount of light entering will cause the pupils to attain a larger diameter, all other stimuli remaining equal. This can be demonstrated by covering one eye of a subject and then noting that the uncovered pupil dilates slightly. Both pupils are dilating, but the pupil under cover cannot, of course, be seen. This type of observation led Marcus Gunn to describe the relative afferent pupillary defect (RAPD), which is now routinely tested by the swinging flashlight technique. Marcus Gunn's original observation, made in 1904, was that when an eye has an optic nerve lesion, covering it causes relatively little dilatation of the pupil because almost all the light-induced signal comes to the midbrain from the opposite eye. As the cover is switched to the normal eye, however, the pupils dilate strikingly because all the light information now comes from the eye with the defective afferent function. This variance of pupil size with alternating occlusion (when one eye is providing most of the brightness signal) is the basis of the swinging flashlight test.

Rather than alternately covering each eye in bright ambient light as Marcus Gunn did, the RAPD now is tested by illuminating each eye separately with a focal light source. Both pupils dilate as the light is swung to the defective eye, and both pupils constrict as it is swung to the normal eye. The test is best done in the dark, and only the eye illuminated by the flashlight can be seen at any one time. The unseen fellow eye, however, is undergoing the same pupillary constriction and dilatation that can be observed in the illuminated eye. The swinging flashlight technique provides a sensitive means of comparing afferent function in the two eyes. If one eye is totally blind and the other has normal visual acuity and fields, the difference in magnitude of the direct light reflex between eyes will be evident without the swinging flashlight technique. The test becomes useful when the difference in direct light reflex between the eyes is less, in which case observation of the extent and velocity of pupil constriction may seem the same when either eye is stimulated alone. Nonetheless, a clear difference is usually apparent when the eyes are stimulated alternately in rapid succession.

Under the best circumstances, an afferent pupillary defect is easy to detect, even when small. However, certain variances of pupil function among normal individuals sometimes make interpretation of the swinging flashlight test difficult. The presence of a Marcus Gunn pupil, or RAPD, indicates a lesion in the afferent pupillary reflex arc between the eye and the midbrain, although the type of lesion is not directly specified by the test.

One should not conclude, however, that the RAPD has no specificity as to the cause of visual loss in the defective eye. Cataracts and other opacities in the ocular media do not produce a significant RAPD even with major visual loss. This is probably true because such opacities diffuse light within the eye and degrade the visual image but do not significantly reduce the total quantity of light that reaches the retina until the cataract becomes brown (brunescent) in its late stages. Dark or brown cataracts can induce a mild RAPD. Visual loss resulting from opacities in the media of the eye is not generally a major diagnostic problem because these are seen easily on ophthalmoscopic examination.

There is greater difficulty in distinguishing among macular lesions, optic nerve lesions, and childhood amblyopia. In any of these cases, the fundus appearance may not give a clue as to which is causing the visual loss. Although macular lesions usually cause an observable change in the optic fundus, the findings may be subtle and may even require adjunctive examinations, such as fluorescein angiography, to demonstrate them.

The usefulness of the afferent pupillary defect in this type of situation lies in the relationship between the degree of afferent defect and the degree of visual dysfunction. In the presence of minimal functional impairment (nearly normal visual acuity and fields), a prominent afferent pupil defect signifies a high probability that the lesion is in the optic nerve. A macular lesion must produce a more extensive visual acuity loss than an optic nerve lesion to result in an equivalent RAPD. If the visual acuity is severely impaired from a macular lesion, there may be a fairly prominent RAPD, so the test is specific for optic nerve lesions mainly when visual impairment is minor. Amblyopia (strabismic or anisometropic) may be associated with a mild to moderate RAPD, but oddly enough the degree of RAPD does not correlate well with the level of visual acuity reduction. The afferent pupil defect is decisive in evaluating monocular functional visual loss, which can result from either hysteria or malingering. Most commonly, the differential diagnosis falls between functional visual loss and retrobulbar (behind the globe) optic neuropathy because the fundus is normal in both cases.

If a patient has visual acuity worse than 20/40 in one eye with normal visual acuity and visual field in the other eye without RAPD, it is reasonably safe to conclude that the problem is functional. A problem exists if a person has reduced acuity in one symptomatic eye and an asymptomatic peripheral visual field defect in the other eye. The peripheral field loss may be sufficient to balance the central visual loss in the symptomatic eye, in which case there will be no RAPD. The swinging flashlight technique is a comparative test that uses the fellow eye as an internal control. The phenomenon that has been called Marcus Gunn pupil, therefore, should be referred to as the relative afferent pupillary defect.

It is important to keep in mind that the absence of an RAPD in a patient with symptomatic reduction of visual acuity in one eye is a useful sign of hysteria or malingering only if one has detailed information on the visual function in the fellow eye.

Occasionally, there is confusion between the Marcus Gunn pupil and hippus, which is random, often rhythmic pupillary oscillation that can be observed in many normal individuals during steady illumination of the eyes. The term hippus usually is reserved for those pupils that oscillate with fairly large amplitude; almost every pupil has small sinusoidal oscillations of size with steady illumination. High-amplitude oscillation is a curiosity but not a disease—there are no currently accepted disease associations with the phenomenon. It often complicates the interpretation of the swinging flashlight test, however, because there can be an interaction between the rhythm of flashlight alternation and that of the spontaneous pupil fluctuation. The examiner sometimes swings the light between the eyes in such a way that a false afferent defect is produced on one side or a real afferent defect is masked by the interaction of stimulus alternation and natural oscillation. To avoid this problem, the examiner probably should swing at different rhythms during a single examination, including at least one trial of very slow alternation, changing eyes every 3 to 5 seconds. During the steady illumination of each eye, the examiner can observe whether there is significant hippus; if there is, the results should be interpreted carefully. An apparent afferent defect that is not seen with most alternation rates may be spurious.

A person can see his own pupil oscillate by his sense of the brightness of the stimulus light, which brightens as the pupil widens and dims as the pupil contracts. When you shine a light in your own eye, the pupil first constricts and then dilates slightly. This is normal early release and does not in itself indicate an afferent defect; many normal pupils behave in this manner, although others assume a new smaller size with illumination and do not redi-late. This early contraction and slight redilata-tion should be equal in amplitude between eyes to qualify as a normal variant. If there is significant early release, the swinging flash-light test should be done at slow alternation rates to let the new steady-state pupil size be expressed before changing eyes.

A pupil that dilates right away when it is il-luminated, without any early constriction, strongly indicates a Marcus Gunn pupil. However, an afferent defect may be manifest only in that there is less early constriction in one eye than in the other during the swinging flashlight test. It is not necessary for all early constriction to be abolished in mild degrees of unilateral optic neuropathy. The asymmetry of pupil behavior is the important feature to look for.

Preganglionic Ocular Parasympathetic (Third Cranial Nerve) Lesions

The diagnosis of third cranial nerve lesions based on an abnormal eye position with weak-ness of the extraocular muscles is discussed in a later section. Here, we will concern our-selves with the involvement or sparing of the pupil in oculomotor nerve lesions because a good deal of clinically important information revolves around this issue. Since the large studies of lesions involving third, fourth, and sixth cranial nerves were published from the Mayo Clinic in the 1950s, 1960s, and 1990s, the importance of the pupil in etiologic diag-nosis of third cranial nerve lesions has been recognized. In these studies, and in subse-quent clinical investigations, it has become well established that paralysis of the pupillary sphincter is the rule in third cranial nerve le-sions resulting from aneurysms (Fig. 23.11). However, older patients (generally older than age 65 years) who develop third cranial nerve palsies on the basis of presumed microvascu-lar occlusive disease within the nerve itself seldom have major pupillary involvement. Many patients in this latter category have risk factors for accelerated atherosclerosis, includ-ing diabetes mellitus or hypertension, but the lack of these factors should not rule out the diagnosis. These "medical" lesions tend to improve and most often make a nearly full re-covery within 3 to 6 months.

Although there are only a few pathologic studies of third cranial nerve ischemia, con-sistent morphologic changes have been ob-served. The lesion is dominated by demyeli-nation in the acute stages, and the lesion shrinks with fibrosis in the late "recovery" stages. In both the acute and chronic phases there is relatively little, if any, disruption of axons as they pass through the lesion. This correlates well with the usual clinical out-come in which complete or near-complete re-covery of function occurs over several weeks or months.

Because axons are not disrupted, there is no opportunity for the development of aberrant or misdirected regeneration of fibers in the late stage of recovery. This contrasts with the outcome when the third cranial nerve is dam-aged by hemorrhage from aneurysms in which there is often loss of axonal continuity. A fairly high incidence of aberrant regenera-tion tends to be seen in the late stages of re-covery from aneurysmal third nerve palsy. The most commonly observed clinical mani-festation of this is inappropriate contraction of the levator palpebrae muscle linked with activation of either the medial rectus or infe-rior rectus muscle on attempted adduction or depression of the eye. This causes the striking appearance of lid elevation as the affected eye moves inward (adduction) or downward (de-pression). These phenomena are caused by a misdirection of axons that had been destined originally for one of the extraocular muscles but which on regrowth attain the wrong chan-nel in the peripheral portion of the nerve and end up at the wrong muscle.

Both the medical third cranial nerve palsies and surgical cases caused by aneurysms tend to present acutely with considerable pain in the eye and orbit at the onset. There is a ten-dency to accept painful third cranial nerve palsy caused by aneurysms without much need for explanation. The cause of pain in mi-crovascular occlusive lesions, however, is not readily apparent. On close examination, the cause of pain in the presence of aneurysms is not entirely explained. Although there is often evidence for enlargement of an aneurysm prior to the occurrence of small hemorrhages into the nerve, this is by no means always the case. Whether or not the aneurysm has enlarged, it is always possible that a direct irritation of pain-carrying afferent pathways from the artery wall at the site of the aneurysm is responsible for the pain. The important point is that pain is characteristic both of aneurysmal third cranial nerve lesions and of those secondary to ischemia within the nerve substance. The criterion of pain, therefore, should not be used to differentiate between medical and surgical causes.

The importance of making a differential diagnosis prior to angiography is that patients with an intraneural lesion caused by small-vessel disease are at high risk for angiographic procedures, and the angiogram does not lead to any beneficial therapy. It is, therefore, optimal to avoid angiography in these patients. Fortunately, sparing of the pupil is sufficiently reliable evidence of a medical cause that most of these patients can be managed without angiography.

Although this seems simple and clearcut in abstract discussion, the evaluation of individual cases presents ambiguities. Because all biologic phenomena tend to fall along continua rather than in all-or-none fashion, it is not surprising that this occurs in relation to pupillary involvement with third cranial nerve lesions. The safest formulation is that in aneurysm-induced third cranial nerve palsies, the pupil is strongly involved, whereas in microvascular lesions, the pupil is relatively spared. This means that the degree of pupillary involvement in relation to the degree of extraocular muscle involvement is the critical factor. There is little difficulty in diagnosis when a person presents with a total involvement of all extraocular muscles, including complete ptosis, while the pupil is only slightly larger than that of the other eye and remains reactive to light. This would be the profile of a clearcut medical third cranial nerve palsy. Unfortu-

nately, some patients present with partial involvement of the extraocular muscles, and then, although the pupils are normal, or nearly so, it is difficult to exclude an aneurysm. Newer methods—such as intravenous (IV) or intraarterial digital subtraction angiography, rapid-sequence spiral CT with bolus IV contrast injection, magnetic resonance angiography (MRA) (i.e., a type of angiogram), or duplex scanning methods—all have the capacity to visualize larger aneurysms. In the author's experience MRA using a 3-Tesla magnet can have enough resolution to reliably rule out a berry aneurysm at the circle of Willis, but more experience with this tool is needed before firm conclusions are reached. Presently there is no widely available, definitive test to exclude smaller aneurysms except standard angiography, and some patients with non-aneurysmal third cranial nerve palsies have to be studied using this invasive technique when the characteristics of the cranial nerve involvement are not definitive.

Pupillary involvement in slowly progressive third cranial nerve compressive lesions such as meningioma, pituitary adenoma, and nasopharyngeal carcinoma is much less predictable. The onset and course of the third cranial nerve dysfunction may be the most valuable clue to the presence of one of these other compressive lesions. The onset is generally much less explosive than that resulting from aneurysms or microvascular infarction. Furthermore, the lesions caused by aneurysm or infarction are usually complete within hours or days, whereas the level of pupillary and extraocular muscle dysfunction caused by tumor compression tends to be slowly progressive over weeks or months.

It would seem practical to undertake a small-scale workup on each patient in whom the diagnosis of microvascular infarction of the third cranial nerve is considered. CT or MRI of the sella turcica, cavernous sinus, ethmoid sinus, and sphenoid sinus regions may follow laboratory screening, especially for diabetes, depending on the degree to which alternate diagnoses are suspected. If the patient is hypertensive and diabetic and in the mid- to late 60s, it may be appropriate to stop testing after the blood studies. If the patient is without risk factors for accelerated atherosclerosis, or is younger than age 55 or even 60, it is wise to proceed to MRI or CT scan with special attention to the parasellar and posterior orbital areas. Angiography remains the definitive test for an aneurysm.

Herniation Syndromes

Supratentorial masses large enough to cause herniation of the medial temporal lobe over the tentorium cerebelli bring pressure to bear against the midbrain and third cranial nerve, which results in pupillary dilatation. Once the stage of third cranial nerve dysfunction has commenced in the course of the transtentorial herniation syndrome, there is often only a matter of minutes or hours until irreversible brain damage occurs, and this is clearly a medical emergency. As with more distal third cranial nerve lesions—caused by aneurysms, infarcts, and tumors—the pupillary involvement is on the motor side of the reflex arc. Although it is axiomatic that a lesion on the afferent side of the reflex arc does not cause anisocoria, lesions on the motor side of the arc do so routinely. It is also the rule that a lesion in the efferent pupillary pathway will result in a sluggish pupillary response to either direct or consensual light stimulation on the involved side. It is thus always possible to distinguish an afferent pupillary lesion from one at or distal to the Edinger-Westphal nucleus in the third cranial nerve complex. In the latter instance, the neural message from the midbrain is not conducted on one side only—that is, on the side of the eye being stimulated with light. In other words, both the direct and the consensual light response are diminished on the side of a third cranial nerve lesion.

Depending on the location of the supratentorial mass lesion causing herniation, one can distinguish central and lateral herniation syndromes.

Central herniation, caused by lesions near the midline, commonly in the parasagittal regions, tends to present with symmetric pupillary paralysis in both eyes. In these cases, the entire substance of the diencephalon and midbrain are shifted downward, with a tendency for bilateral dysfunction from the onset. It is not uncommon for both pupils to be small and sluggishly reactive in the early stage of central herniation. The lateral herniation syndrome occurs in conjunction with laterally placed supratentorial masses, commonly in the temporal lobe. The third cranial nerve findings tend to be unilateral until the final stages of global midbrain dysfunction.

In both central and lateral herniation syndromes, there is sufficient disruption of function in the ascending reticular activating system that the patient usually is obtunded by the time that pupillary signs emerge. The end stage of both central and lateral herniation is bilateral pupillary paralysis, which is accompanied by large non-reactive pupils, probably caused by severe ischemia, often with hemorrhages (Duret) in the midbrain and pons. At this stage, it is usually not possible to determine whether the antecedent herniation was of the central or the lateral type.

It is worthy of repeated emphasis that the patients who are in the midst of cerebral herniation syndrome do not present to the office or hospital complaining of pupillary dilatation, or of anything else for that matter. They are usually severely obtunded by the time the pupillary phenomena have begun. Gradual somnolence and outright stupor evolve during the earlier diencephalic phase of herniation, when the level of functional compromise is at the thalamus, above the midbrain level.

POSTGANGLIONIC PARASYMPATHETIC LESION (ADIE'S SYNDROME, TONIC PUPIL, AND VARIATIONS)

Confusion often occurs when an ostensibly healthy, alert patient presents to the emergency room complaining of a dilated pupil, which is not a rarity. This clinical presentation, therefore, must be dealt with effectively in the emergency department, and a firm differential diagnosis of the monosymptomatic dilated pupil is important for all emergency room physicians to keep in mind. Tonic pupil with or without Adie's syndrome and pharmacologically blocked pupil sphincter (atropine-like substances) are the two most common disorders to present in this way.

Adie's Pupil

In 1932 Adie published findings concerning a group of generally healthy young women who presented with a unilaterally dilated pupil. He found that the affected pupil had a peculiar tonic light reaction—it responded slowly to light stimulation and had a more brisk, although still pathologically slow, response to near-vision effort. The pupil seemed totally fixed or unresponsive to light in the usual examination setting—a dim environment with a bright light flashed into either eye briefly (Fig. 23.12). When the patient was observed in a bright environment for several minutes, the "tonic" pupil gradually would decrease in diameter. When the environment was dimmed again, the normal pupil would dilate briskly and the "tonic" pupil would remain small for several minutes, although it would redilate slowly, given enough time.

The absolute diameter of the affected pupil, therefore, depends on the immediate past light experience of the individual: the tonic pupil may be, at a particular time, smaller or larger than the normal pupil, depending on the ambient illumination and the immediate past illumination. It is important to keep this in mind because the tonic pupil usually is described in textbooks as being pathologically large. The average diameter of a tonic pupil generally decreases as months and years go by. These pupils tend not to recover their normal function once the tonic state has begun. An old tonic pupil is often small and does not dilate in dim light over any period of time.

Adie observed that there was a high incidence of areflexia in his group of patients. Many had lost all of their deep tendon reflexes, although others retained some reflexes in a patchy manner. The etiology of this syn-

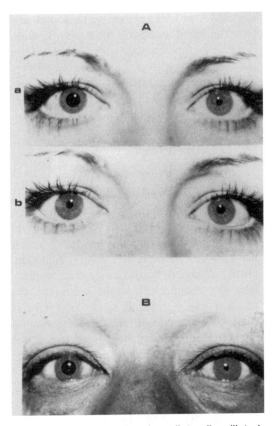

FIG. 23.12. The isolated, unilaterally dilated pupil. **A:** Adie's syndrome. **a:** The right pupil is widely dilated and unreactive to light. There is no ptosis or extraocular muscle weakness. **b:** The right pupil is constricted to a greater extent than the left after instillation of "weak" 1/8% pilocarpine in either eye. **B:** Atropinized pupil. The right pupil was widely dilated and fixed to light. It failed to constrict on instillation of "strong" 4% pilocarpine.

drome has never been elucidated; it remains an idiopathic dysautonomic state.

The presence of normal deep tendon reflexes does not rule out the diagnosis because a significant percentage of patients have normal reflexes, at least when the syndrome first presents, and the features of the pupil syndrome do not distinguish between those with reflex loss and those without. Any of the limb reflexes may be diminished, and asymmetric loss is found in nearly half the patients. The reflexes generally become less active as time passes, although in some patients they become a little more brisk.

Aside from simply noticing the large pupil in the mirror, occasionally symptoms lead the patient to be indirectly aware of the problem. The pupil normally limits the amount of light entering the eye by reacting to variations in ambient illumination. When too much light enters the eye, it creates the sensation of glare. Furthermore, the large pupil alters the optics of the eye toward a state in which there is a shallower depth of focus and an increased spheric aberration. This tends to cause a sensation of blurred vision in both bright and dim environments. The accommodative mechanism also is affected in Adie's syndrome: The change in diopteric power (convexity) of the lens to accommodate for near vision takes many seconds to occur, and then the focus remains for many seconds after the patient has shifted his gaze from a near to a distant object. Vision from the affected eye, therefore, will be blurred for the first few seconds of any near-vision effort and will remain blurred for several seconds as the patient subsequently attempts to use his eyes for distant viewing. The tonic accommodation with a sustained effort at near vision occasionally causes a ciliary spasm, which is manifested as pain in the eye, usually in the vicinity of the brow and inner canthus during close work.

The patient with an Adie's pupil is completely alert without any of the CNS signs that accompany transtentorial herniation. Nonetheless, many such patients are subjected to needless cerebral angiography, often as an emergency procedure.

The tonic pupil is caused by a postganglionic parasympathetic lesion. Some authors believe that this is a viral infection of the ciliary ganglion; however, no definitive data exist as to the cause of the lesion. The lesion is in the postganglionic parasympathetic system because there is denervation supersensitivity to weak cholinergic substances. This seems to follow the same principles as denervation supersensitivity in skeletal muscle that has lost its direct innervation. Normally, the muscle can be activated only through its motor end plate; however, 4 or 5 weeks after an acute loss of direct nerve supply, the functional muscle end plate begins to expand until nearly the entire sarcolemmal membrane becomes responsive to circulating or experimentally applied acetylcholine. This procedure forms the basis of a definitive test for Adie's pupil. Because acetylcholine is unavailable as a pharmaceutical solution, the physician can choose another direct-acting cholinergic such as methacholine chloride (Mecholyl) or pilocarpine for the test. The physician must select a solution that is too weak to cause a normally innervated sphincter muscle to contract. For these purposes, we have selected 1/16% pilocarpine because we found that it does not cause a significant contraction of a normally innervated sphincter muscle, unlike 1/8% pilocarpine, which can cause more than 1-mm miosis in some normal persons (unpublished study). Leavitt and coworkers found 1/16% to be ideal, and the author concurs. Methacholine had been advocated earlier for testing denervation supersensitivity of the iris sphincter, but this drug is no longer readily available and it actually has been shown to be less sensitive than 1/8% pilocarpine in demonstrating iris denervation supersensitivity.

The normal pupil serves as an internal control in this test. One drop of 1/16% pilocarpine is placed in either eye, and a second drop is applied 10 minutes later. The pupil size is measured approximately 30 to 60 minutes from the first application. In most cases, the Adie's pupil will become smaller than the fellow pupil under the influence of this weak solution of pilocarpine, thus demonstrating the presence of denervation supersensitivity. This is categorically different from the failure of a contraction to weak pilocarpine that characterizes the dilated pupil of an intracranial third cranial nerve lesion, in which case the postganglionic innervation is intact. Preganglionic lesions of the intracranial third nerve result in a dilated pupil, but there is not significant denervation supersensitivity and the pupil does not constrict in the presence of 1/16% pilocarpine. Ponsford and coworkers found that among 10 patients with aneurysms causing third cranial nerve palsy, 2.5% methacholine caused pupillary constriction equal to that in 14 patients with Adie's syndrome. These authors had no explanation for this finding, and others have not had similar experience, so it is still generally accepted that significantly greater miosis on the side of a dilated pupil is strongly indicative of a post-ganglionic (orbital) lesion.

It should be mentioned that the weakest solution of pilocarpine available commercially is 1/4%. Thus, the interested physician will have to arrange for having it dilated fourfold to 1/16%, possibly by a local pharmacist.

One, therefore, can distinguish the Adie's pupil from the dilated pupil caused by aneurysms, transtentorial herniation, and intracranial mass lesions that directly compress the third cranial nerve. The dilated pupils caused by all of these central lesions, together with all normal (non-dilated) pupils, will remain the same size after the instillation of a weak pilocarpine solution. There is seldom great difficulty in distinguishing Adie's syndrome from compressive lesions of the third cranial nerve even without pharmacologic tests. The intracranial lesions that compromise functions in the third cranial nerve generally cause clinical findings related to the extraocular muscles in addition to the pupil. Some cases of intracranial aneurysms that cause isolated pupillary involvement have been documented. In these rare instances, the extraocular and lid muscles become involved shortly after the pupil, and there are often subtle lid and ocular motility findings even when the pupil seems to be involved in isolation. The author's experience has not included any aneurysms that caused enough denervation sensitivity of the pupil to cause a clearly positive weak cholinergic test. The reader should be aware that the differential value of weak cholinergic testing is being scrutinized.

Up to this point, the discussion has focused on diagnosis of the unilateral denervated pupil in which the normal fellow pupil is used as an internal control. Bilateral denervation may be encountered in patients with auto-nomic neuropathies that occur in diabetes mellitus. Both pupils are affected in these cases, and thus one pupil cannot serve as a control for the other. In testing for bilateral denervation, the pilocarpine solution must be weak enough that it will not cause any constriction of normal pupils. For this type of test, 1/16% pilocarpine is recommended. If there is any contraction of either pupil, denervation probably can be diagnosed without reference to the other pupil.

Atropinized Pupil

The second major category of patients who present to the emergency room with an isolated large pupil is that of postsynaptic sphincter blockade by atropinic substances. The old term belladonna (alkaloid), indicating atropine and its congeners, derives from the use of these agents by women (donna) who wanted to enhance their beauty (bella). It once was considered attractive for one's eyes to appear as bottomless pools, and this was accomplished by dilating the pupils. This seldom adequately accounts for the situation today. Two groups of people end up with atropinics in one eye—those who do so accidentally and those who put the drug in the eye willfully. The first category includes those people whose work involves the use of atropine, such as nurses and other paramedical personnel, and those who manipulate plants. Many plants have naturally occurring atropinics in the sap and on the surfaces of stems, leaves, and roots. The willful application of atropine to one eye is less easy to understand. In many cases, such a person will present to the emergency room with a large pupil and a history of either blurred vision or headaches, as though there were some secondary gain attached to the frequent sequel of cerebral angiography. It stretches the imagination to assume that all these patients are aware of the relationship between pupil size and cerebral herniation syndromes. Some of the patients, however, are medical personnel who are aware of the relationship and its medical implications. It must be concluded that certain individuals are motivated to seek invasive diagnostic procedures, and the physician must be prepared to rule out CNS causes of the dilated pupil in these cases. This is easily done by the instillation of a strong solution (4% to 6%) of pilocarpine in each eye. A potent cholinergic activator of the iris sphincter that will produce a pinpoint pupil in normal eyes, 6% pilocarpine also will constrict all pathologically denervated pupils including the postganglionic parasympathetic lesions of Adie's syndrome and the preganglionic third cranial nerve lesions. The only condition that will cause a failure of the pupil to constrict with 6% pilocarpine is a postsynaptic receptor blockade at the sphincter muscle—atropinization. If the pupil is large because of iris trauma or infection, with muscle atrophy or synechiae causing an adhesion to the lens capsule, there also will be a failure of constriction; however, this situation should not present a diagnostic problem because the anterior segment appears abnormal. It may require slit-lamp biomicroscopy of the anterior segment to observe iris damage or lens capsule adhesions, and an ophthalmologic consultation should be obtained if this is considered a possibility.

The use of strong pilocarpine, therefore, unequivocally segregates those with a large pupil caused by lesions or pharmacologic blockade at the iris sphincter from normal persons and from those with large pupils caused by intracranial lesions of all types. There are few diagnostic procedures in medicine for which such a claim can be made.

It is theoretically possible for an aneurysm or other mass to compress the third cranial nerve in such a way as to cause isolated paralysis of the pupil. The pupillary fibers are superficial in the subarachnoid portion of the nerve and might be selectively disrupted by any lesion that compresses the nerve. Such a presentation is rare, and only a few cases have been documented. In most of these cases, the extraocular muscles and levator palpebrae are affected within days of isolated pupillary involvement. I have found that subtle, often fluctuating lid and oculomotor signs are present in patients who are said to have isolated

pupil dilatation caused by aneurysms. A carefully repeated examination often gives evidence that leads to the proper diagnosis of these cases. Any patient with a dilated pupil that contracts to strong pilocarpine must be observed carefully, therefore, because there may be a serious intracranial cause such as an aneurysm.

OCULAR SYMPATHETIC SYSTEM

The sympathetic system produces a dilator tone in opposition to the iris sphincter. The dilator system functions by way of a reflex arc just as the sphincter system does; however, the afferent arm is much less circumscribed than that of the light reflex, which probably accounts for the fact that the sympathetic system is often not thought of as a reflex circuit.

Afferent stimulation along pain and temperature pathways from the spinal cord generally causes pupil dilatation that is abrupt in onset and lasts on the order of 20 to 60 seconds. More sustained dilatation often attends mental states involving fear, anxiety, or surprise. Because the sympathetic afferent pathways are anatomically ill defined, especially at rostral levels of the CNS, the subsequent discussion will focus on efferent sympathetic pathways.

Anatomic studies have shown sympathetic fiber degeneration in the upper brainstem after experimental lesions in the hypothalamus. These degeneration studies document widely dispersed fiber tracts in the upper midbrain and diencephalon but no reliably demonstrated pathways in the pons and medulla. The descending system is most likely, therefore, a polysynaptic one, although in clinical usage it is referred to as the central neuron in the chain leading to the iris dilator.

Clinical studies have documented that dorsolateral lesions throughout the brainstem often produce ocular sympathetic dysfunction ipsilaterally, whereas medial and ventral lesions do not. This is the basis for the widely accepted view that the polysynaptic descending system is dorsolaterally disposed in the brainstem. This pathway continues into the spinal cord to the C8 through T2 segmental levels, where the "central" fibers synapse with cells in the intermediolateral gray horns; this zone between C8 and T2 is commonly known as the ciliospinal center of Budge and Waller. The central pathways through the cervical spinal cord are located superficially (near the pia) in the lateral columns. The preganglionic cells from the ciliospinal center send axons to the paravertebral sympathetic ganglion chain by way of the C8–T2 ventral roots. These preganglionic fibers travel upward in the sympathetic chain through the stellate (combined upper thoracic and lower cervical ganglion) and the middle cervical ganglion. They synapse with postganglionic cells in the superior cervical ganglion, which usually is found high in the neck, often under the angle of the mandible. This means that the common lesions that cause ocular sympathetic palsy (Horner's syndrome) interfere with preganglionic fibers as they course through the upper thorax. Virtually all the lesions producing postganglionic sympathetic dysfunction are intracranial and intraorbital in location because the superior cervical ganglion is so near the base of the skull.

The postganglionic axons at first travel in the adventitia of the carotid artery. Those supplying vascular and sweat gland structures in the lower face travel with external carotid branches, whereas the ocular sympathetics and those serving vasomotor and sudomotor function for the forehead go with the internal carotid into the middle cranial fossa. A contingent of ocular sympathetic fibers takes a "side path" through the otic ganglion in the middle ear. This apparently explains the occasional occurrence of Horner's syndrome with middle ear infections. The main ocular sympathetic pathway, however, follows the carotid artery through its siphon region and then joins the first division (ophthalmic) of the trigeminal nerve, which carries it into the orbit. A sympathetic contingent passes through the parasympathetic ciliary ganglion, constituting the so-called sympathetic root of the ganglion, but no sympathetic synapses occur there. In the orbit, the ocular sympathetics innervate the iris dilator muscles together with small smooth muscles in the lids, which contributes to upper lid elevation and lower lid depression. Defective contraction of these sympathetically innervated Mueller's muscles causes a low-grade ptosis or a descent of the upper lid. Less well recognized, however, is the fact that the weakness of Mueller's muscle in the lower lid causes the latter to elevate. Upper-lid ptosis and elevation of the lower lid together cause a narrowing of the palpebral fissure. This contributes to an illusion that the involved eye is displaced backward in the orbit, the so-called apparent enophthalmos that has been described with Horner's syndrome. It used to be stated that the enophthalmos was real in Horner's syndrome; however, only frogs have a sympathetically innervated muscle that normally holds the eye forward in the orbit, the weakness of which allows the eye to move backward. Thus, the enophthalmos in Horner's syndrome is truly apparent—an illusion caused by the narrowed palpebral fissure.

Sympathetic fibers serving the skin of the forehead just above the brow travel with the nasociliary branch of the first or ophthalmic division of the trigeminal nerve. With postganglionic sympathetic lesions, a triangular patch of altered vasomotor tone and decreased sweating may present just above the brow extending to the midline.

CLINICAL DISORDERS OF THE OCULAR SYMPATHETICS

The defective function of the sympathetically innervated Mueller's muscle in the upper lid results in the minor degree of ptosis that occurs typically in Horner's syndrome. The position of the upper and lower lids and thereby the width of the palpebral fissure is determined by the relative tone in the orbicularis muscle, which closes the lids, compared with the tone of the levator palpebrae plus Mueller's muscles, which open the eyes. The levator palpebrae, a striated muscle innervated by the third cranial nerve, provides most of the upper lid's elevation, whereas Mueller's muscle produces some upper lid elevation and lower lid depression. Thus, the levator and Mueller's muscle work together and in opposition to the orbicularis muscle, which encircles the palpebral fissure. When assessing lid position, one must be careful of illusions crated by asymmetric skin folds, by altered position of the eye in the orbit (extraocular muscle palsies and strabismus), and even by anisocoria. The observer's eye uses all of these landmarks for assessing where the lid margin is expected to fall and whether its position is the same in the two eyes. Eyelid position and the relation of lid margins to landmarks such as skin folds is often asymmetric for various non-neurologic reasons. It is useful, therefore, to measure the distance between a central corneal light reflex and the upper and lower lids, respectively, and also to compare these for symmetry between eyes. This reflex, produced when a point source of light such as a penlight or handlight is directed toward the eyes from a position in front of the patient, does not move appreciably with a variation in eye position as long as it still falls on the cornea. By convention, the distance from the light reflex to the upper lid margin has been called the margin-reflex-distance-1 (MRD1) and the distance from the reflex to the lower lid margin has been called margin-reflex-distance-2 (MRD2). A useful and succinct way to note this measurement in the chart is shown in Table 23.3.

A pitfall that occurs not uncommonly is the false diagnosis of a facial or seventh cranial nerve palsy caused by apparent widening of one palpebral fissure (orbicularis oculi weakness) when the fissure is really narrowed on the other side from an ocular sympathetic lesion. This error is more likely to occur if the normal range of facial asymmetry produces an apparent flattening of the nasolabial fold on the side of the wider palpebral fissure and if the pupillary miosis is minimal or lacking in the ocular sympathetic palsy. Pharmacologic pupil testing can be a useful arbiter in this setting.

ETIOLOGIC DIAGNOSIS IN HORNER'S SYNDROME

The most common ocular sympathetic palsies are those caused by an interruption of preganglionic fibers in relation to lesions of the lung apex and the neck. The bulk of these lesions are malignant tumors, often primary in the lung or metastases to cervical nodes, that can complicate a wide variety of carcinomas, lymphomas, and leukemias.

Some of these cases of preganglionic Horner's syndrome will be secondary to trauma and usually will include penetrating neck wounds and root involvement in spinal injuries. These cases should be obvious from the history and physical findings. Inflammation, caused by suppurative infections and granulomatous diseases such as sarcoidosis or tuberculosis in cervical lymph nodes, is an occasional non-malignant cause for preganglionic ocular sympathetic palsy.

CNS lesions (e.g., of the hypothalamus, brainstem, or upper cervical cord) are an uncommon cause of Horner's syndrome. They are almost always recognizable by the associated cranial nerve, cerebellar, and sensorimotor long-tract findings. A classic example is Wallenberg's lateral medullary syndrome, which usually is caused by an occlusion of one vertebral artery with an infarction in the distribution of the posterior inferior cerebellar artery. The attendant dorsolateral medullary lesion produces a syndrome that includes ocular sympathetic palsy, along with facial numbness ipsilateral to the lesion, loss of pain and temperature sensation in the contralateral extremities, vertigo, dysphagia, and dysarthria. This typical central lesion is distinct from the usually isolated, frequently asymptomatic Horner's syndrome that accompanies preganglionic peripheral lesions.

TABLE 23.3. *Width of Palpebral Fissures*

	Right Eye	Left Eye
MRD1	4	4
MRD2	5	5

MRD1, margin-reflex-distance-1 (the distance from the light reflex to the upper lid margin); MRD2, margin-reflex-distance-2 (the distance from the light reflex to the lower lid margin).

Postganglionic ocular sympathetic palsy commonly is associated with pain in the ipsilateral orbit and eye. In the early part of this century, a Norwegian ophthalmologist named Raeder reported this combination of pain, miosis, and ptosis as a "paratrigeminal" syndrome with a localizing value for mass lesions in the middle cranial fossa. All four of his patients had, in addition to ocular sympathetic palsy, findings referable to the third through sixth ipsilateral cranial nerves, either singly or in combination. During the past two decades, there has been an increasing awareness of patients with painful ocular sympathetic palsy without demonstrable middle fossa mass lesions. These patients often have histories of episodic retrobulbar and orbital pain that in many cases is typical of cluster or histamine headache. The ocular sympathetic lesion comes about during a cluster of headaches and sometimes resolves spontaneously after the cluster has ended, although it sometimes remains as a permanent sequel. This benign condition, which is considered a migraine variant, has acquired the name Raeder's paratrigeminal syndrome, type II. To qualify for this benign diagnosis, the patient must have no objective neurologic deficit of the third through sixth cranial nerves; the presence of cranial nerve findings strongly favors the presence of a middle fossa lesion. It has been speculated that in type II Raeder's syndrome, the postganglionic ocular sympathetic fibers are affected by edema in the wall of the carotid artery. Vascular wall changes, probably including edema, are presumed to occur during severe migrainous episodes. The exact sequence of events leading to the ocular sympathetic palsy in this setting is, however, unknown.

Figure 23.13 presents the ocular findings in a man 46 years of age who had frequent episodes of steady intense pain in the left orbit. Each headache lasted 45 to 60 minutes and occurred daily, often at predictable times. These findings had been present for 2 weeks prior to the examination. He had had similar bouts of frequent headaches in previous years. These headaches lasted 1 to 3 weeks at a time.

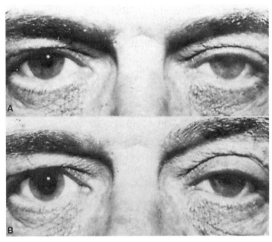

FIG. 23.13. Left ocular sympathetic lesion with ipsilateral orbital headache of migraine type (Raeder's syndrome type II). **A:** The asymmetric position of the upper-lid margin with respect to the overlying skinfold is the most prominent feature of this man's ptosis. The relation of the lid margin to the iris and globe is relatively symmetric between eyes. **B:** The left pupil failed to dilate on instillation of 1% para-OH-amphetamine, indicating a postganglionic ocular sympathetic lesion.

During this symptomatic period, however, a physician had noted left ptosis and miosis of which the patient was unaware. The neurologic examination was otherwise completely normal. This was a typical case of type II Raeder's syndrome with a presumed migrainous etiology. The pupillary pharmacologic aspects of this diagnosis will be discussed later.

PHARMACOLOGIC WORKUP OF OCULAR SYMPATHETIC LESIONS

The objectives of pharmacologic testing in the sympathetic system are twofold. In some cases, the objective is to document the presence or absence of an ocular sympathetic lesion without regard to further localization. A typical example would be a case of isolated anisocoria or isolated ptosis in which the evidence is insufficient for the reliable diagnosis of a sympathetic lesion. The second objective of pharmacologic diagnosis is to identify the level of involvement (preganglionic or post-ganglionic) in a case in which there is reasonable certainty that an ocular sympathetic lesion exists.

There is great practical value in segregating patients with Horner's syndrome into those with preganglionic and those with postganglionic lesions. The group with preganglionic lesions has a high incidence of malignant disease requiring extensive investigation, whereas the group with postganglionic involvement has primarily benign causes (usually a vascular headache).

The physiologic basis of clinically useful pharmacologic tests is noradrenergic transmission at the iris dilator neuromuscular junction, where the sympathetic postganglionic axon terminals contact the muscle cells. The drugs of greatest clinical usefulness are the indirect-acting sympathomimetics: cocaine and para-p-hydroxyamphetamine (Paredrine). The schemes for clinical usage have been worked out primarily by Thompson and co-workers (1971). Transmission in the sympathetic system at the superior cervical ganglion is cholinergic, but there are no clinically useful diagnostic tests for evaluating the function at this level.

At the postganglionic axon terminal, norepinephrine (NE) is maintained in storage vesicles by metabolically active processes. The bound vesicular NE is in equilibrium with a pool of unbound NE in the vesicle and in the cytoplasm of the nerve terminal. A small portion of the vesicular pool is released as each nerve action potential arrives along the postganglionic cell axon. The released NE interacts with specific receptors on the dilator muscle membrane, causing a contraction. As in other adrenergic systems, the effect of the released transmitter is terminated by a metabolically active reuptake from the neuromuscular junction into the postganglionic nerve terminals. Cocaine exerts its primary effect by blocking reuptake at this stage. This potentiates pupil dilator tone as a result of ongoing tonic neural activity and neurotransmitter release in the ocular sympathetic efferents. Failure of this potentiation in the presence of ocular sympathetic

lesions at all levels is useful evidence for Horner's syndrome. The reason that cocaine fails to dilate pupils with central and preganglionic sympathetic dysfunction is related presumably to the fact that the tonic release of NE at the postganglionic terminal is reduced, even with these proximal lesions, so that the blockage of NE reuptake has little effect compared to the normal other eye. A positive cocaine test is defined as relative failure of the pupil to dilate on the side of the lesion with dilatation of the fellow pupil, which is used as an internal control. Cocaine is a weak dilator; thus if neither pupil enlarges, the test must be considered indeterminate and should be ignored.

Para-OH-amphetamine not only blocks reuptake of naturally released NE but promotes the release of any stored NE from the postganglionic axon terminals into the neuromuscular junctions at the iris dilator muscles. This means that regardless of the level of ongoing neural activity in the system, if the postganglionic cell and its terminals at the dilator muscles are intact, para-OH-amphetamine will release the stored NE and then will block its reuptake, both of which actions bring about pupillary dilatation. Para-OH-amphetamine, unlike cocaine, thus will dilate the pupil in the presence of both central and preganglionic Horner's syndrome. Only a pupil with the loss of postganglionic sympathetic fibers and the stored NE at their terminals will fail to dilate in response to para-OH-amphetamine. This is the basis of the localizing value of the para-OH-amphetamine test (Fig. 23.13). It is used primarily to differentiate postganglionic lesions (pupil will not dilate) from preganglionic lesions (pupil will dilate) because central lesions are usually not a problem for localizing diagnosis on account of the associated neurologic findings. Of course, one must be sure that an ocular sympathetic lesion exists before using para-OH-amphetamine because this test will "miss" the central and preganglionic lesions by short-circuiting the neural chain and causing release of the NE stored at the postganglionic terminal, although the level of spontaneous release was diminished because of the more proximal lesion. Para-OH-amphetamine, therefore, should be reserved for the localization of an ocular sympathetic lesion and not for the identification of the lesion. An exception may be a case in which only a postganglionic deficit is suspected—for instance, in a patient with orbital pain plus ptosis and miosis.

A note of caution is in order at this point. Some patients have pain in the orbit ipsilateral to preganglionic ocular sympathetic lesions caused by trauma in the neck. The pathogenesis of this condition is obscure, but it often responds favorably to propranolol (Inderal) with relief of pain. The important point for this discussion is that one should not conclude *a priori* that the sympathetic lesion is postganglionic because of concomitant orbital pain or frontotemporal headaches. If the para-OH-amphetamine test is negative, a cocaine test should be done on another day.

The para-OH-amphetamine and cocaine tests should be done prior to any manipulations that might disrupt the corneal epithelium because any breach of corneal integrity can lead to unequal drug absorption in the two eyes and false-positive or false-negative test results. Thus, corneal reflex testing, ocular pressure measurements (tonometers usually operate through pressure on the cornea), and use of any other topical ophthalmic agents should be done on a separate day or at least after the completion of sympathetic testing. The usual protocol is instillation of one drop of either a 10% solution of cocaine or of a 1% solution of para-OH-amphetamine in each eye, with a second dose 5 to 10 minutes later. The pupil size in standard dim illumination is measured before the first drop and 60 minutes after this dose. An increase in the amount of anisocoria is a positive test result. In other words, selective failure of the involved pupil to dilate as much as the normal eye after an adequate interval is the criterion for a positive test.

DETERMINING THE AGE OF THE LESION

Because malignant disease is such a prominent feature of recently acquired pregan-

glionic ocular sympathetic lesions, it can be helpful to document that a newly observed Horner's syndrome is actually longstanding so that an extensive workup for carcinoma can be avoided. The history is usually not helpful because most patients are unaware of the lesion. The best way to prove that the lesion is not new is to inspect old photographs, which might reveal the ptosis and perhaps even anisocoria.

If the iris of the eye with Horner's syndrome is blue and the other is brown, one can establish that the lesion was probably present at birth or at least during the first year of life. A sympathetic lesion, if present early in life, prevents the development of ipsilateral iris chromatophores in a person who is genetically destined to have brown eyes. This condition is known as heterochromia iridis. The color asymmetry will not be manifest if both eyes are blue.

ARGYLL ROBERTSON PUPIL

A good deal of confusing literature has accumulated concerning the pupillary manifestations of CNS syphilis, most notably that pertaining to the so-called Argyll Robertson pupillary phenomenon. The original report by Argyll Robertson appeared in 1896 under the title "Four Cases of Spinal Myosis: With Remarks on the Action of Light on the Pupil." The thrust of the report centered on the association between spinal cord disease and the peculiar observation of very small pupils that failed to constrict to light but were still capable of response on near-viewing effort. Argyll Robertson noted that although most of the patients had ophthalmoscopic evidence of mild optic atrophy, their vision was not significantly impaired. That is, of course, crucial because a person who is blind from optic nerve disease will have pupils that do not respond to light but that constrict normally to near effort. In this setting, a dissociation between the light and near responses would have no specificity in itself. The differential diagnosis simply would be that of the optic neuropathy. Argyll Robertson was puzzled by the miosis that he felt must have been caused by involvement of the ciliospinal nerves by the spinal disease. When this classic observation first was made, there was neither serologic nor any other method by which the spinal disease could be ascribed to neurosyphilis. In fact, syphilis was not mentioned in the discussion, and only one of the four patients was noted to have previously had syphilis.

In subsequent years, the link between "locomotor ataxia," now called tabes dorsalis, and syphilis came to be well recognized, and Argyll Robertson's sign attained common usage as a powerful diagnostic sign of neurosyphilis. It was noted to be present in 60% to 84% of tabetics and in up to 50% of patients with dementia paralytica or general paresis of the insane.

Much controversy has occurred concerning whether the miosis should be considered essential to the definition of the Argyll Robertson pupil. The problem arose with the observation that diseases other than syphilis can be associated with pupils that are fixed to light but that constrict on near effort in patients with normal vision. This has been reported in a wide variety of disorders, including difficult-to-understand entities such as alcoholism, myotonic dystrophy, and diabetes mellitus. The phenomenon seems easier to accept as specific for the disorder when linked with midbrain lesions such as infarcts, hemorrhages, tumors, and encephalitis lethargica, all of which can produce destructive lesions in parts of the brainstem and spinal cord that are known to participate in pupil function. Most of these non-syphilitic light-near dissociated pupils or Argyll Robertson-like pupils are not miotic, being of average size or larger, and this serves to distinguish the syphilitic from the non-syphilitic cases. It certainly would be a wonderful universe if a differential diagnosis could be so simple and reliable! Irene Loewenfeld has shown by an exhaustive review of the literature and by extensive personal observations that the absolute size of the pupil does not definitely discriminate between syphilitic and non-syphilitic Argyll Robertson pupils. Lawton Smith has shown

that moderately large light-near dissociated pupils occur in many tabetics and paretics, so one cannot rule out syphilis in this setting if a workup fails to reveal an alternative cause. Fortunately, the situation is rendered somewhat academic by the availability of reliable and sensitive serologic markers for past syphilitic infection (e.g., fluorescent treponemal antibody absorption and others), tests that usually remain positive for the life of the patient.

The anatomic pathology leading to the Argyll Robertson pupillary phenomenon still must be considered problematic. It is difficult to imagine a single locus in the nervous system at which the afferents from the retina to the pupillomotor centers (midbrain tectum and Edinger-Westphal nucleus) would be involved together with fibers or centers that oppose the mydriatic tone of the sympathetic system. Kerr (1968) reviewed pathologic studies indicating that syphilis tends to produce a superficial demyelination, or subpial encephalopathy, throughout the neuraxis. He postulated that, in neurosyphilis, subpial demyelination of the superficial pretectal area would affect the light reaction, whereas lesions of the lateral columns just under the pia at the cervical level could produce miosis by interfering with the descending central sympathetic pathways, the combined lesions resulting in the full Argyll Robertson syndrome.

In summary, the Argyll Robertson pupil sign is manifest as a variable miosis but more crucially by fixity of the pupil to light stimulation with preserved ability to constrict on near-viewing effort (with convergence and accommodation) in a patient with normal or near-normal vision. This is most commonly bilateral but may be unilateral when first observed, often becoming bilateral as months or years pass. The phenomenon frequently is associated with neurosyphilis, particularly tabes dorsalis and general paresis, but may occur with all sorts of destructive lesions, suitably situated. Observation of the Argyll Robertson pupil in a patient first should prompt a serologic investigation and an appropriate history to establish or preclude past syphilitic infection. If such infection can be ruled out, a workup for structural lesions, in particular at the midbrain or diencephalic area, should be undertaken.

OCULAR MOTILITY IN NEUROLOGIC DIAGNOSIS

The importance of eye movements for daily visual activity is perhaps intuitively obvious. Humans are foveate: our sharp or high-resolution vision resides in a small area (2 to 3 degrees) of visual field surrounding the fixation point, which is the point in external space at which one is looking. The object of regard then is projected on the fovea centralis of the retina, where high-resolution vision is served. Perception of motion is acute outside the central visual field; however, the resolution of fine spatial details declines rapidly toward the periphery of the visual field. To adequately perceive an extended visual scene (as in daily viewing), therefore, one must "palpate" the environment by moving the fovea from point to point while compiling and storing a central image or engram of the scene. Accordingly, the eye movement system has developed in close association with the sensory or afferent visual system. This is reflected in the anatomy of the oculomotor system, particularly at the cerebral hemisphere level, where major intrahemispheric and interhemispheric connections link the so-called frontal eye fields (area 8 of Brodmann, just anterior to the primary motor strip) with temporal lobe and parietooccipital visual centers. This is of practical significance because lesions in the cerebral hemispheres often produce a diagnostically useful alteration of ocular motility.

SUPRANUCLEAR ORGANIZATION OF EYE MOVEMENT

The supranuclear organization of eye movement is discussed first because it is rich in diagnostically useful signs. Later sections will cover the final common pathway for the accomplishment of eye movement—third, fourth, and sixth cranial nerves, including

their nuclei in the brainstem and their connections with the individual extraocular muscles. Finally, the characteristics of third, fourth, and sixth cranial nerve lesions and of primary disorders of the eye muscles will be discussed.

FUNCTIONAL ORGANIZATION

Images of objects in the visual environment must be brought onto the retinal fovea where a clear neural representation can be generated. This process of foveation is the central issue for the various supranuclear eye movement control systems. In general terms, one must be able to move the eye so as to bring the image of an object onto the fovea and then keep it there despite both object movement in space and head movement—these are unavoidable conditions of daily viewing. The control networks that serve these functions are the saccade system, the pursuit system, and the vestibuloocular system, each with a specific anatomic arrangement in the cerebral hemispheres, brainstem, and cerebellum.

All of the supranuclear systems are concerned with conjugate eye movements, meaning that the visual axes of the two eyes remain parallel during the movement. Dysconjugate eye movements indicate a disorder at or below (peripheral to) the third, fourth, and sixth cranial nerve nuclei or the pathways joining these nuclei.

Saccade System

The saccade system generates high-velocity ballistic movements, or saccades, by which we foveate the elements of a stationary but large or extended visual scene. An adult scans a scene in a highly organized way, extracting data from the highest information areas but directing relatively few saccades to non-specific or uninformative areas in the display. This efficient palpatory behavior is highly learned—it develops progressively during infancy. The efficiency of ocular scanning often is degraded in the presence of cerebral lesions, particularly those associated with dementia, but this type of eye movement alteration is not accessible to bedside examination. It requires elaborate equipment to record exactly where on a visual scene the eyes are fixed at any particular time. This type of ocular motor behavior has organizational elements that encompass the highest levels of whole brain function. This chapter will focus, however, on the motor aspects alone because they can be observed directly at the bedside.

Lesions in the frontal lobes most commonly interrupt saccade function selectively. The system is represented also at the brainstem level where "burst" cells deliver high levels of innervation to oculomotor neurons and produce the high-velocity eye movements characteristic of saccades. The cerebellum also participates in the saccade system: lesions here are associated with abnormal saccade characteristics such as low-velocity or altered metrics (both overshoot and undershoot).

The parameters by which we can measure saccadic eye movement performance include latency, velocity, and metrics or accuracy.

The average normal human takes about 200 msec to generate a refixation eye movement or saccade to a new target presented in his or her visual periphery. The time required for each saccade varies widely, but most saccades occur between 180 and 250 msec. This latent interval includes time for the visual stimulus in the peripheral field to travel along afferent pathways to the cerebral cortex, where the spatial coordinates of the object to be foveated are turned into motor commands or vectors that have both direction and amplitude specifications. This computation of vectors and passage of the efferent commands to the brainstem require additional time. It also has been postulated that the system works by way of intermittent data samples rather than a continuous intake of afferent data. Thus, if a novel visual stimulus occurs just after a sample is taken, it will have to wait for the next sampling interval, which may be 40 to 50 msec later, before entry into the system. This would explain much of the latency variability observed for the generation of individual saccades. The real story is much more complex,

however, and there is considerable controversy as to whether saccade vectors are calculated in an intermittent or continuous sampling way. It is also unclear at present whether saccade motor commands can be modified as the eyes are in motion during a saccade. Under ordinary circumstances, saccades behave as a ballistic movement—as with a thrown ball, the saccade trajectory is not modifiable after the movement begins. Under special test circumstances, however, some individuals are capable of modifying the saccade trajectory in mid flight. These special features of some saccades in normal patients have not yet been explained adequately by existing models of brainstem circuitry.

Saccades have characteristic peak velocities that bear a direct relationship to the size of the eye movement in normal persons. Larger saccades are faster than smaller ones, but it is impossible to perceive these subtle velocity variations by direct observation of the eyes in flight. Fortunately for diagnosis, pathology in the saccade system often slows refixational eye movements sufficiently that the movements are easily perceived to be slow on direct inspection. The best way to observe this is by asking the patient to redirect his gaze to stationary points right and left of primary gaze. A major reduction in saccade velocity generally indicates cerebellar or brainstem disorders, although minor slowing that usually requires electronic eye movement measurement to document can accompany cerebral hemisphere pathology, particularly if it involves the frontal lobes.

Another aspect of saccade abnormality is dysmetria, in which there is altered excursion amplitude—eyes either fall short of their goal (hypometric saccades) or overshoot the target (hypermetric saccades). When saccades are hypometric, the eyes achieve the target by a series of small saccades (usually three or more). This gives the movement a "jerky" or ratchetlike quality that is observed easily. It is useful to count the number of saccades necessary for the eyes to achieve a target 25 degrees or 30 degrees to either side of center (primary gaze). Normal people often require two and occasionally three saccades, but a patient who consistently uses three or more saccades to make a 30-degree refixation can be considered abnormal. It is easier to be sure that saccade hypometria is significant if the number of saccades used for refixation to one side of primary gaze differs markedly from the number required to make an equal distance excursion to the other side.

Overshoot or hypermetric saccades also are observed easily. The eyes overshoot and attain the target by way of a series of decreasing amplitude reversals, each of which overshoots to a smaller degree than the preceding one. Each corrective saccade is separated from the last by the normal obligatory intersaccadic interval of approximately 200 msec. This gives the movement a discontinuous quality as opposed to a smooth to-and-fro, or pendular, appearance. In the acute stages of vascular lesions—infarctions or hemorrhages—of one frontal lobe, the eyes usually are deviated tonically to the side of the lesion because of the suddenly unopposed tonic influence of the normal hemisphere. It can be deduced from this that the normal tonus of a particular hemisphere, and perhaps of the frontal eye field specifically, brings about contralateral eye movements. This contraversive functional orientation also is observed in the disordered saccadic behavior that accompanies chronic frontal lobe lesions. In these cases, after the tonic eye deviation of the acute stage wears off and the patient is able to deviate the eyes fully in both directions, there remains a subtle disorder in which saccades directed away from the side of the lesion are hypometric. As an example, a male patient with right frontal lobe infarction will have trouble looking volitionally to the left. During the first 4 or 5 days after the acute event, his eyes may be strongly deviated to the right, sometimes along with a forceful head and even torso deviation in the same direction. He gradually will be able to direct his gaze further to the left, and finally, full deviation will be possible. He also may require an abnormally long latency before initiating leftward eye movements during the acute stages. This directional latency effect must be distinguished from bidirectional increased latency, which may represent an altered mental function rather than a specific disorder of the saccade system. In the chronic stages of this right-hemisphere vascular lesion, leftward refixations may continue to evoke numerous hypometric saccades, while normometric single saccades are generated for rightward refixations.

This contraversive organization is peculiar to the saccade system because the pursuit system operates in an ipsiversive mode, controlling eye movements toward the hemisphere that is active. This fact of opposing functional orientation in the saccade and pursuit systems at the cerebral hemisphere level greatly enhances the diagnostic usefulness of eye signs related to these subsystems.

Pursuit System

The task of the pursuit system is the maintenance of a target on the fovea with motion of the target in space. If the viewer's head remains stationary, the tracking of a moving target is achieved by matching the angular velocity of the eyes turning in the orbits to the angular velocity of the target moving across visual space.

The visual system is oriented about the retinas, which are on the spherical back surfaces of the eyes, and angular measurements in degrees or minutes of arc are more convenient than the tangent measure, which would have to include the distance traveled in the frontal plane and the distance of that plane from the viewer to define the appropriate pursuit eye movement. The pursuit movement also would be awkward to specify in tangent measure because it involves rotation about a vertical axis rather than translational movement in a flat plane.

The normal behavior of the pursuit system can be specified as the gain (G), and $G = I/O$, where I is the input or target velocity in visual space (deg/sec) and O is the output, in this case pursuit eye velocity (deg/sec). Normal tracking involves a gain of 1.0 such that the eyes stay on the target as it moves.

The most frequently observed abnormality of pursuit is subnormal gain, in which the eyes fall progressively behind the target. The examiner cannot perceive the velocity of a patient's pursuit movements by inspection. Fortunately, the visual system will not tolerate the error that develops as the eyes fall behind the target, and an easily observed saccade is generated as soon as the eye is sufficiently far behind to generate a position error signal. Thus, low-gain pursuit is interrupted by a series of catchup saccades aimed at refoveating the target. These inserted saccades occur rhythmically because it requires about the same amount of time to generate the necessary position error throughout the course of the pursuit movement. Normal pursuit is smooth with no inserted saccades. Low-gain pursuit is indicated to the observer by the presence of rhythmic saccades rather than the slowness of the pursuit movement itself.

This pursuit abnormality, which is best referred to as low-gain pursuit with catchup saccades, has engendered various descriptive names including saccadic pursuit and even cogwheel pursuit in patients with Parkinson's disease. This movement, however, should not be linked to the pathophysiology of parkinsonian cogwheeling. The saccadic pursuit of parkinsonism is the manifestation of low gain in the pursuit system with a relatively normal saccade function so that forward saccades achieve refoveation during defective tracking. This does not differ from low-gain pursuit in other pathologic conditions.

The pursuit system is highly susceptible to degraded function, and bidirectional low-gain pursuit may be a non-specific abnormality in various clinical settings in which the finding has no localizing value. Fatigue and the effects of many drugs bring about bidirectional symmetric low-gain pursuit. Bidirectional low-gain pursuit is common in the elderly and has little prognostic or localizing value.

Unidirectional low-gain pursuit, however, is highly specific for a lesion of the horizontal gaze pathway on one side. The pursuit function in the cerebral hemisphere is ipsiversive, and a unidirectional defective pursuit

suggests a lesion of the parietooccipital convexity on the side toward which pursuit gain is low. For instance, a right-sided posterior hemisphere lesion will cause low-gain pursuit with catchup saccades rightward, but it will leave leftward pursuit unaffected.

Large hemisphere lesions may involve both saccade and pursuit functions, in which case there will be hypometric saccades in one direction (opposite the lesion) and low-gain pursuit in the other (toward the lesion). Low-gain pursuit also can be observed as part of the supranuclear conjugate gaze disorder that accompanies lesions of the rostral pons and midbrain, usually in conjunction with altered saccade parameters, but here the saccades and pursuit are defective in the same direction.

A fundamental distinction therefore must be made between cerebral hemisphere and brainstem conjugate gaze syndromes. At the cerebral level, the direction of the saccade abnormality (contraversive) is opposite to the direction of the pursuit abnormality (ipsiversive), whereas at the brainstem level both are ipsilateral to the lesion side. Clinical evidence tells us that the saccade control pathways cross somewhere caudal to the diencephalon but rostral to the pons, whereas the pursuit pathways either do not cross at all or they cross and recross such that their functional direction is ipsilateral to the disordered hemisphere. I have published a case in which a small hematoma at the posterior thalamus resulted in contraversive hypometric saccades and ipsiversive low-gain pursuit with catchup saccades. This indicates that the hemisphere bidirectionality is preserved as far caudal and as deep as the thalamus. This may indicate that the pursuit and saccade pathways both operate by way of the ipsilateral frontal eye field outflow through the thalamus. Alternatively, the pursuit system may have pathways in the corona radiata separate from the saccade system outflow, but these may funnel through the same region in the thalamus as the frontal system. Clinical evidence does not as yet discriminate between these two possibilities. The fact that some frontal lesions are associated with an ipsidirectional pursuit defect in conjunction with a contraversive saccade disorder supports the idea of a pursuit system outflow by way of a common frontothalamic brainstem pathway. The repeated observation of frontal lesions with isolated contralateral saccade disruption and normal pursuit weigh against a common pathway. Further clinical observations are required to specify more precisely how this might operate.

Saccade versus Pursuit Testing

Proper testing means the separate elicitation of saccade and pursuit-type eye movements. The examiner should stand about 1 meter in front of the patient. Visually guided saccades are tested by asking the patient first to look at the examiner's nose and then to look at an object about 30 degrees to either side of the midline. Appropriately placed objects will be provided if the examiner holds his arms semiextended (elbows about 90 degrees flexed) with hands slightly in front of his own facial plane. The patient should keep his head stationary in a straight-ahead position during this type of testing to avoid introducing vestibuloocular components. He is asked to refixate his gaze from the examiner's nose to one of his hands, then back to his nose, and finally to his other hand and back again. It is often useful to wiggle the fingers of the hand you want the patient to look at as an added stimulus for a visually guided saccade.

The clinical setting sometimes suggests the need to test for saccades without visual targets. This has to do with the ability to imagine coordinates for the saccade system, which can be selectively defective in some cases of higher cortical function abnormality with diffuse or widespread lateralized hemisphere lesions. In this case, simply ask the patient to "look left" or "look right" without providing any target.

A selective examination for pursuit system defects involves providing a slowly moving target for the patient to view. One can infer that pursuit function is pathologic if the normally smooth following or pursuit eye move-

ment is interrupted by a series of "jerky"-appearing saccades. The target should not be moved too rapidly because the pursuit system in normal people falls behind when target velocities reach 40 to 50 degrees/second, producing saccadic pursuit at faster target speeds. A target excursion that carries the patient's eyes from extreme right to extreme left gaze should take about 5 seconds.

Vestibuloocular System

The vestibuloocular system maintains the fixation of objects in visual space in the presence of head movement. The afferent arm of this reflex is initiated by acceleration receptors in the inner ear. A mathematic integration is performed on the acceleration data by virtue of the mechanics of the semicircular canal and cupula, and information on head rotational velocity in space is supplied to the vestibular nuclei by way of the eighth cranial nerve. The information is relayed from there to the brainstem gaze centers, where slow eye movements with velocity equal to and direction opposite head rotation are generated. For instance, if the head rotates rightward at 10 degrees/second, the vestibuloocular reflex produces a leftward eye movement at 10 degrees/second and the image of a viewed stationary object remains fixed on the fovea. The operation of this system, like that of the pursuit system, is expressed conveniently as "gain"—that is, eye movement velocity divided by head rotation velocity in degrees per second. Naturally, a gain of 1.0 is needed to maintain foveation with head rotation. It turns out, however, that the vestibuloocular reflex does not supply the entire eye movement drive because in total darkness the gain of this system falls to about 0.6 in normal people. This means that the vestibuloocular reflex normally works together with the pursuit system, which optimizes function, because the vestibuloocular reflex has no retinal feedback by which to monitor its performance and keep its output accurate. Any inappropriate velocity drive from this "open loop" vestibuloocular system is adjusted by the "closed-loop" pursuit system, which receives direct retinal afferent feedback for fine control of the foveal position on the visual environment.

The key symptom of pathologic underactivity in the vestibuloocular reflex is oscillopsia, which is an illusory sense of movement in the visual environment as the head moves. This is a direct consequence of foveal image motion engendered specifically by head movement. The illusion ceases when the head is immobile. Vertigo, another common symptom of vestibular disorders, often is present when the head is still, although head movement usually aggravates it. Vertigo is a rotational illusion that often is accompanied by rhythmic oscillopsia as a consequence of nystagmus, in which case the rhythm probably is imposed by the regular fast phases of the nystagmus.

Nystagmus is defined as a repetitive bidirectional or multidirectional ocular oscillation in which the slow-phase movement is the pathologic one. When caused by vestibular disease, the nystagmus is created by tonic imbalance or bias in the vestibular subsystems on either side of midline, including the central connections and the peripheral labyrinthine apparatus. Tonic vestibular system imbalance passes a tonic directional bias to the brainstem gaze centers, which causes the eyes to drift toward the side with reduced activity. The tonic influence of each side is contraversive and a lesion creates underactivity of the ipsilateral system, with relative overactivity of the opposite system. The unopposed contraversive tone of the system opposite the lesion imposes eye drift toward the lesion side. This drift is checked by rhythmically occurring saccades in the opposite direction. The ensemble effect is rhythmic jerk-type nystagmus with slow-phase movements toward the side with the lesion and fast phases away from the lesion. This nystagmus is rhythmic because the slow-phase drift is at a constant velocity, determined by the degree of bias or imbalance between the two lateral vestibular subsystems, and the corrective saccades occur whenever a certain fixed amount of retinal position error between the object of regard and fovea occurs.

Vestibular disorders are discussed in Chapter 14. The discussion here is meant to provide the basis for understanding the more important ocular motility aspects of vestibular function.

BRAINSTEM ORGANIZATION OF EYE MOVEMENT CONTROL: THE FINAL COMMON PATHWAY

Zones within the tegmental reticular formation in the brainstem serve to combine the various eye movement commands and to present an integrated set of final motor commands to the oculomotor nuclei. The pontine paramedian reticular formation (PPRF) refers to the zone surrounding the seventh nerve nucleus on either side of midline in the pontine tegmentum. This area is specialized for integration of horizontal eye movement commands. The rostral interstitial nucleus of the medial longitudinal fasciculus (riMLF), the interstitial nucleus of Cajal (iC), the nucleus of Darkschewitsch (nD), the nucleus of the posterior commissure (nPC), and the adjacent portions of the mesencephalic reticular formation probably perform similar integration of commands for vertical eye movement and pass the final innervation pattern to the nuclei of the third and fourth cranial nerves.

Commands for saccades and pursuit come down to the brainstem by way of the supranuclear eye movement pathways outlined previously. In addition, the vestibular nuclei in the medulla and the flocculi and noduli of the cerebellum provide vestibular inputs to both the horizontal eye movement system in the PPRF and to the vertical eye movement zones of the mesencephalic reticular formation, primarily the riMLF and iC.

VERTICAL GAZE

The organization of the vertical eye movement system is complex and is not completely understood. The riMLF appears to contain primarily burst neurons that generate vertical saccades, whereas cells of the iC, nD, nPC, and MRF carry the fully assembled burst–t onic firing pattern needed to perform saccades, ocular pursuit and vestibuloocular movements and to hold the eyes in eccentric positions of gaze. There is evidence that the iC provides vertical gaze–holding signals, whereas the nucleus prepositus hypoglossi (NPH) and medial vestibular nucleus (MVN) provide this function for horizontal eye movements. Nuclei at the pontine and medullary levels are important in the control of vertical eye movements. Bilateral lesions of the medial longitudinal fasciculus (MLF), which carries complex ascending influences from vestibular nuclei, NPH, and PPRF gaze centers to the iC, nD, and nPC, abolish vertical pursuit and vestibuloocular reflex movements but spare saccades. Thus, the riMLF apparently has functional connections with the cerebral hemispheres independent of supranuclear pathways that operate by way of the PPRF. Although vertical saccades are spared with bilateral lesions of the ascending pathways, the eye position signal is abolished and gaze paretic nystagmus occurs with up-and-down gaze effort.

For all practical purposes, there are no clinical disorders in which vertical gaze palsy is caused by cerebral hemisphere disease. Brainstem structures classically thought to mediate vertical gaze are situated in the midbrain tectum and pretectal areas. In this region, lesions commonly cause upward and downward gaze palsies along with certain other classic features, the constellation of which constitutes the midbrain pretectal syndrome, also referred to as the periaqueductal grey matter syndrome, or Parinaud's syndrome. It sometimes is referred to as the syndrome of Koerber and Salus, who documented similar findings in a patient with a mass lesion in the sylvian aqueduct itself, whereas Parinaud described the findings related to pinealomas compressing the midbrain pretectum from the outside. The same clinical constellation results from infarction and hemorrhage involving these same anatomic structures as intrinsic lesions. The syndrome to be described is, therefore, of localizing value but does not provide evidence for a specific etiology in a particular case. For this, the tempo of evolution and the regression of signs and symptoms, along with other clinical details, are needed.

Aside from vertical gaze palsy, the common features of midbrain pretectal lesions include pupillary paralysis with unequal pupils that are sometimes large and sometimes small, loss of pupil reaction to light with preserved miosis on near viewing (light-near dissociation), convergence–retraction nystagmus, and variable degrees of ptosis or pathologic lid retraction. Rhythmic backward movement of the globes into the orbits in a nystagmuslike cycle characterizes retractory nystagmus. In conjunction with globe retraction, there may be convergence movements of the two eyes with respect to one another. This constitutes the classic convergence–retraction nystagmus of midbrain pretectal lesions.

HORIZONTAL GAZE

Efferents from the PPRF on one side connect with large motor cells in the ipsilateral sixth nerve nucleus for abduction of the ipsilateral eye and with small cells in the same nucleus. Axons from the small cells of the abducens nucleus ascend in the MLF and connect with cells in the opposite medial rectus subnucleus of the third nerve for adduction of the contralateral eye. Thus, a contraversive (opposite direction) saccade command from one hemisphere descends to the opposite-side PPRF, then to the abducens nucleus for both abduction of the eye ipsilateral to the active PPRF and adduction of the opposite eye. This produces conjugate gaze contralateral to the hemisphere issuing the command, ipsilateral to the activated PPRF.

Figure 23.14 illustrates schematically the brainstem and hemisphere pathways that participate in conjugate leftward gaze. Beginning at the right cerebral hemisphere, we can follow the path through the deep cerebral white matter and diencephalon to the midbrain, where a proposed crossing occurs just caudal to the third cranial nerve nucleus. This route continues to the PPRF on the left side of the

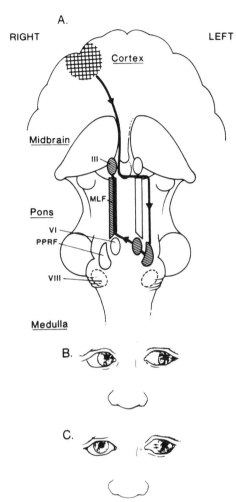

FIG. 23.14. A: Semischematic diagram of the brainstem pathways and centers that serve horizontal conjugate gaze. Multisynaptic pathways from the right frontal cortex decussate in the midbrain and form synapses in the left pontine paramedian reticular formation (PPRF), which relays innervation to two cell populations within the sixth cranial nerve nucleus. The large cells in the nucleus send axons to the lateral rectus muscle to abduct the left eye. The small-cell population gives rise to a pathway that decussates and ascends in the contralateral medial longitudinal fasciculus (MLF) and makes synaptic contact with cells of the medial rectus subnucleus of the third cranial nerve complex. This pathway gives rise to coordinated adduction of the right eye to complete the act of conjugate leftward gaze as illustrated in **B.** A lesion in the MLF causes internuclear ophthalmoplegia, which is characterized by a failure of adduction of the ipsilateral eye during attempted conjugate gaze as illustrated in **C.** The abducting eye often manifests dissociated or monocular nystagmus.

brainstem, probably in the basis pontis. A synapse occurs here with PPRF neurons, which, in turn, make a relay to the ipsilateral sixth cranial nerve nucleus. Activation of the sixth nerve (abducens) nucleus causes abduction of the left eye. It is clear that conjugate leftward gaze will require coordinated adduction of the right eye; thus the next step is a requisite connection between the small-cell population of the left abducens nucleus and the right third cranial nerve nucleus, specifically the medial rectus subnucleus. This connection is served by a paired bundle of fibers that run throughout the brainstem dorsally and just on either side of midline—the MLF. This is the basic connectivity that underlies conjugate horizontal gaze. Of course, there are a great many other contributory connections to and from the other nuclei having to do with the control of saccade, pursuit, and vestibular and gaze-holding functions.

These multidirectional systems admittedly are difficult to follow. However, it will make more sense if you trace the steps carefully from level to level and work out the directions for yourself.

MEDIAL LONGITUDINAL FASCICULUS AND "INTERNUCLEAR OPHTHALMOPLEGIA"

To this point, our discussion has concerned only disorders that bring about conjugate disorders of gaze; that is, if one eye fails to deviate leftward, the other eye also fails in the same direction and to an equal degree. Thus, the eyes in all these lesions remain "straight" with parallel visual axes when viewing objects at a distance. For simplicity, we will ignore the case of near-object viewing with convergence of the visual axes because it is irrelevant for most neurologic diagnoses. After the supranuclear organizational systems supply input to the PPRF for horizontal eye deviation, the neural information must be conveyed to the ipsilateral sixth cranial nerve (lateral rectus nucleus for abduction) and the contralateral third cranial nerve (medial rectus subnucleus for adduction). The MLF provides the pathway that connects these two nuclei, and lesions of this pathway cause a clinical condition known as internuclear ophthalmoplegia (INO).

Lesions affecting the MLF cause failure of the adducting eye to move, whereas the abducting eye deviates laterally to its full extent. This striking pattern of dysconjugate eye movement is called internuclear ophthalmoplegia because the lesion in effect disconnects the sixth and the third cranial nerve nuclei by causing a failure of neural conduction in the internuclear pathway, the MLF.

In addition to failure of the eye on the side of the MLF lesion to adduct, there is usually "dissociated" monocular nystagmus of the abducting other eye in cases of INO. This peculiar monocular nystagmus can be either transitory (one or two beats) or sustained. The clinical importance of diagnosing the MLF syndrome is its exquisite localizing value for lesions deep in the substance of the brainstem tegmentum. This general area in the brainstem contains the ascending reticular activating system, which is necessary for alert consciousness, along with several adjacent cranial nerve nuclei and various ascending and descending sensory and cerebellar pathways. Therefore, the isolated occurrence of an MLF syndrome in an alert individual without other brainstem signs or symptoms suggests the presence of a discrete lesion. For practical purposes, in the adult this is caused by either a small demyelinating plaque of multiple sclerosis or by a tiny infarction resulting from small vessel disease. This type of tiny infarct is called a lacune and occurs mainly in patients with hypertension who are older than age 60 years. An MLF syndrome or INO occasionally is encountered as a result of trauma, and in children it can be the first sign of a brainstem glioma (astrocytoma).

Differentiating between multiple sclerosis and lacunar infarction can be a problem because in either the lesions tend to evolve acutely or subacutely and then resolve slowly over a period of days or weeks. Some generalizations can be helpful, however. The patient with an MLF lesion caused by multiple sclerosis most often will be younger than 40 years of age, whereas the patients at risk for lacunae are generally older than age 60 years. It has been said that a bilateral MLF lesion favors multiple sclerosis because there is nothing to limit a plaque at the anatomic midline, whereas vascular lesions often are limited to one side by the vascular territory of a basilar artery paramedian-penetrating branch.

The clinical appearance of internuclear ophthalmoplegia can be mimicked in most details by myasthenia gravis, which can present with failure of adduction in one eye with dissociated nystagmus of the other eye. It is interesting that the dissociated, unilateral nystagmus of INO also is present in myasthenia, which is, of course, a peripheral disorder. The mechanisms that cause the dissociated nystagmus in MLF lesions are not understood. The practical offshoot is that any patient presenting purely with findings of an MLF lesion, either unilateral or bilateral, without other brainstem signs or symptoms should have an edrophonium chloride (Tensilon) test as part of the workup. If the disorder of eye motility is caused by myasthenia, it will clear dramatically during the time the edrophonium chloride is in effect.

EYE MOVEMENT DISORDERS WITH NUCLEAR AND INFRANUCLEAR LESIONS

Lesions of the oculomotor (third), trochlear (fourth), and abducens (sixth) nerve nuclei and their outflow pathways produce dysconjugate eye movements. The pattern of the movement disorder is highly characteristic of the involved cranial nerve and serves to localize the problem. The medial recti cause adduction of the eye, whereas the lateral recti cause abduction or outward rotation of the eye. The anatomy and physiology of the vertically acting muscles are more complicated.

Elevation and depression are the terms applied to upward and downward rotations of the eyes about a horizontal axis. The term torsion has been applied to rotation of the globe about an anteroposterior axis. Intorsion refers

TABLE 23.4. *Muscle Action by Position*

Muscle	Position	
	Adduction	Abduction
Superior rectus	Intorsion	Elevation
Inferior rectus	Extorsion	Depression
Inferior oblique	Elevation	Extorsion
Superior oblique	Depression	Intorsion

to the rotation of the 12:00 meridian of the iris inward, toward the nose, and extorsion refers to the rotation of this reference point outward toward the ear. The names incyclodeviation and excyclodeviation also have been applied to torsional movements.

The superior and inferior recti function, respectively, as elevators and depressors of the globe when the eye is in abduction. The inferior and superior obliques serve, respectively, as elevators and depressors when the eye is in adduction. The torsional component for each of these muscles comes into play when the optical axis is not in alignment with the axis of pull for the particular muscle (Table 23.4).

THIRD CRANIAL NERVE PALSIES

The third cranial nerve innervates the medial rectus, superior rectus, and inferior oblique muscles, along with the pupil sphincter and the levator palpebrae, which elevates the upper eyelid. The third nerve originates in a rostrocaudally elongated group of subnuclei clustered in the midbrain just rostral to the level of the fourth cranial nerve nucleus. The architecture of this nuclear group has been the subject of intensive study over the years. The most widely accepted anatomic scheme is that of Warwick, which is represented in a stylized view in Fig. 23.15. Warwick conceived of the subnuclei as columns of cells in elongated arrangement along the rostrocaudal dimension. Axons from the more dorsally situated subnuclei pass through the middle and inferior columns of cells on their way to the point of exit from the ventral aspect of the midbrain near the cerebral peduncles. The nuclei for the inferior rectus, inferior oblique, and medial

rectus muscles send axons only to the ipsilateral third cranial nerve. The subnucleus for the levator palpebrae (caudal central nucleus) is a midline structure and sends axons to both nerves. The superior rectus subnucleus sends axons only to the contralateral third nerve trunk. These anatomic details lead to clinical rules by which one can determine whether a lesion is in the third nerve trunk or at the level of the nucleus. Figure 23.15 is set up to illustrate the effects of a right third nerve nuclear lesion. The filled triangles and solid lines indicate uninterrupted neurons from the left subnuclei. The open triangles and dotted lines represent neurons that are affected by the lesion in the right third nerve nucleus. Lesioned neurons include those with cell body damage in the affected nucleus and others with damage primarily to the axons as they pass through the lesioned nucleus. Note that with destruction limited to the right side of the nucleus, there is complete disruption of outflow to the right third cranial nerve. In addition, fibers coming from the left superior rectus and levator palpebrae subnuclei are shown as solid lines changing to dotted lines, indicating axonal disruption as they pass through the right-sided lesion. This is a necessary consequence of the fact that fibers flow through the other nuclear subgroups and almost always are involved in clinical lesions such as infarction or hemorrhage limited to one side. This mixture of crossed and uncrossed axonal involvement leads to the rule that nuclear lesions on one side cause partial bilateral ptosis and failure of elevation of both eyes. The contralateral ptosis is usually incomplete because there are some intact fibers to the levator contralateral to the nuclear lesion supplied by non-crossing neurons in the normal side of the caudal central nucleus.

Nuclear lesions are caused primarily by small infarctions secondary to occlusion of the medial penetrating vessels from the basilar artery. On rare occasions, small hemorrhages in this area may cause nuclear third cranial nerve palsies. More ventral lesions in the brainstem substance may cause a disruption of the fibers emerging from the third cra-

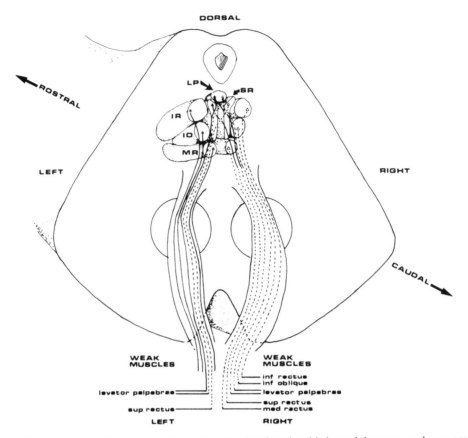

FIG. 23.15. A cross section through the midbrain showing the third cranial nerve nuclear complex. The subnuclei extend in rostrocaudally oriented columns as depicted in this three-dimensional representation modeled on Warwick's schemata. The letters superimposed on each nuclear group indicate the muscle innervated as follows: LP, levator palpebrae; SR, superior rectus; IR, inferior rectus; IO, inferior oblique; MR, medial rectus. A right nuclear third nerve lesion is illustrated. *Open triangles* and *dotted lines* indicate lesioned neurons and their axons. *Filled triangles* and *solid lines* denote normal neurons and their axons. All of the outflow to the right third nerve is lesioned. Crossed outflow from the right SR and LP subnuclei gives rise to paresis of contralateral eye elevation and ptosis. The left ptosis is partial because there is still ipsilateral (uncrossed) outflow from left LP subnucleus to the left LP. The crossed pathway from left LP subnucleus to right LP is affected at the axonal level as the fibers course through the damaged right third nerve complex *(transition of solid lines to dotted);* thus, right ptosis is complete. The contralateral elevator palsy and ptosis thus distinguish nuclear nerve palsy from fascicular palsy in which the findings are limited to the ipsilateral eye.

nial nerve nuclei along with contralateral hemiplegia caused by the involvement of the cerebral peduncle (Weber's syndrome). The characteristics of these fascicular third nerve lesions are the same as those of any distal lesion, affecting only the axons of one nerve.

An important third nerve lesion is caused by aneurysms of the posterior communicating artery that involve the nerve trunk as it passes near this vessel at its junction with the supraclinoid portion of the internal carotid artery near the cavernous sinus. Figure 23.11 illustrates semidiagrammatically the anatomy of the third nerve course in relation to the posterior cerebral artery, the superior cerebellar artery, and the posterior communicating artery. This figure illustrates an aneurysm of the posterior communicating artery at its origin from the internal carotid. The inset shows an aneurysm in cross section and its relationship to the adjacent third cranial nerve. The pupillary fibers from the Edinger–Westphal subnucleus are shown as a black band at the periphery of the nerve. The fact that aneurysms commonly produce dilatation of the pupil on the side of the third nerve lesion was discussed previously. Figure 23.11 shows that the right eye is slightly abducted and depressed on account of a weakness of the medial rectus, superior rectus, and inferior oblique muscles, with unopposed tone in the lateral rectus and superior oblique muscles.

The third nerve often is involved in lesions of the cavernous sinuses, commonly in conjunction with the other cranial nerves that pass in this structure, namely the fourth (trochlear), the sixth (abducens), and the first two divisions of the fifth (trigeminal). The most commonly encountered lesions in this area are inflammatory diseases of unknown etiology, aneurysms of the subclinoid internal carotid artery, and tumors. Granulomatous or primarily lymphocytic inflammation in the cavernous sinus and superior orbital fissure is known as the Tolosa–Hunt syndrome. It is manifest primarily by painful ophthalmoplegia from combined involvement of third, fourth, and sixth cranial nerves, and it nearly always improves with steroid treatment. This relatively benign inflammatory disease must be distinguished, however, from other infiltrating lesions such as lymphomas and carcinomas, which also may respond transiently to steroid administration. Meningiomas of the medial sphenoid ridge and pituitary tumors expanding laterally from the sella also can involve the cranial nerves within the cavernous sinuses. Mucocele of the sphenoid and ethmoid sinuses also can present in this way on rare occasions.

The subject of "medical" third cranial nerve palsy, referring to a microvascular occlusion with infarction in the nerve trunk, already has been discussed in the pupil section. Because the infarction often is limited to the center of the nerve and the pupillary fibers occupy the periphery, the rule for diagnosis of this type of lesion is sparing of the pupil relative to the degree of palsy in the extraocular muscles.

FOURTH CRANIAL NERVE PALSIES

The trochlear nerve innervates the superior oblique muscle. Lesions affecting this cranial nerve produce a failure of the eye to depress in adduction with consequent vertical diplopia. With a right fourth cranial nerve palsy, the vertical diplopia typically would increase in gaze to the left (adduction of the right eye) and in downward gaze (into the field of action of the superior oblique). Because the superior oblique contributes to intorsional tone in primary gaze, the image from the involved eye is tilted. An astute patient with a right fourth nerve palsy may tell you, for instance, that the false image of a horizontal edge is not only below the image from the left eye but also is tilted with respect to the latter. Some patients develop a habitual head tilt, presumably to compensate for this torsional imbalance. A person with a right fourth cranial nerve palsy would tend to tilt his head to the left to bring the extorted eye back to the vertical position. The sound left eye then can increase its intorsional tone to make the two eyes parallel in the plane of rotation around the optic axis (anteroposterior axis). Because some intorsional tone can be contributed by the superior rectus, this muscle may be called into play to overcome the intorsional weakness caused by the fourth cranial nerve palsy. If, for instance, the examiner tilts the head of a person with right fourth nerve palsy to the right, even more intorsion than normal is required. The superior rectus is recruited in an effort to maximize intorsional power. This causes further inappropriate elevation of the right eye because the primary effect of superior rectus contraction is an elevation of the eye.

This is the basis for the Bielschowski test for a fourth nerve palsy. The patient is directed to gaze straight ahead, and the head then is tilted to the right and to the left, making sure that there is no vertical or horizontal deviation away from primary gaze. If the degree of elevation of the eye on the side of the cranial nerve palsy increases as the head is tilted toward the side of the palsied muscle, the test is positive.

The fourth cranial nerve is unique in that it exits from the brainstem dorsally and crosses to the other side before encircling the brainstem on the way to the cavernous sinus. This renders it particularly susceptible to trauma in which forces are brought to bear on the dorsal midbrain. This usually occurs in the setting of severe head trauma in which the brainstem is forced downward and is angulated backward by a sudden shift of supratentorial structures. The dorsal midbrain and both fourth nerves are impacted in the crotch of the tentorium cerebelli, and both nerves tend to be contused together. Because of bilateral injury to the ascending reticular formation, the patient is usually unconscious for a protracted period of time after the injury, following which he complains of vertical double vision. On examination, one finds relative elevation of the right eye in left gaze and relative elevation of the left eye in right gaze. This reversal of vertical deviation indicates bilateral fourth cranial nerve palsies.

Unilateral fourth nerve palsy sometimes follows minor head trauma. There is reason to believe that many of these represent "decompensation" of longstanding or congenital fourth nerve palsies that were never previously symptomatic. Exactly how this comes about is unclear, but it is important to ask these patients to bring in childhood photographs to search for head tilt that would indicate a congenital condition.

Fourth cranial nerve palsies can occur secondary to intraneuronal microvascular ischemic disease as seen in elderly patients, often associated with diabetes and longstanding hypertension. These are presumably similar to the type of third and sixth cranial nerve palsies that one encounters in this same group of patients. The diplopia tends to improve over several weeks or months following the onset. Tumors in the region of the midbrain tectum also occasionally can present with fourth cranial nerve palsies.

SIXTH CRANIAL NERVE PALSIES

The abducens nucleus is medial and dorsal in the brainstem at the pontomedullary junction. Its axons course almost directly ventral and exit from the pons near the midline. The large cells of the abducens nucleus innervate the lateral rectus muscle, while a small-cell population innervates the contralateral medial rectus subnucleus of the oculomotor complex (third cranial nerve) by way of the MLF.

The abducens nucleus is activated by input from the ipsilateral PPRF leading to coordinated abduction of the ipsilateral (to the active PPRF) eye and adduction of the contralateral eye. This yoked deviation of both eyes is horizontal conjugate gaze.

Figure 23.16 illustrates a patient with weakness of the right lateral rectus caused by a sixth cranial nerve palsy. Note that in primary gaze the eyes are slightly crossed or convergent (esodeviated). This is caused by the unopposed tone of the medial rectus that is acting without the normal tonic innervation of the weak lateral rectus muscle. In left gaze, the eyes are parallel, but in right gaze there is a clearcut failure of right eye abduction. In this case it is the right eye that is deviating inward in primary gaze, and it is the right lateral

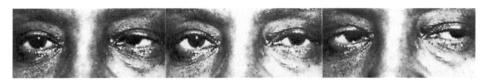

FIG. 23.16. Right lateral rectus palsy. In primary gaze *(center)*, the eyes are slightly inturned with respect to one another (esodeviated). In right gaze *(left figure)*, the angle of esodeviation increases as the right eye fails to abduct fully. In left gaze *(right figure)*, the visual axes are parallel.

rectus muscle that is weak. Be aware, however, that in primary gaze the right eye might be used for fixation of the target, with deviation of the left eye, even with a weak right lateral rectus muscle. Which eye the patient chooses for fixation is a matter of habit that may not be disrupted by muscle paresis, even if the weakness is profound. There is also a strong tendency to fixate with the eye that has better vision.

The degree of esodeviation in primary gaze may be different depending on which eye is fixing. Primary deviation refers to the angle that results from fixation with the "good" eye. Secondary deviation results from fixation with the paretic eye, and it is larger than primary deviation. In primary gaze, the bad eye is "struggling" to abduct even to the midposition against the tone of the medial rectus, and a great deal of rightward innervation is required by the right eye. According to Hering's law of equal innervation, the yoked medial rectus of the opposite (left) eye also will get this large amount of innervation and will adduct a great deal, creating a large-angle esotropia. When the non-paretic left eye is fixing, a standard quantity of rightward innervation is required, and a lesser deviation results from the failure of the right eye to abduct completely.

This difference between primary and secondary deviation is a good clue to the presence of muscle paretic deviation, as opposed to deviation caused by squint or childhood strabismus in which the deviation remains the same whichever eye is fixing. Fixation with one or the other eye can be forced by occluding the fellow eye and then quickly uncovering it to observe the degree of deviation of the covered eye before fixation is shifted.

As with the third and fourth cranial nerves, sixth cranial nerve palsies can occur on the basis of microvascular lesions in patients with hypertension or diabetes, in which case the abduction deficit tends to improve over a 3- to 6-month period. In addition, the sixth cranial nerve is susceptible to all of the local lesions that one could imagine in the pons, including hemorrhage, infarction, demyelination, and neoplasia (e.g., pontine glioma in childhood; metastatic tumor and reticulum cell sarcoma in adults). The sixth nerve also may be involved in inflammatory and infiltrating lesions of the cavernous sinuses, as already mentioned, or of the leptomeninges (e.g., carcinomatous meningitis and chronic or acute infectious meningitis). In addition to these standard lesions, the sixth cranial nerve is susceptible to stretching and distortion in a way that the other cranial nerves are not. This phenomenon results in the so-called false-localizing sixth cranial nerve palsy in which the failure of abduction in one eye or both accompanies lesions that are remote from the sixth cranial nerve or its muscle, the lateral rectus. This occurs most commonly with raised intracranial pressure. Sixth nerve palsy also has been documented occasionally as a transient phenomenon following lumbar puncture. The pathophysiology in these cases is unclear, although presumably a transient shift of the brainstem secondary to cerebrospinal fluid pressure gradients is sufficient to cause the problem. The susceptibility of the sixth nerve to small brainstem displacement may be based on the fact that it is fixed on one end at its emergence from the pons and at the other end at its entry point into the cavernous sinus—Dorello's canal in the petrous bone tip. The sixth nerve is between the proverbial rock and a hard spot.

WEAKNESS OF INDIVIDUAL EXTRAOCULAR MUSCLES

In the preceding sections, we have referred to a weakness of the muscles innervated by the third, fourth, and sixth cranial nerves and to lesions of these cranial nerves as though they were synonymous. This type of thinking should be avoided when one first encounters a patient with a weakness of one or several of these muscles. Disorders of muscle may mimic a lesion in any of these cranial nerves. Myasthenia gravis and thyroid eye disease are frequent offenders because they have a tendency to affect one or several extraocular muscles of one eye or an asymmetric array of muscles in both eyes. The level of the lesion may be difficult to determine when the nerve in question innervates only one muscle. In the case of the third cranial nerve, however, it should be easy to distinguish peripheral muscle disorders from those caused by an involvement of the cranial nerve. It generally is held that a lesion in the nerve trunk or at the nuclear level will involve, to some degree, all of the muscles within the distribution of the third cranial nerve. Isolated weakness of a superior rectus, or an inferior oblique, or a medial rectus muscle should engender suspicion that the disorder is peripheral, in the muscle or the terminal orbital branches of the third nerve, rather than in the more proximal intraorbital or intracranial portion of the nerve. Although an MLF lesion commonly causes isolated medial rectus weakness, the involvement of an inferior oblique or a superior rectus in isolation immediately should lead one to suspect that the disorder is in the orbit involving branches of the third cranial nerve or the muscles themselves. Myasthenia gravis and thyroid eye disease are the most likely etiologies. Myasthenia gravis can mimic INO (an MLF lesion) in all its aspects, including the dissociated monocular nystagmus of the abducting eye. An edrophonium chloride test therefore is warranted in cases in which there are no brainstem signs or symptoms other than the ocular motility disorder of INO. Masses and infiltrating diseases within the orbit may affect one or the other of the muscles in the third cranial nerve group, but in these cases orbital signs (e.g., proptosis, lid edema, and conjunctival chemosis) should be evident.

WHEN TO REFER THE PATIENT TO A NEUROLOGIST

Among the large number of neuroophthalmologic abnormalities described in this chapter, several are of particular importance and complexity to stand out immediately and merit referral to a neurologist. These syndromes are summarized in Table 23.5 with a description of the finding, the timing of recommended referral, and the reason for neurologic concern.

QUESTIONS AND DISCUSSION

1. A 58-year-old man presents with a history of pain in the left orbit. He denies diplopia. The pain is described as intense and "boring" in quality without throbbing. He has no previous neurologic or ophthalmologic history. You have been monitoring him for 5 years for fairly well-controlled adult-onset diabetes mellitus treated with diet restriction alone.

There is a complete left ptosis and the left eye is externally rotated (exodeviated) and depressed (deviated downward, hypodeviated). The pupil is 8 mm and fixed to light (direct stimulation). The patient is able to elevate and depress the eye through only about 10% of the expected range. There is no adduction past midline, but the left eye abducts fully. Your differential diagnosis includes:

A. Myasthenia gravis

B. Thyroid eye disease

C. Third cranial nerve (oculomotor nerve) palsy secondary to diabetes mellitus

D. Third cranial nerve palsy secondary to a tumor in the left cavernous sinus

E. Third cranial nerve palsy resulting from an intracranial "berry aneurysm"

You would order the following:

A. Carotid angiography

B. Skull series

C. Tomograms of the sella turcica region

D. Nothing

As it happens, the patient leaves town because of a family crisis and is away for the next 3 months. When he returns, he is able to open the left lid almost completely, although ptosis still is observed easily. Elevation and depression of the globe are more complete, and he now can adduct the left eye through about 70% of normal range. On adduction and attempted depression (downward rotation), however, there is a peculiar "staring" appearance to the left eye in that the lid elevates farther than its resting position with eyes straight ahead. You now conclude:

TABLE 23.5. *When to Refer the Patient to a Neurologist*

Clinical Condition	When to Refer	Reason for Referral
Ocular parasympathetic syndrome, preganglionic (cranial nerve III palsy with pupillary involvement)	Immediately	This is most commonly from an unstable berry aneurysm (leaking blood or enlarging), and immediate workup and treatment are needed to avoid potentially fatal subarachnoid hemorrhage. If the patient is pathologically drowsy and the pupillary findings are acute, transtentorial herniation from a supratentorial mass is a consideration that demands immediate neurologic evaluation.
Anisocoria with normal pupillary reactivity in both eyes and normal ocular motility	Next available appointment	Referral is appropriate if you are unsure whether the patient has Horner's syndrome and whether to do imaging of the brain, neck, and upper thorax.
Pupillary "light-near dissociation" (pupil reacts to near viewing but not to bright light)	Next available appointment	Argyll–Robertson pupil and neurosyphilis needs to be evaluated, probably including lumbar puncture.
Cranial nerve IV palsy or vertical diplopia	Next available appointment	Workup for upper midbrain tumor and other lesions is needed, especially if it does not resolve spontaneously in several weeks, as do most of the ischemic nerve palsies.
Cranial nerve VI palsy	Depends on associated findings—immediate consultation if there is abrupt onset of drowsiness, vomiting or other localizing neurologic signs with the cranial nerve palsy	Acute cranial nerve VI palsy may be a "false-localizing" sign of elevated intracranial pressure and might be a presenting sign of a serious neurologic condition such as meningitis, encephalitis, intracranial bleeding, or brain tumor.
Internuclear ophthalmoplegia	Immediately	This may be a presenting feature of multiple sclerosis (young patients) or a brainstem infarct (older persons).
Cavernous sinus syndromes	Within 7 days	The most common entity to present this way is inflammation (Tolosa–Hunt syndrome). If you are not comfortable with quantitative assessment of cranial nerve functions to monitor the course of steroid treatment, a referral is advised.
Conjugate gaze syndromes	Depending on acuteness of the presentation	Conjugate gaze palsy in any direction, horizontal or vertical, usually signals a disorder involving the cerebral hemispheres or the brainstem. The associated findings are often complex, and planning the workup requires experience with the differential diagnosis.
Nystagmus syndromes	Depending on acuteness of the presentation and associated neurologic signs or symptoms	Nystagmus may occur with relatively benign disorders of the peripheral vestibular system or secondary to serious brainstem disease, and neurologic experience is needed to decide properly how to plan the diagnostic workup and treatment plan.
Ocular flutter and opsoclonus	Immediately	This can occur as a manifestation of brainstem encephalitis as a paraneoplastic disorder in patients with occult cancer or may be associated with neuroblastoma in childhood. The workup for neuroblastoma would best be managed by a pediatric neurologist. This pattern also may occur in adults with multiple sclerosis, a chronic disease that requires neurologic experience to manage. Immediate referral usually is needed because the patient is quite uncomfortable.
Orbital syndromes	Next available appointment unless onset is acute and the patient is uncomfortable	These may be referred to neurologists, but . typically an ophthalmologic consultation is needed for orbital diseases

A. The danger is over.

B. Despite no change in diabetic management, the lesion has begun to improve; thus no further intervention is warranted.

C. There is an "aberrant regeneration" of fibers.

D. Because there has not been a complete recovery, an aneurysm should be ruled out.

Starting with the first office visit, you can make an educated guess as to the cause of the patient's clinical picture. The problem is not myasthenia gravis because the pupil is involved (internal ophthalmoplegia) as are the extraocular muscles (external ophthalmoplegia). Thyroid eye disease must be considered in a patient with external ophthalmoplegia; however, ptosis and pupillary involvement in this condition is rare, if they occur at all. The combination of ptosis; dilated pupil; weakness of medial, superior, and inferior recti; and weakness of inferior oblique reliably establishes the diagnosis of third cranial nerve (oculomotor nerve) palsy. It is left to decide what is the most likely cause. The differential diagnosis should include (C), (D), and (E) in the first question.

The primary physician commonly is required to make the basic and important decision as to whether a particular patient's third cranial nerve palsy is "medical" or "surgical." Medical third cranial nerve palsies are common in the age group older than age 55 years, and they generally are thought to represent ischemic lesions in the substance of the cranial nerve caused by insufficiency of vasa nervosa. The scant available pathologic material relating to "medical" third cranial nerve palsies shows that healed lesions are characterized by fibrosis and acute lesions are characterized by demyelination. Axons are not disrupted to any appreciable degree in early or late lesions, which accounts for the recovery of function within a few months and which underlies the fact that aberrant regeneration does not occur late in the course. The ischemic lesion also is restricted to the center of the nerve trunk, which is the anatomic basis for another characteristic feature of "medical" third cranial nerve palsies—the pupil is relatively spared. Anatomic studies have shown that the pupillary (sphincter) fibers run in the periphery of the nerve, which is spared from the more centrally distributed ischemia.

These ischemic lesions usually are associated with longstanding hypertension or diabetes mellitus but can occur without these systemic risk factors for atherosclerosis, in which case the cranial nerve palsy is, by default, called idiopathic, although they probably are based on arteriosclerosis in patients older than 60 years of age. These palsies generally clear within 3 to 6 months, and persistence of the deficit beyond this time calls for a further diagnostic workup.

Surgical third cranial nerve palsies most commonly are caused by berry aneurysms, particularly those that originate from the junction of the posterior communicating artery and the internal carotid artery. Observations at surgery or autopsy suggest that small bleeds from the aneurysm break into the parenchyma of the nerve, causing disruption of axons as well as local demyelination. This characteristically causes pupillary dilatation with little or no light reaction because the superficially placed pupillary fibers are disrupted. This pupillary finding is the most reliable differential diagnostic feature to separate medical (ischemic) from surgical (aneurysms) third cranial nerve palsies, at least early in the course of the disease. Sparing of the pupil is most reliable as an indicator of "medical" third nerve palsy when the external ophthalmoplegia is complete. With partial external ophthalmoplegia, one must strongly consider angiography to make the distinction, even with relative sparing of the pupil. This is certainly true if the patient is younger than 60 years of age.

The disruption of axons caused by aneurysmal leakage into the nerve sets the stage for the misdirection of regenerating axons during the recovery phase. As an example of this, fibers destined originally for the medial or inferior rectus sometimes are misdirected to the levator palpebrae. Consequently, when the patient attempts to look down or to adduct the eye, the lid elevates.

Tumors compressing the third cranial nerve also cause pupillary involvement but less frequently than do aneurysms. This patient, therefore, has compelling evidence in favor of an aneurysm as the cause of his cranial nerve palsy, although he has diabetes. One should be highly suspicious of this finding at the first office visit because the pupil was large and fixed to light. After enough time has elapsed for the regeneration of axons and misdirection (aberrant regeneration) to occur, the finding of lid elevation on adduction and downward rotation of the eye further supports the diagnosis of an aneurysm or a tumor as opposed to an ischemic cause.

The best answers for the second question therefore would be (A) and (C). One would be justified in ordering carotid angiography in this case. If this study is negative for aneurysm, it may become necessary to order tomograms of the sella region in search of a meningioma or other tumor in the cavernous sinus or superior orbital fissure area. The angiogram or a routine CT scan is likely to reveal such a lesion but may not if the lesion is an en plaque meningioma, in which case bony erosion or hyperostosis may require thin-section CT with bone windows to be visualized.

The answer to the third question is clearly (C). Response (D) is correct but for the wrong reason.

2. An 18-year-old girl, brought in by her mother, complained that she had transiently gone blind in her right eye. The episode occurred in school and lasted 20 minutes. She noted that the right half of a large word on the blackboard seemed to be missing and that "everything seemed to be shimmering and wavy." She is in good general health, and the physical as well as neurologic examinations are normal. Useful questions you could ask include:

A. Where were you the night before this happened?

B. Did you cover the right or left eye to see if the vision changed?

C. Did you develop a headache during or after these visual symptoms?

D. Do you get sick headaches or sinus headaches?

Which of the following tests would be most appropriate for a workup of this patient?

A. Cerebral angiography

B. Pneumoencephalography

C. Carotid duplex examination

D. CT scan with enhancement, or MRI

E. Visual-field examination

F. Reassurance and a follow-up visit in 1 month or sooner should symptoms recur

Choices (B), (C), and (D) are potentially rewarding in the first part of this question. Patients, even those with reasonable intelligence, often fail to make a simple test of whether a visual defect exists in one or both eyes. People conceptualize vision as a unitary experience and are unaware of binocularity in daily life. As part of this unity of experience, many patients are unwilling to comprehend the concept of a homonymous field defect and doggedly stick to the contention that they lost vision in the right eye when, in fact, they experienced a right homonymous hemianopsia. Careful consideration of this patient's history indicates an inability to see the right half of a word written on the blackboard. This finding was experienced with both eyes open and, therefore, must represent a homonymous binocular loss of vision although the patient's natural reaction was to ascribe the symptom to a loss of vision in the right eye.

It would be comforting in this case to elicit a history of left temporal throbbing headache because this almost undeniably would label this patient's symptom complex as a classic migraine. It is important to realize, however, that many patients with migraine have typical migrainous aura without a subsequent headache. A previous history of severe throbbing headaches with nausea, vomiting, diaphoresis, diarrhea, and vertigo also would identify the individual as one who is prone to common migraine. Such persons occasionally may have classic episodes (i.e., with aura) interspersed among common migraine attacks without aura. Patients with common migraine often will deny that they have migraine because they ascribe their recurring, often unilateral frontal throbbing headaches to "sinus infections."

Choices (C), (D), and (E) certainly would be practical and justifiable non-invasive procedures for the second part of this question. Aside from migraine, which this patient almost certainly has, one should consider the less likely diagnosis of occipital arteriovenous malformation with small volume bleeding or transient steal syndrome and ischemia of the visual cortex, giving rise to the evanescent visual symptoms. Contrast-enhanced CT scan and MRI (D) should identify the vast majority of such lesions.

My choice when confronted with this patient, however, would be to give reassurance that the syndrome is common and would not be expected to produce any serious complications. Teenagers are often easily frightened by diagnostic procedures and actually may develop a functional overlay when confronted with the apparent seriousness of their condition engendered by a flurry of complex and dramatic examinations. The statistical chances of missing a significant structural lesion are small. Return visits are advisable, however, to ensure against missing progressive symptoms and to provide confidence on the part of the patient and family that they are not being abandoned. In treating patients who suffer from headaches, this sense of ongoing commitment is more important than the type of medicine prescribed.

3. A 38-year-old man presents with a 2-week history of frequent severe headaches in the right orbital area. The pain is steady, "boring" in character, and severe, but it lasts only 40 to 60 minutes. It tends to occur two to three times daily and can be anticipated regularly at 10 PM usually just after he retires. On examination, there is right ptosis and miosis but no other physical or neurologic findings. Workup should include:

A. Carotid angiography

B. CT scan including sphenoid and ethmoid paranasal sinuses

C. Instillation of 1% para-OH-amphetamine in either eye

D. Instillation of 4% cocaine in either eye

The answer is C.

The most reliable indicator of a postganglionic lesion is failure of the pupil to dilate on instillation of 1% para-OH-amphetamine, which, like cocaine, blocks the reuptake of norepinephrine into the presynaptic sympathetic nerve terminals in the iris. In addition, however, it causes the release of any existing presynaptic norepinephrine stores. This means that, regardless of a lesion in the oculosympathetic preganglionic or central pathways, para-OH-amphetamine will release stores of norepinephrine and cause pupillary dilatation. Failure of dilatation, therefore, establishes the presence of a postganglionic oculosympathetic neuron lesion in which the normal stores of transmitter are pathologically absent.

Raeder described patients with painful oculosympathetic palsy and space-occupying lesions of the middle cranial fossa. All his patients also had findings referable to one or more of the third through sixth cranial nerves, and he put forth this combination as diagnostic of middle fossa masses. This original, or type I, form of Raeder's syndrome now has been separated from a benign, probably migrainous form, referred to as type II.

The original description of Raeder's syndrome type II included seven patients with painful oculosympathetic palsy. They all had unilateral brief steady headaches that conformed to the pattern of cluster or histamine headache, but they also had an ipsilateral oculosympathetic syndrome. None had findings of third, fourth, or sixth cranial nerve dysfunction. Lawton–Smith's concept that these patients with Raeder's type II have a form of migraine with secondary sympathetic involvement has come to be widely accepted. The patients are generally middle-aged, and men predominate. There must be no associated cranial nerve palsy, and the headache history should be typical of the cluster pattern. The oculosympathetic lesion also should be documented as postganglionic using the para-OH-amphetamine test. The theory is that the sympathetic lesion is caused by edema in the adventitia of the carotid siphon as a consequence of frequent and severe vascular headaches.

The diagnosis of Raeder's syndrome type II relieves the physician of the obligation to consider the patient to be a cancer suspect.

4. A 62-year-old man presents for a routine examination. He has no head or neck symptoms, but an examination reveals 1 to 2 mm of left ptosis. In the examining room, however, the pupils are noted to be equal in size at 3 mm. The patient denies awareness of the lid droop and denies head or neck trauma. A reasonable workup would include:

A. Chest roentgenogram

B. Sputum cytology with acid-fast bacilli (AFB) smear and culture

C. Examination of the pupils in a dim room

D. Instillation of 1% pilocarpine in either eye

E. Instillation of 4% cocaine in either eye

F. Instillation of 1% para-OH-amphetamine in either eye

G. Nothing

H. A request for old full-face photographs

I. Observation of iris color

The answer is C, examining the pupils in a dim room since the pupillary anisocoria may be masked by dominant pupillary sphincter activity even in moderate illumination. If the pupils are still equal then the next test is installation of 4% cocaine to establish that the ptosis is caused by ocular sympathetic dysfunction.

The most serious concern on first observing a patient with Horner's syndrome is the possibility of cancer, which is one of the most common causes of an acquired ocular sympathetic lesion in the adult. Apical carcinoma of the lung (Pancoast's syndrome) is a common type that causes Horner's syndrome, but any neoplasm infiltrating cervical lymph nodes can present this way. Most often the patient is unaware of a change in his facial appearance because the degree of ptosis is small and the onset is insidious without visual or other symptoms. The most practical approach is to determine (a) whether ptosis is actually the result of oculosympathetic dysfunction and (b) the age of the lesion.

Grimson and Thompson (1975) reviewed pharmacologic testing in Horner's syndrome with a logical approach to diagnosis. They found that the use of a weak direct-acting sympathomimetic (1:1,000 epinephrine) was unreliable in clinical diagnosis. Cocaine (4%) blocks the reuptake of norepinephrine into presynaptic terminals at the iris and causes pupillary dilatation in the normal eye. In the presence of Horner's syndrome, the release of norepinephrine is reduced and a reuptake block fails to dilate the pupil as much as it does in the fellow eye, which is used as a control. The cocaine test is useful to identify an oculosympathetic lesion in patients with ptosis and minimal or no anisocoria.

A simple preliminary approach is to observe the eyes for anisocoria in as dim an environment as possible consistent with adequate visualization of the pupils. In bright light, the iris (parasympathetic) sphincter dominates pupil size and can overcome minor asymmetry of tone in the radially oriented, sympathetically innervated dilator muscles. The sphincter relaxes in a dim light, and anisocoria, resulting from weakness of the pupil dilator muscles on the side of the oculosympathetic lesion, may become apparent.

If the ptosis has been present for several years, carcinoma almost certainly can be ruled out as the cause. An examination of old photographs often will settle the issue without an expensive workup by demonstrating the ptosis to be longstanding and unchanged over the years. Furthermore, an oculosympathetic lesion arising before birth, and perhaps in the first 1 to 2 years of life at the latest, will cause failure of iris chromatophores to develop. If the patient has one brown iris contralateral to the ptosis and a blue iris ipsilateral, the Horner's syndrome can be identified as ancient.

If the lesion cannot be documented as old and stable, a workup for carcinoma of the lung or carcinoma metastatic to cervical nodes could be undertaken. This presumes that there is no history of stroke, or of head or neck trauma, to explain the lesion. If the first round of tests is negative, it is important to follow the patient closely for emergence of signs or symptoms of underlying carcinoma. Frequent chest roentgenograms or CT scans with attention to apical regions are usually necessary. MRI probably will be the preferred method for examining the upper chest and neck.

SUGGESTED READING

Asbury AK, Aldridge H, Hershberg R, et al. Oculomotor palsy in diabetes mellitus: a clinicopathologic study. *Brain* 1970;93:555.

Boniuk M, Schlesinger NS. Raeder's paratrigeminal syndrome. *Am J Ophthalmol* 1962;54:1074.

Borchert MS. Principles and techniques of the examination of ocular motility and alignment. In: Miller NR, Newman NJ, eds. *Walsh and Hoyt's clinical neuro-ophthalmology,* 5th ed, vol 1. Baltimore: Williams & Wilkins, 1998.

Chavis PS, al Hazmi A, Clunie D, et al. Temporal crescent syndrome with magnetic resonance correlation. *J Neuroophthalmol* 1997;17(3):151–155.

Giles CL, Henderson JW. Horner's syndrome: an analysis of 216 cases. *Am J Ophthalmol* 1958;46:289.

Girkin CA, Miller NR. Central disorders of vision in humans. *Surv Ophthalmol* 2001;45(5):379–405.

Goldstein JE, Cogan DG. Diabetic ophthalmoplegia with special reference to the pupil. *Arch Ophthalmol* 1960;64:592.

Goodwin J. Disorders of higher cortical visual function. *Curr Neurol Neurosci Rep* 2002;2(5):418–422.

Grimson BS, Thompson HS. *Drug testing in Horner's syndrome,* Vol 8. St. Louis: CV Mosby, 1975.

Hayreh SS. In vivo choroidal circulation and its watershed zones. *Eye* 1990;4:273.

Hayreh SS. The ophthalmic artery: III. Branches. *Br J Ophthalmol* 1962;46:212.

Keitner JL, Johnson CA, Spurr JO, et al. Baseline visual field profile of optic neuritis: the experience of the optic neuritis treatment trial. Optic Neuritis Study Group [see comments]. *Arch Ophthalmol* 1993;111(2):231–234.

Keltner JL, Johnson CA, Spurr JO, et al. Baseline visual field profile of optic neuritis: the experience of the Optic Neuritis Treatment Trial. *Arch Ophthalmol* 1993;111:231.

Kerr WL. The pupil: functional anatomy and clinical correlation. In: Smith JL, ed. *Neuro-Ophthalmology* Vol 4. Hollendale, FL: Huffman, 1968:49–80.

Leavitt JA, Wayman LL, Hodge DO, et al. Pupillary response to four concentrations of pilocarpine in normal subjects: application to testing for Adie tonic pupil. *Am J Ophthalmol* 2002;133(3):333–336.

Leigh RJ, Averbach-Heller L. Nystagmus and related ocular motility disorders. In: Miller NR, Newman NJ, eds. *Walsh and Hoyt's clinical neuro-ophthalmology,* 5th ed, Vol 1. Baltimore: Williams & Wilkins, 1998.

Leigh RJ, Zee DS. *The neurology of eye movements,* 3rd ed. Philadelphia: FA Davis, 1999.

Loewenfeld IE. *The pupil: anatomy, physiology, and clinical applications.* Ames/Detroit: Iowa State University Press/Wayne State University Press, 1993.

Portnoy JZ, Thompson HS, Lennarson L, et al. Pupillary defects in amblyopia. *Am J Ophthalmol* 1983;96(5):609–614.

Rucker CW. The causes of paralysis of the third, fourth and sixth cranial nerves. *Am J Ophthalmol* 1966;61:1294.

Rucker CW. Paralysis of the third, fourth, and sixth cranial nerves. *Am J Ophthalmol* 1958;46:787.

Sharpe JA. Neural control of ocular motor systems. In: Miller NR, Newman NJ, eds. *Walsh and Hoyt's clinical neuro-ophthalmology,* 5th ed. Baltimore: Williams & Wilkins, 1998.

Smith CH. Nuclear and infranuclear ocular motility disorders. In: Miller NR, Newman NJ, eds. *Walsh and Hoyt's clinical neuro-ophthalmology,* 5th ed. Baltimore: Williams & Wilkins, 1998.

Smith JL. Raeder's paratrigeminal syndrome. *Am J Ophthalmol* 1958;46:194.

Thompson HS, Bourgon P, Van Allen MW. The tendon reflexes in Adie's syndrome. In: Thompson HS, ed. *Topics in neuro-ophthalmology.* Baltimore: Williams & Wilkins, 1979:104–113.

Thompson HS, Mensher JM. Adrenergic mydriasis of Horner's syndrome: hydroxyamphetamine test for diagnosis of postganglionic defects. *Am J Ophthalmol* 1971;72:472.

Weber RB, Daroff RB, Mackey EA. Pathology of oculomotor nerve palsy in diabetics. *Neurology* 1970;20:835.

24

Central Nervous System Infections

Larry E. Davis

Central nervous system (CNS) infections can be caused by viruses, bacteria, fungi, and parasites, but bacteria and viruses are the most common causes. Infectious agents enter the body by way of the gastrointestinal tract or respiratory tract or following skin inoculation (animal or insect bite) and set up the initial site of replication in these tissues. The majority of organisms then reach the CNS by way of the bloodstream, but occasional organisms reach the brain by way of peripheral nerves or by direct entry through adjacent bone following open skull fracture or from infected mastoid or air sinuses.

Despite the many infections we develop during our lifetimes, organisms rarely reach the brain. For example, transient bacteremias are common following vigorously brushing teeth, yet the bacteria do not cause meningitis. Important protective systems include the reticuloendothelial system (which efficiently removes bacteria and viruses from blood), cellular and humoral immune responses (which destroy organisms from the blood and primary site of infection), and the blood–brain barrier (which prevents entry of organisms into the brain or cerebrospinal fluid [CSF]). Organisms that do enter the brain or CSF from blood do so by infecting endothelial cells of the cerebral blood vessels (many encephalitis viruses), penetrating the blood–CSF barrier in the meninges or choroid plexus (many bacteria) or occluding small cerebral blood vessels with infected emboli from the heart or lung (brain abscess organisms). Once the invasion has occurred, the brain and CSF have less immune protection than the rest of the body. Normal CSF has about 1/500th the amount of antibody as blood and few white blood cells (WBCs). Thus, individuals who develop a brain or

meningeal infection often die without antimicrobial intervention.

Inflammation of the meninges or brain is the hallmark of CNS infection. Inflammatory cells may be present in the meninges, in perivascular spaces, or within brain parenchyma such as around an abscess. The inflammatory lymphocytes show specific immune activity against the infectious agent.

The signs and symptoms of a CNS infection depend on the site of the infection–not the organism. The organism determines mainly the time course and severity of the infection. In general, the time course to develop CNS signs for viruses is hours to 1 day; for aerobic bacteria it is hours to a few days; for anaerobic bacteria, tuberculosis, and fungi it is a few days to weeks; and for parasites and *Treponema pallidum* (syphilis) it is weeks to years. Follow these steps to diagnose and treat CNS infections:

Determine the site of infection
Obtain appropriate CSF, blood, or tissue specimens for culture and serology to determine type of organism (e.g., bacteria, virus, fungus) and antimicrobial sensitivities.
Begin initial broad spectrum antimicrobial treatment.
Determine specific etiology and antimicrobial sensitivities, and modify treatment if necessary.
Watch for and treat complications.

There are three major sites where infections occur in the nervous system: diffusely in the meninges (meningitis), diffusely in the brain (encephalitis), and locally in the brain (abscess) (Fig. 24.1). Although patients may develop infections at other sites, such as epidural abscess and subdural empyema, this chapter focuses on the most common infec-

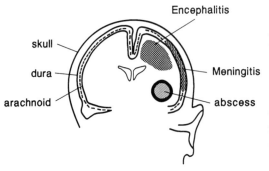

FIG. 24.1. Coronal section of the head demonstrating locations of three major CNS infections.

tions. In addition, prion diseases, a novel infectious agent that breaks conventional rules, will be discussed.

MENINGITIS

A variety of viral, bacterial, fungal, parasitic, chemical, and neoplastic agents may cause inflammation of the meninges. These patients all have common clinical features:

Early features: Prodromal illness, fever, headache, stiff neck, relative preservation of mental status, no focal neurologic signs, no papilledema.

Later features: Seizures, stupor and coma, cranial nerve palsies, deafness, focal neurologic signs may develop.

The time course of the meningitis may give clues as to its etiology. Viral and bacterial meningitis are acute illnesses with symptoms developing over hours to 1 day. Patients with fungal meningitis or tuberculous meningitis develop symptoms over days to 2 weeks.

Common Laboratory Findings

The WBC in blood usually is elevated, as is the erythrocyte sedimentation rate. The CSF examination is the key to the diagnosis of meningitis, ascertainment of the type of infecting agent, establishment of the etiologic agent, and determination of antimicrobial sensitivities (Fig. 24.2). Viral, bacterial, tuberculous, and fungal infections of the meninges have differing CSF profiles (Table 24.1). CSF culture determines the etiology of the infection as well as antimicrobial sensitivities. In general, cultures for bacteria take 1 to 3 days, virus cul-

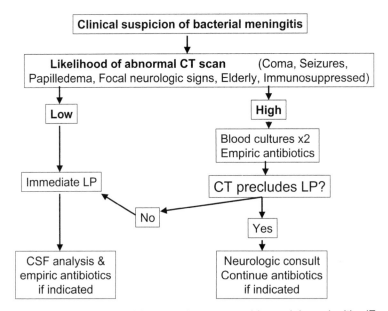

FIG. 24.2. Flow diagram for LP and CSF tests in suspected bacterial meningitis. (From Davis LE. Acute bacterial meningitis. In: Weiner WJ, ed. *Emergent and urgent neurology.* Philadelphia: JB Lippincott, 1992:139, with permission.)

TABLE 24.1. *Spinal Fluid Profiles in CNS Infections*

	Opening Pressure	White Blood Cells	Protein	Glucose	Bacterial or Fungal Culture
Epidural abscess	N or s1 ↑	0–20 (lymphs)	N or s1 ↑	N	Negative
Subdural empyema	↑	10–1,000 (polys)	s1 ↑	N	Negative
Viral meningitis	N or s1 ↑	20–1,000 (lymphs)	s1 ↑	N	Negative
Bacterial meningitis	↑	50–10,000 (polys)	↑	Low	Positive
Fungal or tuberculous meningitis	↑	50–10,000 polys & lymphs	↑	Low	Positive
Meningovascular syphilis	N or s1 ↑	10–1,000 lymphs	↑	N	Negative
Brain abscess	↑	0–10 lymphs & polys	N	N	Negative
Viral encephalitis	s1 ↑	10–200 lymphs	N or s1 ↑	N	Negative

N, normal; s1 ↑, slight increase; ↑, increased.

tures take days to 3 weeks, and tuberculosis and fungi cultures take 1 to 6 weeks. Rapid diagnosis of bacteria can be made by Gram stain of CSF sediment and by testing CSF for common bacterial antigens. The Gram stain will detect bacteria in CSF sediment in more than three-fourths of patients with acute bacterial meningitis and often gives clues for initial antibiotic treatment. Latex agglutination antigen tests are commercially available to detect *Hemophilus influenzae, Streptococcus pneumoniae, Neisseria meningitidis,* and group A beta-hemolytic streptococci. Antigen tests have about the same sensitivity as the Gram stain. The polymerase chain reaction (PCR) diagnostic test is available to rapidly diagnose *Mycobacterium tuberculosis,* enteroviruses, and herpes simplex virus. Many others are available on a research basis. PCR detects tiny amounts of nucleic acids of these infectious agents in CSF. Currently the sensitivity of PCR is equal or slightly better than culturing the infectious agent and can be performed within hours. Of importance, the PCR does not give information regarding antimicrobial sensitivities. Thus, the best diagnostic test is still to culture the CSF and blood for an infectious agent and use the isolate to determine antimicrobial sensitivities.

Viral Meningitis

Enteroviruses (echoviruses and Coxsackie viruses) are the most common cause of viral meningitis. Less common causes include herpes simplex virus type 2, mumps virus, and human immunodeficiency virus. Typically in viral meningitis, the CSF contains a pleocytosis with predominately lymphocytes, mildly elevated protein, normal glucose, and negative Gram stain of sediment. Viruses often can be isolated from CSF early in the meningitis, and PCR analysis of CSF rapidly diagnoses enteroviruses and herpes simplex type 2 viruses. Treatment of viral meningitis is usually symptomatic and may include analgesics for the headache and antiemetics for nausea and vomiting. If herpes simplex virus is identified, use of high-dose acyclovir may shorten the duration of the meningitis. Hospitalization is often not required if the diagnosis of viral and not bacterial meningitis is certain, but the patient should be observed at home by a responsible individual. The prognosis of viral meningitis is excellent, and most patients fully recover within 1 to 2 weeks.

Acute Bacterial Meningitis

Both Gram-positive and Gram-negative aerobic bacteria cause meningitis mainly in children, in the elderly, and in the immunosuppressed. *S. pneumoniae* is the most common bacterium affecting all ages except infants, followed by *N. meningitidis* and *H. influenzae.* Unlike viral meningitis, patients with bacterial meningitis will progress to death if untreated with antibiotics. Therefore, prompt diagnosis and treatment are essential. If bacterial meningitis is suspected, the lumbar puncture (LP) becomes an emergency procedure (Fig. 24.2). Although increased intracranial pressure is common in bacterial meningitis, it rarely poses a risk of brain herniation that would prevent an LP. Thus, it seldom is necessary to perform a computed tomography (CT) or a magnetic resonance imaging (MRI) scan before the LP unless the patient is immunosuppressed; is elderly; or presents with coma, focal neurologic signs, or papilledema that places them at increased risk for a focal CNS mass. If there is to be a significant delay before the neuroimaging can be obtained, broad-spectrum antibiotics may be given before the LP. However, one always should obtain a blood culture before administrating the antibiotics. A blood culture is positive in 60% of patients with bacterial meningitis and thus could yield antibiotic sensitivities.

The key to treatment of acute bacterial meningitis is the prompt administration of appropriate antibiotics. General principles involved in the use of antibiotics include the following: (a) the antibiotic should be given early in the clinical course; (b) the bacteria must be sensitive to the antibiotic; (c) the antibiotic must cross the blood–brain barrier and achieve sufficient CSF concentrations to kill the bacteria. Once the diagnosis of bacterial meningitis is made, one should begin treatment with broad-spectrum antibiotics, which later can be modified when antibiotic sensitivities become available. The choice of an antibiotic for initial treatment depends on several factors: age, immune status, and predisposing medical conditions of the patient; results of CSF Gram stain and bacterial antigen tests; knowledge of the types of drug-resistant bacteria in the community; and whether the patient is allergic to any antibiotic. Table 24.2 gives common initial antibiotic regimens, but one should check references such as the *Medical Letter* for the latest recommendations.

Neurologic injury in bacteria meningitis is not only the result of meningeal inflammation but also to cerebral vasculitis, cerebral edema, cerebral necrosis, and hydrocephalus. Menin-

TABLE 24.2. *Initial Antibiotic Therapy While Awaiting Identification of Infecting Organism[a]*

Setting	Therapy
Preterm and newborn	Ampicillin plus cefotaxime, with or without gentamicin
2 months to adulthood	High-dose ceftriaxone or ceftixamine plus vancomycin, with or without rifampin. The vancomycin and rifampin should be stopped if the bacteria are sensitive to cephalosporins. Ampicillin, with or without gentamycin, can be added if *Listeria monocytogenes* is suspected.

[a]One always should check with references such as the *Medical Letter* for the latest recommendations because resistance patterns are changing.

geal bacteria do not readily penetrate the pia mater and invade the brain. However, interactions between meningeal bacteria and host result in meningeal inflammation; vascular injury; disruption of the blood–brain barrier; vasogenic, interstitial, and cytotoxic edema; and disruption of normal CSF flow. At the molecular level, bacterial cell walls have been shown to induce cerebrovascular endothelial cells, microglia, and meningeal inflammatory cells to release cytokines, chemokines, and reactive oxygen species that damage neurons. Because many of the neurologic sequelae stem from the CSF inflammation, there is a search for adjunctive therapies that will minimize the meningeal inflammation and release of cytotoxic products. At present, corticosteroids have been shown to have a modest benefit in children and adults, particularly in reducing the incidence of hearing loss. Dexamethasone (0.15 mg/kg intravenously in children every 6 hours and 10 mg in adults every 6 hours for 2–4 days) commonly is administered as early as possible. However, dexamethasone should be given only when the illness and CSF findings are highly suggestive of bacterial meningitis in an immunocompetent patient without contraindications for steroid administration.

In general, the CSF becomes sterile 1 to 2 days after antibiotic treatment. The fever usually disappears within a few days but may persist for up to 2 weeks. CSF abnormalities rapidly return toward normal, but the pleocytosis and elevated protein may persist for several weeks. Dead bacteria may be seen on Gram stain of CSF for several days.

Even if the patient is treated promptly with appropriate antibiotics and steroids, serious complications still may develop. Seizures develop in about one-third of patients. The seizures usually occur early in the meningitis and seldom recur after the hospitalization. Causes of seizures in meningitis include cerebral cortex irritation from bacterial toxins or meningeal inflammation, CNS vasculitis, brain infarction, high fever, and hyponatremia from the syndrome of inappropriate antidiuretic hormone coupled with excess fluid administration. Treatment of the seizures is usually with phenytoin until hospital discharge. Focal neurologic signs develop in up to 25% of patients. These include cranial nerve palsies, especially cranial nerves VIII (deafness) and VI and III (diplopia). In surviving children, 15% have language disorders or delayed language development and 10% have mental retardation. Brain damage resulting in hemiparesis, ataxia, aphasia, or visual loss also may occur. CT or MRI of the head is often helpful in the evaluation of these complications and may demonstrate cerebral or cerebellar infarction, brain necrosis, subdural hygromas, or mild ventricular dilatation. Hydrocephalus, subdural empyema, and brain abscess occur but are uncommon. Patients with focal neurologic damage benefit from rehabilitation following acute antibiotic therapy, especially if deafness is identified. Mortality from bacterial meningitis ranges from 5% to 25%, depending on the strain of infecting bacteria, the age group, and predisposing illnesses in the patient.

Some bacterial meningitis requires chemoprophylaxis of immediate family members and close contacts because of their increased risk of developing meningitis. In *N. meningitidis* meningitis, treatment of all close contracts is indicated. Rifampin (600 mg for adults or 10 mg/kg for children twice daily orally for 2 days) or ciprofloxacin (single oral dose of 500 mg for adults) may be given. If the patient has *H. influenzae* type B meningitis, chemoprophylaxis is indicated for children younger than 4 years of age who have been in close contact with the patient and not previously vaccinated with the *H. influenzae* vaccine. Rifampin (10 mg/kg twice daily orally for 4 days) usually is given. All close contacts should be observed carefully for the next week.

Many cases of bacterial meningitis can be prevented by immunizing infants with the *H. influenzae* vaccine and by immunizing high-risk populations and possibly children with meningococcal and pneumococcal vaccines.

Spirochete Meningitis

Spirochetes produce chronic bacterial meningitis. *Borrelia burgdorferi* (CNS Lyme disease) and *T. pallidum* (neurosyphilis) both cause chronic meningitis, and patients develop headaches, cranial nerve palsies (especially Bell's palsy in CNS Lyme disease), and occasionally brain infarctions from thrombosis of cortical blood vessels (meningovascular syphilis). Years later, the spirochetes invade the brain to cause low-grade encephalitis (general paresis or CNS Lyme disease). The CSF contains a lymphocytic pleocytosis, elevated protein, and usually normal glucose level. Spirochetes seldom are isolated from CSF, and the diagnosis is made by serologic tests (CSF-Venereal Disease Research Laboratory or Lyme antibody titers). Workup for subacute meningitis is given in Table 24.3. Treatment is with high-dose penicillin or ceftriaxone for several weeks.

Tuberculous and Fungal Meningitis

Patients with tuberculous and fungal meningitis usually develop subacute meningitis with the onset of CNS signs developing over days to weeks. These infections occur most often in individuals who are malnourished, debilitated, or immunosuppressed. Although initial entry is usually by way of the lungs, less than 50% will have an active pul-

TABLE 24.3. *Evaluation of Subacute Meningitis*

CSF studies: Opening pressure, cell count with differential, glucose, protein, IgG, Gram stain, acid-fast stain, and cytology. CSF serology includes CSF-VDRL, *Coccidioides immitis, Histoplasma capsulatum* antibody titers, and *Cryptococcus neoformans* antigen titer. PCR assays for *M. tuberculosis* and other fungi as available.
Skin tests: Intermediate purified protein derivative tuberculin test and anergy skin tests
Serum antibody tests: Brucella, syphilis, toxoplasmosis, *Coccidioides immitis,* other fungi, Lyme disease, and human immunodeficiency virus
Cultures for bacteria, M. tuberculosis, and fungi: CSF cultures repeated three times; blood, urine, sputum, or gastric aspirate; bone marrow biopsy; and skin lesion biopsy
Magnetic resonance image or computed tomograph of head with contrast
Chest x-ray and computed tomograph of abdomen, if indicated

IgG, immunoglobulin G; VDRL, Venereal Disease Research Laboratory.

monary infection at the time of the meningitis. The best methods to establish the etiology are by (a) culture of the CSF, (b) identification by PCR infectious agents such as *M. tuberculosis,* (c) antigen detection for *Cryptococcus neoformans,* and (d) serologic tests for several fungi. Because tuberculous or fungal organisms may be in low concentrations in the CSF, one should culture a concentrate of 5 ml to 10 ml of CSF on several occasions.

Treatment of tuberculous meningitis usually requires administration of four drugs (rifampin, isoniazid, pyrazinamide, and streptomycin or ethambutol) for 2 months followed by rifampin and isoniazid for another 7 months, depending on the antibiotic sensitivities of the *M. tuberculosis* isolate. Dexamethasone often is added if the patient is comatose or has severe neurologic deficits. Most patients with fungal meningitis are treated with amphotericin B for weeks to months. In patients with cryptococcal meningitis, flucytosine often is added. Fluconazole has been shown to be nearly as efficacious as amphotericin B in the treatment of cryptococcal and coccidioidal meningitis. Fluconazole has the advantage that it can be given orally and has less renal and hematopoietic toxicity. In immunosuppressed or AIDS pa-

tients with fungal meningitis in remission, continued use of fluconazole in a lower dosage may prevent recurrence. Complications are similar to those seen in acute bacterial meningitis. Mortality rates range from 20% to 50% depending on the organism and predisposing factors. Survivors may be left with neurologic sequelae similar to those seen in acute bacterial meningitis.

ENCEPHALITIS

The majority of infectious agents that cause encephalitis are viruses that reach the brain by way of a hematogenous route. Once the virus reaches the brain parenchyma, a widely disseminated infection of neurons and glia ensues. Neuronal necrosis and lysis of glial cells result in secondary cerebral edema. The inflammatory response includes perivascular cuffing with inflammatory cells and infiltration of lymphocytes and macrophages into the adjacent brain parenchyma. The invading immune response often terminates the infection, but the patient may be left with permanent neurologic sequelae.

Viruses cause more than 90% of cases. Worldwide, arboviruses (togaviruses) are the most common cause. Because arboviruses require a vector (mosquito or tick), arbovirus encephalitis often occurs in clusters or epidemics. In winter and early spring when mosquitoes and ticks are absent, herpes simplex type 1 virus is the most common cause of encephalitis. Herpes simplex virus is a latent infection in most individuals following a primary stomatitis infection in childhood. Years later the latent virus can reactivate to cause an encephalitis that occurs sporadically year round. Other causes of encephalitis are the result of spirochetes (*T. pallidum, B. burgdorferi*), parasites (toxoplasmosis or falciparum malaria), and other viruses (cytomegalovirus, varicella-zoster, adenovirus).

Clinical Features

Acute encephalitis is a febrile illness characterized by the abrupt onset of headache and mental obtundation. Other common features include seizures, which may be generalized or focal; hyperreflexia; spasticity; and Babinski signs. Some patients develop hemiparesis, aphasia, ataxia, limb tremors, and cortical blindness. Patients with West Nile virus encephalitis usually develop the typical clinical picture of encephalitis, but 10% develop a myelitis that is similar to paralytic poliomyelitis. Patients often have a prodromal illness, which varies with the infectious agent and can include parotitis (mumps virus) or fever, malaise, and myalgias (arbovirus). Encephalitis differs from meningitis primarily because patients with encephalitis develop prominent mental changes and a minimal or absent stiff neck.

Laboratory Findings

The electroencephalogram (EEG) is always abnormal and usually shows diffuse bilateral slowing with occasional seizure activity. An LP in a patient with early encephalitis will have an opening pressure that is normal or slightly elevated. The CSF contains five to several hundred WBC/mm^3 (predominantly lymphocytes). CSF glucose is normal, whereas CSF protein is mildly elevated. Bacterial and viral cultures are usually sterile. Early in the course of encephalitis, the CT scan may be normal, whereas the T2-weighted MRI scan often shows areas of hyperintensity as a result of edema from cerebral vascular permeability. Later, both scans may demonstrate areas of necrosis or hemorrhage. The presence of T2-weighted MRI lesions in the medial aspect of the temporal lobe is highly suggestive for herpes simplex encephalitis.

The diagnosis of viral encephalitis usually is made by serologic tests. Because most arboviruses rarely infect humans in the United States and produce a systemic viral infection before producing the viral encephalitis, immunoglobulin M (IgM) antibodies to the virus often are present early in the encephalitis. The IgM-antibody-capture enzyme-linked immunoabsorbent assay (Mac ELISA) can be used to detect arbovirus antibodies in serum and CSF during the first few days of the encephalitis. Acute and convalescent serum titers can be determined for many viruses. A fourfold increase in antibody titer is diagnostic. Serologic tests are not useful in establishing the diagnosis of herpes simplex encephalitis, but the diagnosis can be made by detection of herpes simplex viral DNA in CSF by PCR. Although herpes simplex virus is almost never cultured from CSF, enough viral DNA leaks into the CSF from the brain infection to be detected by PCR. The CSF PCR test is most sensitive when used in the first few days of the encephalitis.

Management and Prognosis

All patients require excellent symptomatic care to minimize complications. If seizures develop, anticonvulsant medications are indicated. If increased intracranial pressure develops from vascular engorgement and cerebral edema, treatment may require hyperventilation or the administration of mannitol. Use of corticosteroids is controversial. In patients with herpes simplex encephalitis, treatment with acyclovir significantly improves outcome. Acyclovir should be administered early in the encephalitis course. Current recommendations are to give 30 mg/kg/day of acyclovir that is divided into three doses per day for 10 to 14 days. The drug should be delivered intravenously slowly over 1 hour to prevent renal toxicity. Drug complications include transient renal failure, thrombophlebitis, and elevations of serum liver enzymes. Ganciclovir is antiviral for cytomegalovirus, and famciclovir is effective against varicella-zoster virus. For most RNA viruses such as arboviruses, no antiviral treatment is available.

Prognosis of encephalitis depends on the infectious agent. Patients with mumps meningoencephalitis and Venezuelan equine encephalitis have an excellent prognosis. Patients with West Nile, western equine, St. Louis, and California encephalitis usually have a reasonable prognosis (2% to 15% mortality), but up to 25% of patients are left with dementia, seizures, or focal neurologic deficits. Patients with eastern equine, Japanese B, and Murray Valley encephalitis have mortality rates from 20% to 40%. Patients with herpes simplex encephalitis who are treated with acyclovir have a 20% mortality rate, and 55% are left with some neurologic sequelae. Rabies encephalitis is fatal. Patients with cognitive impairment or focal neurologic signs benefit from rehabilitation that may take weeks.

BRAIN ABSCESS

Whereas viruses tend to cause diffuse brain infections, most bacteria, fungi, and parasites cause localized brain disease. Brain abscesses may arise by direct extension from other foci of infection within the cranial cavity (mastoiditis and sinusitis), from infections following skull fracture or craniotomy, or as metastasis carried by the blood from infections elsewhere in the body. The infection usually begins as a localized encephalitis with focal softening, necrosis, and inflammation. As the process continues, fibroblasts proliferate at the edges, forming a capsule wall. A variable amount of cerebral edema surrounds the lesion. If the etiology is bacterial or fungal, the space-occupying lesion slowly expands. If untreated, the brain mass is lethal. Parasites such as cysticercosis develop cysts that usually stop growing after they reach about 10 mm to 15 mm in size.

Anaerobic bacteria are found in more than one-half of brain abscesses. Anaerobic streptococci and *Bacteroides fragilis* are common organisms. Occasionally, multiple bacteria are found in abscesses. Brain abscesses following head trauma or neurosurgery may contain *Staphylococcus aureus*.

Clinical Features

Symptoms from localized brain infections typically are subacute in onset. Early symptoms include headaches, lethargy, intermittent fever, and focal or generalized seizures. Focal neurologic signs may develop depending on the site of the lesion. Thus, lesions in the frontal cortex may produce hemiparesis, whereas lesions in the occipital cortex cause homonymous visual defects. As the mass expands, increased intracranial pressure becomes more pronounced. Psychomotor slowing, lethargy, and confusion increase in severity. Papilledema and horizontal diplopia from a sixth-nerve palsy may be seen. Focal neurologic signs become more prominent. Eventually, the abscess expands to cause brain herniation or ruptures into the ventricle producing ventriculitis. Both usually result in death.

Laboratory Findings

CT and MRI scans are extremely helpful in diagnosing brain abscesses. The CT scan usually demonstrates a lesion with a low-density necrotic center, a well-developed contrast-enhancing capsule, and surrounding cerebral edema (Fig. 24.3). A somewhat similar pic-

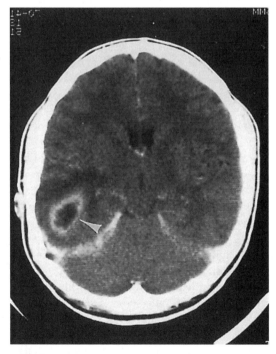

FIG. 24.3. CT scan with contrast demonstrating a brain abscess in the posterior temporal lobe. *Arrow* shows the enhancing capsule with necrotic center. There is some low-density surrounding edema.

ture is seen on MRI scan. Administration of gadolinium will cause the capsule wall to enhance. The EEG is often abnormal, usually producing localized slowing in the region of the abscess. An LP, rarely helpful in establishing the diagnosis, is potentially dangerous because it increases the risk of brain herniation if the intracranial pressure is markedly elevated.

Management and Prognosis

Treatment of brain abscesses usually entails appropriate antibiotic therapy and surgical drainage. Broad-spectrum antibiotics, started as soon as the clinical diagnosis is made, are selected for their effectiveness against all likely pathogens as well as their ability to penetrate brain abscesses and surrounding brain parenchyma. Broad-spectrum antibiotic coverage should be efficacious against both common anaerobic (especially *Streptococcus intermedius* and *Bacteroides fragilis)* and aerobic bacteria. Possible combinations include the use of cefotaxime or ceftriaxone plus metronidazole or chloramphenicol. If staphylococci are suspected or isolated, nafcillin should be given. Once the bacteria are isolated, therapy should be directed by their antibiotic sensitivities. Intravenous antibiotics should be administered for 6 to 8 weeks. Because the most immediate threat from brain abscesses is the mass effect, surgical aspiration of pus often reduces the increased intracranial pressure. The simplest method is aspiration of the pus using a CT-guided stereotactic technique. The received fluid should be Gram stained and cultured for anaerobic and aerobic bacteria, fungi, and tuberculosis. If the brain abscesses are multiple and small or deep involving the basal ganglia and brainstem, they occasionally can be treated only with broad-spectrum antimicrobial agents. However, careful clinical observations and repeated CT scans are needed to determine whether the abscess continues to expand.

Mannitol or corticosteroids may be necessary initially to control cerebral edema. However, corticosteroids should be used cautiously and tapered rapidly because they may interfere with capsule formation and host defenses against the organism.

Mortality from brain abscesses ranges from 30% to 65%, with the lower rates for patients who receive combined therapy with antibiotics and surgery. About 50% of survivors have neurologic sequelae, including seizures and focal neurologic deficits. These patients require rehabilitation.

PRION DISEASES (CREUTZFELDT–JAKOB DISEASE)

Creutzfeldt–Jakob disease (CJD; the most common form, with incidence of 1/1,000,000/ year), Gerstmann-Sträussler syndrome, fatal familial insomnia, and Kuru are classified as human prion diseases. This class of CNS infections breaks all the rules for conventional infections of the CNS. First, no nucleic agent has been identified in the infectious particle. The infectious agent is a protein normally made by neurons that is somehow misfolded into an abnormal infectious particle. Second, patients with the illness do not present with typical signs of an infection. They lack fever and an elevated WBC and have CSF that appears normal on standard tests because an immune response is not made by the host against the infectious particle. Third, the infectious particle is not killed by formalin, ethanol, or boiling (methods that normally destroy infectious agents) but can be destroyed by autoclaving. Fourth, most patients present with a subacute to chronic progressive dementia that is fatal over 6 months to 2 years. The prion infectious agent is present in CSF, brain, pituitary, and peripheral nerves that innervate cornea and dura. The infectious agent does not appear to be present in saliva, urine, sweat, or stool so isolation of the patient is not necessary. Blood should be considered infectious, but no documented human cases have occurred from blood transfusions. Transmission of a prion infectious disease may occur through inoculation via infected human cornea, dura, pituitary, or surgical instruments, or it be hereditary, as in the Gerstmann-Sträussler syndrome and fatal familial insomnia. In the United Kingdom, cases of a variant of CJD (vCJD) appear to be transmitted from infected cattle with bovine spongiform encephalopathy (mad cow disease). However, most cases of CJD appear to be sporadic without a known source of the transmission. Diagnosis may be difficult because there is no simple diagnostic test. CJD should be suspected in an adult with rapidly progressive dementia, myoclonic jerks, and normal CSF. In many patients with CJD, the CSF demonstrates abnormal 14-3-3 proteins on electrophoresis. An EEG may show characteristic abnormalities. MRI shows progressive brain atrophy often with abnormal gadolinium enhancement of the basal ganglia. Pathologically, the brain shows a characteristic spongiform encephalopathy without inflammation. Currently, there is no available treatment to stop disease progression. Patients suspected of having this disease should not donate blood or autopsy organs, but they do not require isolation.

WHEN TO REFER THE PATIENT TO A NEUROLOGIST

At times patients with CNS infections can be difficult to diagnose and manage. If circumstances as noted in the following develop, a neurologic consultation is indicated.

Patient does not fit typical clinical and laboratory picture of meningitis, encephalitis, or brain abscess.
Neuroimaging findings demonstrate brain involvement.
CSF findings are unusual or very abnormal.
CNS complications develop, such as seizures, coma, or focal neurologic signs.
Questions arise regarding best types of neurorehabilitation for the patient.
Diagnosis of a prion disease arises.

QUESTIONS AND DISCUSSION

1. West Nile viral encephalitis:
A. Occurs sporadically all year

B. Is contagious to others for about 1 year
C. Begins with severe headache and a stiff neck
D. Produces widespread death of glia and neurons
E. Is best treated with acyclovir

The answer is (D). West Nile encephalitis virus is an arbovirus that is transmitted to humans from the bite of infected mosquitoes during the summer and early fall. Whereas meningitis begins with a headache and stiff neck, encephalitis usually begins with marked changes in mental status. The virus infects both glia and neurons, producing widespread cell death. West Nile encephalitis virus is not present in urine, saliva, or stool. Therefore, the patient is not contagious and does not need isolation. Acyclovir works as an antiviral drug only against viruses of the herpes family such as herpes simplex. Thus, current treatment is symptomatic and the prevention of severe increased intracranial pressure.

2. In a brain abscess, the best way to establish the etiology is to:
A. Isolate bacteria from CSF
B. Detect specific bacterial antigen in CSF
C. Identify bacteria in CSF by Gram stain
D. Isolate bacteria from abscess pus
E. Isolate bacteria from blood or urine

The answer is (D). In a brain abscess, the bacteria are surrounded by a capsule and confined to the pus. Therefore, the CSF does not contain any bacteria or bacterial products. In a few patients, the blood may contain the bacteria if the organism reached the brain from a bacteremia. Thus, patients with a brain abscess from an acute bacterial endocarditis may have an *S. aureus* bacteremia. The only certain method of isolating the bacteria causing the abscess is to culture the pus. This can be done by stereotactic aspiration of the pus or from a craniotomy and direct surgical aspiration or drainage. The pus should be cultured for anaerobic and aerobic bacteria, fungi, and *M. tuberculosis*.

3. In a right anterior frontal lobe brain abscess, the main signs and symptoms that the patient develops are caused by:
A. Increased intracranial pressure

B. Inflammation of adjacent meninges

C. Disruption of thalamofrontal tracts

D. Destruction of frontal eye fields

E. Compression of the anterior corpus callosum

The answer is (A). Brain abscess produces signs and symptoms by two major mechanisms. If the abscess is located in a critical area of the brain, such as the motor cortex, localized signs develop. The second mechanism is through mass effect. As the abscess expands in size, the mass effect increases intracranial pressure. Increased intracranial pressure causes headache, lethargy, and psychomotor slowing. Eventually, the increased pressure causes brain herniation and death.

4. Treatment of tuberculous meningitis requires multiple drugs. The combination that often is given is isoniazid plus:

A. Streptomycin and para-aminosalicylic acid (PAS)

B. Chloramphenicol and PAS

C. Rifampin and PAS

D. Rifampin, pyrazinamide (PZA), and streptomycin or ethambutol

E. Ethionamide and ethambutol

The correct answer is (D). Most treatment guidelines in the United States and United Kingdom recommend that isoniazid, PZA and streptomycin or ethambutol be continued for 2 months and rifampin and isoniazid be continued for a total of 9 months if the case is uncomplicated and for 12 to 18 months if the patient is immunocompromised. Corticosteroids often are added early in management if the patient is comatose, has obstructive hydrocephalus, or presents with severe neurologic signs such as hemiplegia.

5. Enterovirus meningitis:

A. Is transmitted by a mosquito bite

B. Can be treated with acyclovir

C. Follows a prodrome of cramps and diarrhea

D. Causes cranial nerve palsies in 10% of patients

E. Is the most common cause of aseptic meningitis

The answer is (E). In the United States, enterovirus causes about 75% of cases of viral meningitis and the majority of aseptic meningitis cases. The virus is transmitted to the gastrointestinal tract from infected water. Most patients develop an asymptomatic gastrointestinal infection. In a few patients a viremia occurs that spreads virus to the meninges. No antiviral drugs are available for treatment, but the clinical course is benign, with more than 99% of patients making a complete recovery.

SUGGESTED READING

Anderson NE, Willoughby EW. Chronic meningitis without predisposing illness: a review of 83 cases. *Q J Med* 1987; 63:283–295.

Davis LE. Viral diseases of the nervous system. In: Asbury AK, McKhann GM, McDonald WI, et al., eds. *Diseases of the nervous system: clinical neuroscience and therapeutic principles,* 3rd ed. Cambridge: Cambridge University Press, 2002:1660–1682.

Davis LE, Kennedy PGE, eds. *Infectious diseases of the nervous system.* Oxford: Butterworth-Heinemann, 2000.

DeArmond SJ, Prusiner SB. Etiology and pathogenesis of prion diseases: review. *Am J Pathol* 1995;146:785–811.

Heilpern KL, Lorger B. Focal intracranial infections. *Infect Dis Clin North Am* 1996;10:879–898.

Johnson RT. Acute encephalitis. *Clin Infect Dis* 1996;23: 219–226.

Kastenbauer S, Pfister HW. Pneumococcal meningitis in adults: spectrum of complications and prognostic factors in a series of 87 cases. *Brain* 2003 May;126 (Pt 5): 1015–1025.

Lu C-H, Chang WN, Lin YC, et al. Bacterial brain abscess: microbiological features, epidemiological trends and therapeutic outcomes. *Q J Med* 2002;95:501–509.

Mathisen GE, Johnson JP. Brain abscess. *Clin Infect Dis* 1997;25:763–781.

Peterson LR, Marfin AA. West Nile virus: a primer for the clinician. *Ann Intern Med* 2002;137:173–179.

Skoldenberg B. Herpes simplex encephalitis. *Scand J Infect Dis Suppl* 1996;100:8–13.

Thompson RB Jr, Bertram H. Laboratory diagnosis of central nervous system infections. *Infect Dis Clin North Am* 2001;15:1047–1071.

25

Neurologic Emergencies

Lisa M. Shulman and Tricia Y. Ting

Neurologic emergencies are encountered frequently in the practice of medicine, and, if unrecognized, they may progress rapidly to permanent neurologic disability or death. The topics included in this chapter represent the more common and treatable conditions with which all physicians should be familiar. Cerebrovascular emergencies are discussed in Chapter 6.

CENTRAL NERVOUS SYSTEM

Status Epilepticus

Most epileptic seizures are self-limiting, lasting only seconds to minutes. Seizures that become prolonged or repetitive with impaired recovery of consciousness are at risk of evolving into status epilepticus (SE), a serious medical emergency. SE is not uncommon, affecting approximately 50 patients per 100,000 population yearly with a mortality rate estimated at up to 20% in adults. Long-term morbidity from SE includes chronic epilepsy, cognitive dysfunction, and focal neurologic deficits.

The point at which a seizure may be defined as SE has been a matter of debate over the past decade. Physiologic evidence for neuronal damage in animal studies formerly had led investigators to define SE as any seizure or intermittent seizures without recovery of consciousness lasting for 30 minutes or longer. More recently, clinical experience has led some investigators to broaden the definition of SE to include continuous or repeated seizure activity without return of consciousness for longer than 5 minutes. Although this definition is not yet widely accepted, it reflects a general push to initiate treatment for SE earlier to minimize the potential morbidity

and mortality. Longer seizure duration has been associated with a poorer outcome, and the longer a seizure remains untreated, the more difficult it becomes to control medically.

The most common type of SE carrying the greatest risk of morbidity and mortality is generalized convulsive SE. The seizures are usually easy to recognize clinically as tonic–clonic convulsions of the extremities with complete loss of consciousness. However, generalized convulsive SE may progress over time from overt convulsions to more subtle physical activity such as mild focal twitching or ocular deviation before further evolving to only generalized electrical activity with persistent loss of consciousness but absence of all physical manifestations. There is a risk of delayed recognition of generalized SE when patients present to the emergency room without overt tonic–clonic movements.

Nonconvulsive SE is a more heterogeneous category that includes absence SE and complex partial SE. Both forms of nonconvulsive SE are characterized by confusion or other altered mental status with minimal motor manifestations. Patients may exhibit blinking, automatisms, or fluctuating bizarre behavior. Evidence from an electroencephalogram (EEG) is important to support the diagnosis of nonconvulsive SE and sometimes, but not always, can help differentiate between absence and complex partial SE. EEG findings may vary from generalized epileptiform discharges to focal discharges or generalized activity with a focal predominance. Absence SE is believed to have little long-term neurologic sequelae. Whether complex partial SE carries a risk of significant neurologic morbidity remains controversial. Although several series documented no lasting neurologic deficits in patients following complex partial SE, there are others that reported long-term morbidity, particularly in those whose seizures were precipitated by acute neurologic disorders. Nevertheless, there is widespread agreement that patients with nonconvulsive SE should be treated quickly and aggressively to avoid potential adverse outcomes.

Morbidity and mortality from SE are a result of multiple factors including central nervous system (CNS) damage from the causative illness or acute insult that precipitated SE, the metabolic consequences of prolonged convulsive SE, and the neuronal excitotoxic effects of prolonged electrical seizure activity. It is recognized that continuous electrical activity for more than 60 minutes, even while correcting for SE-associated metabolic derangements, can result in hippocampal damage and probably in more widespread brain damage as well. The chain of events leading to neuronal injury may be induced by lack of gamma-amino-butyric acid (GABA), increased glutamate-mediated excitotoxicity, and calcium-induced neuronal death. These excitotoxic effects are compounded by significant systemic manifestations including hypoxemia, metabolic and respiratory acidosis, hyperglycemia, hyperthermia, and blood pressure fluctuation. With more prolonged SE, rhabdomyolysis may ensue from prolonged muscle activity, and significant sodium and potassium derangements develop. Cardiac arrhythmias may occur from CNS dysregulation, electrolyte abnormalities, or even medications used in the treatment of SE. Laboratory investigations commonly demonstrate a peripheral leukocytosis, an acidotic pH, and a mild cerebrospinal fluid (CSF) pleocytosis.

The general principles that guide a plan to minimize the morbidity and mortality associated with SE are early diagnosis, early intervention, and prompt identification and management of concurrent medical and surgical conditions. Once a diagnosis of SE is suspected, the underlying etiology should be investigated together with seizure control measures to ensure adequate medical or surgical

intervention. The three most common precipitants of SE in adults are withdrawal from anticonvulsive medications, alcohol withdrawal, and cerebral infarction. Metabolic derangements such as hyponatremia, hyperglycemia or hypoglycemia, hypocalcemia, hepatic failure, and renal failure account for 10% to 15% of the cases reported. Other recognized etiologies of SE include anoxia, hypotension, CNS infections (meningitis, abscess, encephalitis), tumors, trauma, and drug overdose.

Treatment of SE

Following the diagnosis of SE, the immediate response should be a timely and organized treatment plan to provide basic life support, terminate the seizure(s), prevent and treat complications of SE, identify the cause of SE, and prevent seizure recurrence (Table 25.1). Generalized convulsive SE is a medical emergency and should be managed in the emergency department or intensive care unit (ICU). The first steps are to assess vital signs and evaluate oxygenation. An oral or nasopharyngeal airway is inserted, nasotracheal suction is performed, and supplemental oxygen is administered if necessary. Oxygenation is evaluated by clinical examination, pulse oximetry, and arterial blood gas determination. Intravenous (IV) access is the next priority. Establishing two IV lines will optimize management by providing a backup IV access as well as allowing parallel delivery of IV glucose, medications, and fluids with IV anticonvulsant therapy. Simultaneously, venous blood is drawn for a complete blood count, electrolytes, glucose, calcium, magnesium, blood urea nitrogen, liver function tests, anticonvulsant drug levels, toxicology screen, and ethanol level. An IV bolus of 50 ml of 50% glucose and thiamine (1 mg/kg) is administered as soon as the IV access is established. Electrocardiographic (ECG) monitoring is instituted immediately, and vital signs are monitored throughout the treatment protocol. Electrographic seizure activity may persist in up to 15% of patients even after anticonvul-

TABLE 25.1. *Management of Status Epilepticus*

Objectives	Time Frame	Intervention
Basic life support	0–10 min	1. Recognize SE. 2. Assess vital signs and oxygenation. 3. Insert oral airway and administer oxygen if necessary. 4. Establish two IV lines. 5. Draw blood for CBC, electrolytes, glucose, calcium, magnesium, BUN, LFTs, anticonvulsant levels, toxicology screen, and ethanol level. 6. Begin ECG and EEG[a] monitoring. 7. Administer IV bolus of thiamine 1 mg/kg and 50 ml of 50% glucose.
Termination of SE	10–20 min	Infuse IV lorazepam at a rate of 2 mg/min to a total of 0.1 mg/kg or IV diazepam at a rate of 2 mg/min until seizures stop or to a total of 20 mg.
	20–60 min	1. Consider transfer to an intensive care unit 2. Infuse IV fosphenytoin 20 PE/kg at a rate of 100 to 150 PE/min. If seizures persist, infuse another bolus of 10 PE/kg at the same rate. Alternatively, use IV phenytoin at 20 mg/kg at no more than 50 mg/min, followed if needed by 10 mg/kg bolus at the same rate. 3. Monitor blood pressure, ECG, and respirations.
	60–90 min	1. If seizures persist, perform elective endotracheal intubation 2. Infuse IV phenobarbital at a rate of 50–100 mg/min until seizures stop or to a loading dose of 20 mg/kg. *Alternatively, proceed directly to treatment of refractory SE (below).*
Treatment of refractory SE	60–90 min	1. If seizures persist, begin midazolam, 0.2 mg/kg load, infusion rate 0.05–2.0 mg/kg/hr, or propofol, 3–5 mg/kg load, infusion rate 1–15 mg/kg/hr, or pentobarbital, 5–15 mg/kg load, infusion rate 0.5–10.0 mg/kg/hr, or thiopental, 75–125 mg load, infusion rate, 1–5 mg/kg/hr. 2. Titrate anesthetic to burst-suppression pattern on EEG for 12–48 hours, then gradually taper infusion rate while monitoring for seizure activity. 3. If clinical or electrographic seizure activity is observed, repeat the anesthetic induction.
Prevention and treatment of complications of SE	Throughout	1. Monitor vital signs. 2. Monitor volume status. 3. Maintain airway and prevent aspiration. 4. Review laboratory information and treat accordingly.
Identification of cause of SE	Throughout	1. Obtain history from relatives and friends. 2. Obtain head CT, when indicated. 3. Perform lumbar puncture, when indicated, following head CT. 5. Initiate IV antibiotic or antiviral coverage when meningitis or encephalitis is suspected.
Prevention of recurrence of SE	Following cessation of seizure activity	1. Monitor anticonvulsant levels. 2. Initiate daily therapy with appropriate anticonvulsant(s). 3. Educate patient and family to ensure medication compliance.

CBC, complete blood count; BUN, blood urea nitrogen; LFTs, liver function tests; PE, phosphenytoin sodium equivalents.
[a]At earliest availability

sant therapy has suppressed all signs of clinical seizure activity. Moreover, seizure activity becomes difficult to assess clinically when patients receive long-acting neuromuscular paralytic agents for endotracheal intubation or when anesthesia is induced for treatment of refractory SE. EEG monitoring, therefore, should begin at the earliest possible opportunity. It should be emphasized, however, that lack of immediate EEG monitoring should never delay therapy for suspected SE.

Termination of seizure activity is the focus of SE treatment, and benzodiazepines are the firstline agents. IV lorazepam should be administered at a rate of 2 mg/min to a total dose of 0.1 mg/kg. Alternatively, IV diazepam may be given at a rate of 2 mg/min, until seizures stop or to a total of 20 mg. Lorazepam is preferable to diazepam because it has a significantly longer duration of action, thus carrying a lower seizure-relapse rate. In case rapid treatment is required in a non-hospital setting, other benzodiazepine formulations available for use by non-medically trained staff include rectal diazepam gel (0.5 mg/kg for ages 2 through 5 years, 0.3 mg/kg for ages 6 through 11 years, and 0.2 mg/kg for older than 11 years of age) and sublingual doses of lorazepam. Infusion of a benzodiazepine should be followed immediately by IV phenytoin 20 mg/kg in non–glucose-containing solutions at a rate no faster than 50 mg/min because of the risk of hypotension and cardiac dysrhythmias. ECG and frequent blood pressure monitoring are essential. If hypotension or bradycardia develops, the rate of administration can be decreased or the infusion can be held until the vital signs stabilize. IV phenytoin should never be delivered by an automatic infusion pump to an unattended patient. If seizures are not controlled, a repeat bolus of phenytoin at 10 mg/kg can be administered.

Phosphenytoin, a prodrug that is converted to phenytoin, is poised to replace parenteral phenytoin. By virtue of its solubility, it does not require the addition of propylene glycol as a vehicle, which is thought to cause most of the clinically significant hypotension, arrhythmias, and local injection reactions of IV phenytoin administration. Absence of these side effects allows for a faster rate of infusion of phosphenytoin, usually at 100 to 150 mg/min, with peak concentrations reached within 10 minutes after infusion. Dosage is expressed in phosphenytoin sodium equivalents (PE), thus requiring a loading dose of 20 PE/kg. Phosphenytoin offers the additional advantage of intramuscular injection in those patients without IV access; therapeutic plasma concentrations are reached within 30 minutes by this route. Phosphenytoin is considerably more expensive than phenytoin, but, in fact, may be more cost-effective as a result

of a reduced need for adverse event management.

If seizures persist, IV phenobarbital traditionally has been used as a secondline agent after benzodiazepines and phenytoin have failed. However, the use of IV phenobarbital may result in respiratory depression, prolonged sedation, or severe hypotension. This adverse side effect profile has relegated the barbiturate to the status of a thirdline agent in some of the more recent SE treatment algorithms. If IV phenobarbital is used, elective endotracheal intubation is recommended before initiation of the infusion, which is administered at a rate of 50 to 100 mg/min until seizures stop or to a loading dose of 2 mg/kg. IV valproate has become available for use in treating SE, with loading doses of 15 to 20 mg/kg infused at a rate of 3 to 6 mg/kg/min. Its safety profile suggests usefulness as a secondline agent, particularly in patients who are hemodynamically unstable. However, clinical experience with IV valproate in this capacity remains limited.

Approximately 30% of patients with SE will have ongoing seizures resistant to standard loading doses of anticonvulsant medications, thus requiring therapy for "refractory SE." Anesthetic doses of benzodiazepines, short-acting barbiturates, or propofol are the thirdline agents used to treat refractory SE, although some investigators have proposed resorting to these drugs as secondline agents in place of IV phenobarbital. Midazolam is a well-tolerated, short-acting benzodiazepine that causes less problems with hypotension. It is loaded at a dose of 0.2 mg/kg and is infused continuously thereafter at a rate of 0.05 to 2.0 mg/kg/hour. An alternative to more costly midazolam is propofol, a non-barbiturate, anesthetic agent. It is loaded at a dose of 3 to 5 mg/kg followed by an infusion of 1 to 15 mg/kg/hour. A disadvantage of this therapy is the potential for developing "propofol-infusion syndrome," characterized by hypotension, lipidemia, metabolic acidosis, renal failure, and cardiovascular collapse. Finally, thiopental sodium and pentobarbital are short-acting barbiturates that may be used in treating refractory SE. Pentobarbital may be loaded at a dose of 5 to 15 mg/kg over 1 hour followed by an infusion of 0.5 to 10.0 mg/kg/hour. IV thiopental is dosed in 75- to 125-mg boluses and infused at doses between 1 to 5 mg/kg/hour. Prolonged elimination and the potential immunosuppressive propensity of these agents are potential disadvantages.

EEG monitoring is important in the management of refractory SE. Although the necessary depth and duration of anesthesia for treatment of refractory SE has not been standardized, anesthetics typically are titrated to produce a burst-suppression pattern on the EEG for 12 to 48 hours. After this time, the infusion rate is decreased gradually. If electrographic or clinical seizures emerge, induction is repeated at progressively longer intervals.

The prevention and management of complications of SE is ongoing throughout the treatment protocol. Hypertension, hyperthermia, and acidosis require attention, but effective treatment of SE should reverse these problems. Hypotension can be a direct consequence of prolonged SE or, alternatively, the effect of anticonvulsant medication, volume depletion, trauma, or cardiovascular disease. The potential risks of rhabdomyolysis, aspiration pneumonia, or traumatic injury as a result of seizure activity also must be recognized and prevented if possible.

The management of SE cannot be separated from the exigency of identifying the underlying cause. Obtaining historical information from the patient's family, friends, or medical records may reveal a pattern of non-compliance with medication or a recurrent history of alcohol withdrawal. Reports of acute neurologic deficits or febrile illness may further help guide appropriate diagnostic evaluation. Computed tomography (CT) of the head is obtained, with and without contrast (if renal function and allergies permit), to exclude the possibilities of neoplasm, cerebrovascular infarction, intracerebral hemorrhage, and traumatic injury. Following CT, lumbar puncture may be indicated. It should be noted that the CSF can reveal a moderate pleocytosis (up to 150 white blood cells) and an increase in CSF protein (up to 100

mg/dl) following persistent seizure activity. Nonetheless, if there is any suspicion of meningitis, antibiotic therapy should be started promptly and appropriate cultures should be sent for evaluation.

Following successful treatment of SE, careful attention to initiating a daily dosing schedule of one or more anticonvulsants and monitoring the total and free serum drug levels will help prevent recurrence of seizure activity. In the coming years, the development of novel routes of administration for established drugs as well as new anticonvulsant and neuroprotective agents holds promise for further reducing the morbidity and mortality of SE.

ACUTE ALTERATION OF MENTAL STATUS

An acute alteration of mental status is the most common neurobehavioral disorder seen in hospitalized patients. It is characterized by a sudden change in cognition with impaired attention that may fluctuate; it is potentially reversible; and it is not a result of preexisting dementia. Studies have demonstrated an incidence of between 5% and 15% in hospitalized patients on medical/surgical floors, 20% and 30% in surgical ICUs, and even higher on geriatric wards. Numerous vague and redundant terms for this disorder (e.g., acute confusional state, organic brain syndrome, acute cerebral insufficiency, organic psychosis, delirium, metabolic encephalopathy, and toxic psychosis) have been used and reflect the difficulty in conceptualizing and categorizing this disorder.

A well-known form of acute alteration of mental status is delirium. The *Diagnostic and Statistical Manual of Mental Disorders,* 4th edition (DSM IV), delineates the following clinical criteria for the diagnosis of delirium: inattention, change in cognition, acute and fluctuating course, and evidence of a medical cause. Patients with delirium are distracted easily and are unable to focus or shift their attention. They may be disoriented with impaired memory, disorganized thinking, emotional lability, disturbance of the sleep–wake cycle, and either increased or decreased psychomotor activity. Their symptoms may take hours or days to develop and fluctuate over the course of the day. Perceptual disturbances may result in illusions, delusions, or hallucinations, which are usually visual and often unpleasant. The sum of these disturbances often is characterized by a clouding of consciousness with reduced ability to sustain attention to environmental stimuli. As a result, the patient is unable to respond to events with the usual clarity, coherence, or speed.

Subtypes of delirium have been described and categorized by overall psychomotor activity and arousal level. These subtypes include hyperactive, hypoactive, and mixed delirium. Hyperactive delirium is dominated by hyperarousal, hallucinations, and agitation, whereas hypoactive delirium is characterized by lethargy, confusion, and sedation. Although specific etiologies do not consistently coincide with certain subtypes, there do appear to be some trends associating causes with clinical subtypes. For instance, patients with alcohol and benzodiazepine withdrawal typically appear more hyperaroused, whereas those with metabolic encephalopathy tend toward hypoactivity. Categorizing patients into general subtypes may be helpful prognostically. Investigators found that patients with hypoactive delirium had longer hospitalizations with increased risk of developing pressure ulcers, whereas their hyperactive counterparts incurred an increased risk of falls.

The differential diagnosis of a patient with an unexplained acute alteration of mental status is extensive and can be divided into three broad etiologic categories: structural lesions, toxic–metabolic causes, and psychiatric disorders. Structural lesions often distinguish themselves with focal or asymmetric findings on neurologic examination, a more abrupt onset, and less fluctuation in consciousness than seen in metabolic disorders. Inconsistencies on repeated examinations and atypical, nonanatomic findings may raise the suspicion of an underlying psychiatric problem.

Common causes of acute alteration in mental status are acquired metabolic encephalop-athies, a diverse group of neurologic disorders defined by an alteration of mental status resulting from failure of organs other than the brain. Cerebral dysfunction may result from three basic mechanisms: deficiency of a necessary metabolic substrate (e.g., hypoglycemia), disruption of the internal environment of the brain (e.g., dehydration), or the presence of a toxin or accumulation of a metabolic waste product (e.g., drug intoxication or uremia). Hepatic and uremic encephalopathies are common metabolic causes of mental status change in hospitalized patients. Disorders of glucose regulation; osmolarity/sodium homeostasis; and derangement of calcium, magnesium, and phosphorous levels are also frequent offenders. Endocrine encephalopathies seen in Cushing's syndrome, Addison's disease, and thyroid disease are less common and may be overlooked.

A patient with a metabolic encephalopathy may evolve through stages of inattentiveness, disturbed memory, and confusion to lethargy, somnolence, obtundation, and coma. The earlier stages of encephalopathy may go unrecognized because of a patient's concurrent loss of insight and judgment. Of note, an alteration of personality, behavior, cognitive function, or level of alertness may be the only symptom that brings a patient with a metabolic derangement to medical attention.

Drug intoxication and withdrawal are particularly common causes of acute alteration in mental status. At-risk patients typically are taking drugs that have anticholinergic properties, including many antidepressants, neuroleptics, antihistamines, antiparkinsonian agents, and over-the-counter cold preparations. High-dose steroids, narcotic pain medications, and sedatives also may cause acute alterations in mental status, especially in elderly patients. Abused street drugs associated with violent delirium include amphetamines, cocaine, hallucinogens, tranquilizers, sedatives, and alcohol.

Alcoholic patients commonly present to the emergency department with mental status alteration, which should be distinguished clinically from intoxication. A blood ethanol level of 80 to 100 mg/dl correlates with a change in mental status. Sharp declines in blood ethanol levels 12 to 24 hours after intake can result in tremulousness followed by alcohol withdrawal seizures. These seizures are usually brief with return to normal neurologic function. Prolonged or focal seizures, a prolonged postictal state, or a focally abnormal neurologic examination should initiate a search for other causes of seizures. Alcoholic patients are particularly prone to head injury, and brain imaging may reveal epidural or subdural hematomas, intraparenchymal hemorrhage, or traumatic subarachnoid hemorrhage. CNS infection also should be considered, potentially warranting a diagnostic lumbar puncture. Coexistent hepatic failure, hypoglycemia, hyponatremia, or drug ingestion should be screened with appropriate testing. Likewise, non-convulsive SE should prompt EEG monitoring when suspected. The clinician should be particularly alert to the possibility of Wernicke's encephalopathy, a manifestation of thiamine deficiency. It is clinically characterized by an apathetic-confusional state, oculomotor dysfunction (at times evidenced by a subtle nystagmus), and ataxia. Thiamine should be administered routinely, before glucose, at 100 mg/day IV to prevent precipitation and progression of Wernicke's encephalopathy to irreversible amnesia. B vitamins also should be supplemented because many patients have concurrent nutritional compromise. Benzodiazepines are the mainstay of management of both alcoholic withdrawal and alcoholic seizures. Although chlordiazepoxide, diazepam, and lorazepam commonly are used, oxazepam may be preferable in patients with liver insufficiency because its clearance is less dependent on hepatic metabolism than other benzodiazepines. Dehydration commonly is seen in alcoholic withdrawal and is best managed acutely with IV fluids. Magnesium may require repletion, and electrolytes should be monitored. Hyponatremia should be corrected slowly, at a rate no faster than μmol/L/24 hours because rapid correction may lead to the development of central pontine myelinolysis.

The general approach to the patient with an acute alteration in mental status involves identification and treatment of the underlying cause, environmental modification, and symptomatic treatment. This approach begins with a thorough history, physical and neurologic examination, and appropriate diagnostic testing. Historical information should be sought about systemic illness, drug or alcohol use, recent trauma, toxin exposure, baseline mental status, and the temporal course of symptoms. A history of dementia, mental retardation, or preexisting brain injury may predispose a patient to acute mental status alteration, particularly in the face of undue physical or psychologic stress. Unfamiliar surroundings with loss of daily routine, disruption of sleep–wake cycles, and sensory understimulation or overstimulation are common precipitants for these patients. Both the very old and the very young are at special risk, especially older patients with hip fractures (up to 65% incidence) because these patients tend to be more frail; advanced in age; taking multiple medications; and sensitive to electrolyte or metabolic disturbances, infection, and hypotension.

A thorough physical examination includes inspection for stigmata of hepatic, renal, or endocrine disorders. Scrutiny of the state of hydration and nutrition provides important information. Alterations in vital signs may provide clues to a wide diversity of problems, ranging from hypoxia to sepsis to elevated intracranial pressure. Signs of head trauma should be sought in the obtunded or comatose patient.

Examination of mental status should be performed in a reproducible manner to guide subsequent reevaluations of progression and efficacy of therapy. A patient's level of consciousness is best described with a few well-recognized descriptors, such as alert, lethargic (easily aroused), stuporous (difficult to arouse), and comatose (little response to external stimulation). Documentation of patient performance on standardized tests of arousability, orientation, attention, and memory are more reproducible and allow for quantitative comparison. The Folstein Mini-Mental Status Examination and the Glasgow Coma Scale are convenient quantitative scales for this purpose.

The neurologic examination includes tests of pupillary response and ocular motility as well as motor responses to stimulation. Oculocephalic reflexes, oculovestibular reflexes, and respiratory patterns should be noted in comatose patients. Demonstration of intact brainstem function makes a structural lesion of the brainstem, including elevation of intracranial pressure, less likely. Hyperreflexia may be seen in association with metabolic encephalopathy, but other evidence of upper motor neuron dysfunction is usually not demonstrated until advanced stages of disease. Asterixis, generalized tremor, and spontaneous myoclonus often are observed. Toxic encephalopathies should be considered in patients with dysarthria, nystagmus, ataxia, tremor, or dilated pupils.

Diagnostic testing can screen for metabolic abnormalities and toxin exposure. Laboratory tests should include a blood count, platelet count, prothrombin time, partial thromboplastin time, chemistry profile (electrolytes, glucose, blood urea nitrogen, creatinine, calcium, magnesium, phosphorous), liver function tests, ammonia level, thyroid function tests, arterial blood gas, urinalysis, and drug and toxicology screen. Drug levels of prescription medications that may alter mental status should be checked (e.g., anticonvulsants, lithium, theophylline, barbiturates, digoxin). Information gathered during the history and physical examination will guide the choice of additional studies: serum osmolality, plasma cortisol level, syphilis serology, erythrocyte sedimentation rate, antinuclear antibody, vitamin B_{12}, folate, human immunodeficiency virus, ceruloplasmin, serum copper, urinary copper, and urinary porphobilinogen.

Neuroimaging is recommended following an acute change in mental status to exclude a structural lesion resulting in increased intracranial pressure or focal abnormalities. Patients with fluent aphasias from dominant temporoparietal lesions or with nondominant parietal injury can be misdiagnosed as psychotic in the absence of appropriate brain imaging. CSF abnormalities are rare in metabolic encephalopathies. Nevertheless, there should be a low threshold for performing a lumbar puncture to diagnose meningitis or encephalitis when previous evaluations have failed to reveal a cause or when there is clinical suspicion of a CNS infection. Brain imaging is recommended prior to lumbar puncture to evaluate for increased intracranial pressure as a result of the risk of provoking herniation.

An EEG can be helpful in patients with metabolic encephalopathy or altered mental status of uncertain etiology. It can provide an objective evaluation of the degree of CNS dysfunction. Disorganization of the normal EEG patterns and generalized slowing are the most commonly observed changes. Seizure activity, particularly nonconvulsive SE, as well as focal abnormalities may be identified. Often, serial EEG studies are valuable to quantitatively and objectively gauge the degree of cerebral dysfunction.

TREATMENT OF ACUTE ALTERATION OF MENTAL STATUS

The management of acute alteration in mental status involves medical or surgical treatment targeted at the identified etiologic process. Even with appropriate therapy, mental status alterations, when reversible, can take weeks to months to improve. Controlling a patient's environment can facilitate reorientation. Environmental modifications include instituting regular wake and sleep schedules, diurnal exposure to natural and artificial light, use of clocks and calendars, and frequent reorientation by staff and visitors.

Patients with disorientation, emotional lability, delusions, hallucinations, paranoid ideation, or intoxication may be agitated, aggressive, violent, and resistant to medical evaluation and treatment. Although it is best to avoid the use of drugs that may result in sedation and CNS depression in these patients, symptomatic therapy for delirium is warranted in instances where behavior poses a significant risk to patient or staff safety.

Pharmacologic intervention should be individualized and directed at the specific problem (anxiety, depression, insomnia, disturbance of sleep–wake cycles, agitation, hallucinations, delusions, and aggression). The most commonly used agents are benzodiazepines and neuroleptics. Neuroleptics should be avoided in long-term management of behavior because of the risk of developing irreversible tardive dyskinesia. Moreover, clinicians should be watchful for the symptoms of neuroleptic malignant syndrome, a rare but potentially fatal idiosyncratic drug reaction. For the patient with acute agitation with psychotic features, haloperidol may be administered in a dosage of 5 mg intramuscularly (IM) every 4 to 8 hours to a maximum of 15 to 30 mg/day. Neuroleptic-induced extrapyramidal symptoms are a significant risk in all patients, particularly the elderly. The atypical neuroleptics, including quetiapine and olanzapine, are less likely to precipitate parkinsonism, acute dystonic reaction, or tardive syndromes (quetiapine 25–300 mg/day, olanzapine 2.5–10 mg/day). When the predominant feature is anxiety, benzodiazepines (e.g., diazepam, 5–10 mg IM) are often sufficient. Rarely, patients may develop paradoxical agitation with benzodiazepines, requiring withdrawal of medication.

Neuroleptics or sedatives should be used cautiously in patients with mental status alteration, particularly when the underlying etiology is unclear because these drugs can mask evidence of clinical deterioration. Sedation should be avoided especially when a patient's level of consciousness is worsening. Intoxication and drug overdose, structural lesions with elevated intracranial pressure, and infections should be excluded. In some situations, the patient's behavior may be a critical index of disease progression, and the use of physical restraints is preferable to sedation.

Although the diagnosis and treatment of delirium may be challenging and difficult in patients with multiple system failure or irreversible brain injury, a significant proportion of these patients are found to have reversible processes. These encounters, when approached with proficiency, can be especially rewarding.

ACUTE INTRACRANIAL HYPERTENSION

The main components of volume in the skull are the brain (1,400 ml), blood (1,400 ml), and CSF (150 ml). Any increase in the volume of one of these components without a corresponding decrease in the volume of the other two will result in increased intracranial pressure (ICP), or intracranial hypertension. Because volume in the cranium cannot change, any volume increase will result initially in a compensatory reduction in intracranial blood volume and displacement of CSF into the lumbar cistern. Once brain compliance is exhausted, small increases in ICP will result in herniation of the brain through the foramen magnum. The prompt recognition and treatment of acutely raised intracranial pressure is, thus, vital to preserve brainstem function and life.

Intracranial hypertension poses a risk of cerebral hypoperfusion as well as herniation. Cerebral blood flow (CBF) normally is maintained over a wide range of cerebral perfusion pressures (CPPs). CPP is defined as the difference between mean arterial blood pressure (MAP) (normally 50 to 150 mmHg) and ICP (normally 3 to 15 mmHg). A CPP greater than or equal to 70 mmHg ensures adequate cerebral perfusion. In disease states, the CPP will approximate the CBF in a linear fashion as a result of loss of vascular autoregulation; therefore, any elevation of ICP or decrease in MAP will result in cerebral hypoperfusion.

Understanding the neuroanatomic shifts that evolve with progressive increases in ICP enables better clinical recognition of pending herniation. The cranial vault is divided incompletely into compartments by thick, fibrous bands of dura mater. The tentorium cerebelli is clinically the most important of these structures. It separates the lower brainstem and cerebellum from the cerebral hemispheres and diencephalon, delineating the infratentorial and supratentorial spaces. The midbrain lies within an opening in the tentorium called the tentorial notch and is bound laterally by fascicles of the oculomotor nerve and the medial portion of the temporal lobes (the uncus). Under conditions of increased intracranial pressure, the downward displacement and herniation of the midbrain and uncus can result in compression of the brainstem, compromising vital functions including respiration, maintenance of consciousness, and cardioregulation. Coma and death may ensue.

The two main types of herniation syndromes are uncal and central. Central herniation occurs when diffusely raised supratentorial pressure compresses central brainstem structures and produces a progressive impairment of consciousness, respiratory irregularities, abnormal motor responses (posturing), and symmetric midposition unreactive pupils. Uncal herniation, however, occurs as a unilateral supratentorial mass lesion displaces the medial temporal lobe toward the tentorial notch. Some of the mass lesions that can lead to herniation are listed in Table 25.2. Early on, the oculomotor nerve becomes compressed between the encroaching uncus and the edge of the tentorial opening, producing a larger and less reactive pupil on that side. Hemiparesis may occur ipsilateral to the herniating uncus because of the compression of the contralateral cerebral peduncle against the far edge of the tentorial notch as the midbrain is displaced laterally (Kernohan's notch syndrome). More commonly, however, the hemiparesis is contralateral to the herniating uncus. In either case, hemiparesis is not a good clinical sign for localizing the side of the herniation. The abducens nerve, by virtue of its extensive intracranial course, is particularly

TABLE 25.2. *Mass Lesions Associated with Brain Herniation*

Neoplasm
Subdural hematoma
Epidural hematoma
Intraparenchymal hemorrhage
Abscess
Infarction

TABLE 25.3. *Causes of Diffuse Intracranial Hypertension with Less Risk of Herniation*

Hypoxia
Meningitis
Encephalitis
Head trauma without subdural or epidural hematoma
Subarachnoid hemorrhage
Malignant hyperthermia
Cerebral-vein thrombosis
Pseudotumor cerebri
Lead encephalopathy

susceptible to traction injury when the intracranial pressure is elevated. Therefore, sixth nerve palsies are frequently seen but have little localizing value. A dilated pupil (oculomotor nerve palsy) is ipsilateral to the herniation 95% of the time and is a more reliable clinical indicator.

Unlike the situation that occurs with mass lesions, raised ICP can be distributed equally among the intracranial compartments with little risk of herniation and brainstem compression. Some of the more common causes of diffuse intracranial hypertension are listed in Table 25.3.

Symptoms and signs of intracranial hypertension are variable and depend on both the etiology and the rapidity with which the pressure increase develops. Intracranial pressure may increase gradually over an extended period or suddenly in a matter of minutes. Headache is more likely to be a prominent symptom in more acute problems, whereas papilledema may be present in subacute or chronic conditions. Patients with large acute hemispheric infarctions may develop signs of herniation between 2 to 5 days of stroke onset, when brain edema typically peaks.

TREATMENT OF ACUTE INTRACRANIAL HYPERTENSION

The primary goal in the management of raised ICP is to reduce ICP while maintaining an adequate CPP (70 mmHg). Therefore, judicious manipulations of systemic MAP is warranted, as well as reliable measurements of ICP. Although estimations of ICP can be deduced from clinical signs, this is unreliable. The gold standard for ICP monitoring is by direct ventricular pressure measurement through a ventriculostomy. This method is precise and allows for therapeutic CSF drainage to reduce ICP. There are risks, however; parenchymal damage may result from direct penetration during placement of the ventriculostomy, and there is a high incidence of infectious ventriculitis with prolonged insertion of ventricular catheters (particularly after 5 days). Other methods are safer, with fewer infectious complications, but also less precise. They include subarachnoid bolts, epidural transducers, and intraparenchymal fiberoptic transducers. Noninvasive methods with transcranial Doppler are promising but not yet reliable.

The evaluation of patients with suspected intracranial hypertension should begin with a brief history from available informants and a brief physical examination. Patients who are unresponsive and in danger of herniation should be intubated immediately, and emergency treatment should be initiated before diagnostic investigation. Mechanical hyperventilation is the fastest way of reducing intracranial pressure. It is desirable to keep the $PaCO_2$ between 25 and 30 mmHg. The decreased $PaCO_2$ causes cerebral vasoconstriction, thereby reducing cerebral blood volume and intracranial pressure. Excessive hypocarbia may cause deleterious vasoconstriction. It is also important not to compress the jugular veins with the tape used to secure the endotracheal tube.

Osmotic agents such as mannitol are given to reduce the water content of the brain. The starting dose is 500 ml of 20% mannitol given IV for 20 to 30 minutes (approximately 1 mg/kg). A urinary catheter is recommended. Serum electrolytes and osmolality are monitored closely, using the latter as a guide to further dosing. A mannitol dose of 100 to 250 mg (0.25 mg/kg) can be given every 4 hours as necessary to maintain serum osmolality at 300 to 320 milliosmoles (mOsm) per liter.

Corticosteroids may be administered if vasogenic edema is present. Vasogenic edema oc-

curs in conditions with breakdown of the blood–brain barrier and often is seen with brain neoplasms. Steroids are generally not effective for the type of edema that accompanies cerebral infarction (cytotoxic edema) and thus are not indicated in large hemispheric strokes. Steroids do not begin working for several hours, so they usually are given concurrently with hyperventilation and hyperosmolar agents in acute situations. Methylprednisolone (Solu-Medrol) 250 mg or dexamethasone (Decadron) 10 mg IV can be used immediately, followed by dexamethasone 4 mg IV every 6 hours.

In situations with rapidly progressing intracranial hypertension, emergency neurosurgery may be necessary. Sizable cerebellar hemorrhages or rapidly expanding epidural or subdural hematomas often require lifesaving evacuation and surgical decompression. Ventricular drainage of CSF can also rapidly decrease ICP and may be performed at the bedside. Decompressive craniotomy for cerebral edema in acute ischemic infarction has shown promise for markedly reducing mortality and morbidity from an otherwise devastating condition. Randomized controlled clinical trials of this treatment are under way to provide more definitive evidence of efficacy. Moderate hypothermia (33–36° C) also has been shown to reduce ICP and improve mortality in patients following massive middle cerebral artery infarction. However, increased ICP may rebound with rewarming. Pentobarbital-induced coma may be helpful in the management of refractory intracranial hypertension; but potential adverse effects, including hypotension, reduced cardiac performance, and severe infection, limit its use.

There are a number of other general therapeutic measures that should be undertaken. IV or enteral fluids should be isotonic or hypertonic. Hypotonic solutions such as 5% dextrose or half-normal (0.45) saline can aggravate cerebral edema. Serum osmolarity of less than 280 mOsm/l should be corrected, and mild hyperosmolarity greater than 300 mOsm/l is desired. The composition of fluids replenished is a greater determinant of cerebral edema than the amount of fluids. Blood pressure should be modified to maintain a CPP of 70 to 120 mmHg. When CPP is greater than 120 and ICP is greater than 20, short-acting antihypertensive medications such as labetalol should be used. Nitroprusside may worsen cerebral edema by dilating the cerebral vasculature. In patients with increased ICP and low CPP, an adequate MAP should be maintained to avoid hypoxic–ischemic injury. Vasopressors sometimes are used in this situation. Sedation may be needed in ventilated patients who become agitated. In these patients, raised intrathoracic pressure may elevate ICP by increasing venous resistance to CSF outflow. Short-acting sedatives are preferred; propofol is gaining popularity in this setting because of its very short half-life, which allows rapid discontinuation, and thus reliable, serial neurologic examinations.

Only after the patient's clinical status has been stabilized should further evaluation with a head CT scan proceed. Because of the risk of precipitating herniation, a lumbar puncture generally should be avoided in a patient suspected of having increased ICP until a mass lesion is excluded by neuroimaging.

ACUTE SPINAL CORD COMPRESSION

Acute compression of the spinal cord often presents insidiously with pain, mild sensory disturbance, weakness, or sphincter or sexual dysfunction, but it may progress rapidly to irreversible paralysis if not corrected. Spinal cord compression is a common complication of metastatic disease, affecting 5% to 10% of patients with cancer, but it also occurs with other conditions (Table 25.4). The most frequent metastatic tumors causing spinal cord compression include multiple myeloma; lym-

phoma; and carcinomas of the prostate, lung, breast, kidney, and colon.

Pain is the earliest symptom in the vast majority of patients and may be localized to the involved spinal area (96%) or may radiate in a dermatomal pattern (90%) if the dorsal spinal roots also are involved. Pain may be intensified by actions that increase intrathoracic pressure and consequently CSF pressure, such as coughing, sneezing, or straining at stool. Percussion tenderness over the spine is often a valuable clinical sign aiding localization. Thoracic cord compression is the most frequent site of involvement (70%) because it is the narrowest area of the spinal canal. It is followed in frequency by the lumbosacral (20%) and cervical (10%) areas. Up to one-fifth of patients have multiple sites of cord compression.

The development of weakness, sensory loss, or erectile or sphincter dysfunction may progress quickly. The distribution of weakness can aid in localizing the level of the lesion. Typically, lesions in the cervical spine region result in paralysis of the legs and varying degrees of weakness in the upper extremities. Less commonly, patients may exhibit weakness that is disproportionately more impaired in the upper extremities than in the lower extremities with bladder dysfunction and varying degrees of sensory loss characteristic of an acute central cervical spinal cord injury. This lesion often results from traumatic hyperextension of the neck causing anterior and posterior cord compression within the spinal canal and subsequent injury to the central substance of the cervical spinal cord.

A rapid diagnosis of acute spinal cord compression is essential for appropriate management and optimal prognosis. This begins with a detailed clinical examination, cervical spinal X-rays to assess vertebral column injury in cases of trauma, and timely magnetic resonance imaging (MRI) of the spinal cord directed at the suspected lesion level(s) to evaluate for intrinsic injury or compression. Plain X-rays of the spine are abnormal in 84% to 94% of cases and may show evidence of bony erosion from metastatic disease, partic-

TABLE 25.4. *Common Causes of Acute Spinal Cord Compression*

Metastatic cancer
Herniated disk
Abscess
Hematoma

ularly loss of vertebral pedicles; however, they are of little help in imaging the soft-tissue structures that are invading the epidural or subdural spaces and compressing the spinal cord. MRI is the procedure of choice for visualizing the extent of anatomic involvement and spinal cord compression. It is superior to myelography in most instances because it is noninvasive and yields better resolution of anatomic structures. Spinal CT and bone scans play an important role in the diagnostic evaluations of these patients as well.

TREATMENT OF ACUTE SPINAL CORD COMPRESSION

Treatment should be started at the first sign of myelopathy. A very high dose of corticosteroids, such as dexamethasone 100 mg IV, is given immediately to reduce the edema caused by the compressing lesion, and this often provides dramatic pain relief and return of some neurologic function. In metastatic epidural cord compression, dexamethasone is continued at 24 mg IV every 6 hours for 24 hours, and then it is tapered over the next 48 hours to 6 mg every 6 hours, until more definite treatment is completed. Lower doses may be as effective. Gastric prophylaxis should be provided concurrently. An indwelling bladder catheter should be inserted. Bladder and bowel function should be monitored, with stool softeners and laxatives given as needed. Patients may require management in the ICU in cases with pulmonary, cardiac, or blood pressure instability.

Specific treatment directed at the underlying process can begin once the etiology and location are defined. In metastatic disease, radiation therapy is started immediately and is especially valuable for the more radiosensitive tumors such as multiple myeloma and lymphoma. Surgical decompression is the treatment of choice for disc disease, epidural abscess, and hematoma, and it sometimes is indicated for metastatic disease in situations in which a tissue diagnosis is needed, spinal stabilization is necessary, or further radiotherapy is not warranted. For acute central cervical spinal cord injury, surgical reduction is warranted for fracture-dislocation injuries, but the benefit of early decompressive surgery is still under investigation.

The prognosis for meaningful functional recovery depends in large part on the functional state of the patient at presentation. Whereas 80% of patients who are able to walk when they come to medical attention remain ambulatory after treatment, only 30% to 40% of non-ambulatory persons with antigravity leg function regain ambulation, and only 5% of people without antigravity leg strength are able to walk after therapy.

A high index of suspicion is required to make the diagnosis of epidural abscess, and a history of recent bacteremia or IV drug use often is obtained. The patient may or may not appear septic at the time of presentation. If epidural abscess is suspected, high-dose IV antibiotics should be given immediately (after sending blood and other appropriate cultures for analysis), while awaiting radiologic procedures and surgical decompression.

PERIPHERAL NERVOUS SYSTEM

Myasthenic Crisis

Myasthenia gravis is an autoimmune disorder directed against the postsynaptic acetylcholine receptor of striated muscle. Neuromuscular transmission is impaired resulting in weakness and fatigability of voluntary muscles. Classically, a diurnal variation in strength is noted, with strength waning as the day progresses. Diplopia or ptosis is the initial symptom in about one-half of the cases. Dysphagia, chewing difficulty, nasal speech, and regurgitation of fluids are the presenting features in one-third of patients, reflecting the involvement of bulbar musculature. Proximal limb weakness, without bulbar or ocular involvement, is the least common presentation and is easily misdiagnosed.

Myasthenic crisis occurs when muscle weakness interferes with vital functions such as breathing and swallowing. Emergency intervention is required. The mortality rate remains approximately 5% to 6%, with cardiac complications and aspiration pneumonia being the leading causes of death. A crisis may be precipitated most commonly by infection, but emotional stress, hypokalemia, thyroid disease, or (rarely) certain drugs (Table 25.5) may trigger a crisis; however, in one-third of patients, no precipitant is identified. A crisis also may be caused by overmedication with anticholinesterase agents, the so-called cholinergic crisis. A cholinergic crisis may be heralded by an increase in muscarinic symptoms such as abdominal colic and diarrhea, with more severe muscarinic signs such as vomiting, lacrimation, hypersalivation, and miosis indicating impending danger. The differentiation of myasthenic from cholinergic crisis may be more academic than practical, however, because the emergency management is the same—protect the airway and maintain adequate ventilation. Following respiratory stabilization, medications may be adjusted and precipitating factors may be investigated further.

Hospitalization, preferably in an intensive care setting, should be considered in any patient with myasthenia who complains of shortness of breath or difficulty swallowing. Frequent monitoring of the vital capacity is important, with endotracheal intubation performed when the vital capacity is less than 800 to 1,000 ml or less than 15 ml/kg or if dysphagia is so severe that there is a serious risk of aspiration. Maximal inspiratory pressure and maximal expiratory pressure are more sensitive for detecting ventilatory weakness than vital capacity. A reduction of maximal inspiratory pressure to less than 30% of that predicted for age and weight should alert the physician to impending respiratory failure and the need for mechanical ventilation. Arterial blood gases are not good predictors because they may be normal up to the onset of respiratory failure. When endotracheal intubation is required, nondepolarizing muscle relaxants should be avoided in patients with myasthenia who often have marked sensitivity to these agents leading to difficulty weaning from the ventilator. For this reason, some anesthesiologists depend on deep inhalational anesthesia (i.e., halothane, isoflurane, or sevoflurane) for tracheal intubation. An alternative to mechanical ventilation, bilevel positive airway pressure (BiPAP), may be a useful non-invasive option for the management of acute respiratory failure in patients with myasthenia. Preliminary data suggest that BiPAP may prevent intubation in patients with myasthenia who are not hypercapnic ($PaCO_2$ >50mmHg). In addition to respiratory monitoring, oral anticholinesterase agents should be discontinued in all patients and withheld for 48 hours even if cholinergic crisis is not suspected. An increased response to these drugs may occur after this "drug holiday," and often less medication may be needed once resumed.

Treatment of Myasthenic Crisis

Treatment begins with a shorter-acting drug, neostigmine (Prostigmin), 0.5 mg IM or 15 mg per nasogastric tube every 2 to 3 hours using the vital capacity or muscle strength as a guide to dosage titration. Once the optimal dose of neostigmine is found, the switch to the longer-acting agent pyridostigmine (Mestinon) can be made. Approximately four times the neostigmine dose is required every 3 to 4 hours. Corticosteroids also may be helpful in ending myasthenic crisis, but they should be used cautiously in the presence of infection. Moreover, steroids initially may worsen weakness and result in respiratory failure, particularly in the first few days of use. For this reason, corticosteroids initially should be administered in a hospital setting, particularly if a high-dose regimen is elected. Because

TABLE 25.5. *Drugs That May Exacerbate the Weakness of Myasthenia Gravis*

Aminoglycoside antibiotics
Quinine
Cardiac antiarrhythmics (e.g., quinidine, procainamide, propranolol, lidocaine)
Polymyxin
Colistin

steroids usually are required for several weeks or more following a crisis exacerbation, alternate-day steroid therapy is recommended to minimize long-term side effects. Prednisone 100 mg, or its equivalent, is given on alternate days, with a gradual taper beginning after the patient's status is clearly stabilized, usually several weeks after the crisis is over. Some authors favor giving high-dose IV corticosteroids on a daily basis early in the course before switching to alternate-day prednisone therapy.

Intravenous immune globulins (IVIG) or plasmapheresis are useful adjunctive therapies in myasthenic crisis. Plasmapheresis is directed at removing the acetylcholine receptor antibody that causes myasthenia gravis. However, for unclear reasons, even patients seronegative for the acetylcholine receptor antibody may improve with plasmapheresis. The effects of plasmapheresis alone are temporary, rarely persisting more than 4 to 11 weeks, and may not occur for several days. Thus, concomitant immunosuppressive therapy usually is recommended for more lasting treatment effect. Although plasmapheresis is generally safe, potential complications include hemodynamic instability, hypocalcemia, and dilutional coagulopathy.

IVIG is administered at 400 mg/kg daily for 3 to 5 consecutive days. It has complex immune-modulating effects, potentially involving downregulation of antibody production. Plasma exchange and IVIG have similar effectiveness, but the ease of administration of the latter makes it the more commonly used modality. Although IVIG is expensive, costs are comparable with plasma exchange. Moreover, IVIG may be a safer alternative in patients with hypotension, sepsis, or autonomic instability. Potential complications of IVIG include hyperviscosity with possible cardiac or cerebral ischemia, mild aseptic meningitis, acute renal failure, or an allergic reaction. It is important to draw serologic titers before IVIG administration because many of these will be altered by the administration of pooled IVIG. In particular, quantitative immune globulins and a history of upper-respiratory infections should be obtained because immune immunoglobulin A (IgA)-deficient individuals can become sensitized and develop adverse responses to repeat administration of IVIG.

Because any infection may precipitate a crisis, an infectious source should be sought and treated aggressively. Many patients with myasthenia are iatrogenically immunosuppressed and are highly susceptible to infection. If an infection is suspected, empiric therapy with broad-spectrum antibiotics is started at once after cultures have been sent. The change to more specific drugs is made when the cultures' sensitivities are available. The aminoglycosides are known to interfere with neuromuscular transmission but may be used when necessary. Chest roentgenogram and blood, urine, and sputum cultures on all patients with myasthenia presenting with exacerbation should be checked routinely. In addition, a diligent search for infections is required in elderly or steroid-treated patients who may not manifest the usual systemic signs of infection.

GUILLAIN-BARRÉ SYNDROME

Acute inflammatory polyradiculoneuropathy, commonly referred to as the Guillain-Barré syndrome (GBS), is a rapidly progressive, demyelinating polyneuropathy that in its most fulminant form may lead to sudden respiratory failure and autonomic instability. It therefore should be considered a neurologic emergency. The mortality rate remains at 3% to 5% despite modern intensive care management.

The classic presentation is a symmetric, ascending, flaccid paralysis that usually begins in the lower extremities (10% begin in the upper extremities) and progresses upward, with the maximum deficit attained by 4 weeks and partial or complete recovery occurring over weeks to months. In contrast to other more slowly progressive polyneuropathies in which a distal weakness predominates, the greatest weakness in GBS is in proximal muscles. Areflexia is the rule and may precede weakness. Many patients complain of distal paresthesias or dysesthesias initially, but formal testing rarely demonstrates a significant sensory loss. Facial weakness is seen in about one-half of the cases. A prior history of a recent (within 4 weeks) respiratory or gastrointestinal illness is obtained in about one-half of the patients; however, a fever at onset is atypical. A previous inoculation, surgery, hematologic malignancy, and hepatitis B or mycoplasma infection also have been associated with the syndrome. CSF analysis within the first week may be normal—the classic albuminocytologic dissociation (elevated CSF protein and <10 mononuclear cells) usually appears after the second week of illness.

Nerve conduction studies may be entirely normal early in the course if the proximal root segments are not studied. The F and H responses, measuring the motor and sensory proximal segments, respectively, may be the only abnormality noted early on. Profound slowing of nerve conduction velocity may appear on routine studies after several weeks of illness. Those cases that show evidence of secondary axonal degeneration with denervation on an electromyogram generally will have a more protracted recovery.

GBS should be differentiated from other causes of rapidly progressive flaccid paralysis (Table 25.6). A brief description of these disorders and their general management follows.

Acute intermittent porphyria can cause a rapidly ascending flaccid paralysis with respiratory and autonomic involvement, but it usually is associated with severe abdominal pain, seizures, and psychosis. Urine porphobilinogen and delta-aminolevulinic acid are elevated. Unlike in GBS, the CSF protein is usually normal. Attacks of acute intermittent porphyria may be precipitated by certain drugs such as barbiturates, phenytoin, sulfonamides, and some benzodiazepines. Acute attacks are managed supportively. A high carbohydrate intake may help further by suppressing porphyrin synthesis.

Diphtheric neuropathy occurs 1 to 2 months after a characteristic pharyngitis. The onset of weakness usually follows pronounced cranial nerve involvement by several weeks, and it may be associated with myocarditis. Unfortunately, by the time neurologic symptoms appear, specific therapy with antitoxin is ineffective. Thus, the mainstays of treatment are respiratory support and good nursing care.

Botulism may present early on, with blurred vision and diplopia as well as gastrointestinal symptoms. Unlike in GBS, pupillary reflexes are lost and the CSF is normal. Sensation remains intact. The diagnosis is supported by nerve conduction studies with reduced amplitude of compound muscle action potentials and an incremental response following rapid repetitive nerve stimulation. Specific treatment with trivalent botulinum antitoxin is recommended. Nasogastric suctioning and enemas may help remove toxin from the gastrointestinal tract early in the illness. Wound botulism is managed with surgical debridement and penicillin. In foodborne botulism, the role of antibiotics is controversial because of the concern that rapid bacterial destruction might increase the release of toxin.

Tick-bite paralysis is caused by a natural endotoxin that interferes with the release of acetylcholine at the neuromuscular junction. It presents as a rapidly ascending paralysis with respiratory and bulbar involvement. A dramatic improvement can occur after removal of the offending tick.

Poliomyelitis can produce a flaccid paralysis with respiratory involvement. However, the weakness of poliomyelitis is characteristically asymmetric, and the disease usually presents as a febrile illness with gastrointestinal symptoms, myalgias, meningismus, and a CSF pleocytosis. Arsenical neuropathy can present as rapidly developing weakness and areflexia, with CSF and nerve conduction

TABLE 25.6. *Disorders That Can Mimic Guillain-Barré Syndrome*

Acute intermittent porphyria
Diphtheria neuropathy
Botulism
Tick-bite paralysis
Poliomyelitis
Arsenic intoxication

studies indistinguishable from those of GBS. However, the neuropathy usually is accompanied by gastrointestinal, hepatic, and hematologic manifestations of arsenic poisoning. The patient with arsenical neuropathy often complains of burning dysesthesia, a feature not common in GBS.

TREATMENT OF GUILLAIN-BARRÉ SYNDROME

GBS is a neurologic emergency because of the life-threatening complications of respiratory failure and cardiovascular collapse that sometimes occur within 24 hours of symptom onset. The patient, therefore, should be monitored in an ICU or an intermediate care unit until the plateau phase of maximal deficit is reached. The vital capacity should be checked every 4 to 6 hours; if it is less than 60% of the predicted value, endotracheal intubation should be considered. Artificial ventilation may be required in up to 23% of patients. Autonomic instability may be severe, with marked fluctuations in blood pressure, tachycardia, and malignant arrhythmias. Cardiac arrhythmias are probably the main cause of death in the acute period, thus warranting continuous cardiac monitoring. Hypotension is usually mild and can be controlled with IV fluids; vasopressor agents rarely are needed. Extreme caution should be used when treating hypertension. Because of the marked lability in blood pressure, only short-acting, easily titratable drugs such as IV nitroprusside should be used. Sustained tachycardia can be treated with small doses of beta blockers if necessary. Corticosteroids, previously widely used in the acute phase of GBS, are no longer advocated because of compelling evidence of slower recovery and an increased relapse rate associated with steroid use. However, methylprednisolone in combination with IVIG has shown promise in GBS therapy.

IVIG remains the cornerstone of treatment for GBS. Studies comparing high-dose IVIG with plasma exchange indicated a beneficial effect from prompt institution of IVIG, comparable to that seen with plasmapheresis.

IVIG has become the treatment of choice for GBS in many centers because of its ease of administration, safety profile, and comparable cost. Despite concerns of early recurrences with IVIG treatment (compared with plasmapheresis), most centers use IVIG as initial treatment of GBS.

Plasmapheresis, if performed within 2 weeks of the onset of symptoms, can significantly shorten the time it takes to attain a functional recovery; however, it does not decrease the incidence of respiratory failure. It is, moreover, contraindicated in patients with severe autonomic instability. Thus, plasmapheresis often is used in patients who do not respond first to IVIG. Waiting 2 weeks before changing to the alternative modality is recommended because the effects of either may not be immediately apparent.

GBS is a self-limiting disease with many patients attaining full recovery; however, some suffer severe residual disabilities including loss of independent ambulation. Studies have identified several clinical predictors of poor outcome for GBS, including advanced age, preceding *Campylobacter jejuni* gastrointestinal illness or cytomegalovirus infection, ventilation requirement, and low compound muscle action potential amplitudes. Whereas the majority of patients with GBS have a demyelinating polyneuropathy, a minority develop axonal degeneration, which carries a poorer prognosis. Evidence suggests that in those patients positive for anti-ganglioside autoantibodies (anti-GM1 IgG) typically associated with the axonal variant, clinical outcome may be further predicted by IgG subclass. The IgG1 subclass, for instance, appears to correlate with slower recovery and more severe residual disability.

NEUROLEPTIC MALIGNANT SYNDROME

Neuroleptic malignant syndrome (NMS) is a potentially lethal complication associated with the use of dopamine-blocking agents that act in the CNS. Although NMS is not exclusively associated with neuroleptic drugs, this syndrome continues to bear a name that reflects the class of drugs in which it was recognized originally. Phenothiazines, butyrophenones, and thioxanthenes are the most commonly implicated agents (Table 25.7). In general, drugs with greater antidopaminergic potency harbor a greater potential for inducing NMS. Thus, haloperidol, chlorpromazine, and fluphenazine have been associated more frequently with NMS than other less potent dopamine-blocking agents. Even olanzapine, an atypical antipsychotic, has been reported, albeit infrequently, to induce NMS. In addition, the use of a dopamine-depleting agent such as tetrabenazine as well as the abrupt discontinuation of antiparkinsonian dopaminergic medication rarely has been associated with NMS.

Because of a scarcity of reliable epidemiologic data, the incidence of NMS is not clearly established. Retrospective studies have documented the incidence of NMS among all patients exposed to neuroleptic drugs to be between 0.5% and 1%. NMS has been reported in all age groups and in both sexes. It is related neither to the duration of exposure to neuroleptics nor to toxic overdoses of neuroleptics; however, numerous predisposing factors in affected patients have been identified. NMS is associated with the initiation of neuroleptic medications at high doses, the rapid upward titration of dose, as well as the use of long-acting depot neuroleptic preparations. Metabolic factors such as dehydration,

physical exhaustion, and acute agitation with excessive sympathetic discharge also have been implicated. Active investigation is under way to identify genetic polymorphisms in patients (e.g., for neurotransmitter receptors and drug-metabolizing enzymes) that may be associated with NMS susceptibility.

The four cardinal features of NMS are hyperthermia, muscle rigidity, altered mental status, and autonomic instability. An interruption of dopaminergic pathways is believed to be the primary etiology. A blockade of dopaminergic receptors in the striatum is thought to cause tonic contraction of skeletal muscles, which generates heat, and a similar blockade in the hypothalamus may disrupt thermoregulatory function. It is further proposed that an analogous disruption of dopaminergic function in the mesocorticolimbic system may underlie the alteration of mental status, and a blockade of dopamine receptors in the spinal cord may be responsible for dysautonomia.

Hyperthermia is present in all cases of NMS; however, the height of the temperature elevation is variable. Body temperature higher than 38°C (100.4°F) was noted in 92% of patients with NMS, and higher temperatures, higher than 40°C (104°F), were recorded in 40%. Muscular rigidity, commonly described as "lead pipe" rigidity, is generalized in distribution and may be severe enough to compromise chest wall compliance, causing hypoventilation and the need for ventilatory support. Dysphagia may occur as a result of the rigidity of the pharyngeal musculature, placing the patient at risk for aspiration. Other commonly reported motor abnormalities include akinesia, bradykinesia, and involuntary movements, such as tremor and dystonia. Mental status changes, often described as fluctuating states of consciousness, occur in 75% of affected patients. Progression through stages of agitation to alert mutism, stupor, and coma may be observed. Autonomic dysfunction is universal. Frequently reported manifestations are tachycardia, diaphoresis, blood pressure instability, urinary incontinence, cardiac dysrhythmias, and pallor or flushing of the skin. Infrequent findings include Babinski

TABLE 25.7. *Causes of Neuroleptic Malignant Syndrome*

Dopamine-blocking agents
  Haloperidol (Haldol)
  Chlorpromazine (Thorazine)
  Fluphenazine (Prolixin)
  Clozapine (Clozaril)
  Thioridazine (Mellaril)
  Thiothixene (Navene)
  Trifluoperazine (Stelazine)
  Metaclopramide (Reglan)
Dopamine-depleting agents (tetrabenazine)
Abrupt discontinuation of antiparkinsonian
  dopaminergic medications
Lithium

sign, hyperreflexia, seizures, opisthotonos, oculogyric crisis, chorea, and trismus. The clinical features of NMS typically develop over a 24- to 72-hour period and continue for approximately 5 to 10 days even when the offending agents are discontinued. Symptoms may persist two to three times longer with depot preparations of neuroleptics.

Although NMS is largely a clinical diagnosis, laboratory investigations can provide supportive data and reveal metabolic alterations that mandate diligent monitoring and treatment. An elevation of the blood creatinine phosphokinase (CPK) level and a polymorphonuclear leukocytosis consistently are found. Myonecrosis resulting from intense sustained muscle contractions underlies a mild to marked increase in CPK. White blood cell counts between 10,000 and 30,000 cells/mm^3 are present in the majority of cases. Electrolyte levels may reveal dehydration, and elevations of muscle enzymes commonly are seen. Lumbar puncture, when performed, demonstrates either normal CSF parameters or nonspecific changes. CT of the head is typically negative, and EEG studies are either normal or consistent with a nonspecific encephalopathy.

The differential diagnoses of CNS infection (meningitis, encephalitis, postinfectious encephalomyelitis), malignant hyperthermia, acute lethal catatonia, and anticholinergic toxicity must be ruled out in patients with suspected NMS. Other disorders with a similar presentation include thyrotoxicosis, heat stroke, tetanus, and drug-induced parkinsonism.

TREATMENT OF NEUROLEPTIC MALIGNANT SYNDROME

Management of NMS begins as soon as the diagnosis is suspected with the immediate withdrawal of neuroleptic medications or other dopamine antagonists. In the acute setting, IV fluids may be indicated for volume repletion, and metabolic abnormalities may need correction. Ice packs and cooling blankets can aid in reducing hyperthermia. The two most commonly used medications for treatment of NMS are dantrolene sodium and bromocriptine. Dantrolene sodium is a muscle relaxant, and bromocriptine is a centrally acting dopamine agonist. These two medications used alone or in combination promote a reduction of body temperature and serum CPK by reducing skeletal muscle rigidity. If NMS is caused by orally administered neuroleptics, treatment with dantrolene and/or bromocriptine should be continued for at least 10 days because recurrence may develop with early withdrawal from therapy. Treatment may be required for 2 to 3 weeks if depot neuroleptics were used. During the treatment period, supportive care is maintained, with careful monitoring of nutrition, fluid balance, and metabolic parameters. Both dantrolene and bromocriptine have been shown to significantly shorten the time of clinical response to therapy as compared with supportive care alone.

Approximately 40% of patients with NMS suffer from medical complications. Respiratory complications arising from diminished chest wall compliance and prolonged immobility include ventilatory failure, aspiration pneumonia, pulmonary edema, and pulmonary embolism. Cardiovascular complications such as phlebitis, dysrhythmias, myocardial infarction, and cardiovascular collapse may be seen. There is a significant risk of renal failure as a result of the combined effects of volume depletion and myoglobinuria due to rhabdomyolysis.

Mortality may result from the cumulative effects of medical complications. Morbidity and mortality from NMS have decreased over the years: reports document a mortality rate of 25% before 1984 and 11.6% since 1984. The improvement in prognosis is attributed more to early recognition and treatment of the syndrome than to the use of any specific therapeutic agent.

Because many patients who recover from NMS continue to require the use of dopamine-blocking agents, the safety of reintroducing neuroleptics often is raised. Experience has shown that neuroleptic agents can be reintroduced safely in the majority of cases. Studies have demonstrated that a recurrence of NMS can best be avoided by waiting for a complete resolution of NMS before reintroducing low doses of low-potency neuroleptics and ensuring that the patient is well hydrated and metabolically stable.

The diagnosis of NMS should come to mind when encountering any individual taking neuroleptics who develops unexplained fever with muscle rigidity. Although there are numerous alternate diagnoses, the life-threatening potential of NMS demands that treatment should not be delayed if there is significant clinical suspicion.

QUESTIONS AND DISCUSSION

1. A 21-year-old woman is seen in the emergency room complaining of a feeling of tingling in her feet and hands for 1 day. She has no other neurologic complaints. She denies shortness of breath, exposure to drugs or toxins, or a recent viral illness. An examination reveals diffuse hyporeflexia with absent ankle jerks. Very careful sensory testing is normal despite the patient's complaints. The best course of action would be:

A. Discharge the patient with the diagnosis of "functional disorder" because of a paucity of objective findings.

B. Admit her to the hospital for close observation, watching carefully for signs of developing weakness or respiratory difficulty.

C. Perform a lumbar puncture in the emergency room, suspecting early GBS, with plans to discharge the patient if the results are normal.

The answer is (B). Paresthesias without objective sensory findings occur commonly and early in GBS, often before clinical weakness develops. The key features in this case are the sensory complaints in the presence of diffuse hyporeflexia. The typically high CSF protein concentration without pleocytosis may not occur until after a few weeks of illness.

The next day, she complains of difficulty in walking and on examination shows a pulse of 120, diffuse areflexia, and bilateral proximal lower-extremity weakness. The best management at this time would be:

A. Admit her to an ICU for cardiac monitoring, frequent vital capacities, and lumbar puncture.

B. Observe her in a general medical ward with daily vital capacities and steroids.

C. Admit her to an ICU for cardiac monitoring, with monitoring of the vital capacity only if respiratory problems occur.

D. Admit her to an ICU for vital capacity and cardiac monitoring, and give high-dose steroids.

The answer is (A). With weakness now developing, it is clear that the patient has GBS. She should be monitored in an ICU setting, and she should be watched closely for the development of cardiac arrhythmias and respiratory compromise. Vital capacities should be checked every 4 to 6 hours, with intubation done if there is less than 60% predicted value. Steroids have not been shown to be effective in GBS.

2. The following statement about generalized SE is true:

A. Generalized SE should be diagnosed in a patient who within a 2-hour period has a series of seizures, between which he is fully oriented and able to clearly state his medications and dosages.

B. Generalized SE should be diagnosed in a patient who has had continuous twitching of his left hand for 6 hours but no impairment of consciousness.

C. A patient in generalized SE should be immediately intubated and paralyzed with neuromuscular blockade to prevent rhabdomyosis from intense muscular contractions.

D. A patient in generalized SE should be treated with a fast-acting benzodiazepine followed immediately by a loading dose of a long-acting anticonvulsant such as phenytoin.

The answer is (D). Generalized SE is defined by prolonged seizure activity with loss of consciousness or repeated seizures without recovery of consciousness between episodes. Neuromuscular blockade will abolish the motor activity but will have no effect on the underlying persistent ictal activity. Following preservation of an airway, drawing labs, and the establishment of intravenous access, first-line therapy is aimed at abolishing electrographic seizure activity with anticonvulsants.

3. Spinal cord compression should be considered in all of the following situations except:

A. Sudden onset of right arm and leg weakness, accompanied by sensory loss

B. Gradual onset of paraparesis associated with a loss of bowel and bladder function

C. Subacute proximal leg weakness associated with a beltlike sensation across the chest that increases with lifting heavy objects

D. Back pain associated with paraparesis

The answer is (A). In this case, the hemineurologic deficit is most likely secondary to a contralateral hemispheric infarct.

4. All of the following statements regarding the management of acute intracranial hypertension are true, except:

A. Reduction of $Paco_2$ is the quickest way of reducing intracranial pressure.

B. Corticosteroids are especially helpful in reducing the edema associated with infarction.

C. Emergency surgery is the preferred treatment for cerebellar hemorrhages.

D. Osmotic agents are helpful in reducing intracranial hypertension from any cause.

The answer is (B). Steroids are useful when considerable tumor edema (vasogenic edema) is present, but they are not particularly effective on the type of edema associated with cellular damage (cytoxic edema) such as occurs with infarction.

5. All of the following statements concerning the treatment of myasthenic crisis are false, except:

A. Aminoglycoside antibiotics are contraindicated.

B. It is not necessary to differentiate a myasthenic from a cholinergic crisis because the emergency management is the same.

C. Anticholinesterase drugs are withdrawn for 48 hours only if a cholinergic crisis is suspected, then they are restarted at twice the previous dose.

D. Plasmapheresis is an important treatment modality because its effects are always immediate.

E. Although vital capacity monitoring is important prior to intubation, it is not helpful in assessing a patient's progress after he has been placed on a mechanical ventilator.

The answer is (B). Emergency management of a crisis is the same regardless of etiology—the maintenance of adequate ventilation and the withdrawal of anticholinesterase medications. These drugs then are restarted after 48 to 72 hours at smaller doses. Aminoglycoside antibiotics can exacerbate myasthenia gravis, but they may be used cautiously if necessary. Plasmapheresis may be helpful, but its effects often are delayed for several days. Vital capacity monitoring may be a useful tool in assessing the adequacy of therapy in the crisis situation.

6. A 45-year-old man presents to the emergency department confused with an unsteady gait. No additional history was attainable. Neurologic examination further revealed intermittent upbeat nystagmus, horizontal gaze palsy, and severe ataxia. Laboratory evaluation revealed an elevated gamma-glutamyl transpeptidase, serum amylase, and serum lipase, but drug and alcohol testing was negative.

The best course of action would be:

A. Immediately request an EEG to evaluate for non-convulsive seizure activity while simultaneously initiating a loading dose of intravenous phenytoin.

B. Stabilize the patient's cervical spine, order cervical spine plain films, and request a psychiatry consultation for further evaluation.

C. Immediately administer intravenous thiamine followed by glucose and intravenous fluids, while considering the need for neuroimaging and lumbar puncture.

D. Order serial neurologic examinations to be done by nursing staff while attempting to contact family members for further historical information.

The answer is (C). This patient presents with the classic triad of clinical features for

Wernicke's encephalopathy—ophthalmoplegia, ataxia, and confusion. Immediate infusion of thiamine is warranted because the symptoms are potentially reversible with early treatment. Glucose should be administered for potential hypoglycemia, but it should be given only after thiamine because of the risk of precipitating encephalopathy in those with borderline nutritional status. Pursuing additional evaluative testing including neuroimaging, lumbar puncture, EEG, and cervical spine plain film series may be warranted based on the clinical picture but should not delay early administration of thiamine.

7. All of the following statements about NMS are true, except:

A. The cardinal features of NMS are hyperthermia, muscle rigidity, and circulatory collapse associated with induction of general anesthesia.

B. The most common therapy, dantrolene and/or bromocriptine, typically is required for 10 days up to 3 weeks.

C. Rarely, NMS may result from the abrupt discontinuation of antiparkinsonian dopaminergic medication.

D. The reintroduction of neuroleptics is not contraindicated in patients who have had NMS.

The answer is (A). Hyperthermia, rigidity, and circulatory failure in the setting of general anesthesia are characteristic of malignant hyperthermia. Similarities in therapy for malignant hyperthermia and NMS include dantrolene, intravenous hydration, and body cooling.

SUGGESTED READING

Byrne TN. Spinal cord compression from epidural metastases. *N Engl J Med* 1992;327:614.

Charness ME, Simon RP, Greenberg DA. Ethanol and the nervous system. *N Engl J Med* 1989;321:442.

DeLorenzo RJ. Status epilepticus: concepts in diagnosis and treatment. *Semin Neurol* 1990;10:396.

Devinsky O, Leppik I, Willmore LJ, et al. Safety of intravenous valproate. *Ann Neurol* 1995;38:670.

Dickey W. The neuroleptic malignant syndrome. *Prog Neurobiol* 1991;36:425.

The Dutch Guillain-Barré Study Group. Treatment of Guillain-Barré syndrome with high-dose immune globulins combined with methylprednisolone: a pilot study. *Ann Neurol* 1994;35:749.

Factor SA, Singer C. Neuroleptic malignant syndrome. In: Weiner WJ, ed. *Emergent and urgent neurology.* Philadelphia: JB Lippincott, 1992.

Gajdos P, Chevret S, Clair B, et al. Clinical trial of plasma exchange and high-dose intravenous immunoglobulins in myasthenia gravis. Myasthenia Gravis Clinical Study Group *Ann Neurol* 1997;41:789.

Grant R, Papadopoulos SM, Sandler HM, et al. Metastatic epidural spinal cord compression: current concepts and treatment. *J Neurooncol* 1994;19:79.

Hadley M. Management of acute central cervical spinal cord injuries. *Neurosurgery* 2002;50(3 Suppl):S166.

Kawanishi C. Genetic predisposition to neuroleptic malignant syndrome: implications for antipsychotic therapy. *Am J Pharmacogenomics* 2003;3:89.

Koga M, Yuki N, Hirata K, et al. Anti-GM1 antibody IgG subclass: a clinical recovery predictor in Guillain-Barré syndrome. *Neurology* 2003;60:1514.

Kogoj A, Velikonja I. Olanzapine induced neuroleptic malignant syndrome—a case review. *Hum Psychopharmacol* 2003;18:301.

Kokontis L, Gutmann L. Current treatment of neuromuscular diseases. *Arch Neurology* 2000;57:939.

Leppik IE. Status epilepticus. In: Wyllie E, ed. *The treatment of epilepsy: principles and practice.* Philadelphia: Lea & Febiger, 1993.

Manno EM. New management strategies in the treatment of status epilepticus. *Mayo Clin Proc* 2003;78:508.

Mayer SA, Dennis LJ. Management of increased intracranial pressure. *Neurologist* 1998;4:2.

Meagher DJ. Delirium: optimizing management. *BMJ* 2001; 322:144.

Rabinstein A, Wijdicks EF. BiPAP in acute respiratory failure due to myasthenic crisis may prevent intubation. *Neurology* 2002;59:1647.

Reid RL, Quigley ME, Yen SS. Pituitary apoplexy. *Arch Neurol* 1985;42:712.

Ropper AH. The Guillain-Barré syndrome. *N Engl J Med* 1992;326:1130.

Steiner T, Ringleb P, Hacke W. Treatment options for large hemispheric stroke. *Neurology* 2001;57(5 Suppl 2):S61.

Thomas CE, Mayer SA, Gungor Y, et al. Myasthenic crisis: clinical features, mortality, complications, and risk factors for prolonged intubation. *Neurology* 1997;48:1253.

Van der Meche FG, Schmitz PI, and the Dutch Guillain-Barré Study Group. A randomized trial comparing intravenous immune globulin and plasma exchange in Guillain-Barré syndrome. *N Engl J Med* 1992;326:1123.

26

Neurologic Complications of Human Immunodeficiency Virus Infection

Meriem K. Bensalem and Joseph R. Berger

In the spring of 1981, the Centers for Disease Control and Prevention (CDC) in Atlanta reported on the occurrences of uncommon opportunistic infections and malignancies among previously healthy young homosexual men in New York and California. This newly recognized immunodeficiency state was referred to as the acquired immunodeficiency syndrome, or AIDS. In 1983 the etiologic agent, a retrovirus, subsequently referred to as the human immunodeficiency virus, or HIV, was isolated initially. Soon afterward, a second major class of HIV was identified in West African patients with an AIDS-like illness; this virus was referred to as HIV-2, and the previously identified AIDS virus received the designation HIV-1.

More than 50% of people infected with HIV will develop symptomatic neurologic disease, but neuropathologic abnormalities are observed in as many as 90% of autopsies of patients dying with AIDS. With respect to the neurologic complications of HIV infection, there are several key points. First, neurologic manifestations are observed far more frequently in the setting of significant immunosuppression, specifically when CD4 lymphocyte counts are less than 200 cells/mm^3. However, neurologic disease may be seen with fairly robust immunity and a limited spectrum of neurologic disease tends to occur very early in the course of infection. Second, the spectrum of illnesses affecting the nervous system may be the consequence of either a direct effect of HIV, or it may occur as a secondary consequence of the infection. The latter is typically, but not always, the result of the associated immunosuppression permitting a recrudescence of latent or persistent infec-

tion. Other neurologic illnesses may result from malignancy, metabolic and nutritional disorders, or cerebrovascular complications related to HIV infection. Third, no part of the central or peripheral nervous system is exempt from the possible neurologic complications accompanying HIV infection. The entire neuraxis from the brain to the muscles may be individually or collectively affected. Fourth, the coexistence of two or more neurologic disorders is not uncommon in any given patient, vastly complicating their diagnosis and management. Thorough neurologic assessment may play a pivotal role in the care and treatment of patients with AIDS, and referral to a neurologist should be considered when a neurologic complication is suspected or confirmed.

This chapter reviews the clinical features, the diagnosis, and the treatment of neurologic disorders associated with HIV-1 infection. The illnesses affecting the central nervous system (CNS) are discussed first, followed by the involvement of the peripheral nervous system. Tables 26.1 and 26.2 contain a summary of the pharmacologic treatments that are cited in this chapter. Table 26.3 is a review of the prophylactic treatment of opportunistic infections in patients infected with HIV.

HIV

The virus known as HIV is a member of a unique family of RNA viruses characterized by the presence of RNA-dependent DNA polymerase or reverse transcriptase. The reverse transcriptase is an enzyme that enables these RNA viruses to produce a DNA copy of the genome, which then can be incorpo-

TABLE 26.1. Selected Antiretroviral Drugs

Drug Name	Dose	Selected Adverse Reactions	Selected Drug Interaction
Zidovudine (AZT)	300 mg twice daily or 200 mg 3 times/day on empty stomach	Headache, fever, nausea, vomiting, anemia, neutropenia, thrombocytopenia, myopathy, hepatitis, hyperpigmented nails (adjusted dose for hepatic failure)	Ganciclovir and interferon alpha may increase the risk of hematologic toxicities. Phenytoin may decrease its clearance. Phenytoin plasma levels may decrease.
Lamivudine (3TC)	150 mg twice daily; if weight <50 kg: 2mg/kg twice daily	Headache, insomnia, fatigue, nausea, vomiting, diarrhea, peripheral neuropathy, depression, fever, rashes, anemia, neutropenia, elevated AST/ALT, pancreatitis	Lamivudine may increase AZT concentrations. Trimethoprim/sulfamethoxazole increases its AUC and decreases its renal clearance.
Abacavir	300 mg twice daily	Hypersensitivity reactions (fever, fatigue, nausea, vomiting, rash), which may be fatal. Do not restart abacavir in patients who have experienced this.	Ethanol may increase the risk of toxicity. Methadone concentration may be decreased by abacavir.
Didanosine (ddI)	For tablet formulation; Weight <60 kg: 125 mg twice daily Weight 60 kg 200 mg twice daily	Hyperglycemia, hypertriglyceridemia, nausea, vomiting Peripheral neuropathy, pancreatitis, diarrhea, rash, pruritus, myopathy, neuritis, retinal depigmentation, anxiety, abdominal pain	Allopurinol may increase ddI toxicity. Ganciclovir may increase ddI concentration. Concomitant use of other drugs that have the potential to cause peripheral neuropathy or pancreatitis may increase the risk of these toxicities.
Zalcitabine (ddC)	0.75 mg every 8 hours	Peripheral neuropathy, oral/esophageal ulceration, rash, nausea, vomiting, diarrhea, myalgia, pancreatitis, anemia, seizures	Magnesium/aluminum-containing antiacids and metoclopramide may reduce ddC absorption. Avoid use of concomitant drugs, which have the potential to cause peripheral neuropathy. It is not recommended to use ddC with ddI, stavudine, or 3TC due to overlapping toxicities, virologic interaction, or lack of clinical data.
Efavirenz	600 mg once daily	Dizziness, insomnia, fatigue, inability to concentrate, vivid dreams, psychiatric symptoms (hallucinations, confusion), rash, nausea, diarrhea, elevated AST/ALT	Cisapride, midazolam, triazolam, astemizole, and ergot alkaloids may result in life-threatening toxicities. This drug may increase or decrease warfarin effect. Phenobarbital, rifampin and rifabutin may decrease serum concentration of efavirenz
Saquinavir (use in combination with nucleoside analogue)	Fortofase 1200 mg 3 times/day within 2 hours after meal Invirase 600 mg 3 times/day within 2 hours after a full meal	Rash, hyperglycemia, dyslipidemia, diarrhea, nausea, headache, paresthesias, weakness	Rifampin may decrease its plasma levels and AUC. Phenobarbital, phenytoin, dexamethasone, and carbamazepine may induce its metabolism. Saquinavir may reduce the metabolism of cisapride and ergot derivatives. Avoid use with simvastatin and lovastatin (increased risk of myopathy).
Ritonavir	Escalation: 300 mg twice daily for 1 day, 400 mg twice daily for 2 days, 500 mg twice daily for 1 day, then 600 mg twice daily. If used with saquinavir, dose is 400 mg twice daily.	Anemia, leukopenia, nausea, vomiting, taste perversion, dyslipidemia, diarrhea, anorexia, circumoral, and peripheral paresthesia	Antiarrhythmics toxicity may be increased; concurrent use of ritonavir is contraindicated. Benzodiazepines toxicity may be increased: concurrent use of midazolam and triazolam is contraindicated Cisapride, ergot derivatives are contraindicated.
Indinavir	800 mg every 8 hours Dose adjustment with certain medications	Hyperbilirubinemia, nephrolithiasis/urolithiasis, headache, insomnia, dyslipidemia, nausea, vomiting, hyperglycemia, increased AST/ALT	Concurrent use of rifampin and rifabutin may decrease the effectiveness of indinavir. Avoid use of astemizole and cisapride. Indinavir inhibits the metabolism of HMG-CoA reductase inhibitors. Prolonged sedation may occur if used with benzodiazepines.

AST/ALT, aspartate aminotransferase/alanine aminotransferase; AUC, area under the curve; HMG-CoA, 3-hydroxy-3-methylglutaryl coenzyme A.

TABLE 26.2. *Prevention of opportunistic infection in persons infected with HIV*

Pathogen	Indication	Drug and Dose	Selected Drug Interaction
Mycobacterium tuberculosis	TST reaction = or > 5 mm or prior positive TST without treatment or contact with a case of active TB	Isoniazid 300 mg daily for 9 months and Pyridoxine 50 mg daily for 9 months Or Isoniazid 900 mg twice a week for 9 months and Pyridoxine 100 mg twice a week for 9 months Or Rifampin 600 mg daily for 2 months and Pyrazinamide 20 mg/kg daily for 2 months The latter regimen is recommended for Isoniazid-resistant pathogens	Decreased effect of INH and aluminum salts Increased hepatic toxicity with alcohol or with rifampin and INH INH may increase toxicity of oral anticoagulants, carbamazepine, meperidine and hydantoins Pyridoxine may decrease serum levels of levodopa, phenobarbital, and phenytoin Rifampin induces liver enzymes which may decrease the plasma concentration of calcium channel blockers, methadone, digitalis, cyclosporine, corticosteroids, oral anticoagulants, haloperidol, theophylline, barbiturates, imidazole antifungals, oral or systemic hormonal contraceptives, benzodiazepines, hydantoins, beta-blockers, zidovudine, protease inhibitors, and non-nucleoside reverse transcriptase inhibitors.
Mycobacterium avium complex	CD4+ <50/microliter	Azithromycin 1200 mg once weekly Or Clarithromycin 500 mg twice daily	Azithromycin may increase levels of tacrolimus, phenytoin, ergot alkaloids, bromocriptine, carbamazepine, cyclosporine and digoxin Avoid use with pimozide Clarithromycin may increase serum I levels of benzodiazepines metabolized by CYP34A4, bromocriptine, buspirone, calcium channel blockers, carbamazepine, cyclosporine, digoxin, ergot alkaloids, indinavir, oral contraceptives, phenytoin, pimozide. Rotonavir increases clarithromycin levels
Toxoplasma gondii	IgG antibody to *Toxoplasma* and CD4+ <100/microliter	TMP-SMZ 1 Double-strength tablet daily	Trimethoprim increases toxicity/levels of phenytoin. May increase levels of digoxin. Increases myelosuppression with methotrexate. Increased toxicity of sulfonamides with diuretics, indomethacin, probenecid and salicylates Increased toxicity of oral anticoagulants, oral hypoglycemic agents, hydantoins, uricosuric agents, methotrexate when administered with sulfonamides

TABLE 26.3. *Treatment Regimens for Infectious Conditions Leading to Neurologic Complications in Patients Infected with HIV*

Neurologic Complication	Drug Name	Dose	Selected Drug Interactions
CMV encephalitis	Ganciclovir	*Induction therapy:* 14–21 days	Increases didanosine concentrations and excretion in the urine.
		5 mg/kg IV every 12 hours	Hematologic toxicity may be increased with concomitant use of zidovudine.
		Maintenance therapy: 5 mg/kg/day IV	Immunosuppressive agents may increase cytotoxicity of ganciclovir.
		Adjust dose with renal impairment	Its renal clearance is decreased with probenecid.
	Foscarnet	90 mg/kg IV every 12 hours with the induction therapy	Pentamidine increases hypocalcemia.
		90–120 mg/kg/day IV for the maintenance therapy	Concurrent use with ciprofloxacin increases seizure potential. Nephrotoxic drugs should be avoided to minimize additive renal effects
		Adjust dose with renal impairment	(renal impairment has been reported with concurrent use with ritonavir and saquinavir).
Cerebral toxoplasmosis	Sulfadiazine	2–4 g daily divided every 4–8 hours for 3–6 weeks then 500–1,000 mg 4 times daily, in conjunction with pyrimethamine and folinic acid	There is increased effect of oral anticoagulants and oral hypoglycemic agents. There is decreased effect with procaine and sunscreens.
		Adjust dose with renal impairment	
	Pyrimethamine	Loading dose 200 mg orally once, then 75 to 100 mg daily for 3–6 weeks, then suppressive therapy 25–75 mg orally daily Folinic acid 10–25 mg daily is added with pyrimethamine	Its effectiveness is decreased by acid. There is increased effect of pyrimethamine with sulfonamides (synergy). Methotrexate. TPM/SMX may increase the risk of bone marrow suppression.
	Clindamycin, if allergies to sulfa drugs	600 mg orally IV every 6 hours. For suppressive therapy 300–450 mg every 6–8 hours with pyrimethamine and folinic acid as above	Mild hepatotoxicity may occur with lorazepam. Increased duration of neuromuscular blockade from tubocurarine, pancuronium occurs.

(continued on next page)

TABLE 26.3. (Continued)

Neurologic Complication	Drug Name	Dose	Selected Drug Interactions
Cryptococcal meningitis	Amphotericin B for at least 2 weeks, then use fluconazole	0.7–1 mg/kg daily IV for 2 weeks then switch to fluconazole, as indicated below	Increased nephrotoxicity with aminoglycosides and cyclosporine may occur. Potentiates hypokalemia with corticosteroids and corticotropin may occur. Increased digitalis and neuromuscular blocking agent toxicity due to hypokalemia may occur. Decreased effect if given with azole antifungal drugs may occur. Increased effect/toxicity with concurrent amphotericin use may occur.
	Flucytosine (can be added to the amphotericin B)	50–150 mg/kg daily divided doses every 6 hours	
	Fluconazole	Start 400 mg daily for 10 weeks total then switch to 200 mg daily indefinitely	It may decrease the effect of oral contraceptives. Concurrent use with cisapride is contraindicated. Rifampin and cimetidine decrease concentrations of fluconazole Fluconazole may inhibit warfarin, phenytoin, cyclosporine, theophylline, zidovudine and sulfylureas clearance Increases toxicity of tacrolimus
Tuberculous meningitis	INH	300 mg daily	Hepatic toxicity is increased with concomitant use of alcohol or rifampin. It increases toxicity of oral anticoagulants, carbamazepine, cyclosporine, meperidine, and hydantoins. Its effect is decreased with aluminum salts. It decreases effect of ketoconazole.
INH+RIF+PZA for 2 months, then INH+RIF for 4 months. May treat up to 9 months Adjust doses if using concomitant protease inhibitors.		Add pyridoxine 25–50 mg daily	
	RIF	10 mg/kg/day	Rifampin induces liver enzymes, which may decrease the plasma concentration of calcium channel blockers, methadone, digitalis, cyclosporine, corticosteroids, oral anticoagulants, haloperidol, theophylline, barbiturates,

Condition	Drug	Dose	Interactions
	PZA	25 mg/kg daily Dose adjustment in renal and hepatic impairment	imidazole antifungals, oral or systemic hormonal contraceptives, benzodiazepines, hydantoins, beta blockers, zidovudine, protease inhibitors, and non-nucleoside reverse transcriptase inhibitors.
Syphilitic meningitis	Penicillin G	24 million units daily hours for 14–21 days	Heparin and parenteral penicillins may result in increased bleeding. Probenecid, disulfuram may increase penicillin levels. It may reduce efficacy of oral contraceptives It may increase effects of warfarin
Listeria meningitis	Ampicillin	2 g IV every 4 hours	Tetracyclines may decrease penicillin effectiveness. It may reduce efficacy of oral contraceptives. Probenecid, disulfuram may increase penicillin levels. It may increase effects of warfarin.

IV, intravenous; TPM/SMX, trimethoprin/sulfamethoxazole; INH, isoniazid; RIF, rifampin; PZA, pyrazinamide.

TABLE 26.4. *Neurologic Complications of HIV-1 Infection*

Table 1: Antiretroviral drugs.

Nucleoside and non-nucleoside reverse transcriptase inhibitors and protease inhibitors, usual dose in the adult, selected adverse reaction, and drug interaction. All of the drugs listed are nucleoside reverse transcriptase inhibitors except for efavirenz, which is a non-nucleoside reverse transcriptase inhibitor, and saquinavir, ritonavir, and indinavir, which are protease inhibitors. All these drugs need a renal dose adjustment with renal impairment.

Table 2: Usual dose and selected drug interaction for antiviral, antiprotozoan, antifungal, antimycobacterial, antispirochetal and antibacterial infections associated with HIV-infection discussed in this chapter.

Table 3: Drugs for prevention of opportunistic infections in persons infected with HIV.

Early

Acute syndromes associated with initial infection
Multiple sclerosis–like illness
Aseptic meningitis
Demyelinating neuropathies

Late

AIDS dementia complex
Vacuolar myelopathy
Peripheral neuropathy
Myopathies
Cerebrovascular complications
Seizures
Opportunistic infections and neoplasms
    Cerebral toxoplasmosis
    Cryptococcal meningitis
    Progressive multifocal leukoencephalopathy
    Cytomegalovirus infections
    Syphilis
    Primary central nervous system lymphoma
    Meningitis lymphomatosis

TABLE 26.5. *Incidence of Neurologic Complications in AIDS*

Cerebral toxoplasmosis	10–20%
Cryptococcal meningitis	2–10%
Progressive multifocal leukoencephalopathy	2–5%
Cytomegalovirus polyradiculopathy	2%
Cytomegalovirus encephalitis	<1%
Primary central nervous system lymphoma	2–13%
Meningitis lymphomatosis	0.5–3%
Aseptic meningitis	<5%
AIDS dementia complex	5–33%
Vacuolar myelopathy	20–30%
Polyneuropathy	10–35%
Myopathy	<10%

HIV AND THE CNS

The involvement of the CNS will be categorized into brain disease without mass effect and brain disease with mass effect, followed by a discussion on meningeal involvement and disease of the spinal cord.

BRAIN DISEASE WITHOUT MASS EFFECT

The most common causes of intracranial lesions without mass effect in patients infected with HIV are HIV encephalopathy, cytomegalovirus (CMV) encephalitis, and progressive multifocal leukoencephalopathy (PML). Of these disorders, only PML typically presents with focal neurologic disturbances.

HIV DEMENTIA

One of the most important neurologic syndromes in patients with AIDS is HIV dementia. Several appellations have been used to describe this unique, progressive, dementing illness, including subacute encephalitis, AIDS dementia complex (ADC), HIV encephalopathy, and HIV-associated major cognitive/motor disorder. The exact incidence of this encephalopathy in individuals infected with HIV is unknown. By the time of death, more than one-third of patients with AIDS will exhibit this dementia, but since the use of zi-

rated into the host genome. Other characteristics of this family of viruses are their large size, their ability to produce cytopathic changes in the infected cells, and their long incubation times before the development of clinical illness (typically, immunologic or neurologic disease). Any part of the neuraxis can be involved, and some of the neurologic complications occur in the early stages of the disease, whereas others are associated with advanced HIV-1 infection, as illustrated in Table 26.4. The incidence of neurologic complications in AIDS is given in Table 26.5.

dovudine and the introduction of highly active antiretroviral therapy (HAART), the incidence of this disorder appears to have declined.

The symptoms of HIV dementia can be subdivided into three main categories: cognitive, motor, and behavioral. The onset is usually insidious, developing over several weeks to months. Forgetfulness, decreased concentrating, slowness of thoughts, difficulty reading, and the slow performance of a wide variety of tasks often are reported by patients or their relatives. Other complaints include fatigue, malaise, headaches, increasing social isolation, and loss of sexual drive. Some patients may become socially withdrawn, often mistakenly attributed to depression. Motor symptoms include clumsiness, tremor, poor balance, and unsteady gait. Psychosis, such as, mania may develop in some patients and may be a primary manifestation of HIV dementia.

A general physical examination may reveal the typical findings of advanced AIDS, including wasting, alopecia, seborrheic dermatitis, and generalized lymphadenopathy. Performance during cognitive testing typically is slow. Because cortical symptoms such as aphasia, alexia, and agraphia are absent or do not appear until very advanced stages of the disorder, tests such as the Folstein Mini-Mental State Examination are not particularly helpful. However, assessments of attention and executive function are useful. Ocular motility examination often reveals that saccadic and pursuit eye movements are slowed and inaccurate. Muscle tone may be normal or increased. Fine motor movements and rapid alternating movements generally are slow and imprecise. Frontal release signs, such as the snout and glabellar response, frequently are elicitable. Deep tendon reflexes may be normal or brisk, but ankle jerks often are depressed as a consequence of concomitant peripheral neuropathy. Worsening of psychomotor slowing may progress to severe dementia with akinetic mutism, paraparesis, and incontinence.

Diagnostic studies are important to exclude treatable conditions of the dementia, such as metabolic or infectious causes and tumors. Laboratory studies should assess renal, liver, and thyroid function; electrolytes; syphilis serologies; and vitamin B_{12} and folate levels. The computed tomography (CT) scan and magnetic resonance imaging (MRI) of the brain may be normal, but in most instances they reveal cortical atrophy and enlarged ventricles or both. Usually the degree of central atrophy as reflected by ventricular enlargement exceeds the degree of cortical atrophy. The brain MRI also may reveal patchy or diffuse increased signal intensity on T2-weighted images, usually located in the periventricular white matter and centrum semiovale and always without associated mass effect (Fig. 26.1). The neuroradiologic abnormalities correlate poorly with the degree of dementia and may be seen in patients infected with HIV without evident dementing illness.

Examination of cerebrospinal fluid (CSF) may reveal a mononuclear pleocytosis (with counts typically less than 20 cells/microliter)

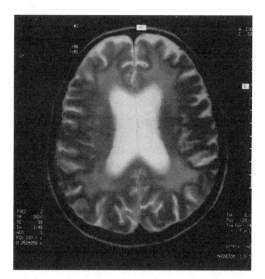

FIG. 26.1. HIV dementia. T2-weighted MRIs showing mild central atrophy and diffuse confluent white matter hyperintense signal abnormalities.

and increased proteins (usually less than 65 mg/dl). HIV-1 itself may be cultured from the CSF in up to 30% of patients, and HIV-1 p24 core protein in CSF, which is independent of HIV-1 antigen in serum, is detectable in 50% of patients with HIV dementia. Neither test is a particularly useful diagnostic tool for this disorder. A variety of surrogate markers, chiefly indicators of immune activation, such as quinolinic acid, neopterin, and β-2 microglobulin, have been proposed to assist in the diagnosis of HIV dementia, but none has been broadly applicable clinically.

Neuropsychologic testing is extremely helpful in determining the presence of associated depression, measuring the degree of cognitive impairment, and evaluating the response to therapy.

This illness is characterized pathologically by cerebral atrophy. Meningeal fibrosis may be observed. Histopathologic examination typically reveals pallor of the cerebral white matter, perivascular macrophages, and multinucleated giant cells. As with the neuroradiologic features, there is a poor correlation between the clinical features of the disorder and the observed pathology.

Controlled trials of individuals with HIV dementia have demonstrated the value of high-dose zidovudine, also known as AZT. Zidovudine crosses the blood–brain barrier, and treatment has been found to be associated with decreasing HIV-1 antigen levels in serum and CSF. More recent data suggest that HAART may substantially improve the manifestations of HIV dementia. HAART regimens consist of a combination of one protease inhibitor with two reverse transcriptase inhibitors (Table 26.1). New modes of treatment for HIV dementia include not only the antiretroviral drugs but also neuroprotective agents and, possibly, antiinflammatory agents. Symptomatic treatment is an important adjunct to antiretroviral treatment. Hypnotics and anxiolytics should be avoided because individuals with HIV dementia are extremely susceptible to the side affects of those drugs.

CYTOMEGALOVIRUS ENCEPHALITIS

As with the other infections that occur in the setting of AIDS, CMV is typically the result of reactivation of a latent infection. CMV most frequently presents in AIDS with retinitis, which may cause severe visual loss. No part of the neuraxis is impervious to CMV infection, although CMV encephalitis is the most frequent neurologic manifestation. The latter often is accompanied by evidence of CMV infection of other organs, particularly the adrenal glands.

The clinical recognition of CMV encephalitis may be difficult. Neurologic symptoms develop relatively abruptly and may include meningeal signs, disorientation, short-term memory deficits, apathy, dementia, coma, seizures, or brainstem involvement with cranial nerve palsies. CSF analysis may be normal but more often reveals a pleocytosis and increased protein. A clue to the diagnosis may be the predominance of polymorphonuclear cells in the CSF. Rarely, CMV can be isolated from CSF by viral culture, but as with many other pathogens that are difficult to isolate by culture, polymerase chain reaction (PCR) for CMV in the CSF can be quite helpful diagnostically. CT scan of the brain may reveal subependymal enhancement consequent to the associated ventriculitis.

The median survival of individuals with CMV encephalitis is about 5 weeks. Effective therapeutic regimens include the use of ganciclovir and foscarnet (Table 26.2). Both are known to penetrate very well into the CSF. Therapy should be initiated promptly if CMV encephalitis is suspected. The duration of maintenance therapy is a matter of debate.

PROGRESSIVE MULTIFOCAL LEUKOENCEPHALOPATHY

PML is a demyelinating disease of the CNS that occurs as a consequence of a reactivation of a ubiquitous papova virus, JC virus. After infection, the virus remains latent in the reticuloendothelial system and the kidneys. Reactivation of JC virus may result in a productive infection of oligodendrocytes, resulting in multifocal demyelination of the brain. Before the AIDS pandemic, PML was a rare disease that was seen most often in individuals immunosuppressed from lymphoproliferative disorders. With the AIDS pandemic, PML is no longer a rare disorder. It is estimated that approximately 5% of all patients with AIDS ultimately will develop PML, and in approximately one-fourth of these patients, PML is heralding manifestation of AIDS.

The onset of PML is insidious. Hemiparesis is the most common presenting symptom. Other common clinical manifestations include headaches, speech disturbance, cognitive dysfunction, visual impairment, limb ataxia, and sensory loss. Seizures can be seen in 10% of patients. These signs and symptoms are not different from the ones seen in PML complicating other immunosuppressive conditions, although their relative proportions may differ.

The diagnosis is strongly supported but not confirmed based on radiographic imaging. CT scan reveals single or multiple confluent, non-enhancing (less than 10% of lesions show faint enhancement), hypodense white-matter lesions without mass effect. The lesions are located in the centrum semiovale, predominantly in the parietooccipital white matter, and the cerebellum. Cranial MRI shows non-enhancing (as with CT scan, enhancement is an exception) hyperintense lesions on T2-weighted images in the affected regions (Fig. 26.2).

The CSF analysis is usually normal. CSF abnormalities that may be encountered include a slight pleocytosis (<25 mononuclear cells/mm³), mildly increased proteins, increased myelin basic protein, and increased CSF immunoglobulin G (IgG). The presence of an increased opening pressure or significant CSF pleocytosis should raise serious concerns about the diagnosis. Depending on the laboratory, PCR for JC virus genome in the CSF of affected patients may be positive in as many as 75%. Diagnostic confirmation requires either brain biopsy or a positive CSF

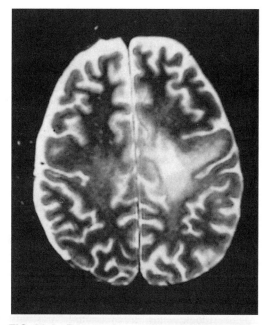

FIG. 26.2. Progressive multifocal leukoencephalopathy. T2-weighted MRI with extensive hyperintense signal abnormality in the right hemisphere from progressive multifocal leukoencephalopathy (PML).

PCR for JC virus coupled with the appropriate clinical and radiographic findings.

The pathology of PML is characterized by the triad of demyelination, large intranuclear inclusions in oligodendrocytes, and large bizarre astrocytes with hyperchromatic nuclei. Pathologic evidence of JC virus includes its demonstration by electron microscopy or by immunohistochemical techniques.

The average survival from the time of diagnosis is 3 to 6 months, although occasional, prolonged survivals with near-complete neurologic recovery have been reported. Low CSF titers of JC virus by quantitative PCR, PML as the heralding manifestation AIDS, contrast enhancement on radiographic imaging, a high CD4 count (>300 cells/mm³), and inflammatory infiltrates on histopathology appear to predict prolonged survival. Survival is unaffected by cytosine arabinoside administered either intravenously or intrathecally. HAART significantly increases survival, presumably by restoring the cytotoxic T-lympho-cyte response to JC virus (Table 26.1). The antiretroviral drugs do not appear to have any effect on JC viral replication *in vitro.* No other therapy has been systematically demonstrated to prolong survival in PML.

BRAIN DISEASE WITH MASS EFFECT

Toxoplasma encephalitis is the most common cause of focal intracranial mass lesion in HIV infection, followed in frequency by lymphoma. Less common causes of intracranial lesions include opportunistic infections (pyogenic abscess, syphilitic gumma, candida abscess, nocardia abscess, cryptococcoma and cryptococcal pseudocysts, other fungal and parasitic diseases) and vascular-occlusive lesions. In the patient infected with HIV with focal neurologic signs, either cranial MRI with gadolinium or a contrast-enhanced CT scan is mandated. The former is more sensitive.

CEREBRAL TOXOPLASMOSIS

Toxoplasma gondii is an intracellular protozoan that has a worldwide distribution. The infection is frequently subclinical and results in seropositivity and chronic, latent infection in immunocompetent individuals. The seroprevalence in adults varies geographically and depends on certain risk factors (e.g., eating habits). Between 5% and 25% of patients with AIDS in the United States will develop *Toxoplasma encephalitis,* although these numbers may be declining as a result of primary prophylaxis in patients infected with HIV with positive toxoplasmosis serology and profound immunosuppression. The variation in the frequency is largely a consequence of the number of immigrants from high-risk regions in the underlying population. Therefore, south Florida, with its sizable population of Haitian immigrants, exhibits a high prevalence of toxoplasmosis.

The onset of the neurologic illness may be heralded by fever and malaise for several days to weeks. Hemiparesis is the most common focal finding. Aphasia, seizures, homonymous hemianopsia, confusion, lethargy, and brainstem and cerebellar symptoms and signs may be seen. The combination of focal abnormalities and signs of a global encephalopathy is highly suggestive of cerebral toxoplasmosis. Furthermore, the appearance of chorea in patients with AIDS is believed to be virtually pathognomonic of toxoplasmosis because the organism has a propensity to involve the basal ganglia.

Brain CT scan usually reveals single or multiple, hypodense, nodular or ring-enhancing lesions with edema and mass effect. Most lesions occur in the basal ganglia and the cerebral hemispheres, particularly the frontoparietal lobes. They appear as discrete areas of increased signal intensity on T2-weighted images (Fig. 26.3). A single lesion suggests primary CNS lymphoma (PCNSL). A thallium 201 single-photon emission computed tomographic scan (SPECT) may help distinguish toxoplasmosis from PCNSL. As a result

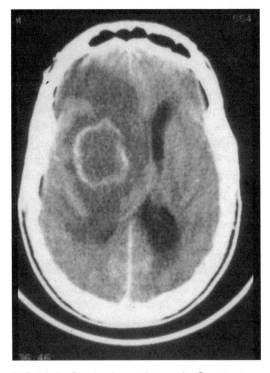

FIG. 26.3. Cerebral toxoplasmosis. Contrast-enhanced T1-weighted MRI with mass lesions in right frontal lobe and left basal ganglia secondary to toxoplasmosis.

of the metabolic activity of the PCNSL, increased activity is seen on SPECT.

Serology is rarely diagnostic at the time CNS toxoplasmosis develops.

Lumbar puncture may be relatively contraindicated because of the presence of brain edema and mass effect. If performed, CSF abnormalities are non-specific. One-third of infected patients show a mononuclear pleocytosis (usually not exceeding 100 cells/microliter; higher counts suggest the presence of another disease.) An elevation of the CSF protein (50 to 200 mg/dl) is seen in the majority of cases, and PCR for *Toxoplasma gondii* may be diagnostic.

If cerebral toxoplasmosis is suspected in patients with AIDS, based on clinical and imaging findings, empirical treatment is justifiable, reserving brain biopsy for atypical or refractory cases. A reliable presumptive diagnosis can be made based on response to sulfadiazine and pyrimethamine (Table 26.2), given as a trial therapy of 2 weeks duration with careful clinical and radiographic monitoring for resolution of the lesions. Of patients with toxoplasmosis, 90% respond within 2 to 4 weeks. Pyrimethamine, a dihydrofolate reductase inhibitor, is administered orally along with sulfadiazine. Oral folinic acid is required with the use of pyrimethamine to prevent hematologic side effects. The increasing difficulty in obtaining sulfadiazine and the high frequency of its side effects, mainly skin rash and nephrotoxicity, have lead to the adoption of sulfisoxazole. In case of rash resulting from sulfadiazine use, clindamycin may represent an alternative therapy.

As with other opportunistic infections occurring with AIDS, the risks of relapse is high, warranting the use of lifelong prophylaxis. For this maintenance treatment, the pyrimethamine/sulfamethoxazole combination is effective.

PRIMARY CNS LYMPHOMA

PCNSL is a non-Hodgkin's lymphoma that arises within and is confined to the nervous system. In the setting of HIV infection, the incidence of PCNSL increases dramatically. Up to 0.6% of patients will present with PCNSL concurrent with the diagnosis of AIDS, and ultimately 2% to 13% develop this malignancy. PCNSL is the second most frequent CNS mass lesion in adults with AIDS and is the most frequent cause of brain mass lesions in children with AIDS.

Clinically, PCNSL presents in descending order of frequency, with confusion, lethargy, memory loss, hemiparesis, speech and language disorders, seizures, and cranial nerve palsies. On CT scan, a solitary mass, or multiple masses, hyperdense or isodense, with variable surrounding edema and with diffuse or ring or nodular enhancement may be seen. The lesions show a predilection for the corpus callosum, basal ganglia, and periventricular areas. PCNSL may not be distinguishable from toxoplasmosis, especially if it presents as a solitary mass. Tl SPECT studies are often diagnostically useful in distinguishing PCNSL from infectious mass lesions, such as toxoplasmosis. CSF examination is often not possible because of the presence of mass effect. However, if performed, up to 25% of patients with PCNSL demonstrate positive cytology, eliminating the need for a diagnostic stereotaxic brain biopsy. CSF analysis by PCR for Ebstein-Barr virus is diagnostically helpful in PCNSL as well. It is important to be aware that corticosteroid administration can reduce the size of the tumor seen on imaging studies and can render the seeming response to a trial of antitoxoplasmosis therapy difficult to interpret. Therefore, when PCNSL is a diagnostic consideration, corticosteroids should be withheld while antitoxoplasmosis therapy is administered and the response to therapy is assessed.

Once the diagnosis is established, radiotherapy is the treatment of choice and median survival can be prolonged by 4 to 5 months. Patients with PCNSL may respond both clinically and radiologically to whole-brain radiotherapy (4,000 Gy). If possible, a boost of 1,500 cGy to the tumor bed can be added. Leptomeningeal lymphoma should be treated with intrathecal chemotherapy: methotrexate or cytosine arabinoside, using an Ommaya reservoir. Systemic chemotherapy may be of value but is generally poorly tolerated by the patient with AIDS.

CEREBROVASCULAR DISEASE

The spectrum of cerebrovascular disease that has been reported in association with AIDS is broad and includes both ischemic and hemorrhagic disorders. In autopsy series, rates as high as 19% have been reported. Sometimes these cerebrovascular complications occur as a result of an underlying opportunistic infection or lymphoma, or occasionally they are secondary to marantic endocarditis. Infectious vasculitis, especially meningovascular syphilis, always must be considered in the differential diagnosis of these disorders. Vasculitis secondary to HIV infection has been reported. In many cases, no underlying condition for the stroke is identified. Increasingly, it appears that some patients infected with HIV have a hypercoagulable state as the cause of their cerebrovascular disease. Anticardiolipin antibodies may be found in patients infected with HIV. Additionally, treatment with protease inhibitors may cause a lipodystrophy and potentially accelerate the development of atherosclerosis in the cerebral vasculature. Treatment is no different from that used in the patient who is not infected with HIV.

MENINGITIS

Meningitis is a frequent occurrence in the patient with HIV infection (Table 26.6). Shortly after the initial infection with HIV, an aseptic meningitis may occur and actually may herald the infection. If unsuspected, the etiology is not identified. The most important meningeal infection in patients with AIDS is caused by *Cryptococcus neoformans.* Other common etiologies of meningitis include tuberculosis, syphilitic meningitis, *Listeria* meningitis, and meningeal lymphomatosis (non-Hodgkin's lymphoma). CSF studies are

TABLE 26.6. *Meningitis in HIV-1 Infection*

HIV-1 meningitis
Cryptococcal meningitis
Tuberculous meningitis
Syphilitic meningitis
Listeria meningitis
Meningitis lymphomatosis (non-Hodgkin's lymphoma)

required for a precise identification of the etiology, and these studies are incomplete without thorough microbiologic and cytologic evaluations. These CSF studies should include PCR for *Mycobacterium tuberculosis,* herpes simplex viruses 1 and 2, CMV, and varicella-zoster virus.

HIV MENINGITIS

HIV meningitis is seen infrequently clinically. It may present as acute or chronic aseptic meningitis. In a small number of patients, acute meningitis may accompany the primary infection with HIV. The acute viral illness develops within 3 to 6 weeks of infection, before seroconversion to HIV, and it is not distinguishable from many other viral illnesses. With this acute infection, a meningitis or meningoencephalitis may present with fever, headache, meningismus, photophobia, altered mental state, and generalized seizures. Involvement of cranial nerves may be seen, especially of cranial nerve V, VII, and VIII. CSF analysis shows a mononuclear pleocytosis (<200 cells/mm), slightly increased protein, and normal or mildly depressed glucose content. This meningitis is presumed to result from direct infection of the meninges by HIV because p24 antigen in the CSF or amplification of HIV RNA can be demonstrated. As a rule, mild CSF abnormalities are seen in individuals infected with HIV, even in the absence of neurologic symptoms, and their interpretation requires caution.

CRYPTOCOCCAL MENINGITIS

Cryptococcal meningitis is the most common mycotic infection involving the nervous system in patients with HIV infection. Meningitis results from hematogenous dissemination of *C. neoformans* frequently following an asymptomatic pulmonary infection. The estimated incidence of cryptococcosis with AIDS varies between 2% and 10%. It is a feature of advanced HIV disease, and most patients have CD4+ counts of less than 50 cells/mm^3.

Clinically the illness manifests as a subacute or chronic meningitis with headache, altered mental status, photophobia, blurred vision, nausea, vomiting, and fever. Neck stiffness frequently is absent. Papilledema (occasionally accompanied by visual loss) and sixth cranial nerve palsy often are present. Hemiparesis, seizures, cerebellar symptoms, language disturbances, and psychosis are observed less frequently.

Radiographic studies are usually normal. Mass lesions from cryptococcomas and cryptococcal abscesses may be observed in up to 10% of patients, and cerebral edema may be seen in another 3%. Additionally, cryptococcal meningitis uncommonly may result in stroke. The CSF opening pressure usually is increased, and the opening pressure should be measured routinely in all patients with suspected meningitis because it is useful both diagnostically and prognostically. CSF analysis shows variable mononuclear pleocytosis, with mildly elevated protein and low glucose; however, these CSF parameters may be normal in up to 50% of affected patients. India ink study may be positive in more than 70% of these individuals. Cryptococcal polysaccharide capsular antigen is nearly always positive in the CSF and serum, as are fungal cultures of CSF.

The current recommendation regarding treatment of cryptococcal meningitis is to use amphotericin B (0.7 mg/kg/day) with or without flucytosine (100 to 150 mg/kg/day). At the completion of 2 or more weeks, this therapy may be replaced by oral fluconazole at 400 mg/day for 8 to 10 weeks (Table 26.2). If at the end of this time the CSF culture is negative for *C. neoformans,* the fluconazole dose may be reduced to 200 mg/day and continued indefinitely as secondary prophylaxis to prevent relapse. Oral fluconazole is better tolerated than intravenous amphotericin and is effective in preventing relapses. Amphotericin B treatment is limited because of its side effects such as fever, renal insufficiency, and the rare occurrence of leukoencephalopathy. The liposomal form of amphotericin B has fewer side effects.

TUBERCULOUS MENINGITIS

Infection with *M. tuberculosis, Mycobacterium avium-intracellulare,* and rarely other atypical mycobacteria occurs frequently in AIDS and is often extrapulmonary.

Clinically, altered mental status, fever, signs of meningeal irritation, and seizures may be seen. CT scan may show hypodense areas or ring-enhancing lesions. In contrast to *M. tuberculosis,* which often presents as meningitis, *M. avium-intracellulare* typically causes single or multiple mass lesions. In addition to meningitis, the clinical spectrum of CNS tuberculosis associated with HIV infection includes cerebral and spinal abscesses and tuberculomas. The CSF analysis may be unremarkable or acellular. When a mass lesion is suspected, brain biopsy is necessary to confirm the diagnosis.

All HIV-seropositive patients should receive a skin test for tuberculosis and, if positive, should be treated. Patients respond well to the standard therapy for *M. tuberculosis,* which includes isoniazid, rifampin, and pyrazinamide (Table 26.2).

SYPHILITIC MENINGITIS

Even in the absence of neurologic disease, neurosyphilis always must be considered in patients with HIV infection. In some populations, between 1% and 6% of all patients infected with HIV have neurosyphilis as defined by a positive Venereal Disease Research Laboratory (VDRL) test in the CSF, but this test is relatively insensitive. Acute, symptomatic, syphilitic meningitis during the course of secondary syphilis is not uncommon. Other unusual manifestations of syphilis that have been reported in association with HIV infection include fever, bilateral optic neuritis with blindness, Bell's palsy and bilateral sensorineural hearing loss, syphilitic meningomyelitis, syphilitic polyradiculopathy, and syphilitic cerebral gumma presenting as a mass lesion.

Because the CSF VDRL is not highly sensitive, diagnosing neurosyphilis may be quite difficult. Of all patients infected with HIV, 40% to 60% may display a CSF pleocytosis, elevated protein, an elevated IgG synthesis rate, and oligoclonal bands, rendering it impossible to use these CSF parameters as indicators of neurosyphilis. Second, the signs and symptoms of the clinical syndrome caused by neurosyphilis infection (meningitis, stroke, myelopathy, and dementia) also may be the consequence of HIV infection. Third, the CSF serologic tests for neurosyphilis, such as the VDRL, may be negative in individuals infected with HIV with viable *Treponema pallidum* in their CSF.

A proposed approach to the diagnosis of neurosyphilis is as follows: (a) a reactive CSF VDRL in the absence of gross blood contamination of CSF; or (b) a reactive CSF fluorescent treponemal antibody absorption (FTA-ABS) test in the absence of blood contamination occurring in association with a CSF pleocytosis (>5 cells/mm), increased protein (>50 mg), an increased IgG index (>6), or oligoclonal bands in the absence of HIV infection or identifiable neurologic illness; or (c) a reactive CSF FTA-ABS in association with neurologic illness compatible with neurosyphilis, unexplained by other disease, and responding to penicillin therapy; or (d) *T. pallidum* isolated from the CSF by animal inoculation.

Neurosyphilis always should be considered in the differential diagnosis of neurologic disease patients infected with HIV. CSF examination should be performed in all persons infected with HIV with neurologic complaints and a history of syphilis or serologic evidence of syphilis, regardless of prior treatment.

Treatment of syphilis requires the administration of intravenous, high-dose aqueous penicillin G administered over 10 to 14 days (Table 26.2). Whether secondary prophylaxis needs to be used remains unanswered. CSF examinations following treatment should be repeated at 6-month intervals over the succeeding 2 years. The CSF VDRL titer should decline, but the CSF VDRL may remain reactive in low titer.

LISTERIA MENINGITIS

Listeria monocytogenes is a gram-positive, rod-shaped, aerobic bacterium that is widespread in nature. Despite a profound impairment of cellular immunity, the incidence of *L. monocytogenes* infection appears to be less with AIDS than with other causes of impaired cell-mediated immunity. Listeria infection may result in meningitis or brain abscess and appears to have a predilection for the brainstem. In any case of meningitis of unknown cause occurring in a patient with AIDS, the antibiotic regimen should include agents effective against *L. monocytogenes,* such as intravenous ampicillin or penicillin or trimethoprim/sulfamethoxazole.

LYMPHOMATOUS MENINGITIS

Approximately 5% of patients with AIDS ultimately will develop systemic lymphoma (usually high-grade B-cell neoplasms). The most common form of neurologic illness occurring in association with AIDS-related systemic lymphoma is lymphomatous leptomeningitis, which may be either asymptomatic or symptomatic. Symptomatic lymphomatous leptomeningitis may present with headache, altered mental status, seizures, cranial neuropathies, hydrocephalus, and radiculopathies. An otherwise unexplained cranial polyneuropathy in a patient with AIDS is not infrequently the result of lymphomatous (usually large-cell lymphoma) infiltration. A differential diagnostic list of the potential causes of cranial neuropathy in AIDS is presented in Table 26.7. The frequency of asymptomatic lymphomatous meningitis occurring in AIDS-related lymphoma approaches 20%; therefore, CSF analysis should be performed in all patients with AIDS with systemic lymphoma as part of the staging evaluation.

TABLE 26.7. *Etiologies of Cranial Nerve Palsies with HIV-1 Infection*

Infectious meningitis
  Fungal (cryptococcus)
  Bacterial (*Mycobacterium tuberculosis, Listeria monocytogenes, Treponem pallidum*)
  Viral (HIV-1)
Neoplastic meningitis
  Meningitis lymphomatosa
Compression from a mass lesion
  Infectious (toxoplasmosis)
  Neoplastic (central nervous system lymphoma)
Vasculitis
Inflammatory
  Guillain-Barré syndrome
  Chronic inflammatory polyradiculopathy
Miscellaneous
    Malignant otitis externa

TABLE 26.8. *Myelopathies in HIV-1 Infection*

HIV-1–associated vacuolar myelopathy
Cytomegalovirus polyradiculopathy
Varicella-zoster virus radiculopathy
HTLV-1–associated myelopathy
Lymphoma (epidural or intradural)
Vascular insults
Vitamin B_{12} deficiency

HTLV, human lymphotrophic virus.

The neurologic manifestations of AIDS-associated lymphomatous meningitis, particularly cranial neuropathy, may be exquisitely responsive to the administration of corticosteroids. Appropriate treatment requires intrathecal chemotherapy with methotrexate (or cytosine arabinoside). An Ommaya reservoir should be placed. Radiotherapy can be added to the symptomatic region.

MYELOPATHY

Spinal cord disease is observed frequently in HIV infection. The chief cause of myelopathy has been ascribed to HIV infection and referred to as HIV-associated vacuolar myelopathy. The diagnosis of this condition, like that of HIV encephalopathy, is one of exclusion. Multiple other conditions associated with HIV infection can cause myelopathies. These are infectious myelopathies (CMV, herpes simplex virus type 2, herpes zoster, human T-lymphotropic virus type I, mycobacteria, *T. pallidum,* and epidural abscesses seen frequently in abusers of parenteral drugs with *Staphylococcus aureus* being the most common organism isolated), vascular myelopathies, epidural and intramedullary tumors, and demyelinating myelopathy (Table 26.8).

It is useful to categorize spinal diseases occurring with HIV infection into those occurring in the absence of mass lesion and those that are the result of a mass lesion. MRI of the spinal cord is the single most useful study for this purpose. CSF analysis is required to search for treatable infectious pathogens.

HIV RELATED MYELOPATHY

HIV-1–related vacuolar myelopathy is seen at autopsy in more than 20% of patients with AIDS. This condition occurs with advanced immunosuppression, and it often is associated with AIDS dementia complex, but it may occur in isolation.

It begins insidiously with leg weakness and paresthesias, gait impairment, and bladder and bowel incontinence. On examination there is evidence of a spastic paraparesis (leg involvement may be asymmetric) and hyperreflexia of the legs, except in the presence of a concomitant peripheral neuropathy. Gait ataxia with impaired sensation with vibratory and position sense may be seen. A discrete sensory level is unusual. MRI of the spine is frequently normal, although occasionally spinal cord atrophy and hyperintense signals on T2-weighted images may be seen.

Pathologic changes are most prominent in the thoracic cord and closely mimic the findings of subacute combined degeneration of the spinal cord seen with vitamin B_{12} deficiency. There is loss of myelin and spongy degeneration (probably from swelling within the layers of myelin) with relative axonal preservation. These changes mainly affect the dorsal and lateral columns. Microglial nodules and HIV-laden multinucleated giant cells can be detected, but the role of HIV-1 in the pathogenesis of this myelopathy remains unclear, and a disturbance in vitamin B_{12} metabolic pathways has been suggested. No treatment has demonstrated unequivocal value in the treatment of this myelopathy. Trials with high dose S-adenosyl methionine are under investigation.

Other spinal cord disorders attributed to HIV infection include an acute myelopathy occurring at the time of primary infection, spinal myoclonus, and a relapsing-remitting myelopathy that may be associated with optic neuritis.

HIV AND THE PERIPHERAL NERVOUS SYSTEM

The neuromuscular complications of HIV-1 infection are considered to be common (Table 26.9).

PERIPHERAL NEUROPATHY

Some studies suggest that as many as one-half of patients with advanced HIV infection have evidence of peripheral neuropathy. The exact role of HIV in the etiopathogenesis of these neuropathies remains obscure. Concomitant infections, nutritional deficiencies, metabolic disorders, and side effects of drugs may be responsible, however, for some of these neuropathies. It is useful to categorize the neuropathies occurring with HIV into three major groups: a distal symmetric peripheral neuropathy, an inflammatory demyelinating peripheral neuropathy, (mononeuritis multiplex), and autonomic and toxic neuropathies.

TABLE 26.9. *Neuromuscular Complications of HIV-1 Infection*

Neuropathies
   Distal symmetric polyneuropathy
   Inflammatory demyelinating polyneuropathy
     (acute and chronic)
   Mononeuropathy multiplex
   Autonomic polyneuropathy
   Toxic neuropathies
Myopathies
   HIV-1–associated polymyositis
   Zidovudine-associated myopathy
   HIV wasting syndrome

Distal Symmetric Polyneuropathy

Distal symmetric polyneuropathy, or HIV-associated predominantly sensory polyneuropathy, is the most common polyneuropathy associated with HIV, seen in as many as 35% of patients. It tends to occur late in HIV infection. Patients complain of painful dysesthesias and numbness of the feet. When present, distal weakness is generally mild. Clinically, ankle reflexes are depressed or absent; the sensory loss is greatest for vibratory perception, but other sensory modalities may be affected. The hands are affected less often. Electrophysiologic studies show a polyneuropathy with mainly axonal involvement, although features of demyelination also may be seen. Nerve biopsy may reveal epineural and endoneural perivascular inflammation with primarily axonal degeneration. HIV has been isolated from peripheral nerves. Possible mechanisms include direct viral infection or cell-mediated immune attack on components of peripheral nerve. Symptomatic therapy with anticonvulsants (such as carbamazepine), tricyclic antidepressants, mexitiline, and topical capsaicin are of variable benefit. HAART, lamotrigine, and recombinant nerve growth factor have been demonstrated in some studies to be of benefit.

Inflammatory Demyelinating Polyneuropathies

Inflammatory demyelinating polyneuropathies tend to occur late in the course of HIV infection, and it may occur acutely or chronically. An autoimmune process probably is involved. The HIV-associated acute inflammatory demyelinating polyradiculopathy is similar to Guillain–Barré syndrome in patients not infected with HIV. Patients complain of progressive weakness. Clinically depressed or absent muscle stretch reflexes and minor sensory signs are found. CSF analysis may reveal (in the acute form or in the HIV-1–associated chronic inflammatory demyelinating polyneuropathy) a mild mononuclear pleocytosis with elevated protein. In contradistinction to typical Guillain–Barré syndrome, CSF albuminocytologic dissociation very seldom is found. Electrophysiologic studies demonstrate features of primary demyelination with axonal loss. The clinical course is variable, but most patients improve and some recover spontaneously. Plasmapheresis may be beneficial in patients with chronic relapsing polyradiculopathy, and high-dose intravenous immunoglobulin may be associated with remarkable improvement.

Mononeuropathy Multiplex

Mononeuritis multiplex is seen rarely in patients infected with HIV. This condition has been attributed to immune complex deposition leading to a necrotizing vasculitis. Sensory and motor deficits may be seen in the distribution of multiple spinal, cranial, and peripheral nerves. CSF studies show both pleocytosis and elevated protein content. Electrophysiologic studies suggest axonal involvement. Other causes of mononeuropathy (herpes zoster, CMV, and lymphomatous nerve root involvement) must be excluded.

Autonomic Neuropathy

Autonomic neuropathy is a rare condition in HIV infection and tends to occur late in the disease. Patients present with postural hypotension, bowel and bladder dysfunction, impotence, sweating abnormalities, presyncope, and arrhythmias with risk of sudden death. These symptoms are frequently the result of small-fiber peripheral neuropathy, with both parasympathetic and sympathetic dysfunction demonstrated by autonomic testing in up to one-half of affected patients. Treatment is purely symptomatic. Agents such as fludrocortisone can stabilize blood pressure.

Toxic Polyneuropathies

A painful peripheral neuropathy has been associated with the use of the dideoxynucleoside analogues, dideoxyinosine (ddI), dideoxycytidine (ddC), and d4T. Patients complain of burning pain and tingling in the feet and legs, which starts 2 to 6 months after initiating the treatment and may be related to the cumulative dose of the drug. Some patients have reported marked improvement in symptoms shortly after discontinuing the offending drug, but progression may be observed for several months after its discontinuation—a phenomenon referred to as "coasting." Electrophysiologic studies are consistent with a distal axonopathy primarily affecting sensory fibers. Treatment of this condition is symptomatic.

CYTOMEGALOVIRUS POLYRADICULOPATHY

CMV polyradiculopathy, or polyradiculitis, generally occurs with advanced immunodeficiency. It is characterized at onset by involvement of the legs and by sacral paresthesias. Progressive paraparesis follows, with ascending mild sensory loss and sphincter dysfunction. Examination reveals absent muscle stretch reflexes. CSF examination reveals polymorphonuclear pleocytosis. CMV can be detected in the CSF by culture or PCR. Rarely, cytomegalic cells may be seen in the CSF. Myelography and contrast-enhanced spinal MRI may show thickened adherent lumbar nerve roots. Pathology reveals extensive multifocal necrosis, acute inflammatory infiltrates, and vasculitis of spinal roots. Typical CMV inclusions are seen.

A painful neuropathy has been attributed to CMV-associated dorsal root ganglionitis, and CMV may result in an acute demyelinating polyneuropathy, resembling Guillain–Barré syndrome. This condition is potentially treatable with ganciclovir or foscarnet. The ganciclovir regimen recommended is 5 mg/kg intravenously every 12 hours for 2 to 3 weeks, followed by maintenance therapy, 5 mg/kg/day, 5 days per week.

MYOPATHIES

Several myopathies have been recognized in association with HIV infection. The most important are HIV-1–associated polymyositis and zidovudine-associated myopathy.

HIV-associated polymyositis or myopathy is undistinguishable from idiopathic polymyositis, and it can be seen at all stages of HIV infection. Patients present with proximal muscle weakness (leg and neck flexors predominantly), myalgias (mainly of the thighs), and fatigability. High serum creatine kinase (CK) is found. Electrophysiologic studies are similar to the one seen with idiopathic polymyositis. Muscle biopsy shows fibrous tissue proliferation, necrosis, and phagocytosis of muscle fibers associated with intense inflammation. Pathology also may reveal nemaline rod bodies, cytoplasmic bodies, and mitochondrial abnormalities. This myopathy may respond to corticosteroids.

Zidovudine-associated myopathy tends to occur in patients who have been treated with high doses of this drug for 6 or more months. It has been postulated to be the result of zidovudine on muscle mitochondria. This condition presents with proximal weakness and muscle wasting, preceded by CK elevation. Pathology reveals ragged-red fibers (indicative of abnormal mitochondria) and inflammatory changes. Zidovudine withdrawal is the key to management.

Special Concerns for Hospitalized Patients

Infection Control and Infection Precautions

In general, guidelines for infection control must be thorough, reasonable to apply, and protective of patients, visitors, and staff. The guidelines for isolation precautions in hospitals proposed by the CDC include the following:

Standard precautions, which combine universal and body substance isolation. These precautions should be applied to all patients with or without HIV. Only standard precautions are required for immunocompromised patients with CMV, Epstein-Barr infection, fungal and tuberculous meningitis, and syphilis.

Transmission-based precautions are additional precautions beyond standard precau-

tions. For instance, patients with meningococcal and *haemophilus influenzae* meningitis should be subject to additional droplet precautions for 24 hours after initiation of effective therapy.

The infection control professionals are encouraged to modify or adapt these recommendations to local conditions.

Prejudice Within the Hospital

Unfortunately patients with HIV infection are subject to prejudices within the hospital, and very few of us are free of all prejudices. It is an obligation to provide unbiased, high-quality care to all patients. Educational programs can be very helpful for this purpose.

ALTERNATIVE TREATMENTS

From the inception of the AIDS pandemic, the affected community in general has been very keen on using alternative therapies for the treatment of the infection as well as the complications associated with HIV infection. These alternative therapies have been chiefly, although not exclusively, with vitamins (B vitamins) and minerals (zinc and magnesium). With respect to HIV-related neurologic complications, none of the alternative therapeutic regimens proposed has been demonstrated in a rigorous scientific fashion to be associated with an improvement in symptoms or an amelioration of the underlying condition. For AIDS dementia, vitamin B_{12} has been proposed in light of the frequency of B_{12} deficiency seen in association with HIV infection consequent to altered absorption and metabolism. Low B_{12} levels have been correlated with cognitive deficits related to information processing speed and visuospatial problem-solving skills in an HIV-infected population as well as with the presence of peripheral neuropathy and myelopathy. However, no convincing studies have demonstrated the efficacy of vitamin B_{12} repletion or megadoses on any of these neurologic complications. Altered B_{12} metabolism as a result of an interference with the methyl transferase cycle by macrophage products rather than an absolute deficiency of the vitamin has been proposed as a cause of HIV-associated myelopathy. This has led to a trial of S-adenosyl methionine in the treatment of this condition. However, the results of this study are currently unavailable.

REFERRAL TO A NEUROLOGIST

As indicated in the opening paragraphs of this chapter, neurologic disease in the setting of HIV infection has many characteristics, including the following:

Neurologic disease is a common complication of HIV infection. Neurologic disease may be the heralding manifestation of AIDS in 10% to 20% of patients and ultimately will affect two-thirds or more when careful assessment is performed.

HIV-related neurologic diseases are among the most debilitating consequences of the infection.

The spectrum of neurologic diseases is broad.

No part of the neuraxis (brain, spinal cord, nerve roots, peripheral nerves, or muscle) is immune to involvement.

Not infrequently, two or more neurologic disorders exist in the same individual.

Diagnosis of the neurologic disorders complicating HIV infection is often difficult.

Effective treatment strategies require not only therapy of the underlying process but also the institution of secondary prophylaxis for a wide variety of opportunistic infections when appropriate.

In light of these facts, neurologic consultation generally is warranted in any person infected with HIV with symptoms and signs suggestive of neurologic disease.

QUESTIONS AND DISCUSSION

1. A patient with AIDS presents with fever and very severe headache. Neurologic examination reveals no abnormalities (not even neck stiffness). Give a differential diagnosis and diagnostic approach.

Answer: Physicians should remember that the presence of headache alone in a person infected with HIV seldom indicates a serious underlying pathology. However, in a patient with AIDS (usually severely immunosuppressed) who presents with new-onset, severe headache with fever in the absence of focal neurologic abnormalities, cryptococcal meningitis is the most likely diagnosis. This meningitis often results in very severe headaches as a result of raised intracranial pressure, without focal abnormalities, and in two-thirds of patients without meningeal signs. When there is any doubt about focal abnormalities, CT or MRI should precede lumbar puncture. Other causes for meningitis include HIV-1, *M. tuberculosis, L. monocytogenes, T. pallidum,* and lymphomatous meningitis. HIV-1 (aseptic) meningitis usually occurs early in HIV-1 infection, and the others occur less frequently than cryptococcal meningitis. CSF analysis almost always will provide the conclusive answer.

2. A patient with AIDS presents with apathy, slowness, and forgetfulness. He has no headache or fever. Can we conclude that the diagnosis is AIDS dementia complex?

Answer: No, we cannot. The diagnosis of AIDS dementia complex is one of exclusion. Clinically, this patient presents with frontal lobe dysfunction, so CT or MR should be performed. Frontal lobe toxoplasmosis, PML, and PCNSL have to be excluded. Chronic meningitis (syphilis, *M. tuberculosis,* Listeria) also must be excluded by CSF examination. If CT or MRI and CSF are negative, further support for the diagnosis of AIDS dementia complex can be obtained by neuropsychologic examination, which may show abnormalities compatible with "subcortical dementia" and may help to exclude depression. CT or MRI and CSF examination may give additional support for a diagnosis of AIDS dementia complex. CT or MRI may show atrophy and diffuse white matter abnormalities; CSF analysis may reveal HIV-1 p24 antigen and increased levels of beta-2-microglobulin, neopterin, and quinolinic acid. The diagnosis of AIDS dementia complex can be extremely difficult to make. Sometimes longer follow-up is necessary to make a definite conclusion.

3. A patient infected with HIV presents with headache, fever, aphasia, and a slight right-sided hemiparesis. The day before, he had a seizure. His illness developed in 1 week. What is the most likely diagnosis?

Answer: The most likely diagnosis in an HIV-infected individual who presents with focal abnormalities is cerebral toxoplasmosis. This is the leading cause of cerebral mass lesions in patients with HIV infection. A CT or MRI scan was performed, which showed multiple ring-enhancing lesions with surrounding edema, compatible with cerebral toxoplasmosis. Because of its high incidence and the fact that toxoplasmosis is easily treatable, empiric treatment is usually justifiable. When the lesion is radiographically observed to be single and the toxoplasmosis serology is negative, the likelihood of it being toxoplasmosis is low and the physician should proceed to brain biopsy. The presence of a lesion that enhances in thallium SPECT is suggestive of PCNSL. A positive PCR for Epstein-Barr virus in the CSF is felt by many investigators to be diagnostic of PCNSL. If antitoxoplasmosis therapy is used, most patients react favorably, both clinically and radiologically, within 5 days and almost invariably within 2 weeks. Among the differential diagnoses of focal abnormalities in AIDS are PCNSL (the second most common brain mass lesion in AIDS) and PML. PCNSL is clinically and radiologically indistinguishable from toxoplasmosis and has to be confirmed by brain biopsy. PML presents with a more protracted course and is radiologically different (white matter lesions, usually without contrast enhancement or mass effect). Patients with AIDS with focal lesions, without a favorable response to empiric antitoxoplasmosis treatment, require a brain biopsy to make a definite diagnosis.

4. A patient with AIDS presents with slowly progressive gait disturbances. On neurologic examination, he has a spastic paraparesis and a sensory ataxia. Give a differential diagnosis.

Answer: A slowly progressive spastic paraparesis with a sensory ataxia usually is caused by a myelopathy. There are several etiologic possibilities in a patient with AIDS. Medullary compression (e.g., an epidural tuberculous abscess or lymphoma) has to be excluded by MRI. CSF examination should exclude infectious agents, of which the most important are CMV, varicella-zoster virus, human T-lymphotropic virus type I, and *T. pallidum*. Vitamin B_{12} deficiency should be ruled out. If the MRI and CSF are negative for the previously mentioned causes, the most likely diagnosis is HIV-1–related vacuolar myelopathy. This is a slowly progressive myelopathy that is related to HIV infection and often is associated with AIDS dementia complex but may occur without dementia. Its pathogenesis is poorly understood, and zidovudine has no clear efficacy. The diagnosis is one of exclusion.

5. An AIDS patient with CMV retinitis presents with subacute low back pain and radicular pain in the left leg. Do you think this patient has a herniated lumbar disk?

Answer: HIV infection does not protect against herniated disks. But be careful—a very aggressive polyradiculomyelopathy caused by CMV has been described in patients with AIDS, and this syndrome may present as if it were a herniated disk. In this syndrome, in days to weeks after the initial lumbago and radicular pain, a rapidly progressive flaccid paraparesis with sphincter disturbances may develop. The CSF reveals a pleocytosis with predominance of polymorphonuclear leukocytes. CMV may be cultured from the CSF, or CMV may be detected by immunohistochemistry or *in situ* hybridization. Treatment with ganciclovir, started early, may stop progression or even cause some improvement. In every patient with AIDS with radicular pain in the legs who develops a paresis, a lumbar puncture should be done; when the previously mentioned CSF abnormalities are found, ganciclovir should be started while awaiting CSF culture.

SUGGESTED READING

Anduze-Faris BM, Fillet AM, Gozlan J, et al. Induction and maintenance therapy of cytomegalovirus central nervous system infection in HIV-infected patients. *AIDS* 2000;14: 517–524.

Beach RS, Morgan R. Plasma vitamin B_{12} level as a potential cofactor in studies of human immunodeficiency virus type 1-related cognitive changes. *Arch Neurol* 1992;49:501–506.

Berger JR, Levy RM. *AIDS and the nervous system,* 2nd ed. Philadelphia: Lippincott-Raven, 1998.

De Luca A, Giancola ML, Ammassari A, et al. Cidofovir added to HAART improves virological and clinical outcome in AIDS-associated progressive multifocal leukoencephalopathy. *AIDS* 2000;14:117–121.

Antinori A, Ammassari A, Giancola ML, et al. Epidemiology and prognosis of AIDS-associated progressive multifocal leukoencephalopathy in the HAART era. *J Neurovirol* 2001;7:323–328.

De Luca A, Giancola ML, Ammassari A, et al. The effect of potent antiretroviral therapy and JC virus load in cerebrospinal fluid on clinical outcome of patients with AIDS-associated progressive multifocal leukoencephalopathy. *J Infect Dis* 2000;182:1077–1083.

Di Rocco A, Bottiglieri T, Werner P, et al. Abnormal cobalamin-dependent transmethylation in AIDS-associated myelopathy. *Neurology* 2002;58:730–735.

Geschwind MD, Skolasky RI, Royal WS, et al. The relative contributions of HAART and alpha-interferon for therapy of progressive multifocal leukoencephalopathy in AIDS. *J Neurovirol* 2001;7:353–357.

Martin C, et al. Antiretroviral therapy may improve sensory function in HIV-infected patients: a pilot study. *Neurology* 2000;54:2120–2127.

Maschke M, Kastrup O, Diener HC. CNS manifestations of cytomegalovirus infections. *CNS Drugs* 2002;16(5): 303–315.

Maschke M, Kastrup O, Esser S, et al. Incidence and prevalence of neurologic disorders associated with HIV since the introduction of highly active antiretroviral therapy (HAART). *J Neurol Neurosurg Psychiatry* 2000;69: 376–380.

McArthur JC, Yiannoutsos C, Simpson DM, et al. A phase II trial of nerve growth factor for sensory neuropathy associated with HIV infection. AIDS Clinical Trials Group Team 291. *Neurology* 2000;54:1080–1088.

Sacktor NC, Skolasky RL, Lyles RH, et al. Improvement in HIV-associated motor slowing after antiretroviral therapy including protease inhibitors. *J Neurovirol* 2000;6:84–88.

Simpson DM, Olney R, McArthur JC, et al. A placebo-controlled randomized trial of lamotrigine in the painful HIV-associated peripheral neuropathy. *Neurology* 2000;54: 2115–2119.

Spina M, Vaccher E, Juzbasic S, et al. Human immunodeficiency virus-related non-Hodgkin lymphoma: activity of infusional cyclophosphamide, doxorubicin, and etoposide as second-Line chemotherapy in 40 patients. *Cancer* 2001;92:200–206.

Tan SV, Guiloff RJ. Hypothesis on the pathogenesis of vacuolar myelopathy, dementia, and peripheral neuropathy in AIDS. *J Neurol Neurosurg Psychiatry* 1998;65:23–28.

27

Neurologic Disorders in Pregnancy

Kathleen M. Shannon

The majority of women who become pregnant do so at times in their lives of relative health and physical fitness. Fortunately, concomitant diseases are relatively rare in this population. However, the childbearing years overlap periods of increased risk for neurologic disorders such as migraine headache, vascular malformations, multiple sclerosis, and myasthenia gravis. Pregnancy enhances susceptibility to some conditions, such as venous and arterial thrombosis, or it may be the setting for conditions such as eclampsia, which do not occur in the nongravid state. An understanding of the physiologic changes of pregnancy and how they are likely to influence neurologic diseases forms the foundation on which decisions about diagnostic and therapeutic interventions are made.

The focus of this chapter is on the evaluation and treatment of neurologic disorders that commonly are encountered during pregnancy. For those conditions that commonly occur in the nongravid population as well, the reader is referred elsewhere in the text for more comprehensive discussion of the disease entities.

TERATOLOGY

Teratologic concerns weigh heavily on the minds of pregnant patients and their physicians. The result is a reluctance to perform neurodiagnostic tests, particularly ones in which ionizing radiation is used. There is also a popular perception that the risk of malformation consequent to drug ingestion may be as high as 25%, even with drugs not known to be teratogenic. This perception commonly leads to noncompliance with prescribed medications.

Malformations are detected in 2% to 3% of live births; less than 5% are thought to result from exposure to teratogens. The effects of a teratogen depend on the dose reaching the fetus, the duration of exposure, the gestational age of the fetus at the time of the exposure, and simultaneous exposure to other agents. Two major classes of teratogens are of concern to the treating physician: ionizing radiation and drugs.

The effects of radiation on the developing fetus depend on the dose and duration of radiation absorbed by the conceptus and the stage of development at which exposure occurs. With the exception of myelography and fluoroscopy, less than 0.1% of neuroradiographic examinations properly performed with abdominal shielding expose the fetus to levels of radiation greater than 1 rad, a level that is not felt to pose significant risk to the fetus. In general, if a radiographic study is indicated for the diagnosis or management of a pregnant woman, the benefits far outweigh the risks to the fetus. Head computed tomography (CT) is relatively safe and is the procedure of choice for the evaluation of head trauma. Cervical spine films are permissible, although thoracic or lumbar plain films, myelography, or CT should be avoided if possible. Intravenous contrast crosses the placenta and should be avoided.

The risks of magnetic resonance imaging (MRI) to the fetus are not known. However, limited studies have not shown teratogenic potential, and it is believed to be safe for use during pregnancy. Contrast agents, however, should be avoided.

Reports of drug teratogenicity most often are based on animal studies, anecdotal reports, or case-control studies. Unfortunately, few drugs are known to be entirely without risk in pregnancy and few are known to be teratogenic. For the majority of compounds, the actual risks to the fetus are unknown.

Because organogenesis occurs mainly during the first trimester, drugs should be avoided whenever possible during this time. Throughout pregnancy, prudent assessment of risk-to-benefit ratios is encouraged.

PERIPHERAL NERVOUS SYSTEM AND MUSCLE DISORDERS IN PREGNANCY

Back pain is almost universal during pregnancy and relates to changes in posture and relaxation of spinal joints and ligaments as well as to posterior pelvic pain. The pain usually is localized to the back and buttock, or it radiates into the thighs. The cumulative incidence of back pain increases with the duration of pregnancy. Women contemplating pregnancy can help to prevent this symptom by strengthening the back before pregnancy or during its early course. Musculoskeletal back pain is treated with bed rest, analgesia, heat, and massage. Using a cushion to support the lower back when sitting, putting a foot on a footstool when standing, changing position frequently, taking warm baths, and walking can all effectively reduce symptoms.

Disc disease in pregnancy is rare. When it occurs, the complaint is usually of unilateral low back pain radiating through the buttock into the foot. L5 and S1 radiculopathies are most common. Treatment should be conservative—with the same recommendations as for back pain. Steroid injections may benefit some who are refractory to conservative management. Surgery should be used only in refractory cases or when there is objective evidence by electromyography or examination of nerve compromise. About 1% of vaginal deliveries are complicated by lumbosacral complaints or injury. The risk of this is increased in multiparous women and those with a prolonged second stage of labor. The symptoms generally resolve after a mean duration of 2 months.

PLEXUS DISORDERS, POLYNEUROPATHIES, AND MONONEUROPATHIES

Pregnancy-associated brachial plexus neuropathy may be familial or sporadic. The clinical syndrome consists of pain followed by weakness of the shoulder and arm. Neurologic examination points to a plexus lesion rather than a root or nerve lesion. Recovery usually begins 4 to 8 weeks after onset, irrespective of the time of onset relative to the pregnancy. Recovery is complete in 60% of patients at 1 year and nearly 100% at 3 years. The syndrome may recur during subsequent pregnancies. Treatment is supportive.

Lesions of the lumbosacral plexus or nerves exiting the plexus most commonly are related to traumatic or forceps-manipulated delivery. Most are self-limited, although complete recovery may take many months.

Pregnancy-associated polyneuropathies can result from nutritional deficiencies and resemble those seen in the nonpregnant malnourished population.

Acute idiopathic demyelinating polyneuropathy (AIDP, or Guillain–Barré syndrome) occurs in women of childbearing age, but pregnancy does not seem to confer added risk of this disorder. AIDP presents as rapidly ascending motor neuropathy with autonomic dysfunction. The presentation and course do not differ from that in the nonpregnant population. AIDP does not adversely affect pregnancy outcome. Depending on the functional status of the patient at term, it may be necessary to assist delivery with forceps or vacuum extraction. Plasmapheresis has been shown to shorten the duration of severe symptoms in AIDP when instituted early in the course of the illness, and it is permissible during pregnancy. Special attention should be given to avoiding extreme fluid shifts during pheresis.

Chronic idiopathic demyelinating polyneuropathy (CIDP) shares an inflammatory etiology with AIDP. Patients have a chronic motor and large sensory fiber neuropathy with a remitting and relapsing course. CIDP may begin or relapse during pregnancy. For unknown reasons, the relapse rate is increased during pregnancy. Treatment with plasmapheresis, as described for AIDP, may be helpful. Alternative strategies include use of chronic corticosteroids and human immune globulin administration.

Mononeuropathies in pregnancy result from hormonal and fluid changes as well as disruptions in body mechanics secondary to the gravid uterus. Bell's palsy is an acute, idiopathic unilateral weakness of muscles innervated by the facial nerve. Retroauricular pain commonly is associated. The etiology is obscure, but viral infection, nerve edema, and hormonal influences have been implicated. Most cases occur in the third trimester. The prognosis for complete recovery is good, but some patients with very severe involvement may have residual paralysis. Treatment remains controversial. Prednisone, 40 to 60 mg daily for 10 days, has been said to improve long-term outcome.

Carpal tunnel syndrome, presenting as nocturnal pain and burning in the first three digits of the hand, is the most common peripheral neuropathy of pregnancy. The symptoms relate to compression of the median nerve as it traverses the carpal canal. Symptomatic treatment with splinting of the wrist at night and analgesics as needed is adequate for most patients. Because aspirin has been associated with fetal malformations and with complications during labor and delivery, acetaminophen is the preferred analgesic in pregnancy. Persistent carpal tunnel symptoms may require treatment with steroid injection into the tunnel. Some patients may need surgical release of the compressed nerve. Prospective studies show slightly more than one-half of pregnant women with carpal tunnel syndrome have persistent symptoms 1 year later. Onset of symptoms early in the pregnancy portends persistent symptoms. Meralgia paresthetica is seen in conditions that place undue pressure on the lateral femoral cutaneous nerve as it passes the inguinal ligament. As in the nonpregnant population, weight gain is largely responsible. Typically, patients notice symptoms beginning in the third trimester. Pain and burning affect the middle third of the lateral thigh. Treatment consists of losing weight if possible, avoiding binding garments or belts, taking acetaminophen, and, if needed, receiving local injections of analgesics or transcutaneous nerve stimulation. Most patients recover after the pregnancy.

DISORDERS OF THE NEUROMUSCULAR JUNCTION OR MUSCLE

Myasthenia gravis (MG) is a disease of women of childbearing age and older men. MG is an autoimmune disorder of neuromuscular junction transmission that manifests as fatigable weakness in skeletal muscle. MG rarely presents during pregnancy, but in patients with treated MG, worsening can be expected in about 19% of cases; 22% of patients improve, and 59% are unchanged. When worsening occurs, it is most likely to happen in the first trimester of pregnancy and the first postpartum month. The clinical course is not predicted by the clinical severity before conception or by the behavior of the illness in prior pregnancies. Although malignant thymoma is no more common during pregnancy than in the general MG population, pregnancy has been associated with an increased risk of widespread metastases. MG is not associated with prematurity, low birthweight, or an increased perinatal death rate. Management of the patient with MG who desires to become pregnant should include stabilization of the medication regimen. Anticholinesterase drugs are safe to use during pregnancy. Corticosteroids may be continued during pregnancy, but immunosuppressants should be discontinued in favor of non-teratogenic therapies. Plasmapheresis and gamma-globulins are safe and effective during pregnancy. Should thymectomy be indicated, it is best to perform this prior to pregnancy. When pregnancy occurs in the course of therapy, the risks and benefits of continuing the preexistent management plan should be weighed. There is little to be gained by discontinuing immunosuppressants once the patient has passed the phase of organogenesis, but such patients may be offered ultrasound imaging studies to assess malformations. Thymectomy may be undertaken if indicated, but the patient should be prepared for this with a course of plasmapheresis, which also may be needed for disease exacerbations occurring during pregnancy. They may be particularly helpful and may be given parenterally during labor and parturition. It may be necessary to assist delivery with low forceps and vacuum extraction. It is wise to remember that patients taking long-term corticosteroids may have adrenal suppression with a blunted response to stress, so they may require supplemental corticosteroids for delivery. Special attention must be focused on the infant of the mother with MG following delivery. Nearly half of all infants of mothers with MG have antiacetylcholine receptor antibodies, and up to 20% show signs of neonatal myasthenia secondary to transplacental antibody transfer. There is no correlation with the severity of the maternal disease or the mother's antibody titer. Affected infants are floppy, with poor suck and cry and ventilatory insufficiency. They should receive ventilatory assistance as indicated and may require tube feeding. Anticholinesterases may be required in some instances. The disease is self-limited and resolves as antibody titers decrease, usually within 30 days of birth.

The course of muscular dystrophies is not altered by pregnancy. Muscular dystrophies do not adversely affect pregnancy outcome, but labor and delivery may be hindered by weakness and fatigability. It may be necessary to assist in the second stage of labor with forceps or vacuum extraction.

Polymyositis is a subacute T-cell mediated inflammatory myopathy with characteristic proximal muscle weakness. Tenderness and proximal muscle weakness, sometimes with rash (dermatomyositis), are accompanied by striking increases in creatinine phosphokinase and erythrocyte sedimentation rate. Other autoimmune diseases may be associated. Treatment is usually with corticosteroids or immunosuppressants. Adverse fetal outcome has been reported in half of pregnancies in patients with polymyositis/dermatomyositis, and some infants have been reported to have persistent elevations of creatinine phosphokinase. Treatment of the pregnant woman with polymyositis/dermatomyositis stresses avoidance of teratogenic immunosuppressants, attention to steroid replacement peripartum, and support of the second stage of labor, as indicated.

CENTRAL NERVOUS SYSTEM DISORDERS IN PREGNANCY

Headache

Headache is the most common neurologic symptom in pregnancy, and rarely does its presence reflect serious underlying pathology. Indications for diagnostic evaluation include headaches that present during pregnancy and are severe or atypical, persistently unilateral, or associated with focal findings or papilledema. The most common headache encountered in the gravid patient is the tension or muscle-contraction headache. Such headaches are dull and persistent with bandlike or viselike pain lasting days to years. They commonly are associated with tension or spasm in the muscles of the scalp and neck, and they may respond in part to nonpharmacologic measures such as relaxation training, massage, and heat. When headaches are disabling, they may be treated with acetaminophen or codeine, which have been found to be safe analgesics in pregnancy.

Migraine headaches are severe, throbbing, often unilateral headaches that may be preceded by a visual or sensory aura. They often are associated with nausea and vomiting. Migraine headache affects 5% to 10% of the general population and a higher percentage of women in the childbearing years. Of women with migraine, 50% to 74% experience some decrease in the frequency of severity of migraine during pregnancy. However, some are worsened, and migraine rarely may present during pregnancy, usually during the first trimester.

Infrequent migraine headaches are treated with analgesics. Acetaminophen and nonsteroidal antiinflammatory drugs are safe to use during pregnancy, although the latter should be discontinued in the last trimester. Adjunctive caffeine may be useful. Metoclopramide is safe, if needed for nausea. Patients with more severe headaches may require narcotic analgesics such as codeine; barbiturates also may be useful for pulse therapy. These agents should not be used chronically. The triptans have been given to many pregnant patients and are associated with a higher incidence of preterm delivery and low birthweight but no teratogenic effects. Ergot drugs are contraindicated during pregnancy because of their propensity to cause uterine contraction.

When disabling headaches occur more frequently than once weekly and adequate control is not achieved with analgesics alone, prophylactic therapy may be indicated. Propranolol 80–320 mg daily is the treatment of choice for migraine prophylaxis, but this drug may be associated with fetal growth retardation, prematurity, respiratory depression, hypoglycemia, and hyperbilirubinemia. Relatively low doses of antidepressants, such as amitriptyline 25 mg, also may be helpful.

Pseudotumor cerebri, a syndrome of headache associated with increased intracranial pressure, occurs rarely in the pregnant population. Patients must be evaluated for intracranial mass lesion or cerebral vein thrombosis. Because visual loss may result from compression of the optic nerves, visual fields and acuity must be followed. Analgesics may help the headache. Corticosteroids or repeated lumbar punctures (LP) may be required for progression of the syndrome with threatened loss of vision.

MULTIPLE SCLEROSIS

Multiple sclerosis (MS) is an inflammatory demyelinating disorder of the central nervous system (CNS) that usually presents in young adulthood and more commonly affects women. The signs and symptoms of MS relate to the location of demyelinating lesions. Retrospective studies suggest that the relapse rate decreases during pregnancy, although it may increase again postpartum. MS does not affect the outcome of pregnancy. Treatment should be reserved for significant exacerbations; mild exacerbation should be managed conservatively. When treatment is needed, short-term high-dose corticosteroids should be used. Immunosuppressants should be avoided, although immunoglobins or copolymer 1 can be considered for more severe cases.

EPILEPSY

One in every 200 pregnancies occurs in a woman with epilepsy, and 80% of these women are taking anticonvulsants at the time they become pregnant. Management issues include the effects of pregnancy on seizure frequency and anticonvulsant pharmacokinetics, the effects of epilepsy on pregnancy and fetal development, and the effects of anticonvulsants on fetal development.

Seizure frequency is increased in 5% to 46%, decreased in 19% to 44%, and unchanged in 35% to 55% of patients. Patients whose epilepsy has been poorly controlled prior to pregnancy are more likely to be poorly controlled during pregnancy. Increased seizure frequency is most likely to occur during the first two trimesters, and it often is related to changes in serum drug levels (as a result of altered pharmacokinetics or noncompliance) or to sleep deprivation.

Total concentrations of all anticonvulsants decrease during pregnancy. This reflects changes in dose, body weight, and plasma protein binding (Table 27.1). Decreased levels are apparent during the first trimester but become more pronounced throughout pregnancy and may be associated with exacerbation of seizures. Changes in protein binding make total drug levels unreliable in monitoring of patients with epilepsy because free levels may remain unchanged or may increase. The clinician should use the patient's clinical condition, frequency of seizures, and drug levels to monitor epileptic drug therapy. Whenever possible, free anticonvulsant levels should be used to monitor drug levels.

In prospective studies of women with epilepsy, complications of pregnancy, includ-

TABLE 27.1. *Factors Affecting Drug Pharmacokinetics During Pregnancy*

Absorption
  Slowed gastric emptying
  Increased mucus production
  Decreased acid secretion
Distribution
  Increased intravascular volume
  Increased extravascular volume
  Increased tissue volume
Changes in plasma protein binding
  Decreased plasma protein concentration
  Decreased binding capacity of albumin
  Increased concentration of endogenous inhibitors
    of protein binding
Liver metabolism
  Induction of microsomal enzymes by circulating
    steroid hormones
  Centrilobular bile stasis
Renal excretion
  Increased renal plasma flow
  Increased glomerular filtration rate

ing preeclampsia, hemorrhage, placental abruption, and preterm labor, occur 1.5 to 3 times as frequently as in controls. Stillbirth, prematurity, intrauterine growth restriction, and cesarean delivery occur with increased frequency in the pregnancies of patients with seizure disorders, and these are associated with increased neonatal morbidity. There has been no association found between antiepileptic drug therapy and these complications. Although severe and prolonged convulsions may cause fetal heart decelerations, obvious neonatal sequelae of convulsions are rare, even in the case of status epilepticus.

The risk of major congenital malformations in children of mothers with epilepsy is 4% to 8%. These defects consist mainly of congenital heart malformations, facial clefts, and neural tube defects. Although there is conflicting information about the effect of uncontrolled seizures on the outcome of pregnancy, it is clear from many studies that anticonvulsant treatment increases the risk of major fetal malformation. Polytherapy increases the risk of embryopathy. The incidence of neural tube defect in women being treated for epilepsy is about 1%, which is more than 10 times that in the normal population. Prospective studies suggest the use of valproic acid, carbamazepine, or oxcar-

bazepine is an independent risk factor for major malformation in infants of treated mothers with epilepsy. Lower levels of education and low serum folate levels also have been implicated. With the exception of the association between valproic acid and neural tube defects, there is no specific association with a particular drug and resulting malformation. Controlled studies have shown an excess of minor malformations in offspring of women with epilepsy. The anomalies, which are seen in up to 11% of infants exposed in utero to anticonvulsants, include epicanthal folds, hypertelorism, small nose with anteverted nars, low nasal bridge, long philtrum, abnormal ears, low hairline, nail hypoplasia, distal phalangeal hypoplasia, and increased dermal arches. Similar abnormalities have been shown to occur in children of women with epilepsy who have not been exposed to anticonvulsant drugs, which suggests that some of them may be genetically linked to epilepsy. Proposed mechanisms of anticonvulsant teratogenicity include folate deficiency induced by the agents themselves and the effects of toxic intermediate metabolites. Traditional thinking is that up to 10% of infants exposed to anticonvulsants in utero will develop hemorrhagic complications. These relate to induction of fetal hepatic enzymes by anticonvulsants with secondary development of vitamin K deficiency and reduced circulating vitamin K–dependent coagulation factors. Prospective studies, however, suggest that, although there is some evidence of deficiency of vitamin K–dependent coagulation factors, the risk of bleeding in the infants of women with epilepsy does not differ from that in the infants of control subjects. Bleeding is usually within the first 24 hours of life and can be prevented in most instances by administering parenteral vitamin K to the infant immediately after delivery. Fresh frozen plasma can be used for acute hemorrhage, if needed. Current recommendations also include treating pregnant women with epilepsy with vitamin K during the last month of pregnancy.

Patients in the childbearing years should be encouraged to inform the physician when they begin trying to have children. They should be counseled about the risks of anomalies in their offspring as well as the importance to fetal outcome of careful seizure control during pregnancy. It should be stressed that the likelihood they will have a normal infant is 90%. Vitamin replacement should begin before pregnancy. Prospective studies have shown that folic acid supplementation in a dose of 0.4 mg daily does not reduce the rate of major malformation. Although folate supplementation is recommended, the appropriate dose remains unknown. When possible, seizures should be managed with monotherapy and should be monitored closely to establish the level at which optimal control is achieved. Valproic acid and trimethadione should be avoided in patients likely to have children. With the exception of these two agents, the evidence that one anticonvulsant is less teratogenic than the others, is not strong enough to justify removing a patient from a drug regimen under which her seizures are well controlled.

When patients with epilepsy present after they have become pregnant, there is little to be gained from changing the anticonvulsant regimen because malformations may have occurred already. Patients who have been exposed to valproic acid during the first trimester should be offered ultrasound and amniocentesis with quantitation of alpha-fetoprotein levels at the 20th week of gestation to detect neural tube defects.

The previously well patient who has a noneclamptic seizure during pregnancy should have its cause investigated. Most represent coincidental onset of idiopathic epilepsy, but an underlying structural lesion should be excluded. The choice of anticonvulsant medication should be dictated by the seizure type. Most physicians elect not to initiate anticonvulsants for a single uncomplicated seizure. When anticonvulsants are indicated, monotherapy is desirable; the dose should be optimized to the lowest dose that maintains seizure control. Experience with newer anticonvulsants indicates a low teratogenic potential in animal models, but there is little clinical information.

Pregnant women taking anticonvulsants should have serum levels (preferably free drug levels) monitored on a monthly basis, and the dosage of medications should be adjusted to maintain levels in the range of those that controlled seizures before the pregnancy. Free drug levels more accurately reflect concentrations of active drug, and they are useful when seizures prove difficult to manage despite therapeutic serum drug levels. Important aspects of the management of epilepsy before and during pregnancy are listed in Table 27.2.

TABLE 27.2. *Management of Epilepsy During Pregnancy*

Before pregnancy
  Counsel about effectiveness of oral contraceptives with anticonvulsants
  Prescribe folate supplementation
  Provide monotherapy when possible
  Withdraw valproic acid
  Obtain baseline total (and free) anticonvulsant levels
First trimester
  Reassess drug regimen for possibility of simplification
  Perform monthly total (and free) anticonvulsant levels if seizures are uncontrolled or total levels fall
  Determine levels once during the first trimester in uncomplicated pregnancies
Second trimester
  Perform monthly total (and free) anticonvulsant levels if seizures are uncontrolled or total levels fall
  Determine levels once during this trimester in uncomplicated pregnancies
  Perform high-definition ultrasound/amniocentesis if needed
Third trimester
  Perform monthly total (and free) anticonvulsant levels if seizures are uncontrolled or total levels fall
  Adjust anticonvulsants to therapeutic total (free) levels
  Determine levels once during this trimester in uncomplicated pregnancies
  Prescribe daily vitamin K (10 mg/day) for mother during last month
Labor and delivery
  Prescribe parenteral benzodiazepines for intrapartum seizures
Postpartum care of the child
  Inform about safety measures in the home
  Watch for signs of hemorrhage, anticonvulsant-induced sedation
  Watch for evidence of teratogenesis
  Watch for developmental delay

CEREBROVASCULAR DISEASE

The differential diagnosis of stroke in pregnancy is listed in Table 27.3.

Ischemic Cerebrovascular Disease

Whether pregnancy increases the risk for stroke remains poorly understood. Of ischemic cerebrovascular events in pregnancy, 60% to 80% result from arterial occlusion. Most occur during the second and third trimesters and the first postpartum week, and they are related to cervical or cranial arterial disease or to cardiac disease with cardiogenic cerebral embolization. Patients with preexisting hypertension, diabetes mellitus, cigarette smoking, and familial hyperlipidemia are at particular risk for atherosclerotic disease of the cervical and intracranial arteries. Cranial arterial disease also may result from infectious or noninfectious vasculitis or from long-

TABLE 27.3. *Differential Diagnosis of Stroke During Pregnancy*

Hemorrhagic
  Subarachnoid hemorrhage due to:
    Aneurysm
    Arteriovenous malformation
  Intracerebral hematoma
    Hypertension
    Eclampsia
    Clotting disorder
Ischemic–arterial strokes
  Embolism due to:
    Cardiac disease
    Valve disease
    Arrhythmia
    Cardiomyopathy of pregnancy
  Systemic venous thromboembolism
    Patent foramen ovale
  Thrombosis due to:
    Cervical arterial disease
    Atherosclerosis
    Takayasu's pulseless disease
    Fibromuscular dysplasia
    Carotid artery dissection
  Cranial arterial disease
    Arteritis
    Hypertension
  Hypercoagulable state
Ischemic–venous strokes
  Infectious
  Aseptic
    Idiopathic
    Associated with coagulopathy

standing hypertension. Coagulopathy may be related to changes in coagulation factors during pregnancy, to underlying sickle cell anemia, or to thrombotic thrombocytopenic purpura. Cardiogenic cerebral emboli originate on infected or damaged cardiac valves or from the cardiac chambers in the presence of hypokinetic wall segments or arrhythmias. Rarely, a patent foramen ovale will be the route for cerebral emboli originating in the systemic venous circulation or for fat or amniotic fluid emboli.

The evaluation and treatment of arterial occlusion in the pregnant patient differ little from those in the general population. CT, MRI, and arteriography, if indicated, can be performed without significant risk to the fetus. When diagnostic evaluation indicates infarction resulting from carotid artery disease, a symptomatic, surgically accessible, highly stenosed artery can be approached surgically at a center with acceptably low morbidity and mortality rates. Conservative treatment with daily low-dose aspirin therapy may be advised as initial therapy for patients with surgically accessible lesions, as well as for those with nonsurgical lesions. The only clear indications for systemic anticoagulation are the prevention of recurrent emboli of cardiac origin and the treatment of documented coagulopathy.

Venous infarction in pregnancy and the puerperium may arise from infectious or noninfectious causes, although the incidence of the former is quite small in the antibiotic age. Most venous infarctions occur in the second to fifth weeks after delivery. Typically, infarction is heralded by severe headache, nausea, and vomiting. Weakness of one or both legs may be accompanied by proximal arm weakness. Focal deficits are commonly progressive and may be accompanied by focal or generalized seizures and increased intracranial pressure. Consciousness often is impaired. Mortality during the acute phase approaches 25%, but the prognosis is good for patients who survive, and recovery is often complete. Diagnosis is based on clinical features, characteristic CT or MRI findings, or angiographic studies.

Treatment is conservative and includes hospitalization, hydration, and antibiotic and anticonvulsant therapy when indicated. The role of anticoagulation is controversial, but a trial may be indicated for patients who are showing progressive deterioration, early in the course, without evidence of hemorrhage on imaging studies or LP.

It should be noted that heparin does not cross the placenta, so it is not teratogenic. However, heparin exposure has been associated with an increased risk of prematurity or stillbirth and also with osteopenia and pathologic fracture in the mother. However, it is the anticoagulant of choice prior to the 13th week of pregnancy. Although it is not without risk in the second and third trimesters, warfarin is a superior anticoagulant and is the drug of choice during the time between the 13th and 36th weeks of gestation. After the 36th week, heparin should be used again to minimize the risk of peripartum hemorrhage.

Hemorrhagic Cerebrovascular Disease

Intracranial hemorrhage rarely complicates pregnancy, but its outcome is often catastrophic. Intracranial hemorrhage accounts for as many as 10% of maternal deaths. An underlying arteriovenous malformation or aneurysm can be found in 94% of pregnant patients presenting with subarachnoid hemorrhage, and aggressive and immediate diagnostic evaluation of the pregnant woman presenting with subarachnoid hemorrhage is indicated.

Arteriovenous malformations tend to occur in younger primiparous women; the bleed tends to occur during the second trimester, with rebleed during labor, delivery, and subsequent pregnancies (Table 27.4). It is recommended that the patient with arteriovenous malformations be delivered by elective cesarean section and that the risks of future pregnancy be explained to her. Surgical intervention during pregnancy is avoided when possible.

Aneurysms tend to present in older multiparous women, usually during the last trimester, and the risk of rebleeding is greatest in the first 2 weeks after the initial bleed. Early surgical intervention is recommended. The risk of rebleeding is low during labor and delivery, and vaginal delivery may be allowed. It is recommended that forceps assistance be used in the second stage of labor.

ECLAMPSIA

Although maternal mortality from all causes has declined, preeclampsia and eclampsia continue to account for about 5% of maternal deaths. Eclampsia may have up to 20% maternal mortality and 53% infant mortality. The incidence of preeclampsia ranges from 1:100 pregnancies in some developing countries to 1:23,000 in developed countries. It is largely a disease of nulliparous gravid women. When it occurs in multiparous women, it usually is associated with multiple gestation, chronic hypertension, diabetes, or renal failure. Hypertension (systolic = 140 mmHg, or increase of = 30 mmHg; diastolic = 90 mmHg, or increase of 15 mmHg), usually occurring after the 20th week of pregnancy, is accompanied by proteinuria and edema. Other symptoms include headache, visual disturbance, epigastric pain, hyper-

TABLE 27.4. *Subarachnoid Hemorrhage in Pregnancy*

	AVM	Aneurysm
Decade of presentation	3rd	4th
Presentation trimester	1–2	2–3
Time of rebleeding risk	Intrapartum	Postpartum
Surgery when gravid?	Not recommended	Recommended
Allow labor?	Not recommended	Postoperative

AVM, arteriovenous malformation.

reflexia, and consumptive coagulopathy. Eclampsia is differentiated from preeclampsia by the occurrence of CNS signs, usually seizure or coma. Other neurologic manifestations of eclampsia include lethargy, obtundation, flashing lights, cortical blindness, visual hallucinations, and other focal signs. Seizures may be partial, but are usually generalized. Electroencephalogram may show focal or generalized slowing of epileptiform activity. Neuroimaging studies are often normal but may show cerebral edema or hemorrhages.

The pathogenesis of preeclampsia/eclampsia remains unknown. It is a multiorgan system disorder characterized by vasospasm and endothelial dysfunction. The root cause may relate to failure of the normal development of a low-pressure vascular supply to the fetus, resulting in placental ischemia. Other potential contributors include immunologic, inflammatory, endocrine, or genetic factors and alterations in prostaglandin metabolism. The CNS signs in eclampsia result from hypertensive encephalopathy and vasospasm. The relative vulnerability of the parietooccipital vascular supply to hypertension leads to predominance of pathology in this region.

Gross neuropathologic features of eclampsia include patchy areas of infarction and petechial hemorrhage. Some patients have large hemorrhages in the cortical white matter, deep grey-matter structures, or brainstem. There is microscopic evidence of endothelial cell damage, vasospasm, and medial necrosis.

The treatment of preeclampsia and eclampsia are directed by clinical manifestations. A large clinical trial suggested that magnesium sulfate reduces the development of eclampsia by 58% in women with preeclampsia and possibly reduces maternal mortality. No serious adverse effects were associated with the treatment. Blood pressure must be controlled, usually with intravenous nicardipine, labetalol, or nifedipine. Treatment of refractory seizures uses benzodiazepines, phenytoin, or phosphenytoin. Following the acute eclamptic period, it is recommended that anticonvulsants be continued through the 30th postpartum day to prevent seizure recurrence.

USE OF ALTERNATIVE MEDICATIONS AND REHABILITATION

Alternative therapies for any of the illnesses described in this chapter have not been tested in pregnant women. Women should be counseled that although herbal and other alternative therapies might seem benign, they might pose a risk to the pregnancy or developing fetus. They also may interfere with prescription medications. It is particularly important to stress that substituting alternative treatments for prescription treatments introduces the additional hazard that the treated condition might become unstable, further endangering both the mother and fetus. Rehabilitative therapies may provide a valuable adjunct to management of neuromuscular disorders, the worsening of primary neurologic disorders associated with pregnancy, or the recovery of function after pregnancy associated central or peripheral nervous system injury.

SPECIAL ISSUES FOR HOSPITALIZED PATIENTS

Hospitalized pregnant patients usually require a team approach. Pregnant women with primary neurologic disorders may require hospitalization on medical or neurologic units where staff may have limited experience in monitoring pregnant patients. Staff therefore need to be educated regarding the vascular risks of inactivity and bed rest as well as the potential for pressure neuropathies and enhanced back pain if hospital bed rest is not comfortable. Although some hospitals permit standard admission medication orders, especially for sleep or anxiety, pregnant women should have each medication order scrutinized and nursing personnel must be informed against a general "prn" use of medication in pregnant women.

WHEN TO REFER TO A NEUROLOGIST

The most common neurologic disorders encountered during pregnancy—headaches and back pain—can be managed easily by a primary care physician. Patients with headaches or back pain whose symptoms are refractory to simple management or who develop localizing neurologic signs should be referred to a neurologist. Patients with peripheral nervous signs or symptoms suggestive of plexopathy, carpal tunnel syndrome, or other entrapment should be referred to a neurologist at least for confirmation of the diagnosis. Patients with primary neurologic diseases such as myasthenia gravis, multiple sclerosis, and epilepsy already may have neurologists, and they should follow along carefully. Those who do not yet have neurologists or who newly develop symptoms during pregnancy also should establish a treatment relationship with a neurologist.

SUMMARY

Although as many as 45% of pregnant women are exposed to one or more medications during pregnancy, the majority have uncomplicated pregnancies and deliver normal, healthy infants. The physician must function as diagnostician, medication prescriber, and counselor to pregnant women. A coherent approach to care during pregnancy is founded on comprehension of the effects of pregnancy on acute and chronic disease states, working knowledge of pharmacologic and teratologic principles, and sensitivity to the concerns of the mother about the outcome of pregnancy.

QUESTIONS AND DISCUSSION

1. A 27-year-old primiparous woman has pain in the right shoulder and lower-motor neuron weakness in the right shoulder girdle and proximal arm. What is the most likely diagnosis?

A. Peripheral neuropathy
B. Brachial plexopathy
C. Cerebral infarct
D. Multiple sclerosis

The answer is (B). Inflammation of the brachial plexus during pregnancy may be idiopathic or may reflect a familial predisposition to the disorder. The condition is self-limited, although it may recur in subsequent pregnancies.

2. Pregnancy-related factors contributing to changes in anticonvulsant treatment of epilepsy include all but which of the following?

A. Changes in cortical irritability with lowered seizure threshold
B. Noncompliance
C. Changes in the volume of distribution of anticonvulsant drugs
D. Sleep deprivation

The answer is (A). Difficulties managing epilepsy in pregnancy relate to changes in the pharmacokinetics of anticonvulsants or to noncompliance, rather than to changes in the primary pathophysiology of the convulsions themselves.

3. A 22-year-old primiparous woman in the 16th week of gestation with severe headache and photophobia has a nonfocal examination but shows mild neck stiffness. What is the appropriate management?

A. She should be sent home with instructions to take acetaminophen for any subsequent headaches and should return for a follow-up appointment in 1 week.
B. She should be admitted to the hospital and have a CT scan and LP to evaluate for subarachnoid hemorrhage.
C. She should be started taking magnesium with a presumed diagnosis of eclampsia.
D. She should be referred to psychiatry for counseling to better cope with the stresses of pregnancy.

The answer is (B). The history strongly suggests subarachnoid hemorrhage, likely related to aneurysmal rupture. CT scan should be performed immediately with a follow-up LP if no subarachnoid blood is seen on the CT.

4. A 27-year-old woman in the 10th week of pregnancy complains of 2 weeks of back

pain that radiates into her left buttock, thigh, and great toe. Examination shows some weakness of plantar flexion of the left foot and loss of the left ankle jerk. Which of the following is FALSE?

A. The diagnosis of S1 radiculopathy should be considered.

B. Short-term bed rest, back strengthening, and mild analgesics should be prescribed.

C. Lumbar myelogram should be performed as soon as possible.

D. Back pain is common in pregnancy.

The answer is (C). Back pain is frequent in pregnancy, and it usually responds to conservative management. In this case, S1 radiculopathy is the likely diagnosis. Lumbar myelogram is not considered safe during early pregnancy.

SUGGESTED READING

Batocchia AP, Majolini L, Evoli A, et al. Course and treatment of myasthenia gravis during pregnancy. *Neurology* 1999;52:447–452.

Cook SD. Multiple sclerosis. *Adv Neurol* 2002;90:135–144.

Magpie Trial Collaboration Group. Do women with preeclampsia, and their babies, benefit from magnesium sulphate? The Magpie Trial: a randomised placebo-controlled trial. *Lancet* 2002;359:1877–1890.

Hainline B. Low back pain. *Adv Neurol* 2002;90:9–23.

Hainline B. Migraine and other headache conditions. *Adv Neurol* 2002;90:25–40.

Kaaja E, Kaaja R, Hiilesmaa V. Major malformation in offspring of women with epilepsy. *Neurology* 2003;60:575–579.

Kaplan PW. Neurologic aspects of eclampsia. *Adv Neurol* 2002;90:41–49.

Messina S, Fagiolari G, Lamperti C, et al. Women with pregnancy-related polymyositis and high serum CK levels in the newborn. *Neurology* 2002;58:482–484.

Morrell MJ. Epilepsy in women. *Am Fam Physician* 2002;66:1489–1494.

Padua L, Aprile I, Caliandro P, et al. Carpal tunnel syndrome in pregnancy: multiperspective follow-up of untreated cases. *Neurology* 2002;59:1643–1646.

Palmieri C, Canger R. Teratogenic potential of the newer antiepileptic drugs: what is known and how should this influence prescribing? *CNS Drugs* 2002;16:755–764.

Schwartz RB. Neuroradiographic imaging: techniques and safety considerations. *Adv Neurol* 2002;90:1–8.

Von Wald T, Walling AD. Headache during pregnancy. *Obstet Gynecol Surv* 2002;57:179–185.

Williams J, Myson V, Steward S, et al. Self-discontinuation of antiepileptic medication in pregnancy: detection by hair analysis. *Epilepsia* 2002;43:824–831.

Wilterdink JL, Easton JD. Cerebral ischemia in pregnancy. *Adv Neurol* 2002;90:51–62.

Wong CA, Scavone BM, Dugan S, et al. Incidence of postpartum lumbosacral spine and lower extremity nerve injuries. *Obstet Gynecol* 2003;101:279–288.

28

Principles of Neurorehabilitation

David S. Kushner

The World Health Organization has described disablement in terms of disease, impairment, disability, and handicap (Table 28.1). In this conceptual model, disease is an underlying condition or pathologic process that results in an impairment. Impairment is an abnormality in physical or psychologic capacity. Disability is the limitation an impairment places on an individual's ability to perform necessary routine daily functional activities. Handicap is the social disadvantage that results from disabilities that prevent an individual from fulfilling his or her expected role in society. Handicap is influenced in a society by physical barriers, social and cultural factors, and the attitudes of those involved.

A host of neurologic conditions exist that can result in static or progressive impairments. Neurologic disorders can occur at any point in an individual's lifetime and may be developmental, hereditary, infectious, autoimmune, metabolic, degenerative, vascular, neoplastic, or traumatic. Pathology may involve any part of the nervous system, from the central nervous system (CNS) (including the brain or spinal cord) to the peripheral nervous system and the muscle (resulting in impairments such as disorders of strength, endurance, balance, coordination, mobility, cognition, perception, communication, swallowing, and sensation). The same neurologic impairments can vary in intensity between individuals depending on the pathologic cause or the region of the nervous system affected. Similarly, the prognosis may differ with similar impairments but with different pathologic processes at work. For example, hemiparesis resulting directly from an area of brain infarction would be less likely to resolve than would hemiparesis resulting from demyelination or edema involving the same region of the brain.

Disabilities that may result from neurologic impairments can involve any of the routine daily functions of an individual from ordinary self-care tasks, including grooming, toileting, bathing, dressing, and feeding, to the more complex tasks of independent living, including financial management, shopping, home making, and the ability to use a telephone or drive a car. Pathology at different sites of the nervous system can result in similar functional disability manifestations between individuals. For example, disorders affecting balance, coordination, cognition, or strength all may separately result in the inability of an individual to walk or to effectively perform routine self-care activities. In neurorehabilitation, functional disabilities are the focus of medical, restorative, adaptive, environmental, and social interventions.

Neurorehabilitation encompasses medical, physical, social, educational, and vocational interventions that can be provided in a variety of institutional and community settings. Professionals include specialized physicians, nurses, therapists, psychologists, social workers, dietitians, and orthotists. Goals include the prevention of secondary complications, treatment to reduce neurologic impairments, compensatory strategies for residual disabilities, patient and caretaker education, and maintenance of function (Table 28.2). Anyone with neurologic im-

TABLE 28.1. *Aspects of Disablement*

Disease: a condition or pathologic process that may result in an impairment.
Impairment: an abnormality in physical or psychologic capacity.
Disability: limitations in function resulting from an impairment.
Handicap: social disadvantages that result from disabilities.

TABLE 28.2. *Goals of Neurorehabilitation*

Treatments to reduce neurologic impairments.
Compensatory strategies for residual disabilities.
Prevention of secondary complications.
Maintenance of function.
Patient/caretaker education.

pairments can benefit from neurorehabilitation, but the setting, approach, and limitations of treatment will vary with the type and extent of the disabilities. The objective is to match patient needs with capabilities of available programs. This chapter will focus on principles of neurorehabilitation, including a broad overview of the role of ongoing patient assessment, acute-care intervention, the determination of rehabilitation need and an appropriate setting, the rehabilitation management plan, and issues pertaining to community transition and neurorehabilitation outcomes. In addition, case presentations will be given in the Questions and Discussion section to explore potential benefits and limitations of neurorehabilitation in a variety of neurologic conditions.

ROLE OF ASSESSMENT IN NEUROREHABILITATION

Ongoing and thorough patient assessment is a crucial aspect of the neurorehabilitation process. The goals of assessment change over the clinical course of rehabilitation from the acute hospitalization, to the transfer to a rehabilitation facility or program, to the transition back to the community. Initial concerns often include patient survival, level of consciousness, and response to acute treatments. Later concerns focus on specific neurologic impairments and a patient's functional abilities. Patient evaluation throughout the neurorehabilitation process involves clinical examinations and well-validated standardized measures performed by various members of the interdisciplinary team of rehabilitation specialists. This team often is composed of the physician (neurologist or physiatrist), nurses, a social worker, therapists (including physical, occupational, speech, and recreational/vocational), and a psychologist.

The non-neurologist primary care physician should obtain a neurorehabilitation consultation for evaluation of all patients admitted to the hospital with acute neurologic impairments resulting in functional deficits. In addition, patients with chronic medical or neurologic conditions with functional deficits that may be related to deconditioning weakness, reduced joint mobility, or progression of the condition also may benefit from rehabilitation. In principle, a neurorehabilitation evaluation should be obtained for all hospitalized or ambulatory clinic patients with functional decline in any routine daily functions including mobility; transfers; ambulation; or the ability to dress, bathe, feed, groom, speak, or carry out previously routine duties such as vocational or homemaking responsibilities.

The objectives of neurorehabilitation assessment during the acute hospital admission include documentation of the diagnosis, the impairments, and the disabilities as well as identification of treatment needs. Subsequent reevaluation focuses on response to acute-care treatments and any changes in neurologic or medical status. Once patients are medically stable, the evaluation is geared toward identifying those who will benefit from further rehabilitation intervention and determining the appropriate rehabilitation setting. Recommendation may be made for referral to an interdisciplinary rehabilitation program, in an inpatient or an outpatient facility, or for selected individual rehabilitation services in an ambulatory care setting.

On admission to a neurorehabilitation program, assessment is performed to help develop a rehabilitation management plan with realistic goals and to document a baseline level of function for monitoring progress. Periodic weekly or biweekly reassessment during the rehabilitation program allows patient progress to be monitored, treatment regimens to be adjusted when necessary to maximize patient potential, and discharge planning to be facilitated. Objectives of assessment after discharge include the evaluation of patient adaptation to the home environment and community setting, the determination of the need for further rehabilitation services, and the assessment of caregiver burden and needs.

Standardized assessment instruments in neurorehabilitation complement the neurologic examination in evaluating functional recovery. Standardized measurement scales facilitate reliable documentation of severity of functional disabilities, help to increase consistency of treatment decisions, facilitate communication between therapists, and provide a reliable basis for monitoring progress. Scales exist to measure many areas of neurologic function, such as consciousness, cognition, perception, communication, strength, mobility, balance, coordination, somatosensation, and affective function. For example, the Rancho Los Amigos Cognitive Scale often is used to document levels of cognitive recovery following a traumatic brain injury and the Functional Independence Measure Scale often is used to assess levels of independence in areas of basic daily function. In addition, many other scales exist to help measure and quantify specific functional impairments and disabilities. Limitations of various standardized measurement scales often are counterbalanced by use of other scales and the neurologic examination.

Another important aspect of patient assessment in neurorehabilitation is the clarification of the complex relationship that exists between disease, impairment, and disability in any individual patient. Specific neurologic impairments may play a role in multiple functional disabilities. For example, a patient's inability to adequately self-feed, dress, or propel a wheelchair could separately result from impairments in strength, endurance, cognition, comprehension, perception, sensation, coordination, balance, lack of motivation, or the presence of pain or fatigue. Furthermore, individual impairments may have multiple possible etiologies. For example, fatigue may result directly from a neurologic disease process or it may indirectly result from depression, sedative side effects of various medications, or a lack of adequate sleep. Similarly, a patient's inability to effectively concentrate and attend to therapies may result

from impairments of cognition or perception resulting directly from neurologic disease or indirectly from depression, the side effects of medications, or the distraction of pain. Thus, the role of assessment in neurorehabilitation includes clarification of etiologies contributing to a patient's disabilities so that appropriate therapeutic interventions may be undertaken at any point during the rehabilitation process. In addition, certain treatments may be contraindicated or recovery may be limited by comorbid chronic conditions such as cardiovascular disease, chronic pulmonary disease, cancer, musculoskeletal disorders, or psychiatric conditions. Evaluation and treatment of poorly controlled comorbid medical conditions also will improve neurorehabilitation outcomes.

NEUROREHABILITATION DURING ACUTE CARE

Neurorehabilitation intervention should begin following an acute hospitalization once a neurologic diagnosis has been established and life-threatening problems are controlled. Highest priorities are the prevention of secondary complications, maintenance of general health functions, early mobilization, and resumption of self-care activities (Table 28.3). Immediate neurorehabilitation concerns include the maintenance of homeostasis and the prevention of complications that could result from the particular neurologic condition. Maintenance of homeostasis is a priority in all

TABLE 28.3. *Neurorehabilitation During Acute Care*

Prevention of secondary complications
Deep-vein thrombosis/pulmonary embolism
Skin breakdown
Joint contractures/dislocations/subluxations
Pneumonia
Falls
Autonomic dysfunction
Malnutrition/dehydration
Maintenance of homeostasis
Normalization of sleep
Normalization of bowel/bladder function
Normalization of nutritional states
Promotion of early mobilization and return to self-care

neurologic patients in the acute-care hospital setting. Routine continuous monitoring of basic health functions can help to prevent further disability. Included in any rehabilitation program are efforts to ensure regulation and adequacy of nutrition and hydration, bladder and bowel function, and sleep. In addition, measures usually are undertaken to prevent deep-vein thrombosis (DVT), pulmonary embolism, skin ulcerations, orthostasis, development of joint contractures, and pneumonia, which all may result from impaired mobility. In those patients with disorders of swallowing or cognition, efforts also are undertaken to prevent malnutrition and dehydration. The prevention of recurrent stroke is a concern in those individuals with acute cerebrovascular disorders. Autonomic dysreflexia is of concern in individuals with spinal cord injury or disorders. Autonomic dysfunction including cardiovascular dysfunction is of concern in patients with the acute Guillain-Barré syndrome (acute demyelinating polyneuropathies). In addition, efforts to prevent falls and accidental fractures or joint dislocations are undertaken in all patients who may be at risk.

MAINTENANCE OF HOMEOSTASIS

Dehydration and malnutrition may be consequences of neurologic disorders resulting in dysphagia, inability to self-feed, confusion, or inability to communicate hunger or thirst. Reduction of risk may include monitoring daily intake of liquids and calories, weekly determinations of body weight, and supervision with meals. A formal dysphagia assessment may be indicated in certain patients (see Management of Dysphagia and Aspiration, later in this chapter).

Bladder dysfunction is another possible consequence of neurologic disease. Dysfunction may result from neurologic conditions causing bladder hypertonicity, bladder hypotonicity, and areflexia or hyperactivity of the internal or external sphincters. Often, a urologic consultation and urodynamic testing is necessary. Treatment may involve a program of bladder training that may include intermittent bladder catheterization, certain medications, and toileting at regular intervals. Use of indwelling Foley catheters is avoided with the exceptions of urinary retention that cannot otherwise be controlled, in patients with extensive skin ulcerations, or if incontinence interferes with fluid and electrolyte-balance monitoring.

Bowel dysfunction, and particularly constipation or fecal impaction, may occur in neurologic disease as a result of immobility, inadequate nutrition (food or fluid), cognitive impairment, neurogenic bowel, and even depression or anxiety. Treatment measures include the assurance of adequate intake of fluids and fiber, establishment of a regular toileting schedule, and judicious use of stool softeners or laxatives.

Insomnia may occur as a direct result of a neurologic disorder, or it may result indirectly from comorbidities including depression, agitation, anxiety, the side effects of medications, muscle spasms, pain, inability to move in bed, urinary frequency or incontinence, or interruptions related to the hospital environment. Inadequate sleep can result in daytime drowsiness and inability to fully benefit from rehabilitation therapies. Goals of management include determination and treatment of a specific etiology if one exists; alteration of the environment if necessary to reduce disturbances of sleep; adjustment of type, timing, and dose of offending medications; and if all else fails, limited judicious use of hypnotic medications.

PREVENTION OF DEEP-VEIN THROMBOSIS

Acute prolonged immobility, and particularly the paralysis of one or both legs, places an individual at risk for DVT and pulmonary embolism. Randomized trials have shown effective risk reduction with use of subcutaneous low-dose heparin or low–molecular-weight heparin products. In addition, warfarin, intermittent pneumatic compression, early mobilization, and elastic stockings have been shown to be effective. Management of DVT risk in neurorehabilitation often includes early mobilization; elastic stockings; and, in the absence of contraindications, mini-dose subcutaneous heparin.

PREVENTION OF SKIN BREAKDOWN

Risk factors for skin breakdown include impaired cognition, poor mobility, incontinence, spasticity, and obesity. Steps to maintain skin integrity in those at risk include systemic daily inspection, gentle routine skin cleansing, protection from moisture, maintenance of hydration and nutrition, efforts to improve patient mobility, frequent turning and repositioning of immobile patients, and avoidance of skin pressure or friction. Prior to discharge from the acute-care hospital setting, patients or caretakers should be educated on skin care issues.

PREVENTION OF JOINT CONTRACTURES

A patient's potential for functional recovery may be limited by the restriction of movement or pain that results from joint contractures. The joints of spastic paretic limbs are most at risk for contractures. Simple prolonged disuse of an extremity also can result in contractures. For example, a comatose individual with spastic hemiparesis is at risk for bilateral plantar flexion contractures, with one plantar flexion contracture related to spasticity and the other related to simple disuse. Spasticity often develops in individuals with so-called upper motor neuron lesions that result from disorders involving the brain or spinal cord. Spasticity may involve one extremity (monoparesis) to all four extremities (quadriparesis), depending on the underlying pathologic process. Routine prevention of contractures often includes antispastic limb positioning, frequent range-of-motion exercises with passive or active stretching, and splinting or bracing where necessary. Other treatment options to further limit the effects of spasticity or reduce early contractures may include medica-tions, progressive casting, surgical correction (i.e., tendon-release procedures), motor point blocks, botulinum toxin injections, or an intrathecal baclofen pump. Antispasticity medications exist with various sites of action, ranging from effects at the CNS to effects at the muscle. Patients with early contractures in a monoparesis or hemiparesis pattern may benefit from botulinum toxin injections of involved muscles. Patients with spastic quadriparesis may benefit from placement of an intrathecal baclofen pump. In general, botulinum toxin or intrathecal baclofen may be indicated if reduction of spasticity/early contractures will improve functional independence, hygiene, or comfort or will decrease risk of skin breakdown.

PREVENTION OF PNEUMONIA

Pneumonia is a common complication of neurologic illness. Risk factors include depressed cognition, swallowing disorders, and impaired mobility. Risk-reduction programs include efforts toward early mobilization as well as prevention of aspiration through modification of diet, alteration of means of nutrition intake if necessary, and proper positioning during feedings. Prolonged bed rest can result in poor aeration of the lungs, atelectasis, and a greater likelihood for development of pneumonia. Early patient mobilization can minimize this risk.

MANAGEMENT OF DYSPHAGIA AND ASPIRATION

Dysphagia occurs in certain neurologic conditions and may lead to aspiration pneumonia. Swallowing dysfunction can occur as a result of impaired cognition or from incoordination or weakness of the muscles of deglutition. Thus, swallowing is assessed prior to oral feedings in those patients who may be at risk (patients with strokes, brain injuries, neuromuscular diseases, etc.). Signs of possible dysphagia include dysarthria, confusion, frequent coughing, choking on fluids, nasal regurgitation, and pneumonia. Currently, the gold standard of diagnosis is a modified barium swallow study, which can help clarify the phase of swallowing that may be impaired. Goals of dysphagia management include the prevention of aspiration, dehydration, and malnutrition and the restoration of the ability to chew and swallow safely. Treatment includes oral motor exercises, compensatory feeding strategies, modification of food textures, or alternative methods of feeding such as nasogastric tubes or percutaneous endoscopic gastrostomy tubes.

PREVENTION OF FALLS, FRACTURES, AND DISLOCATIONS

A goal of neurorehabilitation intervention includes ensuring patient safety by preventing falls. The risk of falls is increased in patients with sensorimotor deficits, confusion, or difficulty with communication. Methods to prevent falls vary with the type and severity of the disabilities. A risk-reduction program may include supervision of high-risk patients, toileting at regular intervals, supervision of transfers and ambulation, adapted nurse-call systems, and patient and family education. The use of restraints is avoided whenever possible because restraints may lead to other injuries or cause greater agitation in those already restless.

Another concern is prevention of shoulder dislocations in patients with paretic upper extremities. There is a tendency for subluxation to occur at the shoulder joint capsule as a result of the gravitational pull from the weight of a paretic arm. Preventive measures include maintenance of normal scapulohumeral positioning through physical measures, use of lap trays on wheelchairs, use of pull-sheets during bed positioning, and avoidance of excessive range-of-motion exercises. Caution must be taken with lap trays because improper use can lead to nerve injuries or wrist flexion contractures; furthermore, sling arm supports may promote upper-extremity flexion contractures if used improperly. The differential diagnosis for shoulder pain in those with paretic upper extremities also includes rotator cuff tears, adhesive capsulitis, bicipital tendonitis, reflex sympathetic dystrophy, arthritis, and previous injuries.

PREVENTION IN SPECIFIC NEUROLOGIC DISORDERS

Patients who have had an ischemic stroke are at substantial risk for a recurrent stroke. Often, the acute-care team will determine the need for carotid endarterectomy or anticoagulation with warfarin, ticlopidine, or aspirin. Neurorehabilitation can help with patient and family education regarding potential modifiable risk factors including hypertension, diabetes mellitus, cigarette smoking, alcohol consumption, drug abuse, obesity, high serum cholesterol, coronary artery disease, left ventricular hypertrophy, and atrial fibrillation.

Spinal cord injuries and disorders can result in a potential for autonomic dysreflexia. This is more likely with high-level cord pathology. Autonomic dysreflexia manifests as precipitous drops or elevations in blood pressure or pulse, often accompanied by a pounding headache, hyperventilation, and flushing or sweating above the level of the lesion. The cause is usually a noxious stimulus involving a numb portion of the body detectable only to the autonomic nervous system. Possible causes may include a full bladder, a fecal impaction, tight-fitting clothing or shoes, a skin irritation, a DVT, or an infection. Prevention includes a routine bowel and bladder program, daily skin inspection, and careful dressing. Treatment of acute autonomic dysreflexia includes blood pressure stabilization as well as determination and correction of the etiology.

Autonomic dysfunction also may occur in the setting of acute demyelinating polyneuropathy (Guillain-Barré syndrome). Autonomic symptoms including sinus tachycardia, bradycardia, facial flushing, hypotension, or hypertension; profuse diaphoresis or even anhydrosis can occur. In addition, urinary retention also may occur in some patients. The autonomic dysfunction associated with acute demyelinating polyneuropathies often remits after a few weeks. Treatment is supportive and expectant.

EARLY MOBILIZATION AND RETURN TO SELF-CARE

Another goal of acute neurorehabilitation intervention is early patient mobilization and the encouragement of self-care activities. Early mobilization helps to prevent DVT, skin breakdowns, pneumonia, joint contractures, and constipation; it promotes early ambulation, better orthostatic tolerance, and performance of basic activities of daily living. Early participation in self-care activities can help to increase strength, endurance, awareness, communication, problem solving, and social activity. Mobilization and the encouragement of self-care is beneficial as soon as a patient's medical and neurologic condition is stabilized, and, if possible, within 1 to 2 days of admission to the hospital. Early mobilization is delayed or approached with caution in patients with coma, obtundation, evolving neurologic signs, intracranial hemorrhage, DVT, or persistent orthostasis.

Mobilization may be passive or active at first, depending on a patient's condition. It will progress variably from ability to move in bed, to sitting in bed, to sitting up, to transferring, to operating a wheelchair, to standing and bearing weight, and eventually to walking. Basic self-care activities, including feeding, grooming, toileting, bathing, and dressing, are encouraged as soon as possible. Training in compensatory strategies and use of adaptive devices are offered to any patient with persistent disability with any aspect of mobility or self-care.

DISCHARGE FROM ACUTE CARE

Ideally, acute-care discharge planning should begin shortly after admission. Objectives of rehabilitation involvement in the discharge process include determining need for further rehabilitation services, helping to select the best discharge environment, educating the patient and caretakers regarding pertinent issues, and ensuring continuity of care. Patients or caretakers should be instructed on the effects and prognosis of the neurologic condition, the prevention of potential complications, and the need and rationale for further treatments. The patient and family are included in the discharge decision-making process whenever possible.

DETERMINATION OF REHABILITATION NEED AND SETTING

A patient's medical condition and the extent of functional disabilities are the most important determinants of need for neurorehabilitation services and the choice of an appropriate rehabilitation setting. The neurologic condition, medical comorbidities, ability to tolerate physical activity, and ability to learn are all important considerations. Rehabilitation services can be provided in a variety of programs and settings following discharge from acute care. Neurorehabilitation may continue in an inpatient rehabilitation hospital or the rehabilitation unit of an acute-care hospital, in a nursing home, in the patient's home, or in an outpatient facility. Determination of an appropriate program is based on patient needs and capabilities.

REHABILITATION PROGRAM CRITERIA

Referrals for neurorehabilitation programs usually are made on patients in an acute-care hospital setting, but patients with chronic stable impairments and disabilities also may be referred from ambulatory care settings. The rehabilitation specialist physician often will be consulted to help facilitate the evaluation and transfer process. Determination of the most appropriate rehabilitation setting is based on strict criteria.

Threshold criteria for admission to any active rehabilitation program include medical stability, one or more persistent disabilities, the ability to learn, and the endurance to sit supported at least 1 hour per day. More debilitated patients may benefit from rehabilitation services at home or in a supported living setting. Candidates for intense interdisciplinary inpatient rehabilitation require total to moderate assistance in either mobility or self-care function and are able to tolerate at least 3 hours of active daily therapy. Candidates for outpatient rehabilitation programs include patients with limited mild functional deficits who are otherwise able to live independently and those requiring supervision to minimal assistance with mobility or self-care. Patients having complex medical problems are candidates for inpatient programs with 24-hour medical supervision.

In general, the inability to learn that results from a fixed static lesion is a contraindication to active neurorehabilitation. However, some patients may have cognitive deficits that are temporary and that have the potential to clear over time as a lesion resolves (e.g., some cases of brain swelling, multiple sclerosis, or traumatic brain injury). In such cases, a trial admission to an active rehabilitation program is warranted. Also, some patients who are unable to learn still may benefit from a course of passive rehabilitation, such as those with severe spasticity who recently may have received botulinum toxin injections or an intrathecal baclofen pump. In cases such as those, vigorous passive range-of-motion exercises may further help to reduce early contractures to allow better hygiene, to help decrease pain and discomfort, and to prevent skin breakdown. In addition, families and caretakers of such patients can benefit from education regarding pertinent care issues, including a program of passive range-of-motion exercises as well as other preventive care.

PROGRAMS AND SETTINGS

Freestanding rehabilitation hospitals and rehabilitation units in acute-care hospitals usually offer intense comprehensive programs staffed by a full range of rehabilitation professionals. A physician certified in neurorehabilitation or psychiatry is available at all times for patient management issues. General practitioners and specialist medical consultants are generally available as needed. Weekly interdisciplinary team care plan conferences are held and attended by the physician, nurse, and therapists to establish goals, to develop a plan to achieve goals, to assess patient progress, to identify barriers to progress, and to facilitate revision of goals and the management plan when necessary. These programs are active and require greater physical and cognitive effort from patients than would be necessary in other rehabilitation settings.

Rehabilitation programs also exist at nursing facilities, which also may be hospital based or freestanding. Staff, rehabilitation services, and physician coverage vary between facilities. Usually supportive care and low-level rehabilitation services (so-called subacute rehabilitation programs) are offered. Programs may provide 1 hour of selected rehabilitation services 5 days a week, or they may provide comprehensive therapies that may include physical, occupational, speech, psychology, and recreational therapies several hours per day. Interdisciplinary team care plan conferences usually are held every 2 weeks. These programs can accommodate patients who have the potential to later become suitable candidates for further rehabilitation at an inpatient hospital, at home, or in an outpatient rehabilitation program.

Outpatient rehabilitation facilities also may be hospital based or freestanding and can provide selected rehabilitation therapies or comprehensive programs. Services and intensity vary with patient needs from 1 hour to several hours of therapy per day, from 1 to 5 days per week. Team care plan conferences often are held monthly to review patient progress. These programs allow a patient to reintegrate into home life while providing necessary therapies, rehabilitation equipment, social contact, and peer support.

Home rehabilitation programs vary in capabilities from comprehensive services to selected rehabilitation therapies. These programs are designed for patients who are medically stable. Advantages include that skills will be learned and applied at home where they are most necessary, and some patients may function better in a familiar environment. Disadvantages include absence of peer support (fellow patients), limited availability of specialized rehabilitation equipment, and increased burden on caregivers.

REHABILITATION MANAGEMENT PLAN

On admission to a neurorehabilitation program, a patient management plan is formulated by the rehabilitation physician and the therapy team. The rehabilitation management plan includes a clear description of a patient's impairments, disabilities, and strengths; explicit short- and long-term functional goals; and specification of treatment strategies to achieve goals and to prevent secondary complications. The objective is to devise short- and long-term goals that are realistic in terms of patient potential. Overly ambitious goals can set a patient up for failure, and overly modest goals can limit a patient's potential for recovery. A rehabilitation management care plan is reevaluated on a regular basis based on patient progress, and it may be adjusted as needed to suit patient needs (Table 28.4). Typically, in an intense multidisciplinary inpatient program, the management plan and patient progress are reviewed on a weekly basis; in less intense rehabilitation programs, the care plan is reviewed monthly. Pharmacologic interventions in neurorehabilitation vary based on a patient's condition (Table 28.5).

TABLE 28.4. *Impairments, Disabilities, and Treatments*

Impaired mobility/self-care	*Management of impaired mobility:*
Abnormal muscle strength/tone	Remediation/Facilitation (volitional movement present):
Loss of joint range of motion	Traditional exercises
Psychomotor delay	Resistive training
Abnormal muscle synergy/sequencing	Forced sensory stimulation
Abnormal coordination/balance	Compensatory strategies (volitional movement absent):
Loss of endurance	Use of unaffected limbs
Sensory impairments/pain	Use of orthotics or braces
Abnormalities of cognition	Use of adaptive equipment
	Task-specific retraining (motor apraxias):
	Components of above strategies
	Environmental cues to enhance performance
	Pharmacologic interventions
Impaired cognition	*Management of impaired cognition/perception:*
Poor concentration/attention	Identify/treat causal factors (e.g., sedation)
Disorientation	Cognitive retraining
Impaired memory, perception, executive function	Substitution of intact abilities
Fatigue/apathy/sedation	Compensatory strategies
Emotional dysfunction	Pharmacologic interventions
Distracters (pain, diplopia, anxiety, etc.)	
Impaired communication	*Management of communication disorders:*
Aphasias	Aphasias:
	Enhancement of comprehension/expression
	Compensatory strategies
	Adjustment issues
	Caregiver/patient communication issues
Right-hemispheric language disorders	Right-hemisphere language disorders:
	Increase awareness of deficits
	Reinstate pragmatics of communication
	Compensatory strategies
Dysarthrias	Dysarthrias:
	Oral motor exercises
	Manipulation of vocalization/articulation/respiration/ prosody

TABLE 28.5. *Pharmacologic Treatments in Neurorehabilitation*

Medication Class	Reasons
Antispasticity medications	Tone reduction/contracture prevention; analgesia
Analgesics	Pain relief
Psychostimulants	Enhancement of concentration, attention, arousal
Antidepressants	Depression relief; improvement of motivation; pain relief
Antipsychotics	Enhancement of reality testing; reduction of agitation/hallucinations/delusions
Anticholinergics	Improvement of memory/cognition
Anticonvulsants	Management of seizures/mood disorders/pain
Antithrombotics	Prevention of deep-vein thrombosis/stroke/pulmonary embolism
Dopaminergics	Enhancement of arousal/cognition; improvement of mobility in patients with Parkinson's disease

MANAGEMENT OF IMPAIRED MOBILITY

Disabilities involving mobility may result from impairment that can include muscle weakness, abnormal muscle tone, loss of joint range of motion, delayed response time, abnormal muscle synergy patterns, abnormal muscle contraction sequencing (motor apraxia), abnormal coordination or balance, lack of endurance, pain, and sensory impairments (especially proprioception). Prior to treatment, the specific cause of motor dysfunction and impaired mobility must be determined. Options for treatment may include a program of remediation/facilitation, compensation, or task-specific motor retraining. Some degree of volitional movement is required in an affected limb for remediation/facilitation to be effective. This approach includes traditional exercises, resistive training, and forced sensory stimulation modalities to improve limb strength and function. In the compensation approach, the goal is to improve a patient's level of functional independence in performing self-care activities by teaching compensatory strategies that involve the unaffected limbs. The compensation approach can result in learned non-use of an impaired limb and therefore is reserved for patients with a poor prognosis for recovery of sensorimotor function or those whose motor recovery has reached a plateau. A program of task-specific motor retraining involves some components of both remediation/facilitation and compensation and use of environmental cues to assist in enhancement of performance of specific tasks. This approach may be helpful for patients with motor apraxias. The effectiveness of these functional approaches may be enhanced by treatment of specific causes of impaired mobility, such as spasticity, contractures, or chronic pain, and use of orthotic devices, braces, and adaptive equipment when necessary. Adjunct modalities that also may aid in functional recovery include biofeedback, functional electrical stimulation, and various computerized retraining devices. In summary, patients with some voluntary motor control are encouraged to use an affected limb in functional tasks. Patients unable to use an affected limb are taught compensatory strategies. Adaptive devices are used if more natural methods are not available or cannot be learned, and orthotic devices or braces are indicated if joint or limb stabilization will help improve function or ambulation.

MANAGEMENT OF IMPAIRED COGNITION

Limitations in cognition or perception are important in planning and conducting rehabilitation efforts, in preparing for functional safety on discharge, and in predicting a patient's ability to resume vocational activities. Cognitive deficits may involve difficulties of concentration, attention, orientation, memory, perception, and executive function. Causes may include specific brain lesions and environmental or non-environmental distractors. Non-environmental distractors may include chronic pain, vertigo, lack of motivation, diplopia, visual loss, hearing loss, fatigue, impulsiveness, the side effects of medications, the effect of emotional disturbances (e.g., depression, anxiety, or agitation), or intermittent seizures such as non-convulsive seizures or brief absence or psychomotor seizures. Environmental distractors can include aspects of the hospital routine that may prevent adequate sleep at night such as late medications or busy or noisy therapy areas. Prior to treatment, specific etiologies are identified and a relevant management plan is devised. A cognitive remediation program often includes the efforts of an occupational therapist, a speech therapist, and a psychologist. Treatments emphasize cognitive retraining, substitution of intact abilities, and compensatory strategies. Irreversible cognitive deficits that absolutely preclude learning are a contraindication to active neurorehabilitation (see previous section, Rehabilitation Program Criteria).

MANAGEMENT OF COMMUNICATION DISORDERS

Impairments of speech and language may include aphasias, disorders of pragmatics (right-hemisphere communication disorders), and difficulties related to dysarthria. Management varies with etiology and often involves the services of a speech therapist and a psychologist. Treatment of aphasia targets problems of comprehension or expression. Specific goals variably include improving ability to speak, comprehend, read, or write; developing strategies to compensate for persistent problems; addressing associated adjustment issues; and teaching caregivers to communicate with the patient. Goals of treatment for right-hemisphere language disorders (i.e., right-hemispheric strokes with left hemineglect) include increasing the awareness of deficits, reinstating the pragmatics of communication, and providing appropriate compensatory strategies. Treatment goals for dysarthria include improving intelligibility of speech through special exercises and compensatory strategies such as manipulation of respiration, phonation, resonation, articulation, and prosody.

MANAGEMENT OF EMOTIONAL DYSFUNCTION

Emotional disturbances such as depression, anxiety, apathy, mania, agitation, delusions, hallucinations, personality changes, and obsessive–compulsive behavior may occur in association with certain neurologic conditions. The etiology of emotional dysfunction complicating a neurologic condition may be multifactorial. Possible causes include organic brain damage, exacerbation of a preexisting psychiatric condition or personality disorder, the side effects of medications, acute medical conditions (e.g., electrolyte disturbances, hypothyroidism, or hyperthyroidism), chronic pain, environmental factors (e.g., interruption of sleep), or a reaction to functional loss. Emotional dysfunction can adversely affect participation in active rehabilitation and long-term outcomes. Effective treatment depends on an accurate diagnosis of etiology. A psychiatry consultation may be indicated. Management may include psychotherapy, a brief course of a psychoactive medication, a program of maladaptive behavior modification, and addressing specific etiologies. A behavior-modification program will involve the interdisciplinary team in redirecting and discouraging socially inappropriate behaviors while encouraging appropriate conduct.

MANAGEMENT OF CHRONIC PAIN

The physiologic and psychologic causes and effects of chronic pain are quite complex. Pain occurs in many forms and may involve any portion of the body. The stimulus for pain may arise at the level of the peripheral nerves, the autonomic nervous system, or the CNS. Etiologies may include static or progressive disorders involving soft tissues, joints, bones, the viscera (internal organs), the peripheral nerves or nerve roots, and the CNS. Pain could result from pathology related to the postoperative state, trauma, burns, and a host of other conditions including degenerative, inflammatory, infectious, metabolic, or neoplastic disorders. Environmental factors may interact with internal factors to result in pain. For example, individuals with muscle spasticity, contractures, or decubitus skin ulcers often experience pain when being moved or repositioned. Also, the perception of pain may be modified by certain psychologic factors, which can contribute to the onset, severity, exacerbation, and maintenance of chronic pain. It is known that chronic anxiety or depression can adversely influence the subjective experience of pain, and similarly chronic pain can result in the onset of chronic anxiety or depression. The pattern of behavior resulting from chronic pain may include irritability, anger, dysphoric moods, loss of self-confidence or self-esteem, poor treatment compliance, and deterioration of important social relationships (possibly including the doctor–patient relationship). The subjective experience of chronic pain may also adversely affect cognitive functioning and overall functional recovery outcomes. Concentration, attention, mental alertness, and capacity to perform complex neuropsychologic tasks may be reduced by the direct distraction of pain or may be indirectly impaired by associated fatigue, sleep deprivation, depression, anxiety, poor motivation, or the effects of analgesics. In addition, physical capacity, including mobility and the ability to perform self-care activities, may be diminished by chronic pain.

The treatment of chronic pain involves the identification and correction of causal factors whenever possible. A course of opioid or non-opioid analgesic, anxiolytic, or antidepressant medications may be useful. Long-term use of narcotic or anxiolytic medications should be avoided with few exceptions (e.g., cancer pain). Often, a psychologic evaluation and course of psychotherapy may be beneficial for adjustment issues and associated affective dysfunction. If there are prominent signs of affective dysfunction, a psychiatry consultation may be necessary. Pain and other somatic complaints rooted in emotional dysfunction may be refractive to traditional treatments but responsive to psychopharmacologic intervention. Physical modalities that may be helpful in a pain management program include thermotherapy (hot packs, ultrasound, analgesic creams), cryotherapy (cold packs), transcutaneous electrical nerve stimulation, massage, progressive joint mobilization, acupressure or acupuncture, biofeedback, relaxation exercises, and movement education regarding proper body mechanics. Consultation with an anesthesia or pain specialist for local anesthesia, regional blocks, epidural analgesics, or sympathetic nerve blocks may be helpful to break a cycle of pain. Refractive cases may require a surgical consultation. For example, orthopedic surgeons may be able to replace painful degenerative joints. Neurosurgeons may be able to correct or ablate sources of chronic neuropathic pain. Finally, compensation issues also should be considered in certain cases as a possible source of chronic pain.

DISCHARGE PLANNING

Discharge planning is an integral part of a rehabilitation management plan and involves the interdisciplinary team, the patient, and the family or caregivers. Objectives include the education of the patient or caregivers and the determination of the best living environment if other than home, family or caregiver capabilities, home accessibility, special equipment needs, disability entitlements, the ability to return to work or to school, driving issues including handicap parking needs, need for further rehabilitation therapies such as vocational rehabilitation, and necessary community services including appropriate medical follow-up. Discharge occurs when reasonable treatment goals have been achieved. Reasonable treatment goals can include the progression from one level of functional dependence to a more independent level that is realistic for that patient. For example, discharge may be indicated when a patient who initially required total assistance in certain mobility or self-care activities progresses to a level of moderate or minimal assistance or supervision. In general, inpatients are discharged from intense comprehensive rehabilitation programs when they progress to a level of minimal assistance in mobility, which may include proficiency in wheelchair operation or progression to ambulation with the physical assistance of another person with use of an assistive device, and have the ability to assist caregivers with transfers. Discharge from an outpatient program often occurs when a level of supervision to independence is reached in mobility and self-care activities. Absence of patient progress in mobility or self-care function on two successive care plan evaluations suggests a functional plateau and a need to reconsider the treatment regimen or the rehabilitation setting. Interdisciplinary care plan conferences are held weekly in intense comprehensive inpatient programs and bimonthly to monthly in outpatient or subacute rehabilitation programs. These meetings are held to allow interdisciplinary team members the chance to update one another on patient progress and potential problems. The care plan meetings facilitate the formulation of individualized rehabilitation management plans, modifications of existing plans, and the discharge planning process.

A crucial aspect of the discharge planning process is the determination of the best living environment and family caregiver capabilities. Therapeutic weekend day passes often are encouraged during a comprehensive inpatient rehabilitation program to allow a patient and caregivers the opportunity to test their abilities at home and in the community. Thus, problem areas of community transition may be identified, allowing therapists to focus special attention prior to discharge. In addition, some programs allow therapists to perform home consultations to determine potential safety hazards and special home equipment needs (e.g., wheelchair ramps, grab bars), to help patients and caregivers rehearse the daily routine, and to assess accessibility of community facilities that still may be used by the patient following discharge. Whether a patient is discharged to home or to an alternative living

facility depends in part on patient or caregiver preferences and a realistic assessment of patient or caregiver capabilities. For example, an elderly, chronically ill spouse may not be able to care for the patient unless full-time help is available at home. Also, patients who previously lived independently may no longer be able to do so. In addition, some patients may require temporary placement in a transitional living program in preparation for more independent living. In other cases, the availability of home health care services including a home health aide and a visiting nurse may allow a patient to be discharged to the home setting.

Another important objective of the discharge planning process is patient or caregiver education and training regarding pertinent care issues and community transition. This includes prevention of complications, necessary techniques such as safe car transfers, home exercises, proper use of necessary adaptive equipment or braces, routine care needs such as bladder catheterization or the use of alternative feeding devices, instruction on medication administration or potential side effects, information regarding specific precautions such as driving or the use of machinery, information regarding sexual issues, information regarding available community services that may include vocational or recreational programs and support groups, and instructions regarding discharge follow-up and continued therapy needs. The importance of continuity of care is emphasized. Usually, the team case manager will assist the patient and caregivers in arranging for necessary community services such as home health care and outpatient therapies. In addition, arrangements are made for important medical follow-up that often includes the primary medical physician, the neurorehabilitation specialist, and all other treating specialist physicians. Prior to discharge, a patient's functional baseline is documented to help monitor subsequent progress and maintenance of function. Also, disability entitlements are addressed, such as handicapped parking needs, certification of disabilities, and clarification of a patient's ability to return to work or school. If necessary, arrangements are made for special education or vocational programs. Whenever possible, adaptive equipment or strategies are offered to allow individuals the ability to return to work or school.

NEUROREHABILITATION FOLLOW-UP AND COMMUNITY TRANSITION

Gaps in medical follow-up increase risks for institutionalization of patients with certain disabilities. Therefore, routine medical follow-up is encouraged following discharge from a neurorehabilitation program. The frequency of recommended follow-up varies with patient needs. Responsibility for coordination of outpatient medical care, rehabilitation services, and determination of further rehabilitation needs rests with the primary care physician, who may be the previous treating family physician, internist, pediatrician, or rehabilitation specialist. Goals of follow-up include assessment of a patient's health status, safety at home and in the community, and maintenance of function. In addition, if applicable, the follow-up physician should assess adequacy of family or caregiver interventions. Areas of concern include medical, physical, cognitive, emotional, and social function. Problems may develop once an individual begins to attempt resumption of previous community activities and social relationships. This is when the full impact of disabilities resulting from a neurologic condition may become apparent to the patient or the family. Changes in traditional family roles also may have profound consequences on the patient or the family members. Support groups and psychotherapy may be useful in certain situations. Also, the ability of a family member or caretaker to provide effective care for a patient with severe disabilities must be reevaluated constantly. Even committed caregivers may reach a point of desperation when providing continuous support without relief. Another concern is a patient's ability to maintain functional levels previously achieved during a rehabilitation program. Loss of function

may occur secondary to exacerbation of medical comorbid conditions or the neurologic disorder or from lack of stimulation, lack of self-confidence, physical barriers to activity, or inadvertent suppression of initiation by overprotective caregivers.

The need for continued or additional rehabilitation services also must be considered. Further outpatient rehabilitation needs vary with a patient's progress in an existing program and the extent of remaining disabilities. Goals of further rehabilitation services may include encouragement of recreational activities and the return to work or school. Specific rehabilitation programs exist to assess the capacity to perform certain activities such as the ability to drive or to return to work-related physical activities. Work-capacity assessments are available. In addition, driving programs for handicapped people exist to assess driving safety as well as to teach adaptive strategies. The ability to drive is influenced by an individual's impairments, including visual/spatial and cognitive function. Adaptive driving instruction programs are available for appropriate patients. Another follow-up concern includes sexual function issues. Adaptive strategies, devices, and counseling can enhance sexual function in patients with disabilities and can even allow sexual reproduction for patients with spinal cord injuries. In summary, in an attempt to maximize quality of life and functional independence, neurorehabilitation outpatient follow-up concerns include medical, physical, cognitive, emotional, and social aspects of patient function during the transition back into the community.

WHEN TO REFER A PATIENT TO A NEUROREHABILITATION SPECIALIST

The most common disease processes for which neurorehabilitation interventions are warranted include stroke, multiple sclerosis, traumatic brain injury, and postoperative conditions following neurosurgery. In addition, all individuals with an acute (e.g., stroke), chronic (e.g., multiple sclerosis), or progressive (e.g., Parkinson's disease) neurologic disorder may benefit at least to some degree from neurorehabilitation treatment to enhance function and to improve quality of life. The primary care physician is the usual gatekeeper for patient referrals to the neurorehabilitation specialist. Patient referrals to a neurorehabilitation specialist can be made at any point during an individual's disease process, form the time of the acute hospitalization to the time following discharge to home care. As previously outlined in this chapter, neurorehabilitation can be carried out in a variety of settings, ranging from inpatient to outpatient care settings. Early patient referrals for neurorehabilitation treatment can enhance functional outcomes. For example, studies have shown that beginning rehabilitation as early as possible after a stroke produces better results than if rehabilitation treatment was started later. However, the primary care physician should never consider it too late to refer a patient for an evaluation with a neurorehabilitation specialist to determine whether there may be helpful physical, pharmacologic, or adaptive interventions that may improve function and quality of life for that individual. Primary care physicians always should be aware that patients with impairments and disabilities resulting from neurologic conditions may benefit at least to some degree from neurorehabilitation interventions. Also, it is important that primary care physicians closely monitor their outpatients with neurologic conditions for any deterioration in function either related to the disease process, aging, or other intercurrent illnesses because these patients also may benefit from further neurorehabilitation interventions. Ideally, primary care physicians should request a neurorehabilitation evaluation for all their patients with impairments or disabilities related to a neurologic condition who have not yet undergone rehabilitation treatment and for those patients who have undergone rehabilitation treatment but who have experienced a decline in their level of functional independence.

rologic conditions who may have been undergoing rehabilitation treatment. Functional decline is a common result of any intercurrent illness in patients who already have impairments resulting from a neurologic disorder. For example, individuals with a history of stroke, multiple sclerosis, Parkinson's disease, spinal cord injury, or brain injury who may require hospital treatment for an intercurrent illness such as pneumonia, heart disease, or urosepsis usually will experience a setback in their functional status. In addition, the more prolonged a hospitalization for an intercurrent illness may be, the more profound will be the setback in that individual's functional recovery. Aspects of a rehospitalization that are counterproductive to the functional recovery process include a number of factors. Bed rest and immobility are among the single most damaging factors. The risks associated with bed rest and immobility were discussed at length earlier in this chapter and include the possibility for the development of DVT, joint contractures, skin breakdown, pneumonia, deconditioning weakness, and orthostatic intolerance. Impaired nutritional status resulting from an intercurrent illness may also negatively affect motor function recovery and lead to muscle wasting and worsened weakness. Infections such as pneumonia or urinary tract infections may result in exacerbations of confusion in patients with brain injuries or encephalopathies. Hospitalizations for a second stroke or hospitalizations for exacerbations of multiple sclerosis can have obvious detrimental effects in a patient who had been undergoing rehabilitation treatment. Measures to prevent the complications of immobility should be instituted in all patients with neurologic conditions who may require a hospitalization for an intercurrent illness. In addition, early rehabilitation interventions by rehabilitation specialists and therapists during the rehospitalizations are critical to enhance functional recovery once the patient is stabilized.

SPECIAL CHALLENGES FOR HOSPITALIZED PATIENTS

Hospitalizations for intercurrent illnesses pose special challenges to individuals with neu-

NEUROREHABILITATION OUTCOMES

The effectiveness of a medical treatment may be measured in terms of biologic or functional changes in an individual and cost efficiency. The biologic effectiveness of a medical treatment can be assessed in terms of changes in an impairment rating such as the degree of sensory loss, spasticity, or weakness. The functional effectiveness of a medical treatment may be measured by changes in disability or handicap scores. The cost efficiency of a medical treatment may be measured in terms of relative monetary savings or losses to the payer in relation to the outcome, which may include length of hospital stay or an individual's ability to return to work, school, or independent living. Variables that may complicate the assessment of a specific medical treatment outcome on an individual may include age, sex, social factors such as prior education, coexistent chronic medical or psychologic problems, the effects of other treatments, and patient compliance. Numerous prior and ongoing outcome studies exist regarding the effectiveness of neurorehabilitation in terms of various neurologic impairments, disabilities, handicaps, and cost efficiency. The goal of these studies has been to determine the most effective and cost-efficient neurorehabilitation approaches for a host of specific neurologic impairments or disorders, while considering possible individual variables. Already, a number of specific neurorehabilitation interventions have been shown to be effective for a variety of impairments (e.g., various speech therapy language exercises for certain aphasias or dysphasias and various occupational therapy and physical therapy interventions for certain problems of mobility). In addition, the multidisciplinary rehabilitation team approach has been shown to be effective in a variety of neurologic disorders such as stroke and traumatic brain or spinal cord injury. National collaborative rehabilitation outcome studies should continue to provide useful data for determination of model systems of care for a host of neurologic conditions and disorders.

QUESTIONS AND DISCUSSION

1. A 51-year-old woman with a history of multiple substance abuse developed difficulty swallowing. Two days later, she developed an acute onset of paraplegia and was admitted for an evaluation. She was diagnosed with an extensive retropharyngeal abscess with compression of the cervical spinal cord. She underwent surgical drainage of the abscess and was prescribed broad-spectrum intravenous antibiotics. One month later, she presents for neurorehabilitation with incomplete quadriplegia with four-fifths strength in the both arms and two-fifths strength at both legs. A low cervical sensory level is present, below which there is partial pin prick and light touch sensation to the toes. An indwelling Foley catheter is in place, and there is a small area of superficial skin breakdown at the sacrum involving only the epidermis.

The indwelling Foley catheter should be removed.

A. True
B. False

The answer is (A). This is a middle-aged woman presenting for neurorehabilitation with incomplete quadriplegia secondary to a compressive cervical myelopathy and with an area of superficial skin breakdown at her sacrum. The indwelling Foley catheter should be removed on admission, and a program of bladder training should be started. Initially, bladder catheterizations should be performed at least every 6 hours, and postvoid residuals should be monitored closely. Bladder catheterization frequency may be tapered as postvoid residuals diminish. A urology consultation may be helpful in determining medications that may hasten recovery of bladder function. Superficial skin breakdown is not a contraindication to removal of the Foley catheter. However, if the area of skin ulceration penetrated through the dermis into the soft tissue or muscle, then Foley catheter removal might be contraindicated. Moisture from urine incontinence can contribute to further skin ulceration.

Short-term rehabilitation goals should include:

A. Patient and family education
B. Prevention of secondary complications
C. Compensatory strategies and strengthening

D. All of the above

The answer is (D). Short-term neurorehabilitation goals in this patient would include patient and family education, prevention of secondary complications, strengthening of deconditioned muscles, and provision of compensatory strategies to overcome functional disabilities. Long-term prognosis for recovery of ambulation in this patient is fair because there is already some movement and sensation present in both legs.

2. A previously healthy 49-year-old man developed progressive weakness that started in his legs following a flulike illness. A workup included a lumbar puncture, which demonstrated an elevated protein, and an electromyographic nerve conduction study that showed nerve demyelination with axonal involvement. He was diagnosed with Guillain-Barré syndrome and underwent a course of plasmapheresis. On admission for neurorehabilitation 2 months later, he presents with flaccid quadriplegia, with the ability to shrug his shoulders. Proprioception is intact down to the ankles but is absent at the toes. Reflexes are absent. Bulbar muscles are not involved.

Secondary complications here may include:

A. Dysautonomia

B. Pneumonia

C. Contractures

D. Skin breakdown

E. All of the above

At admission, ambulation should be set as a long-term neurorehabilitation goal in this patient.

A. True

B. False

The answer to the first part is (E), and the answer to the second part is (B). This is a middle-aged man who presents for neurorehabilitation with complete flaccid quadriplegia following an episode of acute demyelinating polyneuropathy with axonal involvement. He is at risk for complications of immobility including pneumonia, contractures, DVT, and skin breakdown. In addition, he is at risk for orthostasis and dysautonomia. The latter is a rare complication of Guillain-Barré syndrome that occurs most often during the acute illness rather than the convalescence. Ambulation would be an unrealistic long-term rehabilitation goal at the time of his admission because he is presenting as a flaccid quadriplegic. However, many patients with acute demyelinating polyneuropathies present for rehabilitation with flaccid quadriplegia 1 to 2 months after onset of their illness and later recover the ability to ambulate. Therefore, ambulation would not be an impossibility in this patient. Short-term rehabilitation goals here would include patient education, prevention of secondary complications, and gradual mobilization with passive range-of-motion exercises to help strengthen deconditioned muscles and prevent development of contractures. Motor recovery may be delayed in this patient because his polyneuropathy involves both demyelination and axonal nerve damage. Motor recovery occurs more rapidly in those individuals with only demyelination.

3. A 70-year-old woman underwent a coronary artery bypass graft and suffered a left-hemispheric stroke 3 days later. Her hospital stay was complicated by pneumonia. Three weeks later, she is transferred for neurorehabilitation with a nasogastric feeding tube in place, expressive aphasia, a flaccid right arm, and two-fifths strength present in the right leg. She is able to follow simple commands. Mood and affect are flat to tearful.

The nasogastric feeding tube should be removed, and a trial pureed diet with thickened liquids should be started:

A. True

B. False

Short-term rehabilitation goals in this patient should include:

A. Compensatory strategies

B. Bracing and splinting to enhance function and prevent contractures

C. Patient and family education

D. All of the above

The answer to the first part is (B), and the answer to the second part is (D). This is an elderly woman presenting for neurorehabilitation 3 weeks after the onset of a left-hemispheric stroke. There is a nasogastric feeding tube in place that should not be removed until a swallowing study is performed to evaluate for aspiration. Previous history of pneumonia is suggestive of aspiration. A modified barium swallow study can be performed to document safety in all phases of swallowing with various food textures. Compensatory swallowing strategies are available for certain types of dysphagia, but a temporary alternative means of feeding may be necessary in patients at high risk for aspiration. Short-term rehabilitation goals in this patient should include compensatory strategies to overcome functional disabilities, bracing and splinting to enhance function and prevent contractures, prevention of secondary complications, and patient and family education. Gradual recovery of some functional abilities is likely in this patient. Prognosis for functional recovery is best in those with the ability to comprehend and learn. Rehabilitation is still possible, although more difficult, in patients with receptive aphasias or hemineglect.

4. A 14-year-old boy was involved in a motor-vehicle accident. He remained comatose for 5 days following admission. He was found to have a left ankle fracture and diffuse axonal brain injury. Three weeks later, on transfer for neurorehabilitation, he is restless and agitated with poor concentration and attention. He is non-verbal but attempts to follow some simple commands. There is diminished movement on the left side. A nasogastric feeding tube is in place, and the left ankle is in a cast.

This patient is at risk for:

A. Falls

B. Inadvertent removal of a medical device

C. Elopement from the rehabilitation facility

Initial measures to ensure safety should include:

A. Redirection

B. Vail bed

C. Medications

D. One-to-one supervision

E. Restraints

The answers to the first part are (A) and (B). The answers to the second part are (A) and (D). This is a young man presenting for neurorehabilitation with a severe traumatic brain injury. He is confused, restless, and agitated, which places him at risk for falls and inadvertent removal of the nasogastric tube. Elopement from the facility is less likely because he is hemiparetic and confused. An initial measure to ensure safety would include one-to-one supervision. Redirection alone is unlikely to be successful because he is confused with poor attention and concentration. A vail bed or restraints most likely would result in further agitation. Medications may be effective if one-to-one supervision fails to ensure safety and to redirect impulsive or aggressive behavior.

Cognitive improvement is expected in this patient:

A. True

B. False

The answer is (A). Cognitive improvement is expected. Cognitive function most likely will improve in patients with traumatic brain injuries in which coma lasted 13 days or less. These individuals generally will have selective impairments on neuropsychologic testing at 1 year following injury. Those individuals in a coma lasting 2 weeks to 29 days are more likely to have impairments in all areas of cognitive function at 1 year following trauma. More than one-half of those individuals with coma lasting more than 29 days will remain severely impaired in all areas of cognitive function 1 year following injury.

SUGGESTED READING

Delisa JA, ed. *Rehabilitation medicine: principles and practice.* Philadelphia: JB Lippincott, 1998.

Dikmen S, Machamer JE. Neurobehavioral outcomes and their determinants. *J Head Trauma Rehabil* 1995;10:74.

Dobkin BH. Impairments, disabilities, and bases for neurological rehabilitation after stroke. *J Stroke Cerebrovasc Dis* 1997;6:221.

Gordon J. Assumptions underlying physical therapy intervention: theoretical and historical perspectives. In: Carr J, Shepherd RB, Gordon J, et al, eds. *Movement science foundations for physical therapy in rehabilitation.* Rockville, MD: Aspen, 1987.

Granger CV, Hamilton BB. UDS report: the uniform data system for medical rehabilitation report on the first admissions for 1990. *Am J Phys Med Rehabil* 1992;71: 108.

Gresham GE, Duncan PW, Stason WB, et al. Post-stroke rehabilitation: clinical practice guideline. Rockville, MD: U.S. Department of Health and Human Services, Agency for Healthcare Policy and Research, 1995.

Hamilton BB, Laughlin JA, Granger CV, et al. Interater agreement of the seven level functional independence measures (FIM). *Arch Phys Med Rehabil* 1991;72:790.

Hobart JC. Evidence-based measurement: which disability scale for neurologic rehabilitation? *Neurology* 2001;57 (4):639–644.

Kesselring J. Neurorehabilitation: a bridge between basic science and clinical practice. *Eur J Neurol* 2001;8(3): 221–225.

Kushner D. Neurorehabilitation. In: Evans RW, ed. *Saunders manual of neurologic practice.* Philadelphia: WB Saunders, 2003.

Kushner D. Neurorehabilitation of brain injuries. In: Evans RW, ed. *Saunders manual of neurologic practice.* Philadelphia: WB Saunders, 2003.

Macdonell RA. Neurologic disability and neurologic rehabilitation. *Med J Australia* 2001;174(12):653–658.

Taub E, Uswatte G. New treatments in neurorehabilitation founded on basic research. *Nat Rev Neuroscience* 2002; 3(3):228–236.

Thompson AJ. Neurological rehabilitation: from mechanisms to management. *J Neurol Neurosurg Psychiatry* 2000;69(6):718–722.

Umphred DA, ed. *Neurological rehabilitation.* St. Louis: CV Mosby, 1990.

Wade DT. *Measurement in neurological rehabilitation.* Oxford: Oxford University Press, 1992.

29

Medical–Legal Issues in the Care of the Patient with Neurologic Illness

Lois Margaret Nora and Robert E. Nora

In recent years, legal aspects of medical practice have assumed greater visibility and importance. This has been particularly apparent in the care of patients with neurologic disease. Although increased attention to medical—all does not welcome legal aspects of patient care, it is unlikely that the emphasis will diminish. Knowledge of, and comfort with, legal aspects of medical practice can contribute to optimal medical care.

Laws from three major sources affect medical practice: case, statutory, and administrative law. Case law (also called common law) is developed in the judicial system through the resolution of various criminal and civil matters. An important role of the courts is to interpret the various statutes passed by different legislative bodies. State and federal courts exist in parallel, and appellate review is available in both systems.

Many physicians are most concerned with this aspect of the legal system because of an increase in malpractice insurance rates. Malpractice cases are civil actions. Most malpractice cases allege that the physician was negligent in the care of the plaintiff. To win a lawsuit alleging negligence, the plaintiff must demonstrate by a preponderance of the evidence (a) that the physician had a duty of care to the patient; (b) that the physician breached that duty; and (c) that the breach proximately caused injury to the plaintiff. Expert testimony must be used in most medical malpractice cases to establish what the physician's duty was and whether it was breached. In addition to proving his case, the plaintiff must also successfully counter any defenses brought by the physician.

It is important to be aware of the other sources of law that affect medical practice. Statutory law is developed by local, state, or federal legislative bodies and applies to persons within the jurisdictions of those legislatures. Federal and state laws on medical malpractice, abortion, living wills, and termination of treatment are examples of statutory laws. Variation in laws among different jurisdictions is common. The court system frequently is involved in interpreting statutes and in resolving conflicts that arise between different jurisdictions.

A third source of rules that may affect health care is administrative law. Some government agencies are empowered to make and enforce rules related to their specific activities; these rules constitute administrative law. The Internal Revenue Service, for example, has broad authority to make and enforce rules about the collection of taxes. Government agencies whose rulings affect medical practice include the Food and Drug Administration (FDA), state and federal drug enforcement agencies, and the Occupational Health and Safety Administration (OSHA), among others. The Health Insurance Portability and Accountability Act (HIPAA) is an example of a federal law that is being implemented by administrative regulations. This Act applies to many individual physician practices as well as hospitals, nursing homes, and home health care agencies. Whereas many aspects of the legislation, and the resulting rules, will affect medical practice, the privacy rules have a particular impact on patient care. Privacy rules will affect the practice of physicians treating patients with neurologic diseases as well as other illnesses. Although physicians are used to maintaining confidentiality, the privacy rules will affect getting information from patients, sharing information in the medical record, and communicating with family members. HIPAA rules also impose substantial penalties for physicians and organizations that are not in compliance with the rules. Hence, physicians should cooperate with privacy procedures in their organizations and make sure that their own practice behavior is in line with the latest regulations.

This chapter addresses three specific areas where medical and legal matters interface in the care of patients with neurologic illness. First, informed consent, a legal doctrine that affirms patient self-determination, is presented. The discussion then turns toward the aspects of brain death in clinical practice. The chapter concludes with a discussion of the common problem of licensing drivers with a seizure disorder.

INFORMED CONSENT

Informed consent has been recognized as a legal requirement for nearly a century. Informed consent doctrine supports individual autonomy and states that patients have the right to understand proposed interventions (diagnostic and therapeutic, including medication) and to voluntarily consent to or reject those interventions. Unfortunate instances demonstrate that, even in recent years, medical and scientific practitioners have not always conformed to these expectations.

Several assurances are necessary for informed consent. First, the patient must be competent. Second, the patient must be provided with understandable and adequate information about a proposed intervention. Third, the patient's consent must be given voluntarily.

A patient must be competent to give informed consent. To be competent to give informed consent, the patient must be both legally and clinically competent. Adults are presumed to be legally competent unless they have been legally declared incompetent. In general, minors are not considered legally competent. However, there are exceptions. A minor who has been legally emancipated is considered legally competent to make medical decisions. Also, some minors are legally competent to provide consent for certain interventions but not for others. For example, in some states, adolescents are legally competent to make reproductive health decisions, despite lacking legal competence to make other medical care decisions. When a person is legally incompetent, the appointed guardian should be approached to obtain consent.

Legal competence, by itself, is not enough. A person also must be clinically competent. Clinical competence implies that the patient can understand information, formulate a decision, and communicate his or her decision. Assistive devices (e.g., hearing aids, communication boards) can be helpful in maintaining a patient's clinical competence. Clinical competence is a medical decision. In some situations, not uncommonly in the setting of neurologic illness, a person may be legally competent but not clinically competent. Dementia, encephalopathy, and other conditions may render the patient incapable of providing informed consent for a variable period.

In the event of clinical incompetence, medical treatment can proceed in an emergency situation. Attempts should be made to contact members of the patient's family to obtain approval for the intervention, although their consent is not legally necessary if the treatment is a medical necessity.

In situations when consent from an incompetent person is not possible, two legal tests have been used to determine whether an intervention should proceed. These tests are *substituted judgment* and *best interest*. The substituted judgment test reviews the patient's prior actions, comments, and beliefs in an effort to determine what decision the patient would have made. The best interest approach looks at all the facts of the case and attempts to identify the action that would be in the best interest of the incompetent patient.

A judgment of legal and/or clinical incompetence for certain medical decision making should not preclude the patient's ability to participate in other decisions. Every attempt should be made to allow continued decision making by the patient (e.g., even as basic as what to eat for dinner).

The second requirement for informed consent is that adequate information be provided to the patient in an understandable fashion. Although other health care personnel may be involved in obtaining consent, the physician remains responsible for ensuring adequate information provision as well as the other aspects of informed consent. Information provided to the patient should include the nature and purpose of the proposed intervention, its risks and anticipated benefits, alternatives to the proposed interventions, prognosis without the intervention, and prognosis with alternative interventions. The patient should be told of his rights to refuse and to withdraw his consent at any time.

The adequacy of information provided to a patient can be an issue in malpractice suits. Two different legal standards of information disclosure are recognized: the professional standard and the material risk standard. The professional standard requires the physician to give the patient information that other physicians of the same specialty, in the same community, would give to patients considering the same intervention. Expert testimony is necessary to delineate what this information consists of. This is the older of the two standards and is currently the choice of most courts.

The material risk standard requires the physician to provide any information that a reasonable person in the patient's position would want disclosed or would use in making a consent decision. Advocates of this standard identify its emphasis on the patient's need for information. Opponents point to its retrospective application as a major disadvantage.

The most appropriate approach is probably a hybrid. Physicians should communicate those risks that occur with great enough frequency or that are so severe, even if infrequent, that a usual patient would wish to know of them. For example, patients should be advised of the possibility of hirsutism and gingival hyperplasia with phenytoin use, and they should be given information about spinal headaches prior to lumbar puncture. In addition, if a physician is aware of a particular characteristic of a patient that would make a potential side effect more important to that patient, this side effect should be communicated, even if not generally discussed. For example, potential teratogenic effects of medications should be discussed with female patients who may become pregnant.

A third requirement of informed consent is that the patient must give consent voluntarily. Coercion invalidates consent. A physician should provide patients with advice and guidance regarding proposed therapies, but this must be done in a non-coercive way. No explicit or implicit threat of loss of medical or nursing care should be linked to a decision.

Consent discussion should be documented in the patient record. A patient-signed consent is not required for valid consent, but it can provide evidence of decision making by the patient. Prepared consent forms can be helpful, but the value of these documents should not be overestimated. Courts and juries are sometimes suspicious of complicated consent documents that appear to be written more to protect the physician than inform the patient.

Care must be taken that interventions remain within the scope of the consent given by the patient. Consent is given for a particular procedure and other procedures that are within the scope of that procedure or that can be reasonably expected. Consent usually is given to a particular individual and those working with that individual. The physician should not overextend the consent to procedures that are not logically associated with the consent or to personnel not reasonably anticipated by the patient.

In certain circumstances, an intervention can proceed without informed consent. Some exceptions to informed consent exist. In emergency situations, when there is significant, immediate risk to the patient, necessary therapy can proceed. A competent patient may waive his right to informed consent: the patient decides to "let the doctor decide." Although courts recognize patient waiver of informed consent, physicians should take care that waiver decisions are documented carefully, and they may wish to have the patient put the waiver in writing.

Therapeutic privilege is another exception to informed consent. This exception is used when the physician determines that an informed consent discussion will prove so detrimental to the patient's health that it should not be done. For example, some physicians have used this exception to justify not disclosing the risk of tardive dyskinesia when neuroleptic medications are prescribed to certain patients who, they fear, will refuse a potentially beneficial medication because of a severe, but unlikely, side effect.

Physicians must be extremely cautious in their use of therapeutic privilege. Courts may not be sympathetic to physicians' defending their use of therapeutic privilege when confronted by an uninformed patient who has suffered severe side effects. If a physician feels the use of therapeutic privilege is absolutely necessary, involving the patient's family in the decision may be beneficial. In addition, complete disclosure to the patient at the earliest opportunity is also advisable. The physician should keep contemporaneous clear documentation of reasons for the decision.

The right of a patient to give informed consent carries with it an obvious recognition of the patient's right of informed refusal. Patients have a legal right to refuse interventions, even if the refusal will result in the patient's death. Education and persuasion of the patient are the tools usually available to the physician confronted by a refusal. Physicians must inform patients of potential problems related to refusing a potential intervention, and this also should be documented.

Informed refusal is not an absolute right. Certain exceptions to the patient's right to refuse an intervention have been recognized, and judicial intervention is possible in certain situations. Courts will not permit informed refusal to be used as a means to commit suicide and may override a patient's refusal if deemed necessary for the protection of innocent third parties. The court may modify a patient's refusal to protect the standards of the medical profession or of an institution.

Legal proceedings against physicians for failure to obtain informed consent may take two forms. A physician may be sued for battery, an intentional non-consented-to touching of an individual (the patient) by another (the physician). As an intentional tort, punitive damages (monetary damages meant to punish the physician, not just recompense the patient) may be available if a physician is found liable. Except in extreme cases when no consent was obtained or when misrepresentation or fraud was used to obtain the consent, it is unlikely that battery will be alleged. The fact that malpractice insurance coverage is usually not available for intentional torts also may limit the use of a battery action by plaintiffs.

More commonly, failure to obtain informed consent will lead to a negligence suit. To win, the plaintiff must demonstrate by a preponderance of the evidence that (a) the injury sustained was a known risk of the therapy, (b) the physician failed to meet the applicable standard of care regarding information about the risk that caused the injury, and (c) the patient would not have consented to the therapy if the information had been provided. If these things are proved, the plaintiff can succeed, even if the sustained injury was a known complication of the intervention and did not result through any fault of the physician.

In summary, physicians remain responsible for informed consent even when others are involved in obtaining it. Information given to patients should be adequate and understandable. Patients must be legally and clinically competent, and assent to interventions must be given voluntarily. Written documentation may help provide evidence of patient decision making, although written documentation is neither required nor guaranteed to relieve the physician of liability.

In the case of legal incompetence, guardians should be approached for consent. When a patient is legally competent but clinically incompetent, medical care can proceed in an emergency situation. Intervention by the courts may be necessary in determining non-emergency care for incompetent patients.

In the case of informed refusal, care must be taken to inform the patient of risks of refusal. Although informed refusal is allowed, even when misguided or life threatening, courts do recognize exceptions to the doctrine. Excellent medical and nursing care should continue regardless of a patient's individual treatment decisions.

BRAIN DEATH

Death traditionally was defined clinically by the lack of cardiac and pulmonary functioning. In recent years, medical and technologic advances make artificial ventilation and continued cardiac rhythm possible even when death of the brain has occurred. As a result, it is necessary to recognize that irreversible and total brain death is an additional means of demonstrating death of the patient.

The concept that irreversible coma was equivalent to death first was articulated by the Harvard criteria in 1968. A National Institutes of Health Collaborative Study in 1977 studied brain death further, and in 1981 the President's Commission for the Study of Ethical Problems in Medicine and Biomedical and Behavioral Research published a treatise on the issue. In 1980 the United States Uniform Determination of Death Act codified brain death as a legally acceptable definition of death, and states were encouraged to adopt this law. These studies and opinions have contributed to a gradual acceptance in the United States of brain death as a medical and legal criterion for death. Practice parameters and diagnosis guidelines for brain death have been developed.

The laws of most states currently define death as either the irreversible cessation of circulation and respiratory functioning or the irreversible cessation of all functions of the entire brain, including the brainstem. This does not imply that there are two types of death. Instead, two mechanisms for determining death in a given patient are delineated.

There are two critical aspects in the determination of brain death: (a) the total cessation of functioning of the total brain (including the brainstem) and (b) the irreversibility of the condition. Potential legal difficulties related to brain death can be avoided by a rigorous medical approach to establishing the condition. In addition, careful and considerate communication with the patient's family members contributes to optimal medical care and the avoidance of legal problems.

The diagnosis of brain death should be made by a physician experienced in the process of making this diagnosis. This usually will be a neurologist, neurosurgeon, or critical care specialist. Any physician with a real or perceived conflict of interest in the diagnosis (e.g., member of a transplant team, relative of a potential organ recipient) should not be involved in making the diagnosis. The brain death discussion in this chapter is focused on adult patients. Specific consultation with experts in pediatric neurology or pediatric critical care should be obtained when diagnosing brain death in a young child.

A diagnosis of brain death is established in three interrelated steps. First, an etiology should be established, and certain conditions that can mimic brain death, but are reversible, must be excluded. The second step is the clinical evaluation of the patient. Third, ancillary laboratory tests may be used provide confirmation of the diagnosis and prognosis. Careful attention to these three steps will ensure that complete cessation of brain functioning and its irreversibility are established. Physicians also should be aware of any specific institutional requirements for establishing brain death. For example, some institutions require certain tests or a formal checklist approach.

The reason for the patient's condition must be known. In general, brain death should not be diagnosed without a clear etiology. Common causes of brain death are head trauma, intracerebral hemorrhage, and anoxia following a cardiopulmonary arrest. A careful history, a careful examination, and various laboratory tests (e.g., magnetic resonance imaging) may be helpful in determining the etiology.

Medical conditions that can mimic brain death must be ruled out prior to making a diagnosis of brain death. These include hypothermia, metabolic dysfunction, and drug intoxication. In the setting of hypothermia, the temperature must be corrected prior to a diagnosis. Barbiturate and anesthetic agents are the most frequently implicated drugs in this setting, but tricyclic antidepressants and other medications also have been reported. In the setting of drug intoxication, endocrine derangement, or metabolic dysfunction, brain death should be established only after correction of the problem or with demonstration of the absence of cerebral circulation.

The second component of the brain death evaluation is the clinical examination. The clinical examination establishes the total absence of brain (cerebral and brainstem) functioning and helps rule out those conditions that may mimic brain death. The patient must be unresponsive to any external stimuli, including pain. Any form of purposeful response, seizure activity, or decerebrate or decorticate posturing is inconsistent with the diagnosis of brain death.

All activities, including reflexes, mediated by the cortex and the brainstem must be absent. Pupils are usually midpoint. The light reflex must be absent. Other brainstem reflexes, including doll's eye, calorics, corneal, gag, swallow, and cough, must be absent.

The brainstem controls respiration, and the evaluation of brain death should include formal apnea testing to rule out the ability of the brainstem to maintain respiration. Formal apnea testing should be done only by individuals familiar with and experienced in this testing. Apnea testing includes preoxygenation of the patient before testing and delivery of oxygen at the level of the carina via an endotracheal tube during the testing. The ventilator is disconnected long enough for the $PaCO_2$ to increase to 60 mmHg or higher. No spontaneous respiratory attempts should be evident with the $PaCO_2$ at this level before it can be said with confidence that the patient has no spontaneous respiration.

Although brainstem reflexes are completely absent with brain death, certain spinal-mediated reflexes can be preserved. The presence of these reflexes does not preclude the diagnosis, and it is important that members of the health care team and the patient's family are aware that such movements do not constitute purposeful activity.

The third component of a brain death evaluation is laboratory testing. Although laboratory tests generally are considered optional, confirmatory tests are mandatory when specific components of clinical testing cannot be reliably evaluated or when an etiology for the diagnosis is not established or when local regulations require that this testing be done. These tests can help rule out conditions that can mimic brain death, confirm the neurologic examination, and establish the irreversibility of the condition.

The electroencephalogram has been used as part of brain death evaluation for many years. Great care must be taken to ensure a high technical quality of these studies. Cerebral blood flow studies, using angiography or radionuclide imaging, can be very helpful in the diagnosis of brain death. Blood flow studies that demonstrate no intracranial circulation for 10 minutes or more provide compelling and conclusive evidence of irreversible brain death.

It is critically important that adequate time be allowed for complete evaluation and serial observations of the patient during the determination of brain death. Repeat clinical examination 6 hours after the first examination is recommended. The time necessary to reach the diagnosis will vary depending on the etiology of the patient's condition, the clinical expertise of the examiner, and the use of various diagnostic tests. Some states and certain institutions also may have local rules about reexamination. Pressure for organ harvesting and other concerns should not prevent the careful and complete process necessary to reach the diagnosis.

Some legal difficulties related to brain death have resulted from poor communication with the patient's family members. Probably the most frequent error in the clinical setting, as well as in literature about brain death, is the suggestion that the brain-dead patient is somehow still alive. This usually is done by referring to the brain as "dead" but the body as "alive." For example, a family member is told the "patient is dead [because of brain death], but we are keeping the body alive [because of desire for organ donor possibilities]." This is confusing information for the family, made more so by the chest movements created by the ventilator and the cardiac rhythm bleeping on a monitor. The situation is complicated further if activities around the patient elicit some form of spinal reflex response.

It is extremely important to communicate that brain death is one way that death is diagnosed and that brain death is death. Families must be helped to understand that their loved one is dead. Continued pharmacologic and technologic supports should be described in terms of perfusing organs (particularly when the specific organs are being considered for donation) rather than keeping the person alive. Pharmacologic and technologic support should be discontinued as soon as feasible following the diagnosis of brain death; allowing families to say their goodbyes prior to discontinuation of machinery may be appropriate, but extended technologic support of dead bodies is not.

It should be recognized that a substantial number of people continue to debate the validity of the brain death definition of death. Particular care must be taken in situations when a patient and/or the patient's family has religious objections to the diagnosis of death using brain death criteria. Some states either have enacted exceptions to the declaration of death using brain death criteria for patients with religious objections to these criteria or mandated that procedures for the reasonable accommodation of persons with such objections.

Brain death determinations sometimes are done in conjunction with a decision on organ donation. Although organ harvesting is possible in the absence of family consent (e.g., when there is a valid donor card), physicians usually will not do so without family consent. From a risk-management perspective, this is appropriate. When there is a possibility of or-

gan donation, it should be discussed with the family early in the care of the patient by persons uninvolved in diagnostic and treatment decisions about the patient. Many organ procurement programs have personnel specially trained to perform these tasks. In no event should undue pressure be exerted on family members to consent to organ harvesting. One institution was sued successfully for refusing to discontinue organ support systems and release the body of a brain-dead teenager to his family while physicians persisted in encouraging the family to consent to organ harvesting.

When there are no organ harvesting considerations, there may be fewer pressures to declare the patient brain dead and discontinue mechanical support. This may be a particularly tempting course of action when there is family dissension about terminating organ support systems. Nonetheless, this course of action must be balanced against the ethics of using limited resources (including nursing and medical support staff) to support a corpse.

EPILEPSY AND LICENSING OF DRIVERS

The licensing of drivers with epilepsy is a complex issue. Driving a car is an important life activity for most adults, and limitations may have important occupational and social impacts. Most patients with controlled seizure disorders can drive safely and without incident. However, some seizures pose a risk of injury and death to a patient who is driving when they occur, and there is a risk to others. Individuals who have uncontrolled seizures of this type should not drive. The laws about epilepsy and licensing vary among the states, and the treating physician should be aware of the requirements in his or her own locale.

Several areas of legal interest occur in the management of the patient with seizures who wishes to drive. First, what should the physician tell the patient with a seizure disorder about driving? How should this be documented? Second, what are the state Department of Motor Vehicle (DOMV) requirements and procedures for licensing people with seizures? How does the physician participate in the patient's obtaining a license? Finally, when a person with an active seizure disorder drives against medical advice, how does the physician balance his duty to maintain patient confidences with his duty to warn others about behavior that places the patient and others in danger?

Physicians should inform patients with seizures of any recommended lifestyle, recreational, or occupational limitations related to the seizure disorder. Physicians commonly recommend that patients abstain from driving following a seizure, particularly those that involve an alteration in consciousness or loss of motor control. Most states have a mandatory seizure-free interval, and physicians must be aware of their own state's regulations regarding licensing. Mandatory seizure-free periods range from 3 months to 1 year in duration in the states, and Puerto Rico mandates a 2-year seizure-free period. Most states with mandatory seizure-free periods either require periodic medical updates or give the DOMV discretion to require periodic medical updates. Restricted licenses are available in many states and may represent a way that patients can drive despite not meeting the statutory seizure-free interval. Examples include licenses that only allow driving in emergencies, driving to and from work, or driving in daylight hours.

Some states do not have a mandatory seizure-free interval prior to licensure; instead, decisions are based on individualized determinations. In such states, important data considered in each decision include the length of time since the last seizure, seizure type, precipitants, and other factors reasonably expected to affect the applicant's ability to control a motor vehicle. The DOMV in these states frequently solicits the recommendation of the treating physician.

The physician should make a medical judgment about necessary driving limitations, incorporating state requirements into his recommendations. If a restricted license or some other exception to the state rules appears appropriate, the physician can work with the patient and the state agency. Recommendations about driving restrictions, as well as other occupational and recreational limits, should be documented carefully in the patient's chart. One effective method of documentation is to have the patient record his understanding of what he has been advised in the chart. This process encourages discussion between the physician and patient and provides clear evidence of patient involvement.

The physician may find that direct interaction with the state's DOMV or similar agency is necessary. In several states, physicians are required to report patients with seizure disorders to the DOMV or another state agency. Mandatory reporting is, however, not common and is considered by many authorities unwise for many reasons. It infantilizes the patient, diminishes patient responsibility, and interposes a third party in the patient–physician relationship. Nonetheless, in these states, physicians can be penalized by the state, and they potentially can be held liable to third parties who are injured as a result of a seizure if this reporting activity is not accomplished. Although the physician is immunized from suit for providing such information to the state, the patient still should be told that the information will be transmitted.

In general, no information about a patient's medical condition should be released without the express consent of the patient. Many states require that the physician fill out periodic reports on persons with seizures who drive. Physicians must fill out these forms honestly and usually are immune from suit for doing so. Nonetheless, it is wise to inform patients that the information is being sent. Office staff should be aware that complying with a state DOMV request does not mean that other requests for information about the patient (e.g., from the patient's employer or family) should be complied with.

Physicians should be aware of the driver's licensing procedures in their state. Typically, applicants for initial or renewal licensure complete forms developed by the DOMV. These forms may ask generally or specifically about seizure disorders. When a seizure disorder is identified, DOMV personnel may act on available information or may ask for more.

Once adequate information is available, DOMV personnel may grant the license, refuse it, or refer the question to a medical advisory panel, a group of experts who advise the state on the correct procedures as well as individual cases. If DOMV personnel refuse a license, a patient may be able to appeal to the medical advisory panel that reviews cases, and it may contact the physician for additional information. Based on its recommendation, the applicant subsequently may be granted or denied licensure. In all states, the denial of a license can be appealed.

Perhaps the most difficult problem that a physician can face occurs when a patient with poorly controlled seizures persists in driving despite medical advice. What is a physician to do in such instances? In states with mandatory reporting, the physician is not only able to report such behavior but may be required to do so. A model driver's licensing statute developed by the Epilepsy Foundation of America in conjunction with physician experts proposes that physicians be immunized for reporting, in good faith, patients with seizures who drive despite loss of consciousness or loss of bodily control. Although the law is not settled, it seems unlikely that a court would find a physician liable for breaching confidentiality if he or she notified the state when a patient refused to comply with medical advice and continued driving despite ongoing seizures that made such driving unsafe.

Concerning a physician's liability to people other than his or her patients, most physicians are aware of the Tarasoff case, in which a health professional was found liable for not notifying the identified potential victim of the patient who threatened her. Plaintiffs have attempted to hold physicians liable for their injuries suffered in automobile accidents with defendant patients. Plaintiffs have sought to hold physicians liable under a number of theories, including telling a patient he or she could drive, failing to warn a patient that he or she should not drive, failing to warn the patient of medication side effects, and failure to comply with statutory requirements. The law is not settled in this area.

Additional information on the status of state and federal laws in this changing area can be obtained from the Epilepsy Foundation of America by phone at 1-800-332-1000 or on their Web site at www.epilepsyfoundation.org.

QUESTIONS AND DISCUSSION

For informed consent to be valid:

1. Without exception, it must be given after information is supplied to the patient in an understandable fashion.

2. It must be given voluntarily.

3. It must be accompanied by a witnessed form.

4. The patient must be competent.

Options:

A. 1, 2, 3

B. 2 and 4

C. 4

D. All the above

The answer is (B). Options (2) and (4) are correct. (1) is correct ordinarily, but there are exceptions, namely when the patient has waived the information provision or when the physician has used the therapeutic privilege exception (which should be used only cautiously). (3) is incorrect—although informed consent should be documented, a specific form and witnessing is not absolutely necessary. Informed-consent forms may be useful in demonstrating consent, but they are not foolproof, and if they are not "user friendly," they actually can do more harm than good.

2. An adult patient is competent to provide consent unless he has been judged incompetent in legal proceedings. True or false?

The answer is false. A patient must be both clinically and legally competent to provide informed consent. An adult patient is presumed to be legally competent unless he has been found incompetent in judicial proceedings. Clinical competence is a medical decision. A patient may be clinically incompetent although legally competent.

3. A 50-year-old man is found collapsed on a city street by paramedics who initiate cardiopulmonary resuscitation and take him to the hospital. One hour later, he is in the emergency room on a ventilator, totally unresponsive to all stimuli and without brainstem reflexes. He has a completed donor card. The most appropriate action at this time is:

A. To pronounce brain death and call the transplant team to come in and recover the organs

B. To call the family to see if they agree with the organ donation

C. To observe the patient in the emergency department for 2 more hours to ensure that there is no change in the examination

D. To transfer the patient to an intensive care setting for further evaluation and workup

The answer is (D). The diagnosis of irreversible and total brain death has not been established. There is no clear etiology for this patient's clinical condition; there is no indication that conditions that can produce this clinical picture, but that might be reversible (e.g., drug overdose), have been ruled out. It is unlikely that a complete examination to establish brain death in this setting, including anoxia testing, has been performed. This patient should receive additional evaluation prior to being declared dead.

Although the family's consent for organ retrieval is not absolutely necessary in the presence of a valid organ donor card, most physicians wish to obtain consent of next of kin prior to organ retrieval.

4. In a state with mandatory reporting of persons with seizure disorders, the physician has a duty to inform the patient's family and employer of the diagnosis. True or false?

The answer is false. Mandatory reporting requirements apply only to the specific state agency mentioned in the statute. Disclosure to any other person or institution is precluded by the physician's duty to maintain patient confidences.

5. Actions to be taken when a patient with uncontrolled seizures continues to operate a motor vehicle include the following:

1. Educate the patient about the risks to himself and others.

2. Carefully document discussions with the patient about driving and have the patient document his understanding of the discussion in the record as well.

3. In states with mandatory reporting, conform to the requirements of the applicable statute.

4. In cases in which patient education has been ineffective and the patient continues to place himself or herself and others at risk by driving despite poor control of seizures, inform the patient of the need to report to the state Department of Motor Vehicles, and do so.

Options:

A. 1, 2, AND 3

B. 2 and 4

C. 4

D. All the above

The answer is (D). Patient education is an important aspect of handling driving restrictions because of uncontrolled seizures. When a patient with uncontrolled seizures persists in driving despite warnings of the risk to self and others, the physician should inform the patient of the need to report to the state. Some states provide immunity for the physician who reports in these instances. Although not all states provide immunities, it is unlikely that a suit for breach of confidentiality would be successful. In some states, a physician may be found liable for failing to report dangerous behavior on the part of a patient.

SUGGESTED READING

A definition of irreversible coma: Report of the Ad Hoc Committee of the Harvard Medical School to examine the definition of brain death. *JAMA* 1968;205:337.

American Academy of Neurology, American Epilepsy Society, and Epilepsy Foundation of America: Consensus statements, sample statutory provisions, and model regulations regarding driver licensing and epilepsy. *Epilepsia* 1994;35:696.

American Medical Association. HIPAA—Health Insurance Portability and Accountability Act. www.ama-assn-assn.org/ama/pbu/category/4234.html.

Buppert C. Safeguarding patient privacy. Establish department compliance with new federal regulations on individually identifiable health information. *Nurs Manage* 2002; 33(12):31.

Brandt AM. Racism and research: the case of the Tuskegee Syphilis Study. *Hastings Cent Rep* 1978;8:21.

Breitowitz YA. The brain death controversy in Jewish law. Jewish Law Articles. Examining Halacha, Jewish Issues and Secular Law. www.jlaw.com/Articles/brain.html. Accessed February 24, 2003.

Canadian Neurocritical Group. Guidelines for the diagnosis of brain death. *Can J Neurol Sci* 1999;26:64.

Health Insurance Portability and Accountability Act of 1996, Public Law 104–191.

Hyman v. Jewish Chronic Disease Hospital, 251 N.Y. 2d 818 (1964), 206 N.E. 2d 338 (1965).

Krauss GL, Ampaw L, Krumholz A. Individual state driving restrictions for people with epilepsy in the United States. *Neurology* 2001;57:1780.

Lustig BA. Theoretical and clinical concerns about brain death: the debate continues. *J Med Philos* 2001;26(5): 447.

National Institutes of Health. A collaborative study: an appraisal of the criteria of cerebral death—a summary statement. *JAMA* 1977;237:982.

New Jersey Administrative Code 10:8-2.3.

New York Compilation of Codes, Rules, and Regulations. Title 10:400.16.

President's Commission for the Study of Ethical Problems in Medicine and Biomedical and Behavioral Research. Defining death: a report on the medical, legal and ethical issues in the determination of death, 1981.

Quality Standards Subcommittee of the American Academy of Neurology: Practice parameters for determining brain death in adults. *Neurology* 1995;45:1012.

Sarno G. Liability of Physician, For Injury to or Death of Third Party. Due to Failure to Disclose Driving Related Impediment, 43 ALR 4th 153 (1986). Standards for privacy of individually identifiable health information, Final Rule, Federal Register, 659250):8246282829, December 28, 2000.

Schloendorff v. Society of New York Hospitals, 211 N.Y. 125, 105 N.E. 2d 92 (1914).

Strachan v. John F. Kennedy Memorial Hospital, 583 A. 2d 346 (N. J. 1988).

Tarasoff v. Board of Regents of the University of California, 17 Cal. 3d 425, 551 P. 2d 334 (1976).

Twelve Uniform Laws annotated 237 Cum. Sups, 1983.

Wijdicks E. The diagnosis of brain death. *N Engl J Med* 2001;344:1215.

Subject Index

Page numbers followed by *f* indicate figures; those followed by *t* indicate tabular material.